MD Anderson Manual of
Psychosocial Oncology

Notice

Medicine is an ever-changing science. As new research and clinical experience broaden our knowledge, changes in treatment and drug therapy are required. The authors and the publisher of this work have checked with sources believed to be reliable in their efforts to provide information that is complete and generally in accord with the standards accepted at the time of publication. However, in view of the possibility of human error or changes in medical sciences, neither the authors nor the publisher nor any other party who has been involved in the preparation or publication of this work warrants that the information contained herein is in every respect accurate or complete, and they disclaim all responsibility for any errors or omissions or for the results obtained from use of the information contained in this work. Readers are encouraged to confirm the information contained herein with other sources. For example and in particular, readers are advised to check the product information sheet included in the package of each drug they plan to administer to be certain that the information contained in this work is accurate and that changes have not been made in the recommended dose or in the contraindications for administration. This recommendation is of particular importance in connection with new or infrequently used drugs.

MD Anderson Manual of Psychosocial Oncology

Edited by

James D. Duffy, MD
Professor
Department of Psychiatry
The University of Texas MD Anderson Cancer Center
Houston, Texas

Alan D. Valentine, MD
Professor
Department of Psychiatry
The University of Texas MD Anderson Cancer Center
Houston, Texas

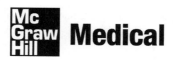

New York   Chicago   San Francisco   Lisbon   London   Madrid   Mexico City
Milan   New Delhi   San Juan   Seoul   Singapore   Sydney   Toronto

MD Anderson Manual of Psychosocial Oncology

1 2 3 4 5 6 7 8 9 0   DOC/DOC   14 13 12 11 10

ISBN 978-0-07-162438-1
MHID 0-07-162438-4

This book was set in Minion by Thomson Digital.
The editors were Jim Shanahan and Christine Diedrich.
The production supervisor was Catherine Saggese.
Project management was provided by Aakriti Kathuria, Thomson Digital.
The designer was Mary McKeon; the cover designer was Anthony Landi. Image credit: Getty.
RR Donnelley was printer and binder.

This book is printed on acid-free paper.

Library of Congress Cataloging-in-Publication Data

MD Anderson manual of psychosocial oncology / [edited by] James D. Duffy, Alan D. Valentine.
   p. ; cm.
  Other title: Handbook of psychosocial oncology
  Includes bibliographical references.
  Summary: "During the past two decades, very significant advances have been made in our understanding and treatment of the psychosocial consequences of cancer. The standard of care in clinical oncology now includes recognition of the psychosocial consequences of cancer, treatment of psychiatric syndromes associated with the disease, and relief of bio-psycho-social-spiritual distress and suffering common to the cancer experience for patients and caregivers. Because the scope of the problem is great and the number of dedicated psycho-oncologists is few, comprehensive cancer care is not delivered by specialists alone. Primary oncologists of all disciplines and the growing interdisciplinary subspecialty of psycho-oncology has done much to help establish this standard of care and to develop a research and clinical framework to support it. Psychosocial oncology is not just another subspecialty. It represents a philosophy of care that seeks to bring together the interdisciplinary team working together to address the particular needs of a patient, family, and community. Implementing such a care delivery model in the culture of our current high technology hierarchical healthcare systems can be a real challenge. However, these barriers cannot be allowed to prevent the implementation of a person-centered model of care that has been demonstrated to improve patient outcomes, decrease costs, and enhance healthcare professional satisfaction. Oncology and psychosocial oncology should take a leadership role in developing and championing this model of healthcare"—Provided by publisher.
  ISBN-13: 978-0-07-162438-1 (pbk. : alk. paper)
  ISBN-10: 0-07-162438-4 (pbk. : alk. paper)
  1. Cancer—Psychological aspects—Handbooks, manuals, etc. 2. Cancer—Social aspects—Handbooks, manuals, etc. I. Duffy, James D. II. Valentine, Alan D. III. University of Texas M.D. Anderson Cancer Center. IV. Title: Handbook of psychosocial oncology.
  [DNLM: 1. Neoplasms—psychology. 2. Neoplasms—therapy. 3. Social Support. QZ 200]
  RC262.M386 2010
  362.196'994—dc22

                                                                 2010033469

McGraw-Hill books are available at special quantity discounts to use as premiums and sales promotions, or for use in corporate training programs. To contact a representative please e-mail us at bulksales@mcgraw-hill.com.

Dedication

For all the remarkable patients and families I have met at MD Anderson
Cancer Center. You have constantly reminded me that healing is
the natural impulse of our universe.

—James D. Duffy

For my family.

—Alan D. Valentine

Contents

Contributors

Julie K. Allen, BA
Graduate Research Assistant
Department of Gynecologic Oncology
The University of Texas MD Anderson Cancer Center
Houston, Texas

Guillermo N. Armaiz-Pena, PhD
Postdoc Fellow
Department of Experimental Therapeutics
The University of Texas MD Anderson Cancer Center
Houston, Texas

Martha Askins, PhD
Assistant Professor
Department of Pediatrics
The University of Texas MD Anderson Cancer Center
Houston, Texas

Walter F. Baile, MD
Professor
Department of Behavioral Science
The University of Texas MD Anderson Cancer Center
Houston, Texas

Laura Baynham-Fletcher, MA
Director
Place of Wellness
The University of Texas MD Anderson Cancer Center
Houston, Texas

Eduardo Bruera, MD
Professor
Department of Palliative Care & Rehabilitative Medicine
The University of Texas MD Anderson Cancer Center
Houston, Texas

Cindy L. Carmack, PhD
Associate Professor
Department of Behavioral Science
The University of Texas MD Anderson Cancer Center
Houston, Texas

M. Alejandro Chaoul, PhD
Adjunct Assistant Professor
Department of General Oncology
The University of Texas MD Anderson Cancer Center
Houston, Texas

Paul Cinciripini, PhD
Professor
Department of Behavioral Science
The University of Texas MD Anderson Cancer Center
Houston, Texas

Lorenzo Cohen, PhD
Professor
Department of Behavioral Science
The University of Texas MD Anderson Cancer Center
Houston, Texas

James D. Duffy, MD
Professor
Department of Psychiatry
The University of Texas MD Anderson Cancer Center
Houston, Texas

Carmen P. Escalante, MD, FACP
Professor
Department of General Internal Medicine, Ambulatory
*   Treatment & Emergency Care*
The University of Texas MD Anderson Cancer Center
Houston, Texas

Michelle Cororve Fingeret , PhD
Assistant Professor
Department of Behavioral Science
The University of Texas MD Anderson Cancer Center
Houston, Texas

M. Kay Garcia, MSN, MS, MPH, DRPH
Advanced Practice Nurse
Integrative Medicine Program
The University of Texas MD Anderson Cancer Center
Houston, Texas

Mark D. Gilbert, MD
Assistant Professor
Department of Psychiatry
University of Arizona College of Medicine
Phoenix, Arizona

Lisa M. Gower, BA
Manager
Integrative Medicine Education Program
The University of Texas MD Anderson Cancer Center
Houston, Texas

Karin Hahn, MD
Associate Professor
Department of General Oncology
The University of Texas MD Anderson Cancer Center
Houston, Texas

Mary K. Hughes, MS, CNS, RN
Advanced Practice Nurse
Department of Psychiatry
The University of Texas MD Anderson Cancer Center
Houston, Texas

David Hui, MD
Fellow
Department of Symptom Control & Palliative Care
The University of Texas MD Anderson Cancer Center
Houston, Texas

David R. Jenkins, DDiv
Chaplin
Department of Chaplaincy & Pastoral Education
The University of Texas MD Anderson Cancer Center
Houston, Texas

Maher Karam-Hage, MD
Associate Professor
Department of Behavioral Science
The University of Texas MD Anderson Cancer Center
Houston, Texas

Benedict Konzen, MD
Assistant Professor
Department of Rehabilitative Medicine
The University of Texas MD Anderson Cancer Center
Houston, Texas

Richard Tsong Lee, MD
Assistant Professor
Department of General Oncology
The University of Texas MD Anderson Cancer Center
Houston, Texas

Ellen F. Manzullo, MD, FACP
Professor
Department of General Internal Medicine, Ambulatory
*   Treatment & Emergency Care*
The University of Texas MD Anderson Cancer Center
Houston, Texas

Diane Novy, PhD
Professor
Department of Pain Medicine
The University of Texas MD Anderson Cancer Center
Houston, Texas

Patricia A. Parker, PhD
Assistant Professor
Department of Behavioral Science
The University of Texas MD Anderson Cancer Center
Houston, Texas

Anis Rashid, MD
Assistant Professor
Department of Psychiatry
The University of Texas MD Anderson Cancer Center
Houston, Texas

Kathie Rickman, DrPH
Advanced Practice Nurse
Department of Psychiatry
The University of Texas MD Anderson Cancer Center
Houston, Texas

Rhonda Robert, PhD
Associate Professor
Department of Pediatrics
The University of Texas MD Anderson Cancer Center
Houston, Texas

Mary Rose, PSYD
Adjunct Assistant Professor
Department of Pulmonary Medicine
The University of Texas MD Anderson Cancer Center
Houston, Texas

Kenneth Sapire, MD
Professor
Department of Anesthesiology & Perioperative Medicine
The University of Texas MD Anderson Cancer Center
Houston, Texas

Eileen H. Shinn, PhD
Assistant Professor
Department of Behavioral Science
The University of Texas MD Anderson Cancer Center
Houston, Texas

Debra Sivesind, MSN, CNS
Advanced Practice Nurse
Department of Palliative Care & Rehabilitative Medicine
The University of Texas MD Anderson Cancer Center
Houston, Texas

Anil K. Sood, MD
Professor
Department of Gynecologic Oncology
The University of Texas MD Anderson Cancer Center
Houston, Texas

Phyddy Tacchi, MS, CNS, RN, LMFT, LPC
Advanced Practice Nurse
Department of Psychiatry
The University of Texas MD Anderson Cancer Center
Houston, Texas

Steven Thorney, MDiv
Chaplain II
Department of Chaplaincy & Pastoral Education
The University of Texas MD Anderson Cancer Center
Houston, Texas

Alan D. Valentine, MD
Professor
Department of Psychiatry
The University of Texas MD Anderson Cancer Center
Houston, Texas

Laura M. van Veldhoven, PhD, MPH
Assistant Professor
Department of Physical Medicine & Rehabilitation
Baylor College of Medicine
Houston, Texas

Jeffrey S. Wefel, PhD
Assistant Professor
Department of Neuro-Oncology
The University of Texas MD Anderson Cancer Center
Houston, Texas

Mariana E. Witgert, PhD
Instructor
Department of Neuro-Oncology
The University of Texas MD Anderson Cancer Center
Houston, Texas

Sriram Yennurajalingam, MD
Assistant Professor
Department of Palliative Care & Rehabilitative Medicine
The University of Texas MD Anderson Cancer Center
Houston, Texas

Preface

During the last two decades, very significant advances have been made in our understanding and treatment of the psychosocial consequences of cancer. The standard of care in clinical oncology now includes recognition of the psychosocial consequences of cancer, treatment of psychiatric syndromes associated with the disease, and relief of biopsychosocial-spiritual distress and suffering common to the cancer experience for patients and caregivers. Because the scope of the problem is great and the number of dedicated psycho-oncologists is few, comprehensive cancer care is not delivered by specialists alone. Primary oncologists of all disciplines and the growing interdisciplinary subspecialty of psycho-oncology has done much to help establish this standard of care and to develop a research and clinical framework to support it.

Psychosocial oncology is not just another subspecialty. It represents a philosophy of care that seeks to bring together the interdisciplinary team working together to address the particular needs of a patient, family, and community. Implementing such a care delivery model in the culture of our current high-technology hierarchical health care systems can be a real challenge. However, these barriers cannot be allowed to prevent the implementation of a person-centered model of care that has been demonstrated to improve patient outcomes, decrease costs, and enhance health care professional satisfaction. Oncology and psychosocial oncology should take a leadership role in developing and championing this model of health care.

Caring for cancer patients and their families is challenging work. Unfortunately, the data indicate that many of us are experiencing burnout and demoralization. Rather than increasing the burden placed on oncology clinicians, an integral interdisciplinary approach offers us an opportunity to bolster our support systems and enhance our job satisfaction.

These support systems also address the fact that cancer occurs within the complex interaction of multiple systems. Although we are developing increasingly detailed molecular models of cancer pathophysiology, it is also clear that the etiology and effects of cancer extend beyond the objective physical realm. The integral biopsychosociospiritual approach outlined in this text provides a framework for beginning to understand how mind, community, and spirit influence the course of cancer and its impact on patients and their relationships. This integral approach does not challenge the importance of objective biological approaches to the treatment of cancer but serves to broaden our perspective of cancer and provides our patients with a wider range of therapeutic options. Importantly, this approach guarantees that we can always provide our patients with therapeutic options, regardless of their physical prognosis.

Cancer is a lived experience, and not simply a disease. Each year, more than 12 million people worldwide receive a new diagnosis of cancer. Although they share a common medical diagnosis, each and every one of these human beings will have a unique experience of cancer and its impact on their lives. These experiences are lived out in the details of their personal stories—not simply in their laboratory investigations. Cancer will inevitably challenge every life narrative and will leave us transformed in ways we cannot predict. Our role as healers is to accompany our patients as they journey through the challenges and terrors of their illness and to create safe spaces in which they can discover their own potential for healing.

This manual, with contributions from multidisciplinary psycho-oncologists at the University of Texas MD Anderson Cancer Center as well as other colleagues working in the field, is designed to assist in that effort. It is not intended to be a definitive text but is intended to provide oncology clinicians with a readily accessible clinical resource that will assist them in identifying and addressing the unique psychosociospiritual needs of their patients.

Acknowledgments

We would like to thank Pat Semmelrogge and Christine Diedrich for all their hard work, persistence, and good humor. Without them, this project would not have been possible.

Thank you to all the members of the Psychiatry Department at MD Anderson Cancer Center for their dedication to their patients and to one another.

Thank you to all the contributors who made this manual a reality. You all walk the walk!

James D. Duffy, MD
Alan D. Valentine, MD

SECTION I

Distress and Cancer

The Clinical Psycho-oncology Assessment

• *James D. Duffy*

This chapter describes a practical, but comprehensive, approach to the clinical psycho-oncology assessment. Rather than representing a skill set that should be relegated only to mental health professionals, this approach has clinical utility for all oncology clinicians and can be incorporated into the comprehensive clinical assessment of any patient undergoing cancer treatment or evaluation. With practice, the initial psycho-oncology assessment can be seamlessly integrated into oncologic practice and does require the allocation of additional resources or referral to mental health professionals. Rather than experiencing the psycho-oncology assessment as an additional clinical burden, clinicians will discover that insights gained from this approach add valuable insights that enhance both the care of the patient and clinicians' satisfaction with their work.

■ THE IMPORTANCE OF THE PSYCHO-ONCOLOGY ASSESSMENT

The psycho-oncology assessment should be considered a vital part of the clinical assessment of *any* patient undergoing cancer evaluation or treatment. As will be described below, psychosocial spiritual factors are important determinants of physical morbidity and mortality. A failure to address these issues will inevitably impact the welfare of our patients and their families.

Emotional distress is common among cancer patients and their families. A recent evidence-based review reports prevalence rates of major depressive disorder of 10–25%

and of anxiety disorders in oncology patients.[1] This prevalence is similar to that reported in other medical disorders such as diabetes and heart disease. However, the risk of depression varies greatly depending on the presence of risk factors (see Table 1-1) and the type and stage of cancer. It is however important to recognize that many patients who are experiencing significant emotional distress do not meet strict Diagnostic Statistical Criteria (DSM)—IVTR criteria for psychiatric disorders.[2] This has led to the development of the concept of *distress* as a distinct psychological state that may occur independently of any specific psychiatric diagnosis. Rather than representing a specific disorder, distress describes a symptom that can be the result of multiple biopsychosociospiritual factors. The development of instruments to assess general distress (eg, the Distress Thermometer,[3] Psychosocial Screen for Cancer[3]) has resulted in more patients being screened for distress and the concept of distress becoming a "sixth vital sign" is gaining increasing acceptance as a valid indicator of psychosocial distress among cancer patients. Numerous psychometric tools are available to assist in the detection of emotional disorders (see Table 1-2). However, although these standardized psychometric instruments may have significant research utility, the clinical psycho-oncology assessment should remain the mainstay for identifying the nature and severity of psychosocial distress in medically ill patients. It is also interesting to note that only approximately one third of those scoring as significantly distressed would like to receive professional help in addressing their distress.[4,5] This further highlights

■ TABLE 1-1. Risk Factors for Depression in Cancer Patients

Psychological	Biological	Social	Spiritual
• Immature ego defenses • Perceived helplessness • Poor communication skills • Anxiety • Ambivalence • Low self-esteem • Avoidant style	• Pain • Fatigue • Substance abuse • History of depression • Family history of depression • Younger age • Certain medications • Disease site (pancreas, head and neck, brain, Hodgkin's lymphoma) • Advanced disease	• Poor social supports • History of abuse • Recent losses	• Existential despair

the importance of identifying patients' distress in the context of an established therapeutic relationship and not as part of an impersonal screening program.

As reported by two recent meta-analyses, psychological distress has a significant negative impact on cancer mortality.[6,7] Based on data from 25 independent studies, Pinquart reported that mortality rates were up to 25% higher in patients experiencing depressive symptoms, and up to 39% higher in patients diagnosed with major or minor depression.[7] In addition to increased mortality, comorbid distress produces a very negative impact on patients' quality of life and the amplification of common somatic symptoms in cancer patients such as fatigue, pain, insomnia, and nausea. In addition, depressed cancer patients have twice the risk of completed suicide versus the general population (see below).[8]

It is important to recognize the impact that cancer exerts over the patient's social network, most particularly their caregivers. In this regard, with the patient's permission and when appropriate, it is important to make every effort to involve family members as part of the assessment. Caregivers will inevitably experience very significant stress associated with the illness of their loved one and are at an increased risk for developing very significant emotional distress. Indeed, caregivers have been reported to experience adverse physical, mental, and social consequences of their role that may actually exceed those of the identified patient.[10] Failure to address the mental health needs of the cancer patient will inevitably raise the burden on their caregiver, resulting in a self-propagating downward spiral for all parties. Clinicians should therefore identify psychosocial resources available to caregivers and be willing to make referrals as necessary.

Patients and their caregivers who are suffering from distress can pose very significant challenges for their physicians and other members of the treatment team. Depressed patients are likely to be less motivated to remember instructions and follow through with treatment recommendations and are more likely to experience treatment-resistant somatic symptoms. In addition, the depressed or anxious patient is more likely to exhibit less adaptive coping mechanisms for dealing with their illness and may manifest behaviors that the clinician will experience as frustrating and/or anxiety provoking.

■ PARTICULAR CHALLENGES OF THE PSYCHOSOCIAL ASSESSMENT IN ONCOLOGY PATIENTS

Several diagnostic barriers make the recognition of psychosocial distress and the identification of specific psychiatric disorders a considerable challenge for even the most experienced clinical oncologist. These potential barriers to diagnostic sensitivity and specificity include:

• The *"normalization of distress."* Unfortunately many clinicians continue to believe that very significant emotional distress is an inevitable and unavoidable consequence of receiving a cancer diagnosis. Cancer patients' distress is therefore interpreted as a normal response to cancer that does not warrant focused

■ **TABLE 1-2. Commonly Used Psychometric Instruments for the Detection of Psychosocial Disorders in Cancer Patients**

Distress
The Distress Thermometer (DT)
Psychological Distress Inventory (PDI)
General Health Questionnaire (GHQ12)
Brief Symptom Inventory (BSI)
Psychological Adjustment to Illness scale (PAIS)
Profile of Mood States (POMS)

Depression
Beck Anxiety Inventory (BDI)
Center for Epidemiologic Studies Depression
  Scale (CESD)
Geriatric Depression Scale (GDS)
Patient Health Questionnaire (PHQ9)
Hospital Anxiety and Depression Scale (HADS)

Anxiety
Beck Anxiety Inventory (BAI)
Impact of Events Scale (IES)
State-Trait Anxiety Inventory (STAI)
Hospital Anxiety and Depression Scale (HADS)

Delirium
Memorial Delirium Assessment Scale (MDAS)
Delirium Rating Scale (DRS)
The CAM

Alcohol and substance abuse
The CAGE
The AUDIT

Spirituality and religion
The FICA

clinical intervention. Furthermore, some clinicians continue to believe that making a psychiatric diagnosis in their patient will "add insult to injury" and further compound the patients' subjective distress as well as their confidence in their clinician.

- *Pathoplastic effects.* Individuals have a limited repertoire of behavioral responses to physical and psychological dysregulation. Pathoplasty describes a situation in which more than one pathophysiological process may produce a similar clinical presentation. In this regard, patients undergoing treatment for cancer are likely to experience considerable somatic symptoms. The "sickness behavior" characterized by lassitude, social withdrawal, and poor appetite that is a natural physiological response to physical illness may be misinterpreted as depression or an existential despair. In addition, several behavioral disorders that frequently occur in cancer patients (ie, fatigue, apathy, demoralization) have clinical signs and symptoms that may mimic depression (particularly diminished goal-directed behavior). The clinician should therefore always attempt to identify the core cognitive symptoms of depression and anxiety (ie, dysphoria, hopelessness, helplessness).

- *Stage-specific stressors and responses.* Each stage of cancer presents very specific challenges for the patient and their families. Although many clinicians believe that suicide risk advances with disease, the first few months following a diagnosis of cancer are the period of greatest risk for suicide. The side effects of chemoradiation therapies may produce neurobehavioral changes in patients who had previously appeared to be coping very effectively with their disease. Patients at the end of life will be confronted with existential and psychological challenges and may begin to question their goals and relationship to physician-assisted suicide (Table 1-3).

- *Multidisciplinary (vs. interdisciplinary) teams and the fragmentation of care.* Unfortunately, many cancer patients receive their care from a wide range of medical disciplines whose only means of communication, if at all, is through the medical record. Within this fragmented and "specialty-blinkered" system, the overall well-being of the patient may be entirely overlooked. In particular, this fragmented care serves to dilute the therapeutic relationship between patients and their treatment providers and lessen the likelihood that patients will feel comfortable discussing their emotional well-being with them. Although every clinician cannot be expected to be an expert in the psychosocial aspects of cancer, they should be able to perform a screen for emotional distress in their patients and have ready access to psycho-oncology resources.

- *Perceived time constraints.* Unfortunately, most clinicians experience themselves to be under severe time constraints and they understandably believe that opening a conversation about the patient's distress will require more time than is available to them. While there is some justification for this concern, with time the clinician who performs a limited psychosocial evaluation of their patients will soon discover how little time is

■ TABLE 1-3. Neuropsychiatric Side Effects of Common Chemotherapeutic Agents

Hormones
Corticosteroids
Insomnia, hyperactivity, anxiety, depression, psychosis, mania, affective lability, akathisia
Tamoxifen
Sleep disorder, irritability, depression

Biologicals
Cytokines
Encephalopathy, depression
Interferon
Depression, mania, psychosis
Delirium, akathisia
Interleukin-2
Dysphoria, delirium, psychosis

Chemotherapy agents
L-Asparaginase
Somnolence, lethargy, delirium
Cisplatin
Encephalopathy (rare), sensory neuropathy
Cytarabine
Delirium
Leukoencephalopathy: syndrome of personality change, drowsiness, dementia, psychomotor retardation, ataxia
5-Fluorouracil
Fatigue, rare seizure or confusion, cerebellar syndrome
Gemcitabine
Fatigue
Ifosfamide
Lethargy, seizures, drunkenness, cerebellar signs, delirium, hallucinations
Methotrexate
(Intrathecal) leukoencephalopathy (acute and delayed forms)
High dose can cause transient delirium
Procarbazine
Somnolence, depression, delirium, psychosis
Tacrolimus
Delirium, psychosis
Taxanes
Sensory neuropathy, fatigue
Thalidomide
Fatigue, depression, anxiety
Vincristine, vinblastine, vinorelbine
Depression, fatigue, encephalopathy

required and how much benefit their patients derive from a thorough psychosocial assessment.

■ THE GOALS OF THE PSYCHOSOCIAL ASSESSMENT

The psychosocial assessment of the cancer patient has several goals that extend beyond simply identifying a specific psychiatric diagnosis:

- *Establishing rapport and the therapeutic relationship.* All therapeutic determinations and decisions are made in the context of the therapeutic relationship between the patient and his or her clinician. The trusting relationship established between them is built upon the rapport established by clear and consistent verbal and nonverbal communication. In particular, patients will be sensitive to evidence that their clinician is authentic, empathic, compassionate, reliable, and nonjudgmental.

- *Obtaining data on specific disorders.* Clear criteria for the diagnosis of mental health disorders have been established. These criteria-based diagnoses assist in determining evidence-based treatment interventions and assessing treatment responses. The clinician should therefore ask specific disorder-centered questions, as well as more open-ended questions intended to explore the patient's subjective experience. With experience, the clinician will learn to move between these two approaches in a seamless fashion and the patients will not experience themselves being bombarded by a symptom checklist.

- *Identifying the patient's strengths.* Unfortunately, most of work in modern medicine focuses almost exclusively on identify and highlighting the patient's weaknesses (both physical and psychological). Clinicians should specifically help patients to identify their strengths and highlight how these can be important to supporting their optimum wellness. Frequently, with the permission of the patient, family members will have very significant strengths that can be recruited to assist the patient through this journey.

■ KEY TERMS IN THE PSYCHO-ONCOLOGY ASSESSMENT

The precise definitions of many terms used in contemporary medicine to describe the subjective aspects of experience are not clearly understood by clinicians. This can sometimes lead to confusion in terminology. Some key terms are given:

- *Empathy.* Empathy describes the ability to be consciously aware of the other person's subjective experience. It involves both cognitive (ie, the ability to have a cognitive appreciation of the other's state) and emotional (ie, the ability to feel the other person's emotional state) components. Unfortunately, most factors that have been demonstrated to impede empathic accuracy (ie, how accurately one is aware of the other's state) have become a routine part of many healthcare interactions. Specific strategies that will increase empathic accuracy include (a) sitting at the same level as the patient, (b) using supportive nonverbal facilitators (eg, mirroring the patient's nonverbal behaviors, providing positive reassurances), and (c) establishing a long-term therapeutic relationship with the patient.
- *Compassion.* Compassion describes one's intention to be of benefit to others. It is different from sympathy that describes feeling sorry for the predicament of another person.
- *Healing.* Although the pursuit of healing is considered to be the goal of medicine, there is no universally accepted definition for the term healing. Derived from the Celtic word *haelon* (wholeness), healing is best described as the process of moving toward psychological, social, and spiritual wholeness. This is very different from curing that describes the resolution of a pathophysiological (ie, disease) state. Given these distinct differences, it is apparent that one may not be cured of a disease but still experience healing.
- *Suffering.* Once again, no universally accepted definition for suffering exists. This author suggests that suffering comes from the experience of being separated from those things that one experiences as being meaningful. This definition implies that suffering is an idiosyncratic experience derived from our particular relationship to the realities of our lives.
- *Illness.* This describes our relationship to our disease and the meaning that one ascribes to it. Once again, each person will experience the disease in a uniquely idiosyncratic way.

■ THE SETTING

Most clinical psychosocial evaluations take place in less than ideal circumstances—typically in a busy clinic or even the emergency room. However, despite the obvious limitations imposed by these settings, the clinician can create an environment that is conducive to discussing the patient's subjective emotional experiences. As a rule, the clinician should always be sitting when talking with the patient and family. Distractions and interruptions should be limited as much as possible and the clinician should avoid taking notes during the examination.

■ THE PSYCHO-ONCOLOGY HISTORY

The Presenting Complaint

The patients' ability to succinctly describe their primary subjective complaint provides valuable information on their relationship to their illness and their coping skills. It is important to provide patients with sufficient time to elaborate on their presenting complaint, and the clinician should resist the impulse to quickly redirect patients to a structured checklist of symptoms. Patients will feel more respected by the clinician who allows them an opportunity to describe their subjective experiences and thoughts and does not impose another clinical agenda. The astute clinician will quickly recognize which patients can benefit from a more structured approach and will assist these patients with a more directive closed-ended questions approach. In patients who exhibit cognitive disorganization the clinician should move quickly to the cognitive examination in order to identify a cognitive deficit that precludes obtaining a meaningful history (eg, delirium).

Past Psychiatric History

Patients with a past psychiatric history are at an increased risk for the psychiatric complications of cancer and its treatment. Particular attention should be paid to the nature and precipitants of previous psychiatric illness. In particular, any history of adverse behavioral effects to medications should be explored (ie, adverse behavioral responses to corticosteroids or antihistamines). Past history of alcohol or other substance use, abuse, and dependence should be explored and documented. Family psychiatric history should be documented. Allergy history should be documented.

Past Medical History

In addition to the routine medical history, the clinician should also inquire about any previous history of head injuries. Family medical history will also provide important

TABLE 1-4. Oncologic Medications Associated with Depression

Asparaginase	Paclitaxel
Corticosteroids	Procarbazine
Cyproterone	Tamoxifen
Docetaxel	Thalidomide
Interferon-alpha	Vinblastine
Interleukin–2	Vincristine
Leuprolide	Vinorelbine

TABLE 1-5. Opiate Risk Tool

Family history (parents and siblings):		
Alcohol abuse	_____(3)	_____(1)
Illegal drug use	_____(3)	_____(2)
Prescription drug abuse	_____(4)	_____(4)
Personal history:		
Alcohol abuse	_____(3)	_____(3)
Illegal drug use	_____(4)	_____(4)
Prescription drug abuse	_____(5)	_____(5)
Mental health:		
Diagnosis of ADD, OCD, bipolar, schizophrenia	_____(2)	_____(2)
Diagnosis of depression	_____(1)	_____(1)
Other:		
Age 16–45 years	_____(1)	_____(1)
History of preadolescent sexual abuse	_____(0)	_____(3)
Total	_____	_____

Scoring:

0–3	low risk:	6% chance of developing problematic behaviors
4–7	moderate risk:	28% chance of developing problematic behaviors
≥8	high risk:	>90% chance of developing problematic behaviors

Adapted with permission from Webster LR, Webster RM. *Pain Med.* 2005;6:432–442.

data about the patient's genetic risk factors as well as their prior experience of disease in loved ones.

Medications

A detailed medication history is a critical component of the psycho-oncology assessment.

Many medications used to treat cancer have adverse neurobehavioral effects (see Tables 1-4 and 1-5). In addition, psychotropic medications may have adverse interactions with many cancer therapies. In particular, the clinician should be alert for potential cytochrome P450 drug interactions between medications.

Complementary Approaches

Although many cancer patients are utilizing complementary therapies, they seldom discuss this with their oncologists. This may lead to unanticipated adverse interactions with medications and/or preventable side effects. Many patients believe that their oncologist will not approve of complementary therapies and they are hesitant to raise the subject. It is therefore important that clinicians feel comfortable and knowledgeable about complementary therapies and encourage their patients to disclose all therapies. Since nutritional factors are an important determinant of the patient's well-being, it is helpful to inquire about the patient's dietary habits and to identify areas that can be improved.

Substance Use

Although the prevalence of substance abuse is relatively low (about 5%) among cancer patients, it does occur with greater frequency among certain cancer patient populations (ie, greater than 25% of patients admitted to a palliative medicine unit were reported to have alcohol-related problems).[10] Unfortunately, clinicians are too often fearful of offending and stigmatizing the patient and they fail to identify this issue in the majority of affected patients. This oversight can have very serious consequences for patients who experience unanticipated and preventable alcohol withdrawal.[10]

It is important to obtain information about the type of substance, duration, frequency, reason for use, periods of sobriety, and any prior history of withdrawal.

The Opiate Risk Tool (ORT) and CAGE are two simple screening tools that are helpful in assessing substance abuse.[11,12] The ORT (see Table 1-5) is designed to be administered prior to starting opiates in patients who are expected to require opiate treatment. Patients are categorized as low, moderate, or high risk for opiate abuse. Rather than stigmatizing the patient or withholding effective analgesia, this allows clinicians to tailor interventions and monitoring schedules to the particular needs of the individual patient.

The CAGE is a simple four-question assessment that effectively screens for alcohol problems and can be administered in just a few minutes.[12] The CAGE questions include:

Have you ever:

1. felt the need to *cut* down your drinking;
2. felt *annoyed* by criticism of your drinking;
3. had *guilty* feelings about drinking; and
4. taken a morning *eye* opener?

A score of 2–3 indicates a high index of suspicion, and a score of 4 is virtually diagnostic for alcoholism.

Nicotine use is a potent risk factor for cancer, and all clinicians should specifically inquire about nicotine use and be knowledgeable about tobacco cessation program.

Social and Developmental History

An informative developmental and social history can be obtained in just a few minutes and often provides powerful insights into the patients' experience of themselves and their illness. Patients with a history of delayed developmental milestones or problems with learning may experience difficulty in navigating the complexity of the modern medical system.

The patients' early life experience of stable parental figures and previous experience of medical illness may have a powerful influence on their relationship to authority figures and how they perceive the role of a patient. It is helpful to identify previous periods of stress in the patient's life and how he or she handled these situations.

It is important to identify and document the patient's current social supports and clarify what role these individuals may play during the patient's treatment. Unfortunately, cancer places a very heavy burden on patients and their families and is often the major cause of their distress. The patient's financial situation should be briefly reviewed, and where necessary, referral to social work and/or financial advisors should be facilitated.

Spiritual and Religious History

Clinicians often feel uncomfortable discussing matters of spirituality and religion with their patients. However, the data clearly indicate that patients want their clinicians to discuss these matters with them during periods of stress and serious illness. Rather than expecting their clinician to act as a spiritual counselor, patients want their clinician to understand and validate their relationship to this critically important aspect of their lives and how they cope with distress. There is no consensus definition of either spirituality or religion. One definition of spirituality is "the person's beliefs and attitude's towards a transcendent purpose." Religion may be described as "those rituals and practices that the individual practices as part of an organized community and its relationship to a transcendent purpose." The concept of spiritual distress describes the subjective suffering that comes from losing meaning in life.[13] Puchalski and Romer have described the simple acronym FICA that can assist the clinician in quickly obtaining very valuable information about a person's spiritual and religious experience[14]:

Faith: "Can you tell me about your religious faith and beliefs?"
Importance: "Can you tell me how important your spiritual life is to you?"
Community: "Are you part of a religious community and how important is that to you?"
Addressed: "How would you like your spiritual issues to be addressed as part of your medical care?"

Advanced Directives and Living Wills

End-of-life care preferences should not be delayed until the terminal phases of disease, and all cancer patients should be provided with an opportunity to discuss their end-of-life care preferences and to complete an advanced directive. At various points through their disease trajectory, patients should be encouraged to complete a living will and to identify their surrogate decision-maker. Most of the resistance to such discussions comes from healthcare providers and not from patients. Failure to address and document patient preferences will result in unnecessary and unwanted burden on the patient, family, and their treatment team.

■ THE CLINICAL EXAMINATION OF THE ONCOLOGIC PATIENT

The astute clinician will have gained considerable information about the patient before their first meeting. Information provided by the referring clinician and a review of the medical record will provide important clues about the patient's risk factors. The patients' ability to schedule appointments, arrive on time, and provide previous medical documentation provides very valuable information about their executive cognitive skills.

General Appearance

The patients' self-grooming provides a lot of information on their organizational skills, comportment, and some insight into their financial situation. Many cancer patients experience significant fatigue and may have difficulty motivating themselves to actively participate in the interview. It is important to realize that patients experiencing significant pain often do not manifest overt physical evidence for their distress. Observing the patient as he or she walks to the examination room can provide very important information on comorbid neurodegenerative disorders or the extrapyramidal side effects of medications.

The Cognitive Assessment

The preponderance of data suggests that a significant percentage of cancer patients experience changes in cognition.[15] These cognitive changes have typically been thought to be secondary to chemotherapy, radiation therapy, and hormonal adjuvant therapy. However, more recent data indicate that these changes may actually antedate the therapeutic intervention in as much as 30% of patients.[15] These patients appear to be at an increased risk for therapy-related cognitive side effects. A thorough cognitive assessment should therefore be a vital and useful part of the psycho-oncology assessment.

The cognitive assessment can also provide very valuable insights on how patients can be expected to self-manage their disease and comply with the myriad expectations inherent to cancer treatment. Specifically, patients with executive cognitive deficits will have difficulty in high-stimulus environments that include large amounts of ambiguous and complicated information (ie, a modern healthcare setting). Such patients will often be wrongly viewed by their healthcare team as resistant or noncompliant with treatment recommendations and will not receive full benefit from their optimum treatment opportunity. Executive cognitive deficits may be caused by multiple etiologies, with by far the most common being subcortical encephalomalacia (associated with the risk factors for vasculopathy), and also frontal-type dementia, traumatic brain injury, normal pressure hydrocephalus, Huntington's disease, and Pick's disease.

The Mini-Mental State Examination has the most commonly employed screening instrument to detect cognitive deficits in almost all clinical settings. Despite its widespread use, the MMSE has very significant limitations in cancer patients. Developed in 1975, the MMSE was originally intended to screen for dementia in the general population. Although it has an 89% specificity for identifying the presence of dementia (at a cutoff of 24/30), the MMSE has only 69% sensitivity for identifying the presence of dementia.[16] Furthermore, since the MMSE does not adequately assess executive cognition, it is an inadequate screen for patients with the risk factors of subcortical encephalomalacia (Binswanger's disease) who are often encountered in the cancer setting. It is important to appreciate that although modular cognitive deficits (eg, memory problems, aphasia) cause significant impairment, patients and families can often develop effective coping strategies to mitigate these deficits. However, although patients with executive deficits may have no overt cognitive deficits, they are typically more incapacitated than modular-deficit patients in novel and ambiguous situations that require insight and problem solving.

Given these limitations of the MMSE, clinicians are strongly urged to utilize a process approach to cognitive assessment (see Table 1-6). This approach recognizes that all cognitive functions require a series of steps that begin with the ability to maintain arousal and appropriately focus, sustain, and redirect attention. Delirium is essentially a disorder of attention and the delirious patient will therefore perform poorly on all cognitive tasks. Tasks of executive function include the ability to manipulate learned material in real time (analogous to the "memory" of a computer processor). Examples include serial reverse days, months, and digit span. Word generation provides a sensitive measure of a person's executive ability to organize and sequence his or her cognitive strategy. Patients are first asked to generate a closed set of words (ie, where task structuring is provided by asking for words from a specific group such as "grocery items"). Patients with good executive skills will demonstrate an orderly approach to this task by starting in the fruit and vegetable section and then shifting to other sections of the store when their productivity is diminishing. Patients with executive deficits typically demonstrate a disorganized approach, skip from one section of the store to another, and may become impersistent or "stuck" in one section. When asked to generate an open set of words (ie, words beginning with the letter F, except for people's names), patients with executive deficits are likely to become overwhelmed and perform very poorly.

While a neuropsychologist may require many hours to perform a very detailed cognitive assessment, the process strategy described in Table 1-6 can be completed in

■ **TABLE 1-6. The Clinical Assessment of Cognition**

Patient: _____ Age: _____

Sex: M   F   Handedness: R   L

Education level: Date: Time: AM/PM

Arousal: Drowsy/Normal/Hypervigilant

Orientation: Day ___ Month ___ Year ____ Person ____ Place ____

Attention:

Days	Forward: Y/N	Reverse: Y/N	(___/2)
Months	Forward: Y/N	Reverse: Y/N	(___/2)
Spell "Radio"	Forward: Y/N	Reverse: Y/N	(___/2)
Digit span	Forward: (6345817)		(___/6)
	Reverse: (63458)		(___/6)
	Total:		(___/18)

Word generation (60 seconds)

Closed set (grocery items) _____   *Open set* ("F") words _____

Motivation: Low/Moderate/High   *Distractibility:* Low/Moderate/High

Preservation: Y/N *Contamination:* Y/N *Impersistence:* Y/N

Recent memory

Trials to learn: ___ Recall after 2 minutes: ___/4 Recall with cues: ___/4

Recall after 5 minutes: ___/4 Recall with cues: ___/4

Remote memory

Autobiographical data: Normal/Impaired

Historical data: Normal/Impaired

Communication

Prosody (Inflection/Rhythmic pattern of language)

Expressive (Show me a happy face)	Normal/Abnormal
Receptive (What kind of face am I making?)	Normal/Abnormal
Paraphasic errors (substituting one word for another) Y/N	
Anemia (Difficulty naming)	Y/N

Aphasia	Repetition	Y/N
	Reading	Y/N
	Writing	Y/N

Praxis (The performance of an action)

Buccofacial (blow out a candle)	On command/Imitation/Fail
Limb (salute like a soldier)	On command/Imitation/Fail
Object use (comb your hair)	On command/Imitation/Fail
Luria three-step (hand: fist, palm, side)	On command/Imitation/Fail

---

Visuospatial performance

Clock face (10 past 11)	Organized	Y/N
	Oriented	Y/N
	Correct hand placement	Y/N
Cube drawing	Organized	Y/N
	3-dimensional	Y/N

Abrastraction

Learned proverb (eg, "Don't cry over spilled milk")	Abstract/Concrete/Fail
Novel proverb (eg, "Hunger is the best gravy")	Abstract/Concrete/Fail

---

just a few minutes and can provide invaluable diagnostic information. Just as importantly, this approach will assist the clinician in identifying what resources the patient will need if he or she is to navigate the healthcare system.

Patients with significant executive deficits will require more intensive case management and a more proactive approach by the treatment team (eg, calling the patient to remind them of scheduled tests, etc).

Mood and Affect

The term *mood* describes the person's predominant and sustained emotional status. *Affect* describes the person's display of emotions. It is important to recognize that not every patient suffering from diminished goal-directed behavior or tearfulness is suffering from a mood disorder. Many patients receiving corticosteroids will manifest pronounced affective lability and a heightened affective response to emotionally provocative stimuli.[17] It is a critical clinical point to recognize that affective lability is a cardinal behavioral sign of delirium. In this regard, patients experiencing delirium are often misdiagnosed as suffering from depression. It is therefore always important to complete a complete review of the criteria for depression before making a presumptive diagnosis of depression in patients with emotional lability or diminished goal-directed behavior. In this regard, cancer therapies may produce apathy and/or fatigue that may mimic depression. Therefore, the clinician should specifically inquire about the motivation and energy levels in all cancer patients.

Thought Content and Process

Specific inquiry should be made into the patient's thought content. The clinician should not be hesitant to ask the patient whether he or she is experiencing any hallucinations, obsessive ruminations, or any particular fears. The form of the patient's thinking is assessed throughout the interview with particular reference to the patient's ability to generate thoughts spontaneously, maintain set, and not become impersistent. Patients suffering from depression or subcortical disease (such as Parkinsonism) will typically exhibit a "dilapidated" cognition that is characterized by poor motivation and a diminished rate of thought production. Once again, delirium may masquerade as virtually any psychiatric disorder and the delirious patient may exhibit overt hallucinosis or delusional thought content that may be misinterpreted as a formal thought disorder. It is important to recognize that the presence of visual hallucinosis strongly suggests the presence of a toxic encephalopathy and possible iatrogenic causes (eg, opiates, anticholinergic drugs) should be explored.

Suicide Assessment

Although only a few of the cancer patients who express suicidal ideation actually go on to commit suicide, the risk of completed suicide is approximately twice the risk in cancer patients compared with the general population. Given the increased risk of suicide associated with cancer, it is important that all clinicians who work with cancer patients feel comfortable screening patients for suicide risk. Self-destructive ideation and behavior varies widely in regard to its severity and the risk that the patient may action it. However, suicidal ideation is of most concern when it is persistent and the patients have a specific plan for harming themselves. Patients with advanced and incurable disease may express self-destructive thoughts that are usually characterized as a desire for hastened death that might include a passive wish to die or the refusal to accept recommended medical interventions. This desire for a hastened death should not be considered an inevitable consequence of the dying process, and any patient who expresses a desire for hastened death should be evaluated for the presence of major depression.

Clinicians may sometimes feel uncomfortable discussing a patient's suicidal ideation and may unconsciously avoid, or inadequately address, this critical area of the psychosocial oncology assessment. Discussing suicidal ideation with patients does not increase the risk of future suicidal behavior by the patient.

The effective assessment and management of suicide risk requires that factors associated with an increased risk for suicide should be explored. These risk factors include:

- *Presence of depression.* At least half of all suicides occur in the context of a major depressive disorder. Depression has been reported to be the most important predictor of desire for hastened death among patients with advanced cancer.[18]
- *Demographic predictors.* Completed suicide is more common among older men who live alone. In addition, males suffering from lung cancer appear to be at the highest risk.[19]
- *Lack of social support.* Lower levels of social support are associated with increased suicidal ideation and a desire for hastened death.[20]
- *Hopelessness.* Helplessness is a stronger determinant of suicidal ideation than the severity of depression experienced by the patient.[18] However, the presence of both depression and helplessness appears to be the strongest determinant of a desire for hastened death.[21]
- *Need for control.* Patients who accept their illness with adaptability and less need for control are less likely to exhibit suicidal ideation.[22,23]
- *Guilty feelings.* Patients who experience themselves as being a burden on their loved ones are more likely to contemplate suicide and request that their death be hastened.[28] Ruminative guilt is cardinal symptom of

depression in cancer patients and its presence should trigger a detailed psychosocial assessment.

- *Pain and physical distress.* Uncontrolled pain and other distressing physical symptoms are a major cause of a desire for hastened death and suicidal ideation and increase the likelihood for the co-occurrence of depression and escalating feelings of hopelessness.[25,26]
- *Substance abuse.* Patients with active substance abuse are at an increased risk for suicide. In particular, such patients are likely to be unpredictable and unreliable based on the effect of alcohol and illicit substances on their impulse control, mood, and judgment. The presence of suicidal ideation in the substance-abusing patient is therefore an indicator for very active involvement by the clinician and the development of a treatment plan that includes aggressive stabilization and treatment of substance abuse.[27]
- *Loss of dignity.* Patients with advanced cancer often experience a loss of dignity and self-respect. This may be further compounded by the guilt they experience from being a burden on loved ones.[28] Discussing the patients' experience of their loss of dignity can be a very important avenue for identifying the determinants of their distress and may provide effective opportunities for clinical intervention.
- *Spiritual and experiential distress.* Patients who express low spiritual or existential well-being are more likely to experience suicidal ideation and a desire to hasten their death.[29]
- *Cognitive dysfunction.* A significant correlation between cognitive dysfunction and suicidal ideation has been reported in cancer patients. Patients with diminished capacity have less cognitive flexibility and a limited repertoire of responses to their personal distress. Clinicians should always assess suicidal patients carefully for evidence of delirium, particularly when the patient is exhibiting affective lability.[30]
- *Previous psychiatric history.* Patients with a prior psychiatric history or personal or family history of suicide are at a significantly greater risk for attempting suicide.[26]
- *Panic disorder.* The presence of a panic disorder is an independent predictor of increased risk for suicide.[31] Clinicians should therefore make sure that they evaluate for the presence of this disorder in patients with suicidal ideation.

Interventions for addressing patients' suicidal risk should be based on the thorough assessment of the nature of the suicidal ideation and risk factors for attempted suicide described above. The findings of this assessment can inform targeted interventions that have a high likelihood of being effective. All patients exhibiting suicidal ideation should immediately be referred to mental health specialists.

Identifying the Patient's Coping Style

Receiving a diagnosis of cancer and undergoing cancer treatment is a terrifying and often overwhelming experience for many people. In this regard, cancer patients are facing perhaps the greatest challenge of their lives and it will test their resilience and ability to cope with stress. The best predictor of the patients' ability to cope is their past pattern of behaviors. It is therefore important to gain some insight into how patients have handled previous challenges in their lives and what resources they have utilized to make it through difficult times. The clinician can ask the patient, "Can you tell me about a time in your life when you faced a difficult challenge? How did you cope with this?" The patient's response to these questions will provide the clinician with some understanding of his or her coping style and, most particularly, the patient's capacity for self-reflection and insight, both critical to navigating the challenges of a cancer diagnosis. Patients with mature ego defenses will fare far better than those with more infantile defenses when faced with severe stressors.

Psychiatrist George Vaillant has developed an empirically validated model of ego defense mechanisms that has great clinical utility. Clinicians who can identify their patient's level of ego defense functioning will become skillful practitioners. Both patients and their clinician will benefit greatly from this approach. According to Vaillant's model, ego defenses can be stratified across four levels of increasing maturity and constructiveness.[32]

Level 1—Pathological Ego Defenses

These describe the defenses of someone who is experiencing life at the level of his or her dyadic relationship with his or her maternal figure. Because such individuals experience themselves as helpless outside the context of an enmeshed nurturing behavior, they are likely to become overwhelmed when confronted with a serious medical diagnosis. Rather than being able to adapt themselves to the new reality of their lives, persons acting at this level will attempt to distort reality to meet their own needs. These defenses are therefore essentially psychotic and always pathological and not beneficial to the patients or their social system. Clinicians working with such patients will therefore find themselves caught in maladaptive closed loops that can rapidly lead to them becoming frustrated, even angry. When working with such patients, it is important to establish clear boundaries with clear communication between all parties. Clearly documented treatment plans and expectations can be helpful. Clinicians must avoid reacting to the patient's distortions with hostility or a need to rescue. Pathological ego defenses include the following:

- *delusional projection*: frank delusions about external reality
- *denial*: refusal to accept external reality because it is too threatening
- *distortion*: reshaping of external reality in order to meet internal needs
- *splitting*: people are idealized or devalued and divided into two (often opposing) categories

Level 2—Immature Ego Defenses

These ego defenses are utilized in an attempt to diminish the person's distress provoked by a particular circumstance. Unfortunately, they do little to effectively address the stressor and typically create nonadaptive and destructive relationships with others. Clinicians will experience such patients as exasperating and difficult to work constructively with in following through with treatment planning and implementation. When clinicians experience uncomfortable emotional reactions to patterns, they should closely evaluate the dynamic of the therapeutic relationship and consider that the patient may be utilizing projective identification as an ego defense. Clinicians working with such patients should establish clear boundaries and clear communication as described above when working with patients with pathological level ego defenses. Immature ego defenses include the following:

- *acting out*: behavior directed by an unconscious wish or impulse
- *fantasy*: retreating into fantasy in order to resolve inner and outer conflicts
- *idealization*: viewing the other person as more positive than reality suggests
- *passive aggression*: exerting control by not doing something
- *projection*: experiencing another person as having our own intolerable emotions
- *projective identification*: behaving in a way that has the other person carry our own intolerable emotions
- *somatization*: transforming our intolerable emotions into somatic experience

Level 3—Neurotic Ego Defenses

These defenses allow the person to experience a sense of control over current stressors. Although they may be helpful in the short term, if they are inflexible, such defenses will result in maladaptive relationships with others. Clinicians working with patients with neurotic defenses may experience challenges relating to their professional authority and may also experience their patients as sabotaging the clinician's attempts to help them. When working with such patients, the clinician should allow the patients to maintain a sense of control and not become confrontational over nonessential clinical details (eg, "Doctor, did you not know about the recent journal article on my disease?"). Neurotic-level ego defenses include the following:

- *displacement*: shifting intolerable emotions from its stimulus to another more acceptable target
- *hypochondriasis*: inappropriate anxiety and preoccupation with a physical complaint
- *isolation*: separating feelings from ideas and events
- *intellectualization*: a form of isolation in which one attempts to utilize cognitive strategies to decrease the intolerable affect
- *rationalization*: creating justifications for one's behavior as a means of avoiding the intolerable emotion provoked by the experience, that is, making excuses
- *reaction formation*: behaving in a manner that is opposite to our unconscious intention
- *regression*: reverting to an earlier stage of ego development
- *repression*: consciously avoiding an intolerable thought and its emotion
- *undoing*: engaging in a behavior that essentially negates the previous action

Level 4—Mature Ego Defenses

These are commonly found among emotionally healthy adults and are likely to support the development of healthy emotional relationships with self and others. By definition, such individuals are consciously aware of their coping strategies and their impact on themselves and others. Clinicians will experience such patients as flexible, resilient, and easy to work with. Mature ego defenses include the following:

- *altruism*: helping others without consideration for one's own rewards
- *anticipation*: planning appropriately for future discomfort

- *humor*: diffusing intolerable emotion through the use of appropriate humor
- *identification*: conscious modeling and behavior
- *sublimation*: transforming intolerable emotions into positive actions
- *suppression*: consciously pushing intolerable emotions out of everyday awareness; the person can however voluntarily access these emotions when necessary

An understanding of ego defenses is critical to working with the so-called challenging patient. It is important to understand that patients with less adaptive coping styles are not consciously attempting to create distress. On the contrary, they are using maladaptive ego defenses as a way of coping with their own intolerable distress. By simply identifying the patient's ego defense style, the clinician can not only manage challenging behaviors but also, more importantly, predict and avoid them. It is also important to appreciate that each of us, patient and clinician, utilizes ego defenses, and that sometimes a challenging clinical relationship may be a manifestation of the clinician utilizing less adaptive coping mechanisms.

The Diagnostic Formulation

A five-axis DSM-related diagnosis should be established for all patients. In particular, when treating cancer patients it is crucial that clinicians first assess all potential biological contributors to the patient's behavioral disorder. A failure to do so can have catastrophic consequences for the patient. However, when formulating a biopsychosociospiritual formulation it is not always possible to determine which of these domains may be producing most distress for the patient. The author has found it useful to ask all patients the following three questions:

"Are you suffering?"
"Can you rate your suffering on a scale of 1 to 10 (with 10 being no suffering)?"
"Can you tell where your suffering comes from?"

Utilizing Neurodiagnostic Technologies

Neurodiagnostic technologies (ie, CT scanning, MRI scanning, EEG, PET/SPECT scanning, and neuropsychological testing) have great diagnostic utility in cancer populations and often provide critical information that ultimately directs treatment decisions. However, it is important that the clinician should have a specific diagnostic hypothesis before requesting a neurodiagnostic study.

KEY POINTS

- The psycho-oncology assessment should be performed on every cancer patient and provides critically important information necessary for providing effective clinical care of the patient and their family.
- Cancer patients and their families experience high psychiatric morbidity that can be effectively treated.
- Behavioral changes in a cancer patient may be the harbinger of significant physical problems.
- Suicide assessment should be performed regularly in all cancer patients.
- Chemotherapeutic agents frequently produce behavioral disorders and can be effectively treated if recognized early.
- All cancer patients should be screened for substance abuse.

REFERENCES

1. Pirl WF. Evidence report on the occurrence, assessment, and treatment of depression in cancer patient. *J Natl Cancer Inst Monogr.* 2004;32:32–39.

2. Barlow DH. *The Diagnostic and Statistical Manual of Mental Disorders.* 4th ed. Washington, DC: American Psychiatric Press Inc, 2007.

3. Ransom S, Jacobsen PB, Booth-Jones M. *Validation of the Distress Scale with bone marrow transplant patients.* Psychooncology. 2006;15(7):604–612.

4. Zabora J, BrintzenofeSzoc K, Jacoben P, et al. A new psychosocial screen for use with cancer patients. *Psychosomatics.* 2001;42:241–246 [the Psychosocial Screen for Cancer].

5. Graves KD, Arnold SM, Love CL, Kirsh KL, Moore PG, Passik SD. Distress screening in a multidisciplinary lung cancer clinic; prevalence and predictors of clinically significant distress. *Lung Cancer.* 2007;55(2):215–224.

6. Baker-Glenn EA, Mitchell AJ. Screening for perceived need for help using the latest screening tools – what do we know about who wants help? *Psychooncology.* 2008;17:S56-57.

7. Pinquart M, Duberstein PR. Depression and cancer mortality: a meta-analysis. *Psychol Med.* 2010;1:1–14.

8. Satin JR, Linden W, Philips MJ. Depression as a predictor of disease progression and mortality in cancer patients. *Cancer.* 2009;115(22):5349–5461.

9. Mellon S, Northouse LL, Weiss LK. A population-based study of the quality of life of cancer survivors and their family caregivers. *Cancer Nurs.* 2006;29:120–131.

10. Bruera E, Moyano J, Seifert J. The frequency of alcoholism among patients with pain due to terminal cancer. *J Pain Symptom Manage.* 1995;10(8):599–603.

11. Lynn R, Webster MD, Webster RM. Predicting aberrant behaviors in opioid-treated patients: preliminary validation of the Opioid Risk Tool. *Pain Med.* 2005;6:432–442.

12. Ewing JA. Detecting alcoholism. The CAGE questionnaire. *JAMA.* 1984;252:1905–1907.

13. Buxton F. Spiritual distress and integrity in palliative and non-palliative patients. *Br J Nurs.* 2007;16(15): 920–924.

14. Puchalski CM, Romer AL. Taking a spiritual history allows clinicians to understand patients more fully. *J Palliat Med.* 2000;3:129–137.

15. Ahles TA, Saykin AJ, McDonald BC. Cognitive function in breast cancer patients prior to adjuvant treatment. *Breast Cancer Res Treat.* 2008;110:143–152.

16. Grut M, Fratiglioni L, Viitanen M. Accuracy of the Mini Mental Status Examination as a screening test for dementia in elderly Swedish population. *Acta Neurol Scand.* 1993;87:312–317.

17. Brown ES, Khan DA, Nejtek VA. The psychiatric side effects of corticosteroids. *Ann Allergy Asthma Immunol.* 1999;83(6):495–503.

18. Chochinov HM, Wilson KG, Enns M, Lander S. Depression, hopelessness, and suicidal ideation in the terminally ill. *Psychosomatics.* 1998;39:366–370.

19. Hem E, Loge JH, Haldorsen T, Ekeberg O. Suicide risk in cancer patients from 1960 to 1999. *J Clin Oncol.* 2004;22:4209–4216.

20. Chochinov HM, Wilson KG, Enns M. Desire for death in the terminally ill. *Am J Psychiatry.* 1995;152(8): 1185–91.

21. Breitbart W, Rosenfeld B, Pessin H, et al. Depression, hopelessness, and desire for hastened death in terminally ill patients with cancer. *JAMA.* 2000;284(22):2907–2911.

22. Hudson PL, Kristjanson LJ, Ashby M. Desire for hastened death in patients with advanced disease and the evidence base of clinical guidelines: a systematic review. *Palliat Med.* 2006;20:693–701.

23. Farberow NL, Schneiderman ES, Leonard CV. Suicide among general medical and surgical hospital patients with malignant neoplasms. *Med Bull.* 1963;9:1–11.

24. Sullivan AD, Hedberg K, Hopkins MS. Legalized physician-assisted suicide in Oregon, 1998–2000. *N Engl J Med.* 2001;344:605–607.

25. Bolund C. Suicide and cancer II. Medical and care factors in suicide by cancer patients in Sweden, 1973–1976. *Psychol Med.* 1991; 21(4):979–984.

26. Breitbart W. Suicide risk and pain in cancer and AIDS patients. In: Chapman CR, Foley KM, eds. *Current and Emerging Issues in Cancer Pain: Research and Practice.* New York: Raven Press; 1993:49–65.

27. Schneider B. Substance use disorders and risk for completed suicide. *Arch Suicide Res.* 2009;13(4):303–16 [review].

28. van der Maas PJ, van der Wal G, Haverkate I. Euthanasia, physician-assisted suicide, and other medical practices at the end-of-life in the Netherlands, 1990–1995. *N Engl J Med.* 1996;335:1699–1705.

29. McClain CS, Rosenfeld B, Breitbart W. Effect of spiritual well-being on end-of-life despair in terminally-ill cancer patients. *Lancet.* 2003;361:1603–1607.

30. Pessin H, Rosenfeld B, Burton L, Breitbart W. The role of cognitive impairment in desire for hastened death: a study of patients with advanced AIDS. *Gen Hosp Psychiatry.* 2003;25:194–199.

31. Brown LA, Gaudiano BA, Miller IW. The impact of panic-agoraphobic comorbidity on suicidality in hospitalized patients with major depression. *Depress Anxiety.* 2010;27(3):310–315.

32. Vaillant GE, Bond M, Vaillant CO. An empirically validated hierarchy of defense mechanisms. *Arch Gen Psychiatry.* 1986;43(8):786–794.

Stress and Cancer

• *Julie K. Allen, Guillermo N. Armaiz-Pena, and Anil K. Sood*

■ INTRODUCTION

Throughout history, scientists have hypothesized that disease can be affected by disposition or behavior. Some observations extend back many centuries when the Roman physician and philosopher Galen stated that "melancholy" women were more likely to develop cancer than women with a "sanguine" disposition.[1] Other historical observations include the doctor who treated the author Alexandre Dumas for stomach cancer. This doctor believed that the principal causes for cancer were "deep sedentary study" and the "anxious agitation of public life."[2] The Buddhist teacher Dogen observed in his *Shobogenzo* that people are less likely to be sick when life is removed of its complications. Although these ideas were primitive in their nature, modern research has started to show that these observations were not far from the truth.

Selye[3] is considered a founder of contemporary concepts of how stress influences the body's ability to cope with disease. In 1936, he defined stress as a state of co-activation of the autonomic nervous system (ANS) and the hypothalamic–pituitary–adrenal (HPA) axis.[3] More modern definitions describe stress as a complex process involving activation of several systems in both the peripheral and central nervous systems (CNS) that, in turn, affect many other body systems and processes.

The overall stress response involves activation of several body systems. The CNS activates the ANS, which in turn activates the sympathetic nervous system (SNS),

causing release of catecholamines (Fig. 2-1).[4] The major catecholamines include norepinephrine, epinephrine, and dopamine. Epinephrine and norepinephrine are responsible for controlling physiological responses and actions including increases in blood pressure and heart rate and causing the release of glucose from energy stores. Dopamine acts primarily as a neurotransmitter and controls the body's ability to feel pleasure or pain.[5]

The CNS also activates the hypothalamic responses that include the release of vasopressin and corticotropin-releasing hormone from the hypothalamus.[6] These, in turn, cause release of adrenocorticotrophic hormone (ACTH) from the anterior pituitary, which results in downstream release of glucocorticoids from the adrenal cortex, and constitute the HPA axis. Virtually all cell types in the body have receptors for glucocorticoids, which control many normal physiological activities such as circadian rhythms, and stress responses such as immune function and restoration of homeostasis.[7]

Although stress can be broken down into many categories such as physical, mental, emotional, social, or biological, there are two overriding types of stress: acute and chronic. Acute stress can be seen as a major event that is short-lived, occurs infrequently, and is beneficial to the body.[8] On detection of the stressor, the body activates stress response systems, releasing catecholamines and glucocorticoids that prepare the body to cope with a threat.[9] Blood pressure and heart rate increase, escalating blood flow to the limbs to prepare the body for the fight-or-flight response. On removal of the stressor, these

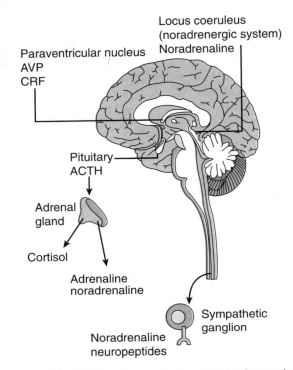

Locus coeruleus
(noradrenergic system)
Noradrenaline

Paraventricular nucleus
AVP
CRF

Pituitary
ACTH

Adrenal
gland

Cortisol

Adrenaline
noradrenaline

Sympathetic
ganglion

Noradrenaline
neuropeptides

FIGURE 2-1. Limbic system activation resulting in catecholamine and glucocorticoid secretion. Detection of a stressor activates the hypothalamus, which secretes corticotrophin-releasing factor (CRF) and arginine vasopressin. These, in turn, stimulate release of adrenocorticotrophic hormone from the pituitary, which signals release of glucocorticoids from the adrenal cortex. Activation of the noradrenergic system signals through sympathetic ganglia for release of catecholamines from sympathetic nerve endings. Reprinted with permission from Macmillan Publishers Ltd: *Nat Rev Cancer.* 6:240–248, copyright 2006.

systems are turned off and the body returns to normal baseline function. Chronic stressors occur frequently and over an extended period of time, typically from months to years. The body remains in a constant state of "overdrive" because the stress occurs so frequently or lasts so long that the body does not have time to reset the stress response systems. This causes a disruption in the body's allostatic load. McEwen defines allostatic load as the "wear and tear that results from chronic overactivity or underactivity of allostatic systems" as the body attempts to account for stress.[4] Over time, this results in increased risk of many diseases and disorders including autoimmune dysfunction, diabetes, cancer, cardiovascular disease, and other signs of premature aging.[4]

Additional neuroendocrine factors are also modulated following stress, including prolactin (PRL), nerve growth factor (NGF), substance P, and oxytocin.[10–13] PRL is a hormone secreted from the anterior pituitary and plays a part in influencing the immune response following stress. NGF is a neurotrophin involved in growth and proliferation of neurons that has also been found to increase following activation of the stress response.[14] It also acts as an angiogenic agent and a survival factor in cancer cells.[15,16] Substance P is a neurokinin involved in pain sensation as well as stress that is highly expressed in areas of the brain associated with behavior regulation and stress response,[17] and acts as a mitogen for cancer cells.[18] Oxytocin is most commonly involved in labor initiation, but has also been implicated in mediating social responses and relieving stress symptoms.[19]

Under chronic stress, the regulation of cellular and systemic functions by stress hormones is augmented. For example, at low, nonstress levels, cortisol has a neuroprotective effect that results from glucocorticoid receptors (GRs) forming complexes with Bcl-2 and translocating to the mitochondria. However, frequent high or stress levels of this hormone result in decreased translocation of this complex, thereby inhibiting Bcl-2-induced apoptosis in neuronal cells.[20] Similarly, short bursts of catecholamines play an essential role in protecting the body as it copes with stress, but long-term exposure causes increased risk for several diseases, most prominently cardiovascular disease.[21]

Effects of catecholamines are mediated through adrenergic receptors (ARs), which are seven transmembrane G-coupled receptors. They are divided into α and β classes; within the β class there are β1-, β2-, and β3-ARs.[22] Several studies have found some classes of these receptors to have increased expression in various tumor types, and other classes to have decreased expression in some tumor types. For example, β2-ARs are increased in oral[23] and liver[24] cancers and β3-ARs in colon cancer,[25] while α1-ARs are decreased in liver[24] and gastric cancers.[26] These receptors are coupled to G proteins, which act as molecular switches to control downstream pathways. In the G protein switching mechanism of control, β2-AR can bind the stimulatory G protein, G_s, or the inhibitory G protein, G_i. Binding of G_s mediates activation of the cAMP-dependent protein kinase A (PKA) system and results in downstream activation of several pathways, resulting in growth and migration of cells,[27,28] while binding of G_i controls multiple signaling cascades, including the MAP kinase pathway, which is frequently overactivated in cancers.

STRESS AND CANCER INITIATION

Human tumorigenesis is a complex multistep process. Several sequential steps must occur in order for a cell to become a cancerous lesion. Hanahan and Weinberg[29] postulated that six steps are required for the transformation of cells: self-sufficiency in growth signals, insensitivity to growth-inhibitory (antigrowth) signals, evasion of programmed cell death (apoptosis), limitless replicative potential, sustained angiogenesis, and tissue invasion and metastasis. Each of these steps requires in some way the avoidance of innate defenses.

Although studies have directly linked stress to cancer progression, the effects on cancer initiation are not as clear. For example, two separate groups have studied women after suspicious lesions were found on mammograms, but before biopsy diagnoses had been made.[30-31] In the first study, women were questioned specifically about their day-to-day stress and stressful events in the previous 5 years, while the other used questionnaires to examine daily stress with no specific time frame. The first study found a significant correlation between malignant lesions and the occurrence of at least one major stressful life event in the previous 5 years.[30] In contrast, the second study found that day-to-day stress actually reduced risk of breast cancer by up to 40%.[31] Other studies have demonstrated that chronically depressed elderly are more likely to develop cancer,[32] and that decreased social support increases incidence of breast cancer by 9-fold.[33] These studies are just examples of the many difficulties that arise in trying to study the effects of stress on cancer initiation. In the case of these studies, the confounding results could be due to many factors including differences in statistical analysis, difficulties in methods of determining stress, or the inability of these methods to differentiate whether the stress actually caused the cancer or was merely responsible for progression of a preinvasive lesion to a malignant lesion. A long-term longitudinal study on a large population would be ideal for eliminating many of these problems. This would allow for continual monitoring of stress levels, rather than a retrospective questionnaire, as well as removing uncertainties about whether the stress levels are aiding in initiation of the lesion or simply causing it to progress to malignancy.

STRESS AND CANCER PROGRESSION

In the last two decades, mounting clinical evidence has cemented the notion that biobehavioral factors can influence cancer progression. A study in ovarian cancer patients demonstrated that those patients who were considered to be under substantial distress had impaired immune function resulting from decreased natural killer (NK) cell cytotoxicity in the tumor-infiltrating lymphocytes (TIL).[34] A study performed in breast cancer patients found similar effects on NK cell activity as well as inhibition of the T-cell response and lymphocyte proliferation,[35] indicating poorer outcome and survival for patients. Additionally, cortisol dysregulation associated with abnormal circadian rhythms or resulting from decreased social support in cancer patients has been associated with increased mortality in women with metastatic breast cancer, suggesting a correlation between social isolation and disease progression.[36,37]

STRESS AND THE IMMUNE SYSTEM

Multiple studies have shown that chronic activation of the stress response can result in decreased immune function. It is known that the CNS, the endocrine system, and the immune system can interact, meaning that variations in one system can affect them all. For example, the CNS controls immunity primarily through control of release of glucocorticoids through the HPA axis as well as release of catecholamines through the ANS. Several factors involved in the stress response are involved in activating or hindering the immune system, which may play a role in allowing tumor cells to escape detection and immune cell elimination.

The role of glucocorticoids in immune function can vary with the concentration of these hormones. For example, it is known that physiological levels of glucocorticoids are immunoregulatory, while levels associated with chronic stress have been shown to be immunosuppressive. Glucocorticoids can elicit direct effects on cells that carry their receptors. Within the immune system, T and B cells, neutrophils, monocytes, and macrophages all carry these receptors, allowing for disruption of both the cellular and humoral immune responses, such as inhibiting inflammation, causing a shift in the balance between Th1 and Th2 cytokines, and causing antigen-presenting cells to cease production of IL-12, which are important in immune adaptation.[38,39] Additionally, glucocorticoids can induce apoptosis in monocytes, macrophages, and T lymphocytes,[40] providing further evidence of their ability to be disruptive to normal immune function.

The humoral immune response, or Th2 immunity, which involves systemic immunity through the production of antibodies, may be enhanced by stress hormones through increased production of cytokines such as interleukin-4 (IL-4), promoting maturation of B cells. This shift increases the Th2 response while stalling the Th1 response, and allows tumor cells to more easily evade immune surveillance.[41] Cellular, or Th1, immunity, which promotes the maturation of surveillance cells, is hindered by stress hormones. Stress inhibits proinflammatory cytokines, such as interferon-γ (IFN-γ), which promotes maturation and differentiation of NK cells, T cells, and macrophages, which are critical for this type of immune response, and are also capable of eliminating tumor cells.[41] Using a restraint stress model, in which mice were confined to a well-ventilated, movement-restricting space for 6 hours per day, one group showed that stressed animals exposed to UVB rays developed tumors in a shorter amount of time and developed more tumors than nonstressed mice, due to immune escape through suppression of type 1 cytokines and protective T cells, and enhancement of suppressor T-cell numbers.[42] Other researchers have provided some evidence that the effects stress has on immune function and DNA repair also play a direct role in initiation of malignant lesions, such as by the increase in oxidative damage[42] and decrease in the DNA repair enzyme methyltransferase, as seen by Glaser and colleagues.[43] These results suggest that chronic stress can indirectly play a role in tumor initiation by suppressing the immune system.

Extending the knowledge gained by previous studies demonstrating the involvement of the hypothalamic–pituitary–thyroid (HPT) axis in chronic stress response,[44] it was found that thyroid hormones also play a role in altering immunity to allow stress-mediated cancer progression. Frick and colleagues showed that chronic restraint stress reduced thyroid hormones, impairing T-lymphocyte proliferation and activation[45] and promoting growth of lymphomas.

Depression can cause systemic disruption in balance of the immune response. A healthy immune system has a balance between type 1 and type 2 responsive elements. In a recent study[48] of patients with epithelial ovarian cancer and benign ovarian neoplasms, patients were evaluated for depressive states and their level of social support prior to surgery. Lymphocytes taken from peripheral blood, tumor, and ascites during surgery were analyzed for IFN-γ and IL-4 in T-helper and T-cytotoxic cells. IFN-γ is a part of the type 1 immune response, and is considered antitumorigenic. IL-4, on the other hand, is a part of the type 2 immune response. The type 1 response has been associated with immune-mediated elimination of tumor cells[46]; therefore, elevation of IL-4 is considered indicative of poorer immune-mediated clearance of tumor cells. Results from this study showed a correlation between depressive mood and systemic inhibition of the type 1 immune response. Prior studies[47] had demonstrated that tumor cells were capable of inhibiting IFN-γ production by TIL. Additionally, TIL taken from ovarian tumors showed increased type 2 response,[48,49] as well as an association between stress hormones and Th1/Th2 response imbalance.[50] Although the mechanisms have not been fully uncovered, it is hypothesized that this effect might be mediated by glucocorticoids, which inhibit type 1 cytokine production and upregulate type 2 cytokines.

■ EFFECTS OF STRESS ON CANCER METASTASIS

Cancer metastasis remains a difficult problem to manage and is responsible for most of the cancer-related mortality. Metastasis is a complex process that requires several steps to be successful.[51] First, growth of a tumor beyond 1 mm in size requires vascularization of the tumor, which also provides a method for dissemination of metastatic cells. Second, a tumor cell must gain the ability to break off from the main tumor, invade through the basement membrane, and embolize into the bloodstream. The cell then arrests in capillary beds and must be able to extravasate from the bloodstream and adhere to the parenchymal tissues. It must also evade immune system surveillance. Once settled, the cell interacts with its microenvironment to grow and ultimately develop its own blood supply. Cells that fail to acquire any one of these characteristics cannot metastasize and the cascade is aborted.[52] Increasing evidence shows that the stress response can affect many parts of this cascade (Fig. 2-2). The following sections present an overview of recent evidence regarding these effects.

Stress and Angiogenesis

Development of a blood supply is critical for tumor growth and metastasis. Neovascularization is a complex process that requires activation of many pathways to induce endothelial cell proliferation and migration. Many factors

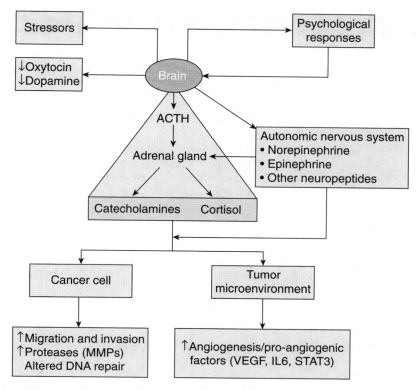

FIGURE 2-2. Effects of stress factors on the tumor microenvironment. On detection of a stressor the brain activates the central and autonomic nervous systems, causing the release of stress hormones, including catecholamines and glucocorticoids. These hormones, in turn, increase tumor cell migration and invasion through enhanced production of MMPs as well as chemoattractive forces, and also hinder DNA repair mechanisms. They also increase secretion of proangiogenic factors in the microenvironment that aid in tumor establishment and growth. Reprinted with permission from Elsevier from Armaiz-Pena GN, Lutgendorf SK, Cole SW, Sood AK. Neuroendocrine modulation of cancer progression. *Brain Behav Immun.* 23(1):10–15, copyright 2009.

promote angiogenesis including vascular endothelial growth factor, interleukin-6 (IL-6), TGF-α and -β, tumor necrosis factor-α (TNF-α), and many others.[53]

First discovered by Dvorak and colleagues[54] in 1983 and originally termed *vascular permeability factor* (VPF), VEGF has been found to be critical for angiogenesis and is produced by both normal and tumor cells. It plays multiple roles, including direct effects on endothelial cells to induce proliferation as well as to protect them from apoptosis.[53] Clinical data have shown a correlation between social support and VEGF expression. In patients with ovarian carcinoma, those with a higher level of social support had lower serum levels of VEGF than those

with poor support, suggesting that stress can stimulate production of VEGF and, therefore, angiogenesis.[55] Further in vitro studies found that norepinephrine and the β-agonist isoproterenol both were capable of inducing VEGF expression in ovarian cancer cell lines.[56] Activation of the β-AR/cAMP/PKA signaling pathway has been seen to result in this downstream increase in VEGF production in both ovarian cancer and adipose tissues.[56,57]

Thaker and colleagues found that tumor-bearing mice undergoing chronic restraint stress (Table 2-1) had increased tissue catecholamine levels, as well as increased tumor burden and invasiveness.[66] The effects of norepinephrine on VEGF were mimicked by the β-agonist

■ **TABLE 2-1.** Effects of Stress and Stress-associated Hormones on Cancer

Experimental Manipulation	Animal	Biological Effect	Tumor Type	Effect on Tumor Growth
Confrontation[58]	Rats	NA	Breast	Increased metastasis of tumor cells to the lung
Restraint stress[59]	Rats	Decreased numbers of T cells	Mammary	Increased growth during stress
Forced swim[60]	Rats	Decreased natural killer cell activity	Leukemia	Increased mortality
Abdominal surgery[60]	Rats	Decreased natural killer cell activity	Mammary	Increased metastasis of tumor cells to the lung
High versus low dopaminergic activity[61]	Rats	Decreased angiogenesis with high dopaminergic reactivity	Mammary	Fewer lung metastases with increased dopaminergic reactivity
Dopamine administration[92]	Mice	Decreased angiogenesis; decreased VEGF–VEGFR2 binding and phosphorylation	Ovarian	Decreased ascites formation
Dopamine administration[62]	Mice	Decreased angiogenesis	Gastric	Decreased growth
Social isolation[63]	Mice	Decreased macrophage activity	Ehrlich	Increased growth
Immobilization stress[66]	Mice	Increased angiogenesis	Ovarian	Increased growth
Restraint stress[64]	Mice	Decreased IL-12, IFN-γ, CCL27 (CTACK), and numbers of infiltrating T cells; increased numbers of suppressor cells	Skin and squamous cell carcinoma	Increased incidence, number, size, and density
Surgical stress[65]	Mice	Increased VEGF	Ovarian	Increased growth

CTACK, cutaneous T cell–attracting chemokine; IL-12, interleukin-12; IFN-γ, interferon-γ; NA, not available; VEGF, vascular endothelial growth factor; VEGFR2, VEGF receptor 2.
Reprinted with permission from Macmillan Publishers Ltd: Nat Rev Cancer. 6:240–248, copyright 2006.

isoproterenol and eliminated by using a β-blocker, thus verifying the importance of the AR in mediating these effects. Stress also caused increases in microvessel density resulting from significantly increased levels of VEGF mRNA and protein compared with tumors from non-stressed animals.

Angiogenesis can also be stimulated by a disruption in the balance between proangiogenic and antiangiogenic factors. IL-6 is a prominent angiogenic factor that disrupts this equilibrium and is produced by tumor cells. It plays an important role in stimulating tumor progression by promoting vascularization both directly by acting on tumor and endothelial cells and indirectly by causing the release of VEGF from tumor cells.[67,68] Additional studies have shown that IL-6 influences ovarian tumor cell proliferation[69] and acts as a chemoattractant to increase tumor cell migration and invasion.[70] Clinically, ovarian cancer patients experiencing chronic stress have higher levels of IL-6, which has been associated with poorer outcome. However, patients with stronger social support had lower levels of IL-6 in circulation as well as ascites.[71,72] Nilsson and colleagues[73] found that norepinephrine was responsible for inducing IL-6 gene transcription through an Src-dependent mechanism, further demonstrating the role of tumor cells in activating pathways critical to their growth.

Recent studies[74] have also shown the involvement of signal transducer and activator of transcription factor-3 (STAT-3) in promoting stress-mediated tumor-associated angiogenesis. STAT-3 is involved in many protumorigenic pathways by activating downstream targets to promote proliferation and inhibit apoptosis. Although STAT-3 can be activated by growth factors and cytokines such as VEGF and IL-6, Landen and colleagues[74] found that it can be activated in a manner independent of IL-6. They found that norepinephrine and epinephrine both are independently capable of inducing STAT3 phosphorylation, leading to translocation to the nucleus and subsequent binding to DNA to promote transcription of genes associated with cell survival, angiogenesis, oncogenesis, and proliferation. They also found that these effects were mediated through the β2-AR and PKA signaling, and IL-6 blockade had no impact on these effects.[74]

Effects on Tumor Cell Migration and Invasion

The second characteristic of a malignant tumor cell is its ability to separate from the main tumor, invade through the basement membrane, and invade the blood supply. The course of progression involved in this process is complex and involves several changes within the tumor cells themselves as well as in the surrounding extracellular matrix (ECM). These changes involve rearrangement of cadherins and integrins found on the cell surface to allow detachment from adherent cells and ECM components; matrix metalloproteinases are released, resulting in proteolysis of the surrounding ECM and basement membrane, and conformational change of the cell to allow invasion of the stroma and basement membrane.[75] Finally, chemoattractive forces can also be involved to provide directional motility for the migrating cells. Stress hormones can affect these processes by increasing MMP production by tumor cells as well as acting as a chemoattractant to induce cell migration.

Work done by Entschladen and colleagues[76–78] has provided evidence that norepinephrine is capable of inducing metastasis in several types of cancers through activation of the β-ARs. Stress levels of norepinephrine increased the in vitro invasive potential of

ovarian cancer cells by 89–198%, which was completely blocked by the β-antagonist propranolol.[57] Additional in vivo and in vitro studies demonstrated that stress hormones norepinephrine and epinephrine significantly increased production of MMP-2 and MMP-9 by ovarian cancer cells[66] through activation of the β-AR pathway.[79] Likewise, daily isoproterenol administration significantly increased tumor cell infiltration in vivo, which was also blocked by propranolol. Yang and colleagues[80] showed that stress levels of circulating catecholamines were capable of producing increases in MMP-2 secretion. Similar studies performed in head and neck cancers had results consistent with these findings, showing that MMP secretion was increased in cell lines following norepinephrine treatment.[57] Additional studies have provided evidence that macrophages and other stromal cells are responsible for release of many of these degradative enzymes. Specifically, Huang and colleagues[81] demonstrated that tumors in mice lacking MMP-9 expression show reduced growth and angiogenesis, suggesting that stroma plays an important role in MMP production. In human studies, Lutgendorf and colleagues[82] showed additional support for this by demonstrating that ovarian cancer patients with depressive symptoms and low social support had increased MMP-9 in tumor-associated macrophages. MMP-2 and MMP-9 are two matrix metalloproteinases that play a critical role in tumor cell invasion. Their expression can be regulated by cytokines, and they are frequently upregulated in cancer cells, with high levels often correlating with increased incidence of metastasis and poorer outcome. On release, MMPs are involved in the proteolytic destruction of the ECM and basement membranes, allowing for tumor cell migration.

In addition to invasion, stress hormones can affect tumor cell migration by allowing cells to migrate toward a blood supply for nutrients and metastasis. Chemotaxis occurs when a chemical in the tumor microenvironment directs the tumor cell's migration by either attracting or repelling it. Norepinephrine was originally shown to induce locomotion in leukocytes; in vitro studies on colon carcinoma have demonstrated that norepinephrine can increase tumor cell migration[77] through activation of the β-ARs. In a breast carcinoma cell line, norepinephrine was capable of not only inducing tumor cell migration, but also attracting the cells.[78] This could play a role in aiding metastasis by increasing cell motility.

With regard to intracellular signaling events, stress hormones activate the cAMP/PKA pathway, which has been shown to have many effects on cell migration. PKA has been seen to affect signaling of several families of the cytoskeletal network, such as integrins, which aid in lamellipodia extension,[83] and myosin, which aids in contracting the trailing edge during migration.[84] It also regulates cell adhesion by activation of the Rho family of small GTPases. RhoA is involved in actin cytoskeleton remodeling, and Rac, a member of the Rho subfamily, is involved in cell adhesion and tail retraction during migration. Activated Rho has been found to be associated with increased metastatic potential in cancer.[85] These GTPases function as switches, flipping between the inactive GDP-bound state and the active GTP-bound state. This switch is mediated by the guanine nucleotide exchange factors (GEFs), which stimulate the GDP/GTP exchange. Enserink et al showed that use of the β-agonist isoproterenol promoted ovarian carcinoma cell spreading and adhesion to laminin-5 in a cAMP/exchange protein directly activated by cAMP (Epac)-dependent fashion.[86] Epac proteins are a family of the GEFs specific for Ras family GTPases that are activated by cAMP and are highly involved in integrin-mediated cell adhesion.

Cell Survival

Circumvention of apoptosis (programmed cell death) is another critical step in the metastatic process. There is evidence that catecholamines may desensitize cells to apoptotic signals in cancer cells. While norepinephrine induced apoptosis in neuroblastoma cells, it did not do so in lung cancer cells.[87] Sastry and colleagues[88] showed that epinephrine is capable of reducing sensitivity of breast and prostate tumor cell lines to apoptosis by interacting with the β2-AR. By treating cell lines in vitro with epinephrine, activation of the β2-AR activates the PKA signaling pathway, leading to phosphorylation of Bcl-2-associated death promoter (BAD). BAD is involved in initiating apoptosis in its unphosphorylated form, which binds antiapoptotic proteins to prevent their localization to sites of activity, but becomes inactive on phosphorylation, thereby releasing Bcl-2 and Bcl-xl that inhibit apoptosis.

Glucocorticoids are also capable of improving cell survival in several ways, although this seems to be cell-type specific. Herr and colleagues[89] showed that while glucocorticoids enhanced proapoptotic effects of cancer

therapies in lymphoid cells, they increased resistance to apoptosis in cervical and lung carcinomas by downregulating elements of the death receptor and mitochondrial apoptotic pathways. Additionally, Wu and colleagues[90] used microarray analysis of GR-mediated pathways to demonstrate that serum and GC-inducible protein kinase-1 (SGK-1) and mitogen-activated protein kinase phosphatase-1 (MKP-1) both increase following GR activation and are involved in survival signaling pathways, and that chemotherapy-induced apoptosis was hindered in breast cell lines when the cells were pretreated with the cortisol-mimic, dexamethasone, through activation of the GRs. These data suggest that chronic stress may increase tumor cell survival by aiding in avoidance of apoptosis.

Furthermore, it has been suggested that glucocorticoids act synergistically with catecholamines in aiding tumor growth.[91] Using lung tumor cells, Nakane and colleagues[91] showed that cortisol is capable of increasing the density of β receptors on the cell surface and markedly increasing the effects of IL-1α, IL-1β, and TNF-α. Additionally, cortisol heightens cAMP accumulation induced by β-AR activation.

■ OTHER STRESS MEDIATORS

Dopamine

Dopamine is a neurotransmitter that has potent effects on tumorigenesis. However, contrary to the other neurotransmitters/stress hormones discussed, such as norepinephrine and epinephrine, dopamine has antitumor effects.[92] These effects are thought to be both direct by inhibition of angiogenic factors such as VEGF and indirect by modulating levels of other hormones. Functional studies[92] seem to agree with the evidence that under conditions of chronic stress, norepinephrine and epinephrine both are increased while dopamine is decreased.

Dopamine can have a direct or indirect effect on the immune response. T cells express dopamine receptors,[93] suggesting it has an important role in immune regulation. For example, Parkinson's disease is associated with damaged dopaminergic neurons, resulting in decreased dopaminergic activity in the CNS. It has also been associated with decreased immune function and response.[94-96] Conversely, schizophrenia is associated with hyperdopaminergic activity as well as increased immune function,[97,98] although these data remain somewhat conflicting due to the immunosuppressive effects of neuroleptics, which are commonly used to treat this disease.[99]

In vivo studies using a dopaminergic neurotoxin have shown that DA depletion decreases T-cell response and increases tumor growth in mice.[100] Decreased levels of dopamine resulting from destruction of the central dopamine system allow for several immune-repressing hormones to be released, including PRL, somatostatin, metenkephalin, and proenkephalin, resulting in decreased T-lymphocyte proliferation, decreased IgG and IgM secretion by B lymphocytes, decreased NK cell activity, and loss of tumor cell killing ability by cytotoxic T cells.[100]

Mounting evidence seems to suggest that dopamine can be a potent antiangiogenic factor. In 2001, Basu and colleagues[92] showed that dopamine treatment of tumor-bearing mice substantially decreased tumor-associated angiogenesis. These effects were mediated by internalization of endothelial cell VEGF receptor 2, resulting in decreased cell proliferation and migration. This group later showed that DA inhibits neovascularization by preventing mobility of endothelial progenitor cells from the bone marrow.[101] Additionally, destruction of peripheral dopaminergic neurons increased angiogenesis, microvessel density, microvascular permeability, and tumor growth,[102] suggesting that local DA depletion surrounding the tumor would be beneficial for tumor growth.

There is also evidence that therapeutic use of dopamine or its analogs in conjunction with traditional antitumor therapies will have an antitumorigenic effect, in a manner similar to the synergism seen with anti-VEGF therapies. Sarkar and colleagues[103] showed that dopamine is effective alone and in combination with chemotherapeutic agents in reducing tumor growth and extending survival of mice bearing human breast and colon tumors. These results suggest that dopamine treatment may prove to be useful when tumors become resistant to traditional antiangiogenic treatments, although more extensive studies are necessary.

Oxytocin

Like dopamine, oxytocin decreases with chronic stress,[13] although it increases under acute stress.[104] Most frequently associated with labor initiation and lactation, oxytocin is now thought to play an important role in mediating social responses, and a positive correlation has been found between high social support and oxytocin levels.[105] It is also capable of ameliorating symptoms caused by stress, such as anxiety, by exerting anxiolytic effects in certain regions of the brain,[19] and also inhibiting growth of some epithelial cell tumors such as breast and endometrial through its modulation of PRL,[106] as well as tumors of neuronal and bone origins. However, studies testing its effects on endothelium tumors found a growth-stimulatory effect.[107]

Prolactin

PRL is another hormone that is secreted during periods of chronic stress. Its release could be due to the decrease in dopamine, the primary negative regulator of PRL secretion. Some epidemiological studies suggest PRL levels may also correlate with risk of breast cancer.[106] PRL can act as a chemoattractant to increase cell motility through activation of the Ras signaling cascade[108] as well as inhibit apoptosis through activation of the Akt pathway in mammary cancer cells.[109] It has also been shown to stimulate proliferation of prostate and endometrial cancer cells.[110] These findings also support potential therapeutic efficacy of dopamine treatment for inhibiting stress-induced cancer progression.

Nerve Growth Factor

NGF is a well-characterized neurotrophic factor that has been found to be involved in neuronal growth and survival. Though most commonly known for this role, it is actually a pleiotrophic factor expressed by several cell types within our bodies and is highly expressed in several types of cancers including breast,[111] pancreatic,[112] and prostate.[113] Its receptors are also present on the tumor cells, suggesting an autocrine feedback loop. NGF has also been identified as an angiogenic factor,[114] and activation of its receptors on tumor cells has been implicated as an antiapoptotic protective pathway in prostate cancer.[15,16] Activation of β-ARs in vitro (such as by norepinephrine) stimulates NGF production, implying that it may be involved in stress-induced tumor growth.[14] There is also a link between social stress and higher NGF expression. Studies performed on primate lymph nodes found an association between low sociability and an increase in lymph node expression of NGF.[115] Together, these data suggest that stress may increase NGF to promote tumor growth. The NGF pathway has been examined as a potential therapeutic target in breast cancer, and it was found that receptor inhibition had proapoptotic and antiproliferative effects on breast cancer cell lines and had an additive effect when used with traditional chemotherapeutic agents.[116]

Substance P

Substance P is an important neurokinin involved in anxiety, depression, and stress, and is highly expressed in areas of the brain associated with behavior regulation and stress response.[17] Several types of tumors express receptors for this peptide, called NK receptors, such as gastric,[117] breast,[118] laryngeal cancers,[119] and neuroblastoma,[18] among others. Substance P acts as a mitogen for these cancer cell lines, inducing proliferation, as well as influencing bone metastasis.[18] It has also been suggested that using NK-1 antagonists may induce tumor cell apoptosis.[119] Although its role in cancer progression is not well understood, the involvement of substance P in the stress response as well as expression of its receptor on many cancer cell types suggests it may play an important role in stress-mediated progression.

■ CLINICAL STUDIES

There is a growing body of literature with mixed results for clinical studies that have examined the efficacy of psychological intervention in prolonging cancer patient survival rates. Some clinical trials have shown that psychological interventions for reducing patient distress can have a marked impact on improving patient health and biobehavioral effects.[120] The study by Andersen and colleagues[120] demonstrated that breast cancer patients who had been placed in small support groups that met weekly for 4 months showed significant decreases in anxiety, improved perception of social support, and improved dietary habits, and all correlated with improved immune responses. Another report[121] from this same group showed that this intervention can also improve health, as measured by accepted measures of patient performance and symptoms of illnesses, laboratory studies, and therapy toxicity.[121] This report also showed that these effects resulted directly from the decrease in patient distress, rather than the improvement in immune response. An updated report of this study[122] demonstrated that, after 11 years of follow-up, patients who had received psychological intervention had reduced risk of both death and recurrence compared

with controls,[122] verifying the substantial impact that reducing patient stress can have on disease progression and outcome.

Studies of cortisol levels in patients following cognitive behavioral stress interventions have demonstrated that the levels of cortisol became lower and remained low for up to 1 year compared with control groups.[123] This form of stress management improved the proliferation response of lymphocytes, which was previously found to be hindered by psychological distress.[124] Furthermore, psychological intervention has been used to fight stress-associated problems exacerbated by cancer. Breast cancer patients who had developed insomnia were assigned to groups for behavioral therapy for 8 weeks. As much as 1 year later the subjects reported better sleeping habits, fewer nights requiring medications to aid sleep, lower levels of anxiety, improved quality of life,[125] and improved secretion of IFN-γ and immune function.[126] These studies suggest that it may be practical to assess the efficacy of cognitive behavioral therapies in discouraging other stress-induced health problems to improve patient health.

Additionally, the active involvement of ARs in stress-mediated cancer progression has also been examined. One epidemiological study looked at the risk of developing prostate cancer in patients who used β-blockers and found that those patients had a reduced risk, suggesting that β-ARs play a role in the development of prostate cancer.[127] A second study found that the use of β-blockers by patients with cardiovascular disease significantly reduced their risk of cancer.[128] Additional studies are needed to further examine the potential protective effects of such pharmacological agents.

■ SUMMARY

Chronic stress and depression affect a substantial portion of cancer patients. These conditions enhance tumor progression and negatively affect outcome by influencing pathways involved in progression and survival of cancer cells. Resultant increases in several neuropeptides and glucocorticoids have multifaceted effects on tumor growth and progression as well as a potential effect on initiation of tumors (Fig. 2-3). Effects on the immune system further permit tumor cells to evade immune surveillance and thereby survive to grow and proliferate. These stress hormones play a role in tumor cell survival and proliferation

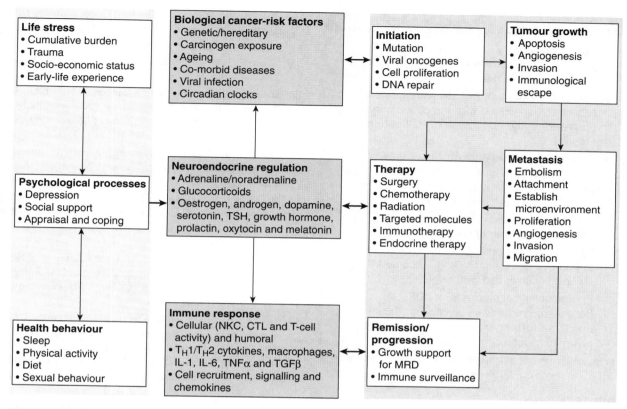

FIGURE 2-3. Overview of stressors, their physiological impact, and ultimate effects on cancer. The blue panel represents biobehavioral factors, which can affect tumor initiation and progression through modulation of neuroendocrine hormones. The red panel represents a summary of the biological cancer risk factors and immune responses that are involved in this process. The green panel represents outcome of these effects. Reprinted with permission from Macmillan Publishers Ltd: *Nat Rev Cancer.* 6:240–248, copyright 2006.

as well as many of the steps required for metastasis such as migration, invasion, and adhesion. Collectively, much of the scientific evidence is converging toward a mechanistic understanding of the deleterious effects of chronic stress on cancer growth and progression. As this mechanistic understanding grows, studies aimed at identifying new therapeutic interventions that interfere with the protumorigenic effects of chronic stress can be rationally designed. It is likely that these interventions may include a combination of pharmacologic and biobehavioral intervention strategies to complement conventional therapies. Such approaches may allow for the development of personalized programs tailored specifically to the needs of the patient and produce more successful clinical outcomes.

■ ACKNOWLEDGMENTS

JKA is supported by the NCI R25E Cancer Prevention Education grant through MD Anderson Cancer Center. GAP is supported by the NCI F31CA126474 Fellowship for Minority Students. Portions of this work were supported by NIH grants (CA110793, CA109298, and CA128797), the Ovarian Cancer Research Fund, Inc (Program Project Development Grant), UT MD Anderson Cancer Center SPORE (P50CA083639), the Zarrow Foundation, the Marcus Foundation, the Entertainment Industry Foundation, the Blanton-Davis Ovarian Cancer Research Program, and the Betty Anne Asche Murray Distinguished Professorship to AKS.

KEY POINTS

- Data supporting a relationship between behavioral risk factors and cancer initiation have been inconsistent.

- Chronic activation of the stress response has been associated with increased cancer progression and decreased overall patient survival.

- Chronic stress can support tumor growth by stimulating various components of the metastatic cascade, such as angiogenesis, invasion, and cell survival.

- Chronic stress and depression affect a substantial portion of cancer patients

- Psychological interventions have been shown to improve quality of life and outcome in chronically stressed cancer patients.

- Pharmacological blockade of ADRB by β-blockers have shown promise in the clinic and merit further examination due to their ability to reduce cancer risk.

REFERENCES

1. Spiegel D, Giese-Davis J. Depression and cancer: mechanisms and disease progression. *Biol Psychiatry.* 2003;54(3):269–282.

2. Kowal SJ. Emotions as a cause of cancer; 18th and 19th century contributions. *Psychoanal Rev.* 1955;42(3):217–227.

3. Selye H. A syndrome produced by diverse nocuous agents. 1936. *J Neuropsychiatry Clin Neurosci.* 1998;10(2): 230–231.

4. McEwen BS. Protective and damaging effects of stress mediators. *N Engl J Med.* 1998;338(3):171–179.

5. Wood PB. Role of central dopamine in pain and analgesia. *Expert Rev Neurother.* 2008;8(5):781–797.

6. Smith SM, Vale WW. The role of the hypothalamic–pituitary–adrenal axis in neuroendocrine responses to stress. *Dialogues Clin Neurosci.* 2006;8(4):383–395.

7. McEwen BS. Physiology and neurobiology of stress and adaptation: central role of the brain. *Physiol Rev.* 2007;87(3):873–904.

8. Cacioppo JT, Berntson GG, Malarkey WB, et al. Autonomic, neuroendocrine, and immune responses to psychological stress: the reactivity hypothesis. *Ann N Y Acad Sci.* 1998;840:664–673.

9. Charmandari E, Tsigos C, Chrousos G. Endocrinology of the stress response. *Annu Rev Physiol.* 2005;67:259–284.

10. Nicoll CS, Talwalker PK, Meites J. Initiation of lactation in rats by nonspecific stresses. *Am J Physiol.* 1960;198:1103–1106.

11. Ebner K, Rupniak NM, Saria A, Singewald N. Substance P in the medial amygdala: emotional stress-sensitive release and modulation of anxiety-related behavior in rats. *Proc Natl Acad Sci U S A.* 2004;101(12):4280–4285.

12. Lakshmanan J. Nerve growth factor levels in mouse serum: variations due to stress. *Neurochem Res.* 1987;12(4):393–397.

13. Young WS 3rd, Lightman SL. Chronic stress elevates enkephalin expression in the rat paraventricular and supraoptic nuclei. *Brain Res Mol Brain Res.* 1992;13 (1–2):111–117.

14. Fabrazzo M, Costa E, Mocchetti I. Stimulation of nerve growth factor biosynthesis in developing rat brain by reserpine: steroids as potential mediators. *Mol Pharmacol.* 1991;39(2):144–149.

15. Miknyoczki SJ, Chang H, Klein-Szanto A, Dionne CA, Ruggeri BA. The Trk tyrosine kinase inhibitor CEP-701 (KT-5555) exhibits significant antitumor efficacy in preclinical xenograft models of human pancreatic ductal adenocarcinoma. *Clin Cancer Res.* 1999;5(8): 2205–2212.

16. Miknyoczki SJ, Wan W, Chang H, et al. The neurotrophin–trk receptor axes are critical for the growth and progression of human prostatic carcinoma and pancreatic ductal adenocarcinoma xenografts in nude mice. *Clin Cancer Res.* 2002;8(6):1924–1931.

17. Kramer MS, Cutler N, Feighner J, et al. Distinct mechanism for antidepressant activity by blockade of central substance P receptors. *Science.* 1998;281(5383): 1640–1645.

18. Mukerji I, Ramkissoon SH, Reddy KK, Rameshwar P. Autocrine proliferation of neuroblastoma cells is partly mediated through neurokinin receptors: relevance to bone marrow metastasis. *J Neurooncol.* 2005;71(2):91–98.

19. McCarthy MM, McDonald CH, Brooks PJ, Goldman D. An anxiolytic action of oxytocin is enhanced by estrogen in the mouse. *Physiol Behav.* 1996;60(5):1209–1215.

20. Du J, Wang Y, Hunter R, et al. Dynamic regulation of mitochondrial function by glucocorticoids. *Proc Natl Acad Sci U S A.* 2009;106(9):3543–3548.

21. Black PH, Garbutt LD. Stress, inflammation and cardiovascular disease. *J Psychosom Res.* 2002;52(1):1–23.

22. Kobilka B. Adrenergic receptors as models for G protein-coupled receptors. *Annu Rev Neurosci.* 1992;15:87–114.

23. Shang ZJ, Liu K, Liang de F. Expression of beta-adrenergic receptor in oral squamous cell carcinoma. *J Oral Pathol Med*. 2009;38(4):371–376.

24. Bevilacqua M, Norbiato G, Chebat E, et al. Changes in alpha-1 and beta-2 adrenoceptor density in human hepatocellular carcinoma. *Cancer*. 1991;67(10):2543–2551.

25. Perrone MG, Notarnicola M, Caruso MG, Tutino V, Scilimati A. Upregulation of beta3-adrenergic receptor mRNA in human colon cancer: a preliminary study. *Oncology*. 2008;75(3–4):224–229.

26. Noda H, Miyaji Y, Nakanishi A, Konisho F, Miki Y. Frequent reduced expression of alpha-1B-adrenergic receptor caused by aberrant promoter methylation in gastric cancers. *Br J Cancer*. 2007;96(2):383–390.

27. Pullar CE, Isseroff RR. The beta 2-adrenergic receptor activates pro-migratory and pro-proliferative pathways in dermal fibroblasts via divergent mechanisms. *J Cell Sci*. 2006;119(pt 3):592–602.

28. Lai LP, Mitchell J. Beta2-adrenergic receptors expressed on murine chondrocytes stimulate cellular growth and inhibit the expression of Indian hedgehog and collagen type X. *J Cell Biochem*. 2008;104(2):545–553.

29. Hanahan D, Weinberg RA. The hallmarks of cancer. *Cell*. 2000;100(1):57–70.

30. Chen CC, David AS, Nunnerley H, et al. Adverse life events and breast cancer: case–control study. *BMJ*. 1995;311(7019):1527–1530.

31. Nielsen NR, Zhang ZF, Kristensen TS, Netterstrøm B, Schnohr P, Grønbaek M. Self reported stress and risk of breast cancer: prospective cohort study. *BMJ*. 2005;331(7516):548.

32. Penninx BW, Guralnik JM, Pahor M, et al. Chronically depressed mood and cancer risk in older persons. *J Natl Cancer Inst*. 1998;90(24):1888–1893.

33. Price MA, Tennant CC, Smith RC, et al. The role of psychosocial factors in the development of breast carcinoma: part I. The cancer prone personality. *Cancer*. 2001;91(4):679–685.

34. Lutgendorf SK, Sood AK, Anderson B, et al. Social support, psychological distress, and natural killer cell activity in ovarian cancer. *J Clin Oncol*. 2005;23(28):7105–7113.

35. Andersen BL, Farrar WB, Golden-Kreutz D, et al. Stress and immune responses after surgical treatment for regional breast cancer. *J Natl Cancer Inst*. 1998;90(1):30–36.

36. Turner-Cobb JM, Sephton SE, Koopman C, Blake-Mortimer J, Spiegel D. Social support and salivary cortisol in women with metastatic breast cancer. *Psychosom Med*. 2000;62(3):337–345.

37. Sephton SE, Sapolsky RM, Kraemer HC, Spiegel D. Diurnal cortisol rhythm as a predictor of breast cancer survival. *J Natl Cancer Inst*. 2000;92(12):994–1000.

38. Miller AH, Spencer RL, Pearce BD, et al. Glucocorticoid receptors are differentially expressed in the cells and tissues of the immune system. *Cell Immunol*. 1998;186(1):45–54.

39. Elenkov IJ. Systemic stress-induced Th2 shift and its clinical implications. *Int Rev Neurobiol*. 2002;52:163–186.

40. Amsterdam A, Tajima K, Sasson R. Cell-specific regulation of apoptosis by glucocorticoids: implication to their anti-inflammatory action. *Biochem Pharmacol*. 2002;64(5–6):843–850.

41. Webster JI, Tonelli L, Sternberg EM. Neuroendocrine regulation of immunity. *Annu Rev Immunol*. 2002;20:125–163.

42. Adachi S, Kawamura K, Takemoto K. Oxidative damage of nuclear DNA in liver of rats exposed to psychological stress. *Cancer Res*. 1993;53(18):4153–4155.

43. Glaser R, Thorn BE, Tarr KL, Kiecolt-Glaser JK, D'Ambrosio SM. Effects of stress on methyltransferase synthesis: an important DNA repair enzyme. *Health Psychol*. 1985;4(5):403–412.

44. Helmreich DL, Parfitt DB, Lu XY, Akil H, Watson SJ. Relation between the hypothalamic–pituitary–thyroid (HPT) axis and the hypothalamic–pituitary–adrenal (HPA) axis during repeated stress. *Neuroendocrinology*. 2005;81(3):183–192.

45. Frick LR, Rapanelli M, Bussman UA, et al. Involvement of thyroid hormones in the alterations of T-cell immunity and tumor progression induced by chronic stress. *Biol Psychiatry*. 2009;65(11):935–942.

46. Olver S, Groves P, Buttigieg K, et al. Tumor-derived interleukin-4 reduces tumor clearance and deviates the cytokine and granzyme profile of tumor-induced CD8+ T cells. *Cancer Res*. 2006;66(1):571–580.

47. Kooi S, Freedman RS, Rodriguez-Villanueva J, Platsoucas CD. Cytokine production by T-cell lines derived from tumor-infiltrating lymphocytes from patients with ovarian carcinoma: tumor-specific immune responses and inhibition of antigen-independent cytokine production by ovarian tumor cells. *Lymphokine Cytokine Res*. 1993;12(6):429–437.

48. Rabinowich H, Suminami Y, Reichert TE, et al. Expression of cytokine genes or proteins and signaling molecules in lymphocytes associated with human ovarian carcinoma. *Int J Cancer*. 1996;68(3):276–284.

49. Goedegebuure PS, Douville CC, Doherty JM, et al. Simultaneous production of T helper-1-like cytokines

and cytolytic activity by tumor-specific T cells in ovarian and breast cancer. *Cell Immunol*. 1997;175(2):150–156.

50. Elenkov IJ, Chrousos GP. Stress hormones, Th1/Th2 patterns, pro/anti-inflammatory cytokines and susceptibility to disease. *Trends Endocrinol Metab*. 1999;10(9):359–368.

51. Fidler IJ. The pathogenesis of cancer metastasis: the 'seed and soil' hypothesis revisited. *Nat Rev Cancer*. 2003;3(6):453–458.

52. Langley RR, Fidler IJ. Tumor cell-organ microenvironment interactions in the pathogenesis of cancer metastasis. *Endocr Rev*. 2007;28(3):297–321.

53. Karamysheva AF. Mechanisms of angiogenesis. *Biochemistry (Mosc)*. 2008;73(7):751–762.

54. Senger DR, Galli SJ, Dvorak AM, Perruzzi CA, Harvey VS, Dvorak HF. Tumor cells secrete a vascular permeability factor that promotes accumulation of ascites fluid. *Science*. 1983;219(4587):983–985.

55. Lutgendorf SK, Johnsen EL, Cooper B, et al. Vascular endothelial growth factor and social support in patients with ovarian carcinoma. *Cancer*. 2002;95(4):808–815.

56. Lutgendorf SK, Cole S, Costanzo E, et al. Stress-related mediators stimulate vascular endothelial growth factor secretion by two ovarian cancer cell lines. *Clin Cancer Res*. 2003;9(12):4514–4521.

57. Yang EV, Sood AK, Chen M, et al. Norepinephrine upregulates the expression of vascular endothelial growth factor, matrix metalloproteinase (MMP)-2, and MMP-9 in nasopharyngeal carcinoma tumor cells. *Cancer Res*. 2006;66(21):10357–10364.

58. Stefanski V, Ben-Eliyahu S. Social confrontation and tumor metastasis in rats: defeat and beta-adrenergic mechanisms. *Physiol Behav*. 1996;60(1):277–282.

59. Steplewski Z, Vogel WH, Ehya H, Poropatich C, Smith JM. Effects of restraint stress on inoculated tumor growth and immune response in rats. *Cancer Res*. 1985;45(10):5128–5133.

60. Ben-Eliyahu S, Page GG, Yirmiya R, Shakhar G. Evidence that stress and surgical interventions promote tumor development by suppressing natural killer cell activity. *Int J Cancer*. 1999;80(6):880–888.

61. Teunis MA, Kavelaars A, Voest E, et al. Reduced tumor growth, experimental metastasis formation, and angiogenesis in rats with a hyperreactive dopaminergic system. *FASEB J*. 2002;16(11):1465–1467.

62. Chakroborty D, Sarkar C, Mitra RB, Banerjee S, Dasgupta PS, Basu S. Depleted dopamine in gastric cancer tissues: dopamine treatment retards growth of gastric cancer by inhibiting angiogenesis. *Clin Cancer Res*. 2004;10(13):4349–4356.

63. Palermo-Neto J, de Oliveira Massoco C, Robespierre de Souza W. Effects of physical and psychological stressors on behavior, macrophage activity, and Ehrlich tumor growth. *Brain Behav Immun*. 2003;17(1):43–54.

64. Saul AN, Oberyszyn TM, Daugherty C, et al. Chronic stress and susceptibility to skin cancer. *J Natl Cancer Inst*. 2005;97(23):1760–1767.

65. Lee JW, Shahzad MM, Lin YG, et al. Surgical stress promotes tumor growth in ovarian carcinoma. *Clin Cancer Res*. 2009;15(8):2695–2702.

66. Thaker PH, Han LY, Kamat AA, et al. Chronic stress promotes tumor growth and angiogenesis in a mouse model of ovarian carcinoma. *Nat Med*. 2006;12(8):939–944.

67. Nilsson MB, Langley RR, Fidler IJ. Interleukin-6, secreted by human ovarian carcinoma cells, is a potent proangiogenic cytokine. *Cancer Res*. 2005;65(23):10794–10800.

68. Cohen T, Nahari D, Cerem LW, Neufeld G, Levi BZ. Interleukin 6 induces the expression of vascular endothelial growth factor. *J Biol Chem*. 1996;271(2):736–741.

69. Wu S, Rodabaugh K, Martinez-Maza O, et al. Stimulation of ovarian tumor cell proliferation with monocyte products including interleukin-1, interleukin-6, and tumor necrosis factor-alpha. *Am J Obstet Gynecol*. 1992;166(3):997–1007.

70. Obata NH, Tamakoshi K, Shibata K, Kikkawa F, Tomoda Y. Effects of interleukin-6 on in vitro cell attachment, migration and invasion of human ovarian carcinoma. *Anticancer Res*. 1997;17(1A):337–342.

71. Kiecolt-Glaser JK, Preacher KJ, MacCallum RC, Atkinson C, Malarkey WB, Glaser R. Chronic stress and age-related increases in the proinflammatory cytokine IL-6. *Proc Natl Acad Sci U S A*. 2003;100(15):9090–9095.

72. Costanzo ES, Lutgendorf SK, Sood AK, Anderson B, Sorosky J, Lubaroff DM. Psychosocial factors and interleukin-6 among women with advanced ovarian cancer. *Cancer*. 2005;104(2):305–313.

73. Nilsson MB, Armaiz-Pena G, Takahashi R, et al. Stress hormones regulate interleukin-6 expression by human ovarian carcinoma cells through a Src-dependent mechanism. *J Biol Chem*. 2007;282(41):29919–29926.

74. Landen CN Jr, Lin YG, Armaiz Pena GN, et al. Neuroendocrine modulation of signal transducer and activator of transcription-3 in ovarian cancer. *Cancer Res*. 2007;67(21):10389–10396.

75. Aznavoorian S, Murphy AN, Stetler-Stevenson WG, Liotta LA. Molecular aspects of tumor cell invasion and metastasis. *Cancer*. 1993;71(4):1368–1383.

76. Palm D, Lang K, Niggemann B, et al. The norepinephrine-driven metastasis development of PC-3 human prostate

cancer cells in BALB/c nude mice is inhibited by beta-blockers. *Int J Cancer.* 2006;118(11):2744–2749.

77. Masur K, Niggemann B, Zanker KS, Entschladen F. Norepinephrine-induced migration of SW 480 colon carcinoma cells is inhibited by beta-blockers. *Cancer Res.* 2001;61(7):2866–2869.

78. Drell TL 4th, Joseph J, Lang K, Niggemann B, Zaenker KS, Entschladen F. Effects of neurotransmitters on the chemokinesis and chemotaxis of MDA-MB-468 human breast carcinoma cells. *Breast Cancer Res Treat.* 2003;80(1):63–70.

79. Sood AK, Bhatty R, Kamat AA, et al. Stress hormone-mediated invasion of ovarian cancer cells. *Clin Cancer Res.* 2006;12(2):369–375.

80. Yang EV, Bane CM, MacCallum RC, Kiecolt-Glaser JK, Malarkey WB, Glaser R. Stress-related modulation of matrix metalloproteinase expression. *J Neuroimmunol.* 2002;133(1–2):144–150.

81. Huang S, Van Arsdall M, Tedjarati S, et al. Contributions of stromal metalloproteinase-9 to angiogenesis and growth of human ovarian carcinoma in mice. *J Natl Cancer Inst.* 2002;94(15):1134–1142.

82. Lamagna C, Aurrand-Lions M, Imhof BA. Dual role of macrophages in tumor growth and angiogenesis. *J Leukoc Biol.* 2006;80(4):705–713.

83. Goldfinger LE, Han J, Kiosses WB, Howe AK, Ginsberg MH. Spatial restriction of alpha4 integrin phosphorylation regulates lamellipodial stability and alpha4beta1-dependent cell migration. *J Cell Biol.* 2003;162(4):731–741.

84. Pfitzer G. Invited review: regulation of myosin phosphorylation in smooth muscle. *J Appl Physiol.* 2001;91(1):497–503.

85. Clark EA, Golub TR, Lander ES, Hynes RO. Genomic analysis of metastasis reveals an essential role for RhoC. *Nature.* 2000;406(6795):532–535.

86. Enserink JM, Price LS, Methi T, et al. The cAMP–Epac–Rap1 pathway regulates cell spreading and cell adhesion to laminin-5 through the alpha3beta1 integrin but not the alpha6beta4 integrin. *J Biol Chem.* 2004;279(43):44889–44896.

87. Chan AS, Ng LW, Poon LS, Chan WW, Wong YH. Dopaminergic and adrenergic toxicities on SK-N-MC human neuroblastoma cells are mediated through G protein signaling and oxidative stress. *Apoptosis.* 2007;12(1):167–179.

88. Sastry KS, Karpova Y, Prokopovich S, et al. Epinephrine protects cancer cells from apoptosis via activation of cAMP-dependent protein kinase and BAD phosphorylation. *J Biol Chem.* 2007;282(19):14094–14100.

89. Herr I, Ucur E, Herzer K, et al. Glucocorticoid cotreatment induces apoptosis resistance toward cancer therapy in carcinomas. *Cancer Res.* 2003;63(12):3112–3120.

90. Wu W, Chaudhuri S, Brickley DR, Pang D, Karrison T, Conzen SD. Microarray analysis reveals glucocorticoid-regulated survival genes that are associated with inhibition of apoptosis in breast epithelial cells. *Cancer Res.* 2004;64(5):1757–1764.

91. Nakane T, Szentendrei T, Stern L, Virmani M, Seely J, Kunos G. Effects of IL-1 and cortisol on beta-adrenergic receptors, cell proliferation, and differentiation in cultured human A549 lung tumor cells. *J Immunol.* 1990;145(1):260–266.

92. Basu S, Nagy JA, Pal S, et al. The neurotransmitter dopamine inhibits angiogenesis induced by vascular permeability factor/vascular endothelial growth factor. *Nat Med.* 2001;7(5):569–574.

93. Basu S, Dasgupta PS, Lahiri T, Chowdhury JR. Uptake and biodistribution of dopamine in bone marrow, spleen and lymph nodes of normal and tumor bearing mice. *Life Sci.* 1993;53(5):415–424.

94. Marttila RJ, Eskola J, Pälvärinta M, Rinne UK. Immune functions in Parkinson's disease. *Adv Neurol.* 1984;40:315–323.

95. Marttila RJ, Eskola J, Soppi E, Rinne UK. Immune functions in Parkinson's disease lymphocyte subsets, concanavalin A-induced suppressor cell activity and in vitro immunoglobulin production. *J Neurol Sci.* 1985;69(3):121–131.

96. Fiszer U, Piotrowska K, Korlak J, Członkowska A. The immunological status in Parkinson's disease. *Med Lab Sci.* 1991;48(3):196–200.

97. Villemain F, Chatenoud L, Galinowski A, et al. Aberrant T cell-mediated immunity in untreated schizophrenic patients: deficient interleukin-2 production. *Am J Psychiatry.* 1989;146(5):609–616.

98. Ganguli R, Brar JS, Chengappa KR, et al. Mitogen-stimulated interleukin-2 production in never-medicated, first-episode schizophrenic patients. The influence of age at onset and negative symptoms. *Arch Gen Psychiatry.* 1995;52(8):668–672.

99. Maes M, Bosmans E, Calabrese J, Smith R, Meltzer HY. Interleukin-2 and interleukin-6 in schizophrenia and mania: effects of neuroleptics and mood stabilizers. *J Psychiatr Res.* 1995;29(2):141–152.

100. Basu S, Dasgupta PS, Chowdhury JR. Enhanced tumor growth in brain dopamine-depleted mice following 1-methyl-4-phenyl-1,2,3,6-tetrahydropyridine (MPTP) treatment. *J Neuroimmunol.* 1995;60(1–2):1–8.

101. Chakroborty D, Chowdhury UR, Sarkar C, Baral R, Dasgupta PS, Basu S. Dopamine regulates endothelial progenitor cell mobilization from mouse bone marrow in tumor vascularization. *J Clin Invest.* 2008;118(4): 1380–1389.

102. Basu S, Sarkar C, Chakroborty D, et al. Ablation of peripheral dopaminergic nerves stimulates malignant tumor growth by inducing vascular permeability factor/vascular endothelial growth factor-mediated angiogenesis. *Cancer Res.* 2004;64(16):5551–5555.

103. Sarkar C, Chakroborty D, Chowdhury UR, Dasgupta PS, Basu S. Dopamine increases the efficacy of anticancer drugs in breast and colon cancer preclinical models. *Clin Cancer Res.* 2008;14(8):2502–2510.

104. Jezova D, Skultetyova I, Tokarev DI, Bakos P, Vigas M. Vasopressin and oxytocin in stress. *Ann N Y Acad Sci.* 1995;771:192–203.

105. Grewen KM, Girdler SS, Amico J, Light KC. Effects of partner support on resting oxytocin, cortisol, norepinephrine, and blood pressure before and after warm partner contact. *Psychosom Med.* 2005;67(4):531–538.

106. Clevenger CV, Furth PA, Hankinson SE, Schuler LA. The role of prolactin in mammary carcinoma. *Endocr Rev.* 2003;24(1):1–27.

107. Pequeux C, Keegan BP, Hagelstein MT, Geenen V, Legros JJ, North WG. Oxytocin- and vasopressin-induced growth of human small-cell lung cancer is mediated by the mitogen-activated protein kinase pathway. *Endocr Relat Cancer.* 2004;11(4):871–885.

108. Maus MV, Reilly SC, Clevenger CV. Prolactin as a chemoattractant for human breast carcinoma. *Endocrinology.* 1999;140(11):5447–5450.

109. Chen WY, Ramamoorthy P, Chen N, Sticca R, Wagner TE. A human prolactin antagonist, hPRL-G129R, inhibits breast cancer cell proliferation through induction of apoptosis. *Clin Cancer Res.* 1999;5(11):3583–3593.

110. Antoni MH, Lutgendorf SK, Cole SW, et al. The influence of bio-behavioural factors on tumour biology: pathways and mechanisms. *Nat Rev Cancer.* 2006;6(3): 240–248.

111. Adriaenssens E, Vanhecke E, Saule P, et al. Nerve growth factor is a potential therapeutic target in breast cancer. *Cancer Res.* 2008;68(2):346–351.

112. Ma J, Jiang Y, Jiang Y, Sun Y, Zhao X. Expression of nerve growth factor and tyrosine kinase receptor A and correlation with perineural invasion in pancreatic cancer. *J Gastroenterol Hepatol.* 2008;23(12):1852–1859.

113. Paul AB, Grant ES, Habib FK. The expression and localisation of beta-nerve growth factor (beta-NGF) in benign and malignant human prostate tissue: relationship to neuroendocrine differentiation. *Br J Cancer.* 1996;74(12):1990–1996.

114. Nico B, Mangieri D, Benagiano V, Crivellato E, Ribatti D. Nerve growth factor as an angiogenic factor. *Microvasc Res.* 2008;75(2):135–141.

115. Sloan EK, Capitanio JP, Tarara RP, Cole SW. Social temperament and lymph node innervation. *Brain Behav Immun.* 2008;22(5):717–726.

116. Naderi A, Hughes-Davies L. Nerve growth factor/nuclear factor-kappaB pathway as a therapeutic target in breast cancer. *J Cancer Res Clin Oncol.* 2009;135(2): 211–216.

117. Rosso M, Robles-Frías MJ, Coveñas R, Salinas-Martín MV, Muñoz M. The NK-1 receptor is expressed in human primary gastric and colon adenocarcinomas and is involved in the antitumor action of L-733,060 and the mitogenic action of substance P on human gastrointestinal cancer cell lines. *Tumour Biol.* 2008;29(4):245–254.

118. Reddy BY, Trzaska KA, Murthy RG, Navarro P, Rameshwar P. Neurokinin receptors as potential targets in breast cancer treatment. *Curr Drug Discov Technol.* 2008;5(1):15–19.

119. Munoz M, Rosso M, Aguilar FJ, González-Moles MA, Redondo M, Esteban F. NK-1 receptor antagonists induce apoptosis and counteract substance P-related mitogenesis in human laryngeal cancer cell line HEp-2. *Invest New Drugs.* 2008;26(2):111–118.

120. Andersen BL, Farrar WB, Golden-Kreutz DM, et al. Psychological, behavioral, and immune changes after a psychological intervention: a clinical trial. *J Clin Oncol.* 2004;22(17):3570–3580.

121. Andersen BL, Farrar WB, Golden-Kreutz DM, et al. Distress reduction from a psychological intervention contributes to improved health for cancer patients. *Brain Behav Immun.* 2007;21(7):953–961.

122. Andersen BL, Yang HC, Farrar WB, et al. Psychoogic intervention improves survival for breast cancer patients: a randomized clinical trial. *Cancer.* 2008;113(12): 3450–3458.

123. Antoni MH, Lechner SC, Kazi A, et al. How stress management improves quality of life after treatment for breast cancer. *J Consult Clin Psychol.* 2006;74(6):1143–1152.

124. McGregor BA, Antoni MH, Boyers A, Alferi SM, Blomberg BB, Carver CS. Cognitive-behavioral stress management increases benefit finding and immune function among women with early-stage breast cancer. *J Psychosom Res.* 2004;56(1):1–8.

125. Savard J, Simard S, Ivers H, Morin CM. Randomized study on the efficacy of cognitive-behavioral therapy for insomnia secondary to breast cancer, part I: sleep and psychological effects. *J Clin Oncol.* 2005;23(25):6083–6096.

126. Savard J, Simard S, Ivers H, Morin CM. Randomized study on the efficacy of cognitive-behavioral therapy for insomnia secondary to breast cancer, part II: immunologic effects. *J Clin Oncol.* 2005;23(25):6097–6106.

127. Perron L, Bairati I, Harel F, Meyer F. Antihypertensive drug use and the risk of prostate cancer (Canada). *Cancer Causes Control.* 2004;15(6):535–541.

128. Algazi M, Plu-Bureau G, Flahault A, Dondon MG, Lê MG. Could treatments with beta-blockers be associated with a reduction in cancer risk? *Rev Epidemiol Sante Publique.* 2004;52(1):53–65.

The Resilient Cancer Patient

• *Mark D. Gilbert*

Whenever one is confronted with an inescapable, unavoidable situation, whenever one has to face a fate that cannot be changed ... such as an incurable or chronic disease ... just then is one given a last chance to actualize the highest value, to fulfill the deepest meaning, the meaning of suffering. For what matters above all is the attitude we take toward suffering, the attitude in which we take our suffering upon ourselves.

Viktor Frankl[1]

■ RESILIENCE AND CANCER: WHAT IS IT?

A cancer diagnosis challenges patients and their caregivers from every conceivable angle: physical, cognitive, emotional, social, spiritual, and financial. To cope with this onslaught and effect the optimal strategy for reestablishing quality and quantity of life, cancer patients are tested for their ability to absorb the impact of this challenge, and then rebound with resilience.

Resilience refers to the ability to successfully adapt to stressors, bounce back from setbacks, and maintain psychological well-being in the face of adversity.[2] The everyday meaning of the word "resilience" extends to anything that bounces back. In psychology it is the word for springing back from serious adversity, such as abuse, war, illness, or natural disasters. In the dictionary, it is explained as an ability to recover from or adjust easily to misfortune or change (from the Latin verb "resilire,"

which means to "jump back" or "recoil").[3] This interactive concept, resilience, refers to a relative resistance to environmental risk experiences, or involves the overcoming of stress or adversity. As such, it differs from both social competence and positive mental health. Resilience also differs from traditional concepts of risk and protection in its focus on individual variations in response to comparable experiences. For the sake of this discussion, we will focus on psychological resilience and the factors that affect it in a cancer patient, although there are many different areas that can be referenced as pertaining to resilience—ranging from biology to the environment, the economy, or sociology.

For the cancer patients resilience is not the result of a fixed attribute, but may come about as the result of either the patient adapting to living with a life-threatening illness, using specific physiologic or psychological coping mechanisms, or having specific traits that allow an advantage for coping. "Bouncing back" may not necessarily involve recovery from cancer, but rather may tap into an opportunity for healing. Through a combination of cognitive, emotional, relational, instrumental, and/or spiritual strategies, the patient may be motivated to explore and act in such a way that the meaning and purpose of life transform suffering, and the individual's perception is that life's harmony and integrity are restored. Medical research over the past 20 years has identified over 30 psychosocial and neurophysiologic components that may contribute to the degree to which a cancer patient is able to be resilient to a life-threatening illness. It would be

■ TABLE 3-1. Some Significant Contributing Factors Towards Resilence.

Early Social Bonding	DHEA Levels and Receptors	Cortisol Levels and Receptors	Hardiness
Positive emotional granularity	Switching cognitive set	Hippocampal volume and HPA axis	Childhood trauma
Stress inoculation	Locus ceruleus and NE levels and receptors	Number of CR-1 and CR-2 receptors	COMT
Neuropeptide Y	Galanin-1 and galanin-2	Dopamine	Serotonin
Neural reward circuitry	Actin-polymerization protein	cAMP response element-binding protein	Brain-derived neurotrophic factor
Fear learning and extinction of amygdala response	Optimism	Hope	Spiritual faith
Psychosocial support	Humor	Family relationships	Financial stability
Life meaning/purpose	Accurate emotional identification and expression	Physical exercise and health-related choices	Active coping style
Artistic expression (art, music, poetry, journaling)	Genetics (5-HTT long-allele transporter genes)		

impossible to discuss each of these components in great detail in this chapter, but a list of significant contributing factors is presented in Table 3-1.

■ TOOLS FOR MEASURING PSYCHOLOGICAL RESILIENCE

Psychologists have used a number of standardized psychological test measures to ascertain resilience over the past decade. The most commonly used measurements have been Wagnild and Young's[4] (1993) 25-item psychological resilience scale, Connor and Davidson's[5] "Connor–Davidson Resilience Scale—2001" (CD-RISC), a list completed by the individual that is used to measure resilience, and "Resilience Scale for Adults," a resilience questionnaire developed by Friborg et al in 2006.[6] Many other scales have been developed, however, as Schaap and colleagues[7] describe the state of the testing field in this area: "the constantly changing context and the differences between and within people make it difficult to pinpoint and measure resilience. Some researchers argue in favor of descriptions of the concept of resilience in terms of risk and protective processes in place of conceptualizations of risk and protective factors."

■ GENETIC RESILIENCE

Genetics has been shown to contribute to an individual being resilient. Roughly one third of the population that carries two long 5-HTT alleles has a significant resilience advantage to those with short serotonin transporter gene alleles. Long-allele pairing seems to provide more protection from the depressed mood and traumatic repercussions of environmental stress, such as occurs in cancer, but only if the patient becomes ill (ie, has a significant stressor that allows gene expression).[8]

However, it has also been shown that a strong adult bond with someone of importance in the patient's life can ameliorate the short allele makeup.[9] Obviously, cancer patients who are equipped with a genetic advantage and have had strong social bonds in their past and present will be best able to withstand the stress of cancer diagnosis and treatment.

■ BIOCHEMICAL RESILIENCE

Although many of these relationships are still highly complex, it is important to note that certain aspects of the cancer patient's history will either enhance or detract from biochemical resilience. The most significant questions on history in this area would include whether patients had a positive emotional bond with a parent in their childhood, whether they experienced mild/moderate rather than severe stress in childhood, whether they were abused, and whether they continue to have strong social connections. As you will see in the following paragraph, the way in which cancer patients cope with their illness is far more complex than simply using a particular cognitive set or attitude.

As seen in Table 3-1, many neuroendocrine processes may affect one's ability to be resilient. Regarding the most studied interactions with resilience, DHEA and cortisol have a complex interaction and contribution. It does appear in general that patients with a higher DHEA/cortisol ratio are likely to have higher resilience measures, excepting in patients who have had early childhood abuse, when higher cortisol levels have been related to resilience.[10] It has been discovered that DHEA enhances cognition and performance under stress. The cognitive effects of positive emotion (increased in resilient patients) are linked to increased dopamine levels and the ability to switch cognitive set quickly. 5-HT1A receptors are anxiolytic and may be linked to adaptive responses to aversive events in resilient patients. Perhaps there is genetic loading for 5-HT1A receptor density. In fact, early life stress may increase corticotropin-releasing hormone (CRH and cortisol, downregulating 5-HT1A).[11,12]

In animal studies, and speculated in humans, the medial prefrontal cortex (mPFC) and the serotonergic neurons of the dorsal raphe nucleus are able to mediate fear responses.[13] Early childhood abuse appears to be a key indicator of resilience in later life, and clinician working with cancer patients should be alert to asking for a past history of abuse. Women abused as children have increased HPA axis and autonomic activity in response to stress compared with controls. Women with severe and prolonged physical abuse in childhood have been found to have smaller hippocampal volumes, and increased HPA axis and autonomic activity in response to stress.[14] However, patients who as children experienced moderately stressful events (family relocation, parental illness) rather than severe abuse seem better equipped to deal with stressors later in life, such as serious illness.[15]

Another neurohormone interfacing with resilience is CRH. Excess stress in childhood can lead to excess CRH activity in the adult brain. CRH-1 receptors have an anxiogenic response, and CRH-2 receptors have an anxiolytic role. Resilient patients appear to have the capacity to regulate CRH levels and the balance of CRH-1 and CRH-2 receptor subtypes.[16] Other contributing neuroanatomical and biochemical features found related to resilience are sufficient levels of testosterone,[17] neuropeptide Y,[18] galanin-1 receptors,[19] and brain-derived neurotrophic factor (BDNF),[20] plus potent mPFC inhibition of amygdala responsiveness.[21] Factors that are inversely related to resilience include high levels of actin-polymerization protein (APP) in the lat.amygdala,[22] cAMP response element-binding protein decreasing reward pursuit in the n. accumbens or in the amygdala,[23] low functioning COMT levels,[24] and a hyperfunctioning locus ceruleus–norepinephrine system[25] (again related to significant childhood stress). Finally, women with higher oxytocin levels seem to have increased social bonding and more resilience to illness.[26]

■ PSYCHOSOCIAL RESILIENCE

The core trilayered foundation of psychosocial resilience, supporting the stable platform from which resilience is manifested, is formed from optimism, hope, and purpose. While each layer of the foundation is somewhat different in character from the other, together they provide the firm stability on which resilience is sustained. We will examine each of these layers in turn.

Optimism

A pessimist sees the difficulty in every opportunity; an optimist sees the opportunity in every difficulty.

Winston Churchill

Optimism is the expectation of positive outcomes.[27] Optimistic style is characterized by the belief that the future will be pleasant because one can control important outcomes.[28] Also of note is that optimists are more likely than pessimists to engage in difficult tasks—optimists work longer on difficult tasks, with greater task engagement, and engage more fully.[29] Task engagement has affective correlates, but is primarily a cognitive and motivational quality. It may be related to active coping in the cancer patient, which is more favorable to positive outcome.

A growing body of research on optimism performed over the past 2 decades has shown that optimism is associated with better health. Dispositional optimists (who hold generalized positive outcome expectancies) have shown less mood disturbance to a number of stressors (eg, breast cancer biopsy and breast cancer surgery),[30,31] and Segerstrom, one of the world's leading researchers on optimism and health, has demonstrated that optimism is associated with mood, coping, and immune change in response to stress. Hers was the first study to show optimism related to enhanced immunity.[31(p27)] With the insult of a stress such as cancer or other life-threatening illness, it has been shown that having high dispositional optimism leads to more problem solving and acceptance, and less disengagement and denial.[32,33] There is strong support for the notion that dispositional optimism protects one from illness,[34] but does optimism lead to better resilience for a patient who has already developed cancer? There are mixed results regarding physical outcome and optimism. For instance, studies have demonstrated decreased mortality rates in optimistic young patients with head and neck cancer but not lung cancer patients.[35,36] Immunity does seem to show improvement over a pessimistic style. For example, pessimistic explanatory style has been found to be associated with lowered immunocompetence (T suppressor CD8 up, relative to T helper cells—elderly men and women pessimists had lower CD4/CD8 ratios).[37]

However, from a perspective of psychophysiologic resilience, Segerstrom's research has replicated a fascinating outcome. She found that when circumstances are easy or straightforward, optimism will be positively related to immunity, because engagement can lead to termination of the stressor; however, when circumstances are difficult or complex, optimism will be negatively related to immunity because it leads to ongoing engagement with persistent stressors.[38] Segerstrom labeled this the "engagement process." She believes that under difficult circumstances, more optimistic people remain engaged, whereas more pessimistic people disengage, or give up, which may be physiologically protective. Cohen et al's[39] work supports this finding, showing that prolonged stress greater than 1 week causes negative effects on immunity, after initial positive effects (NKCC, CD8CD11b T-cell activity in women). In fact, pessimistic women did better after a week. It is Segerstrom's belief that how optimism affects the immune system critically depends on the circumstances being examined—dispositional optimism and specific expectancies appear to buffer the immune system from the effects of psychological stressors, but there is sometimes a physical cost paid for the

optimistic strategy of engaging difficult stressors rather than disengaging and withdrawing (ie, increased cortisol and lower cell immunity). This begs us to wonder, as with the cancer patient, whether resilience is built not just on optimism, but with the flexibility to move back and forth to each leg of the tripod. Resilience for a patient with a life-threatening illness is most likely enhanced by an active coping, positive attitude balanced with the flexibility to change direction or perception based on the external and internal informational inputs of the moment.

With respect to the neuoranatomy and physiology of optimism, the brain generates an optimism bias—humans expect positive events in the future even when there is no evidence to support such expectations.[40] This tendency is related specifically to enhanced activation in the rt. amygdala (simulation of future emotional events) and in the rostral anterior cingulated cortex (RACC). The RACC directs self-reflective tasks and self-referential judgments, reflects on hopes and dreams, indicates preferences, and judges the trustworthiness of others. When imaging positive future events relative to negative ones, the RACC appears to play a key role for areas involved in monitoring emotional salience in mediating the optimism bias. The RACC has been correlated with trait optimism and connected with the ventromedial prefrontal cortex, the dorsomedial prefrontal cortex, and the rt. amygdala, in imagining future events and autobiographical information. It is involved in imaging positive future scenarios as opposed to negative ones, and this effective integration is related to optimism.[40(p41)]

Hope

Hope is not the conviction that something will turn out well, but the certainty that something makes sense, regardless of how it turns out.

Vaclav Havel

Hope is a future-oriented perspective, involving the positive expectation for meaning attached to life events.[41] It is different from optimism: whereas optimism anticipates a positive outcome, hope anticipates a positive meaning. This is a critical difference for a patient struggling with the challenge of cancer, in that when optimism may be lost, hope continues to sustain resilience. In this way, hope is a more fundamentally essential element in the patient's psychological and physical metamorphosis through cancer—it allows for resilience regardless of prognosis.

One may thus conceive of hope underlying optimism, and purpose or meaning underlying hope.

In the case of a patient with cancer onset, hope may be for a cure or prolonged survival, and in terminal illness, it may be defined as a struggle to come to terms with the multiple losses in a changing reality. Hope can transform from a noun (there is always hope) to a verb (I hope), to an adjective (hopeful), or to an adverb (hopefully). Hiding or distorting the truth is not "hope-engendering." Hope is best engineered through honesty and empathy, by framing hope in a wider context through relationships, belief, control, dignity, inner peace, humor, meaningful events, and achievable treatment goals.[42] So while denial may be an effective ego defense mechanism for the cancer patient to deal with the initial existential crisis of a life-threatening diagnosis, it is not a sustainable defense for resilience in the long run. Kim et al[43] note that hope is an experience that is revealed in a dynamic pattern associated with an individual's life situation. In this dynamic pattern is the search for cure, social support, information, and spiritual beliefs, limiting the impact of a trauma/ability to adapt changing capacities, and for living in the moment/self-transcendence.[44] Within the ever-changing dynamic, hopeful experiences shift between dependency and freedom, confidence and insecurity, strength and exhaustion, and desperation and pleasure.[45]

In the end, hope exists as an orientation to future possibilities transcending limits of specific things or materials,[45(p45)] and is an independent condition of mind resulting from a cognitive, evaluative process regarding goal attainment.[46]

Many indirect measures of hope relate to notions of self-efficacy and locus of control.[47] From a neuro-anatomical perspective of hope, studies performed with fMRI testing suggest that people able to manifest hope and being high in psychological well-being (autonomy, environmental mastery, personal growth, positive relations with others, purpose in life, and self-acceptance) effectively recruit the ventral anterior cingulated cortex (ACC) when confronted with potentially aversive stimuli, manifest reduced activity in subcortical regions such as the amygdala, and appraise such information as less salient as reflected in slower evaluative speed.[48]

Hope is a therefore a critical component of the cancer patient's resilience, but the bedrock of hope lies in the patient's connection with his or her own unique life purpose. As Frankl[49] stated, "Hope is a process of human becoming through which one searches for meaning for oneself in relationships outside self."

Purpose/Meaning

How could drops of water know themselves to be a river? Yet the river flows on.

Antoine de Saint-Exupery

What do we mean by meaning? Recker et al[50] define it as "the cognizance of order, coherence and purpose in one's existence, which leads to the pursuit and attainment of worthwhile goals and an accompanying sense of fulfillment." To find purpose or meaning in one's suffering is perhaps the highest and yet ultimate challenge for a human being. For our patients, meaning is enhanced by the finiteness of their life (*appreciating* what they do have), and by the testing of their own strength (*making the most* of what they do have).[51]

Meaningfulness is active—something that one achieves and imposes through choice. It involves the responsibility to find meaning: recognizing one's important role, what life expects of oneself, and a sense of responsibility to others or a task. Actively achieving or imposing meaning leads to transcendence: rising above one's situation through being part of something greater than the self (God, family, profession, community, nature, other).

For the cancer patient, purpose may change through time, or may be branched. Purpose may cover the spectrum from getting one's life "in order" for loved ones, reestablishing relationships, finding forgiveness, searching out new treatment possibilities, caring for one's health in a new way, taking up a new challenge or hobby, establishing faith, or many other possibilities. Purpose, notably, is also part of dying patients' quest as they come to terms with the meaning of their past and present life, and their future transcendence.

Frankl,[51(p1)] author of *Man's Search for Meaning*, said that there are three basic sources of meaning:

1. Creative meaning—actualizing creative values such as art, active causes, and advocacy.
2. Experiential meaning—actualizing valued experiences such as love, social support, and appreciation of beauty, nature, art, and humor (objectivity of one's self).
3. Attitudinal meaning—the attitude with which one bears suffering that is unavoidable (the one freedom Frankl believed that is left to an individual), such as role modeling, using suffering as a catalyst to change (reframing a situation), or dignified coping (as with the dying patient).

For a cancer patient, meaning may be expressed through any or many of the above-mentioned sources, all of which may be linked at the least to better quality of life, and perhaps increased longevity.

■ REBOUND OPPORTUNITIES: RESILIENCE TOOLS FOR PATIENTS WITH CANCER

Our greatest glory is not in never falling, but in rising every time we fall.

Confucius

From the material that has been covered thus far, it becomes clear that patients with cancer have a number of opportunities with which to find resilience, regardless of their genetic predisposition of their prognosis. In this section we will cover the most important, evidence-based tools with which a patient may utilize these opportunities. I choose to label these tools as particular "rebound choices" of life, implying choices to arise to the challenge of cancer. In my youth my hockey coach would always preach that our best chances at scoring were on the rebounds "turn the rebounds into opportunities" he would preach. Based on the research presented, we will look at the most significant rebound opportunities that the cancer patient faces.

Rebound Option 1—Coping Style

Here the cancer patient has the option of a passive or active coping style. For a rebound opportunity, and after the initial diagnosis leads to confusion, angst, and/or denial, patients need to confront their illness with motivation and deliberate intent, that is, educate themselves about their particular cancer and every treatment opportunity available. This means reading, asking questions of their doctors, and searching out a full integrative approach (including questioning fully what life stress(es) they may have not addressed that would hinder their resilience). Again, denial and repression as a means of coping must fade over time, as avoidant, passive coping mechanisms have been associated with poor outcome. This involves acknowledging and accepting problems, facing fears, seeking social support, adopting an optimistic outlook, reframing stressors to a positive light, and exercising; this prevents dysregulation of the serotonergic neurons in the dorsal raphe nucleus (seen in learned helplessness). Resilient individuals are more adept at managing fear, appraising threat, and selecting appropriate action. Active coping, at the time of trauma and on re-exposure to trauma reminders, shapes neural circuits that underlie fear conditioning (redirects activity in the lateral and central amygdala away from the brainstem and toward the ventral striatum motor circuits)—enabling productive action.

Rebound Option 2—Philosophical Approach

The technological approach of contemporary "subspecialty" medical doctors focuses on *fixing* illness. They have a much more difficult time with illness that becomes chronic, or for that matter, has no "fix." This is not just a dilemma for the physician, but for patients and their family as well. It is the dream of almost every patient and physician to "cure" cancer, and this thankfully is happening with more frequency. It is understandable and likely opportunistic for cancer patients to take on the challenge of the cure. However, at the same time it is important for them to learn a concept of "healing," which is not fixing. The definition of healing that I have used with my patients for the past many years is that "healing is an intentional process by which a human being is motivated to accept their authentic life, through the exploration of internal thoughts, feelings, physical, and spiritual connections— in a non-judgmental way and in a trusting environment. As the result of this acceptance, meaning and purpose transform suffering, and the individual's perception is that life's harmony and integrity are restored." There is no discussion of cancer in this definition. Ideally it seems that in rebound option 2, one would be best served by pursuing fixing and practicing healing *at the same time*. It is paradoxical that the more one practices a "healing" approach to cancer, the more one provides oneself a better chance at fixing.

Rebound Option 3—Attitudinal Choice

Optimism has been repeatedly correlated with increased psychological well-being, health, and greater life satisfaction. We have seen that optimism increases immunity if patients retain the flexibility of knowing what they can control and what not. Yet the rebound choice here is not purely optimism, but optimism tempered with hope, not one more than the other. Patients who see themselves as "unlucky," that their cancer "was meant to be," "was God's will," or is a "punishment" of some kind, take on a kind of "negative religiosity" that has been associated with poorer outcome. Patients who choose an optimistic attitude have a better chance at rebounding, yet those who are also hopeful know that regardless of outcome, they will learn to find meaning from their experiences and their suffering, for hope lies in meaning that is attached to life, not in events themselves. Beyond being optimistic for a cure, for sustained healing a patient with a distressing illness may find hope leads to greater connection with others or their faith, rediscovery of meaning, emotional sharing, affirmation, trust, perspective, authenticity, safety, and renewed and more gratifying expectations. Again, this rebound option is *about choosing both paths*. Individuals who can think flexibly, using cognitive reappraisal, produce alternative explanations, reframe positively, and accept challenging situations or distressing events are more psychologically resilient; they find hope by transforming adverse experiences into positive learning through the critical use of meaning and purpose.

Rebound Option 4—Emotional Expression

Cancer patients most natural feel a roller coaster of emotions—at the time of their diagnosis and for some time afterwards. Initial intense existential anxiety, if not panic, may be interspersed with anger ("why me?"), despair (cancer equated with death), or even emptiness (from an unfulfilled life). Sadly, many cancer patients will isolate these feelings often through the ego defenses of denial, displacement, isolation, suppression, and repression. These isolated feelings may have any one of a number of contributing factors. They are often the result of learning to repress trauma from a childhood model, learning that the sick role means being a burden, or that being ill is about not being respected. Whatever the cause, emotional repression is now shown to be a poor prognostic indicator for cancer patients. The rebound option here is for patients to identify their complex set of feelings accurately and to express them in a trusting, nonjudgmental environment. This expression of feeling could take place with their spouse, their friends, their family, a religious counselor, or a psychotherapist, in a group therapy, or through their own personal journaling. This appropriate identification of complex feeling (positive emotional granularity) has been associated with more positive outcome and better resilience, as is the accurate expression of these feelings. Once again, as with the other rebound opportunities, proportion and balance are important. Hope and worry can both be had at the same time, as mixed emotional response leads to coping. This is particularly important for the patient's spouse and family to

understand and encourage. Resilience does not involve denial of the risk of death, which needs expression, but also neither worry overwhelming life. With the right timing and the right setting, practicing emotional expression leads to better adjustment to illness.

Rebound Option 5—Social Support

Significant research evidence now exists in psychosocial oncology demonstrating that cancer patients who have a strong social support network have less mood disturbance, better quality of life, and, in some studies, increased longevity. Social isolation and withdrawal is not linked with rebound opportunity, and those who perceive that they have some support and use that support have a better adjustment. It is patients' choice of who they need for support (instrumental and emotional support may require different people), determine whether they are independence needy, and be offered help to establish supportive networks. Social support causes significantly better outcome in a wide variety of stressors and illnesses. Oxytocin is important for social attachment and bonding and augments anxiolytic effects of social support in stress (perhaps by decreasing HPA axis activity).[51(p26)]

Rebound Option 6—Purpose

A cancer diagnosis could leave an afflicted individual feeling confused and hopeless. The life meaning that arises from a cancer diagnosis often is the result of "taking stock" of one's life. Although the patient did not cause the illness directly, there may be some learning that comes out of it (often involving the meaning of family, community, new causes, appreciation, enlightenment, honesty, or self-care). So often, patients call cancer a "gift," because of an opportunity for transformation—built on new perspective and focused meaning. As noted earlier, life purpose is an underlying foundation for the resilient component of hope. Identifying one's life purpose after a cancer diagnosis is critical for building resilience.

Rebound Option 7—Spiritual Faith

At Brown University's Centre for Gerontology and Health Care Research, spiritual faith is defined as "that which gives meaning to one's life and draws one to transcend oneself."[52] Spirituality is a broader concept than religion, although that is one expression of spirituality. Other expressions include prayer, meditation, interactions with others or nature, and a relationship with God or a higher power. Spirituality is also integral to the dying person's achievement of the developmental task of transcendence. The rebound opportunity here is an option to life being simply material, with no greater purpose than our short time of accomplishments and/or happiness on this earth. Frankl[52(p1)] spoke of three different hierarchal levels of life purpose—willful purpose (creative or altruistic acts), psychological purpose (self-awareness and willful choice), and spiritual purpose. Spiritual purpose transcends individual plight and existential crisis. The benefits of choosing spiritual purpose are inner peace, inner strength, better coping, improved adjustment, and improved quality of life. Many research studies have demonstrated that those who practice spiritual connection have better health outcome and more resilience to setbacks.[53,54] This is just like a trapeze artist for whom, when letting go of the trapeze handle and flying through the air waiting for the next handle to appear, it is comforting to know that there is a net below. For the cancer patient, as one "handle" on life dissolves, knowing a net is below can boost resilience. I would call that net "faith." The balance of the continuum here is not denying the feelings about life being finite, and what that means for each of us personally (not giving up on seizing life) while at the same time finding spiritual and philosophical beliefs that challenge each of us for why life is important.

Resilient individuals have a framework of belief that few things can shatter (adherence to a spiritual system and an altruistic outlook toward others); spiritual or self-transcendent experiences may be associated with density of 5-HT1A receptors in the dorsal raphe, hippocampus, and neocortex; morality has some neural basis intrinsic to human nature (acquired sociopathy can occur with damage to the anterior prefrontal cortex and ant. temporal lobes)—moral judgments are associated with these areas on fMRI and altruism helps resilience (morality leads to action).

Rebound Option 8—Self-Perception

This option requires risk taking, courage, and often the help of a professional counselor. It is the option of either feeling broken, unlovable, and helpless with a life-threatening illness or finding self-compassion, love, and esteem. The difficult challenge comes when a patient has a predisposing problem with ego strengths, as the result of a dysfunctional family upbringing, a history of abuse, little social support, or overwhelming acute and/or chronic trauma. However, low self-esteem may be a problem for any cancer patient as a result of the stigma of being ill

with cancer, change of appearance, decreased physical abilities and activity levels (fatigue), loss of independence and vitality, chronic pain, or role changes in the family or at work. Patients with a predisposing history of mood disorder are particularly at risk, and there is also a higher incidence of depression in cancer patients than in the general population. It is incumbent on the health care professional to screen for depression or anxiety disorders in all cancer patients, and to provide them with a resource for help accordingly. Simple depression screening questionnaires such as the PHQ-9 can be helpful in identifying patients at risk.[55]

Rebound Option 9—Exploration

The patient has the option here of finding every possible way to get better or to be disinterested, unmotivated, and avoidant. Self-efficacy is the belief that one is capable of performing in a certain manner to attain certain goals. Patients throw their ultimate trust in the health care provider, sometimes regressing to a childlike posturing while feeling helpless to their fate. Many individuals naturally may want something or someone to "make it all better." But clinicians are humans, and their art imperfect. Self-efficacious patients would need to want to live as long and be in as good health as possible. In order to do that, they have to find out how. What are their treatment options? What are the possible side effects of treatment? How will their quality of life be affected? Do they need a second opinion? Would their lifestyle be advantageous to change? Who will be their support, and when?

The cancer patient can learn tools to reduce stress in mind and body, such as meditation techniques, imagery, humor, art, journaling, prayer, music appreciation, nutritional awareness, and group support. Increased self-awareness (part of the work of finding psychological purpose) increases quality of life and diminishes fear, anxiety, and depression, along with increasing the likelihood of more supportive social connections.

Rebound Option 10—Humor

Humor diminishes the threatening nature and negative emotional impact of stressful situations by cognitive reappraisal and reframing, and diminishes the threatening nature of events. Mirthful humor activates a network of subcortical regions critical to the DA reward system, and is key component of providing perspective for the cancer patient.

Rebound Option 11—Balance

Resilient individuals are willing to show determination and fortitude when it is called for, and let go when they need to. Homeostasis of physiologic mechanisms seems to mimic the cognitive–behavioral approach that simulates a negative feedback loop. Meditation techniques help to balance alpha and theta brain waves, enhance gamma waves, and improve immunity and parasympathetic drive.

Rebound Option 12—Choosing Optimal Health

In a 2-year research project, Dr Kenneth Pelletier[55] at Stanford University defined health as "a life lived well and fully, a life involved with other people, and with self-exploration of the emotions, the mind, the body and the spirit." With this definition in mind, resilient individuals attend more to the physical, emotional, and spiritual health of themselves and their intimate others than nonresilient individuals; they identify and express their feelings more readily, choose healthier diets, appropriate exercise, and lifestyles, and connect more outside of themselves with purpose and meaning.

■ SUMMARY

For a cancer patient, finding resilience is a complex process involving many interactive biological, psychological, and environmental factors. Yet cancer patients, through will and motivation, can utilize available tools to make appropriate choices in their care, which can improve the quality of their lives, their ability to cope, and their opportunity of finding meaning in life despite or in lieu of their suffering.

KEY POINTS

- Resilience in a cancer patient is defined.
- Tools for measuring psychological resilience are reviewed.
- Components of genetic, biochemical, and psychosocial resilience are described.
- The role of optimism, hope, and purpose is discussed as the foundation of psychosocial resilience.
- Twelve opportunities for cancer patients to develop resilience are detailed.

REFERENCES

1. Frankl VE. *Man's Search for Meaning*. Boston, MA: Beacon Press; 2006 [first publication 1959].

2. Haglund MEM, Nestadt PS, Cooper NS, Southwick SM, Charney DS. Psychobiological mechanisms of resilience: relevance to prevention and treatment of stress-related psychopathology. *Dev Psychopathol*. 2007;19:889–920.

3. *The Merriam-Webster Dictionary*. Springfield, Mass: Merriam-Webster, Incorporated; July 1, 2004:960 pp. [paperback].

4. Wagnild GM, Young HM. Development and psychometric evaluation of the Resilience Scale. *J Nurs Meas*. 1993;1:165–178.

5. Connor K, Davidson JRT. Development of a new resilience scale: the Connor–Davidson Resilience Scale. *Depress Anxiety*. 2003;18(2):76–82.

6. Friborg O, Hjemdal O, Rosenvinge JH, Martinussen M. A new rating scale for adult resilience: what are the central protective resources behind healthy adjustment? *Int J Methods Psychiatr Res*. 2003;12(2):65–76.

7. Alberto NC, van Galen FM, van der Post MJ, Rooze MW, de Ruijter AM. An intervention for primary schools children: the project. *IMPACT, Dutch knowledge & advice centre for post-disaster psychosocial care*. The Netherlands. Available at www.impact-kenniscentrum.nl.

8. Caspi A, Moffitt TE. Gene–environment interactions in psychiatry: joining forces with neuroscience. *Nat Rev Neurosci*. 2006;7(7):583–590.

9. Kaufman J, Charney D. Effects of early stress on brain structure and function: implications for understanding the relationship between child maltreatment and depression. *Dev Psychopathol*. 2001;13(3):451–471.

10. Cicchetti D, Rogosch FA. Personality, adrenal steroid hormones, and resilience in maltreated children: a multilevel perspective. *Dev Psychopathol*. 2007;19(3):787–809.

11. Parker LN, Levin ER, Lifrak ET. Evidence for adrenocortical adaptation to severe illness. *J Clin Endocrinol Metab*. 1985;60(5):947–952.

12. Bauer ME. Chronic stress and immunosenescence: a review. *Neuroimmunomodulation*. 2008;15(4–6):241–250.

13. Amat J, Paul E, Watkins LR, Maier SF. Activation of the ventral medial prefrontal cortex during an uncontrollable stressor reproduces both the immediate and long-term protective effects of behavioral control. *Neuroscience*. 2008;154(4):1178–1186.

14. Heim C, Newport DJ, Heit S, et al. Pituitary–adrenal and autonomic response to stress in women after sexual and physical abuse in childhood. *JAMA*. 2000;284:592–597.

15. Khoshaba DM, Maddi SR. Early experiences in hardiness development. *Consult Psychol J.* 1999;51:106–116.

16. Tache Y, Bonaz B. Corticotropin-releasing factor receptors and stress-related alterations of gut motor function. *J Clin Invest.* 2007;117:33–40.

17. Wirth MM, Schultheiss OC. Basic testosterone moderates response to anger faces in humans. *Physiol Behav.* 2007;90:496–505.

18. Morgan CA 3rd, Wang S, Mason J, et al. Hormone profiles in humans experiencing military survival training. *Biol Psychiatry.* 2000;47:891–901.

19. Holmes FE, Bacon A, Pope RJ, et al. Transgenic overexpression of galanin in the dorsal root ganglia modulates pain related behavior. *Proc Natl Acad Sci U S A.* 2003;100:6180–6185.

20. Berton O, McClung CA, Dileone RJ, et al. Essential role of BDNF in the mesolimbic dopamine pathway in social defeat stress. *Science.* 2006;311;864–868.

21. Herry C, Garcia R. Prefrontal cortex long-term potentiation, but not long-term depression, is associated with the maintenance of extinction learned fear in mice. *J Neurosci.* 2002;22:577–583.

22. Schafe GE, Doyere V, LeDoux JE. Tracking the fear engram: the lateral amygdala is an essential locus of fear memory storage. *J Neurosci.* 2005;25:10010–10014.

23. Josselyn SA, Shi C, Carlezon WA Jr, Neve RL, Nestler EJ, Davis M. Long-term memory is facilitated by cAMP response element-binding protein overexpression in the amygdala. *J Neurosci.* 2001;21:2404–2412.

24. Heinz A, Smolka MN. The effects of catechol-o-methyltransferase genotype on brain activation elicited by affective stimuli and cognitive tasks. *Rev Neurosci.* 2006;17:359–367.

25. Southwick SM, Krystal JH, Bremner JD, et al. Noradrenergic and serotonergic function in post-traumatic stress disorder. *Arch Gen Psychiatry.* 1997;54:749–758.

26. Gidron Y, Ronson A. Psychosocial factors, biological mediators, and cancer prognosis: a new look at an old story. *Curr Opin Oncol.* 2008;20(4):386–392.

27. Segerstrom SC, Taylor SE, Kemeny ME, Fahey JL. Optimism is associated with mood, coping, and immune changes in response to stress. *J Pers Soc Psychol.* 1998;7(6):1646–1655.

28. Kubzansky LD, Sparrow D, Vokonas P, Kawachi I. Is the glass half empty or half full? A prospective study of optimism and coronary heart disease in the Normative Aging Study. *Psychosom Med.* 2001;63:910–916.

29. Nes LS, Segerstrom S, Sephton SE. Engagement and arousal: optimism's effects during a brief stressor. *Pers Soc Psychol Bull.* 2005;31(1):111–120.

30. Stanton AL, Snider PR. Coping with a breast cancer diagnosis: a prospective study. *Health Psychol.* 1993;12;16–23.

31. Carver CS, Pozo C, Harris SD, Noriega V, Scheier MF, Robinson DS, Ketcham AS, Moffat FL Jr, Clark KC. How coping mediates the effect of optimism on distress: a study of women with early stage breast cancer. *J Pers Soc Psychol.* 1993;65(2):375–390.

32. Byrnes DM, Antoni MH, Goodkin K, et al. Stressful events, pessimism, natural killer cell cytotoxicity, and cytotoxic/suppressor T cells in HIV+ black women at risk for cervical cancer. *Psychosomatic Med.* 1998:60:714–722.

33. Schulz R, Bookwala J, Knapp JE, Scheier M, Williamson GM. Pessimism, age, and cancer mortality. *Psychol Aging.* 1996;11:304–309.

34. Maruta T, Colligan R, Malinchoc M, Offord KP. Optimists vs. pessimists: survival rate among medical patients over a 30-year period. *Mayo Clin Proc.* 2000;75:140–143.

35. Allison PJ, Guichard C, Fung K, Gilain L. Dispositional optimism predicts survival status 1 year after diagnosis in head and neck cancer patients. *J Clin Oncol.* 2003;21:543–548.

36. Schofield P, Ball D, Smith JG, Borland R, O'Brien P, Davis S, Olver I, Ryan G, Joseph D. Optimism and survival in lung carcinoma patients. *Cancer.* 2004;100(6):1276–1282.

37. Kamen-Siegel L, Rodin J, Seligman ME, Dwyer J. Explanatory style and cell-mediated immunity in elderly men and women. *Health Psychol.* 1991;10:229–235.

38. Segerstrom S. Optimism and immunity: do positive thoughts always lead to positive effects? *Brain Behav Immun.* 2005;19:195–200.

39. Cohen F, Kearney KA, Zegans LS, Kemeny ME, Neuhaus JM, Stites DP. Differential immune system changes with acute and persistent stress for optimists vs. pessimists. *Brain Behav Immun.* 1999;13:155–174.

40. Sharot T, Riccardi AM, Raio CM, Phelps EA. Neural mechanisms mediating optimism bias. *Nature.* 2007;450:102–106.

41. Cassel EJ. *The Healer's Art.* Cambridge, MA: MIT Press; 1976.

42. Clayton JM, Hancock K, Parker S, et al. Sustaining hope when communication with terminally ill patients

and their families: a systematic review. *Psychooncology*. 2008;17(7):641–659.

43. Kim DS, Kim HS, Schwartz-Barcott D, Zucker D. The nature of hope in hospitalized chronically ill patients. *Int J Nurs Stud*. 2006;43:547–556.

44. Fanos JH, Gelinas DF, Foster RS, Postone N, Miller RG. Hope in palliative care: from narcissism to self-transcendence in amyotrophic lateral sclerosis. *J Palliat Care*. 2008;11(3):470–475.

45. Dufault K, Martocchio BC. Symposium on compassionate care and the dying experience. Hope: its spheres and dimensions. *Nurs Clin North Am*. 1985;20(2):379–391.

46. Stotland NL, Mattson MG, Bergeson S. The recovery concept: clinician and consumer perspectives. *J Psychiatr Pract*. 2008;14(suppl 2):45–54.

47. Davidson P, Dracup K, Phillips J, Daly J, Padilla G. Preparing for the worst while hoping for the best: the relevance of hope in the heart failure illness trajectory. *J Cardiovasc Nurs*. 2007;22(3):159–165.

48. van Reekum CM, Urry HL, Johnstone T, et al. Individual differences in amygdala and ventromedial prefrontal cortex activity are associated with evaluation speed and psychological well-being. *J Cogn Neurosci*. 2007;19(2):237–248.

49. Frankl VE. *Man's Search for Meaning*. Washington, DC: Washington Square Press; 1959.

50. Recker G, Peacock E, Wong P. Meaning and purpose in life and well-being: a life-span perspective. *J Gerontol*. 1987;42:44–49.

51. Greenstein M, Breitbart W. Cancer and the experience of meaning: a group psychotherapy program for people with cancer. *Am J Psychother*. 2000;54(4):486–500.

52. Highfield ME. Providing spiritual care to patients with cancer. *Clin J Oncol Nurs*. 2000;4(3):115–120.

53. Koenig HG, Mc Connell M. The Healing power of faith NY: Simon schuster; 1999.

54. Koenig HG, George LK, Tins P. Religion, spirituality and health in medically ill hospitalized patients. *J. of the American Geriatrics Association*. 2009;52:554–562.

55. Kroenke K, Spitzer RL, Williams JB. The PHQ-9: validity of a brief depression severity measure. *J Gen Intern Med*. 2001;16(9):606–613.

56. An interview with Kenneth Pelletier. *Healthc Forum J*. 1994;37(5):1–5.

The Clinical Assessment of Distress

• *Cindy L. Carmack, Patricia A. Parker, and Eileen H. Shinn*

■ DISTRESS IN CANCER PATIENTS

According to the National Comprehensive Cancer Network (NCCN), distress is:

> a multifactorial unpleasant emotional experience of a psychological (cognitive, behavioral, emotional), social, and/or spiritual nature that may interfere with the ability to cope effectively with cancer, its physical symptoms and its treatment. Distress extends along a continuum, ranging from common normal feelings of vulnerability, sadness, and fears to problems that can become disabling, such as depression, anxiety, panic, social isolation, and existential and spiritual crisis.[1]

The above-mentioned definition looks beyond thinking in terms of diagnosable mood disorders such as major depression, and considers minor and subsyndromal states, such as adjustment disorders. This is notable because individuals presenting with mild-to-moderate levels of distress may also exhibit significant impairment in functioning[2,3] and require psychological treatment just as those with diagnosable disorders do.[3]

Distress is common in cancer patients with prevalence rates for clinical distress varying by disease site ranging from rates as high as 43.4% in lung cancer to 29.6% for gynecological cancers.[4] Rates are likely higher if minor and subsyndromal states are considered. Multiple sources of distress accompany a cancer diagnosis and reemerge at intervals of treatment, changes in disease status, and other markers along the cancer experience.[1,4] Additionally, the needs and concerns of the patient impact the relationships in which the patient is involved.[5,6]

While some distress is normal, it is not benign. Psychological distress in cancer patients must be addressed, as failure to do so may compromise health and quality of life (QOL) outcomes. For example, untreated depression increases rates of noncompliance with difficult and complex chemotherapy and radiation treatment regimens.[7,8] A recent meta-analysis concluded that depressive symptoms were rather consistently associated with a significant but small increase in mortality, independent of other known risk factors.[9] The psychoneuroimmunological literature is replete with studies documenting various aspects of reduced immune function and dysregulated hypothalamic–pituitary axis and noradrenergic stress response activity in distressed patients. For example, patients with even mild-to-moderate levels of depression have reduced natural killer cell activity.[10] Patients treated with interventions for psychosocial distress have been shown to improve quantitative and functional aspects of immunity as well as lower recurrence rates.[11] Untreated psychological distress also may lead to social isolation and reduced QOL. Assessing distress in cancer patients and offering assistance when distress is significant may lower patients' vulnerability to these negative effects.[12,13]

■ RECOMMENDATIONS FOR THE ASSESSMENT OF DISTRESS

The assessment of distress should become an integral part of routine oncological care; results can be used to alert available service staff to patient needs. Patients and their families can be made aware of resources available to assist them as they adjust to diagnosis and treatment. Hospitals and other cancer care facilities have a unique opportunity to intervene in this regard.

The Institute of Medicine (IOM)[14] has established a Standard of Care that acknowledges the necessity to evaluate the psychosocial status of cancer patients and identify those at risk for heightened levels of distress. The report recommends that psychoemotional services should be made available. Furthermore, assistance with life challenges interfering with good health care and with addressing financial and transportation-related issues, as well as help with sustaining normal activities of daily life should be offered. This Standard establishes that cancer care should ensure the provision of appropriate psychosocial health services by:

1. facilitating effective communication between patients and care providers;
2. identifying each patient's psychosocial needs;
3. designing and implementing a plan;
4. following up on, reevaluating, and adjusting plans during the course of care.

The NCCN has established and published practice guidelines in oncology for the clinical identification, assessment, and management of distress in cancer patients. Guidelines stipulate an operating definition of distress and approaches for intervening to support distressed patients and families with psychological, social, and spiritual issues. The Standards of Care for Distress Management specify a range of care that includes steps from recognizing, monitoring, documenting, and promptly treating distress to including the quality of distress management in institutional continuous quality improvement (CQI) projects.[1]

These Standards and Practice Guidelines indicate recognition of the role distress plays in the process of cancer for the cancer patient. They also establish an expectation that care and treatment of distress in cancer patients will become institutionalized within the mainstream of cancer care. Leading researchers in psycho-oncology are proposing the routine practice of making distress the sixth vital sign.[15] In 2004, this was officially recognized by the Canadian Strategy for Cancer Control,[16] and in 2009, it was included in the Canadian Council on Health Services Accreditation as part of its 2009 accreditation guidelines.[17] It has not become routine practice in the United States, although some practice groups have instituted routine screening in their patients.[18]

■ SCREENING FOR DISTRESS

Despite the recommendation of the IOM and NCCN, there is no consensus as to the best screening instrument available. Instruments vary in what they measure with some assessing global distress and others being more specific, such as those assessing depression or anxiety.

Most clinicians prefer brief one to three simple questions or a brief validated questionnaire.[19] However, most screening instruments, including brief screeners, lack specificity and have high false-positive rates. Screening instruments are not widely used in clinical settings.[19] In May 2002, the US Preventive Task Force[20,21] recommended that primary care physicians routinely screen patients for depression. It based its recommendation on the evaluation of new screening studies that were begun after the previous US Preventive Task Force report, which cited lack of evidence regarding routine screening. Based on their evaluation of the research, they concluded that feedback of screening to providers generally increased the recognition of major depression by a factor of 2 to 3. The US Task Force also concluded that feedback of screening results alone is not enough to affect improvements in patient depression. Nevertheless, detection is the first step in improving patient outcomes, and the report concluded that there were a number of accurate screening instruments available to providers.

Ultrashort Screening Methods

Single- and two-item measures are easy to use and may be more appealing to oncology providers who have very limited time during patient visits.

The NCCN Practice Guidelines in Oncology stipulate that all patients will be screened with the single-item Distress Thermometer.[1] The Distress Thermometer asks patients to rate their distress using a scale ranging from 0 ("no distress") to 10 ("extreme distress"). Patients also indicate their source of distress by checking off issues listed on a 34-item problem list. The list includes practical problems, family problems, emotional problems, spiritual/religious concerns, and physical problems. The NCCN recommends those scoring ≥4 should be referred for further evaluation. Research shows this cutoff score has optimal sensitivity and specificity relative to the Hospital Anxiety and Depression Scale (HADS, described below) and the Brief

Symptom Inventory (BSI-18, also described below).[22] An analysis across several studies indicated that the Distress Thermometer had a sensitivity of 77.1% and a specificity of 66.1%. Its positive predictive value was 55.6% and its negative predictive value was 84.0%.[23] Overall, as a screener, it does a good job of ruling out cases of distress, but there are a high number of false positives, validating the need for further professional evaluation.

A March 2002 *Journal of the American Medical Association (JAMA)* meta-analysis of various screening instruments demonstrated good sensitivity and moderately good specificity in detecting depression in primary care settings.[24] Similarly, the instruments performed well with older adults.[25] In a comparison of single- and two-item measures with the Centers for Epidemiological Studies—Depression scale (CES-D) in a sample of 197 terminally ill cancer patients, Chochinov et al[26] found that a single item, "are you depressed?," performed best against the gold standard, with a highly unusual 100% sensitivity and 100% specificity. The two-item prescreening module from the PRIME-MD performed almost as well with 100% sensitivity and 98% specificity. However, others have failed to replicate these results with either the single- or two-item screeners.[27] These two items ask about the two necessary DSM criteria for major depression, depressed mood and anhedonia. Scoring yes on either is counted as having major depression. Other versions of the single-item scale use a visual analog scale, consisting of a 100-mm line with the referent's "worst possible mood" and "best possible mood." Visual analog scales tended to perform relatively poorly as they are confusing to interpret.[26,28]

A two-phase screening strategy has been suggested as a new strategy to decrease the number of false-positive results with ultrashort measures.[27,29] The two-phase screening of Rost et al[30,31] yielded a 76% positive predictive value against a structured diagnosis of major depression in primary care populations, an extremely high value compared to other screening instruments that have yielded PPVs in the ranges of 27% to 35%.[32,33] During the first phase, patients are asked whether they have either of the two core symptoms of depression, depressed mood and anhedonia, either of which must be present to diagnose major depression. If they answer yes to either of the core symptoms, they are then asked about the remaining seven criteria for major depression. The two-phase screening method is efficient in that most patients will only be asked the first phase. Since false-positive depression screening results expend precious clinical staff time to conduct expensive diagnostic interviews for depression, the potential for achieving a high positive predictive value is important.

In general, ultrashort screeners have high rates of false positives, but they are reasonably accurate in terms of ruling out depression, anxiety, or general distress.[27] As Jacobsen[13] notes "… incorrectly identifying a patient as not distressed is likely to have more severe consequences for an individual's QOL and quality of care than incorrectly identifying him or her as distressed."

Multi-item Questionnaires

Multi-item screening instruments are well established, widely used in psychiatric and community samples, and, although brief, range in length between 5 and 30 questions using either true/false or Likert-style response formats. These measures produce a range of possible scores, most of which have cutoff scores that indicate probable clinically significant distress and that additional evaluation is necessary. Three frequently used measures of distress are the BSI-18, the HADS, and the General Health Questionnaire-12 (GHQ-12). The BSI-18 is an abbreviated version of the 53-item BSI that is designed to measure distress in community and medical populations. It is made up of 18, five-point Likert-scale items that measure domains of depression, anxiety, and somatization.[34] Zabora and colleagues[35] have established gender-specific cutoff scores at the upper 25th percentile to identify those experiencing clinically significant distress: ≥10 for men and ≥13 for women. The BSI-18 is currently being used as a routine screening tool at the Sidney Kimmel Comprehensive Cancer Center at Johns Hopkins University (Baltimore, Maryland).[18] The HADS is a 14-item scale that was specifically developed for use with medically ill patients and focuses on cognitive symptoms. Patients report ease in answering the items and administration time is brief. However, in validation studies with female breast cancer patients, the diagnostic performance of the HADS was weak.[28,36] Similarly, the GHQ, a self-report measure for psychological distress that does not include somatic items, reported average sensitivity and specificity, 83% and 76%, respectively.[36] Other studies have adapted traditional screening measures such as the Zung Self-rating

Depression Scale, CES-D, and Beck Depression Inventory (BDI) for primary care use by dropping the somatic items.[37–40] However, these studies did not validate the shortened versions against DSM-based clinical interviews, which are the gold standard for calculating sensitivity and specificity rates.

Other measures include those specifically assessing depressive symptoms in community and in psychiatric samples; they are not intended to diagnose major depression. Two examples of this approach are the CES-D and the BDI FastScreen. The CES-D focuses primarily on cognitive and affective components of depression rather than the somatic symptoms and is a sensible tool to use on medically ill populations such as cancer patients.[41] The CES-D is not a clinical tool; patients scoring 16 or above should receive further evaluation for possible depression.[42] The BDI is a widely used screening tool to measure distress in medical settings.[43] However, the BDI's utility in oncological populations is limited by its inclusion of somatic items (fatigue, lack of appetite), which may contribute to overinflation of its total score. While adopted from the BDI, the BDI FastScreen was specifically developed for evaluating symptoms of depression in patients in primary care and does not contain somatic items.[44]

Structured Clinical Interviews

The gold standard for evaluating psychological disorders is the structured clinical interview based on DSM criteria. While there are several well-validated clinical interviews, the current standard for clinician's diagnosis of adults is the Structured Clinical Interview for DSM-IV (SCID).[45] The SCID's comprehensive approach assesses the patient's past history of psychiatric disorders, comorbid medical disorders, daily functioning and social resources, and longstanding personality patterns. It has been designed so that it can be broken up into modules focusing on certain types of disorders, such as mood or anxiety disorders. Within these modules, decisional skip patterns approximate the decisions that are made in ruling out differential diagnoses (eg, if the death of one's spouse has occurred recently, asking further questions about clinical bereavement, which is not considered to be a depressive disorder). While the SCID accurately identifies psychological disorders, it is time intensive to complete and requires administration by a trained mental health professional.

■ BARRIERS TO THE IDENTIFICATION OF DISTRESS

Despite its prevalence and the potential impact it has on a number of patient outcomes, patient distress is not routinely assessed and managed. In fact, the majority of NCCN member institutions are not following the NCCN clinical practice guidelines for distress management, with only 20% screening all patients as the guidelines recommend. Among those conducting routine screening, 37.5% are relying only on interviews.[46] Similarly, a survey of oncologists who were members of the American Society of Clinical Oncology found that 24.9% reported being "somewhat familiar" with NCCN guidelines. While about two thirds stated that they routinely screened patients for distress, only 14.3% used a screening instrument; most oncologists used direct questions to identify distress in their patients.[47] Use of interviews or direct questions is likely not standardized; thus, the sensitivity and specificity of these methods are unknown. Standardized assessment is important because studies show that patient distress often goes unrecognized by oncologists.[48]

Newell et al[49] assessed medical oncologists' awareness of their patients' physical symptoms, anxiety, depression, and perceived needs in a mixed sample of 240 individuals with cancer. They found that the oncologists had greater awareness of patients' physical symptoms than their distress or psychosocial problems. Not surprisingly, higher levels of awareness were observed when the oncologists felt less pressured by their workloads and for patients they indicated they knew well and with whom they had good rapport. Similarly, Fallowfield and colleagues[48] conducted a study to examine the ability of 143 physicians to detect distress in 2297 patients during outpatient consultations that were videotaped. Before seeing the physician, patients completed the GHQ, a self-report questionnaire that is a screening measure for psychological morbidity. After the consultation, doctors completed ratings of patients' distress. Results showed that physicians were able to identify heightened distress in only 29% of patients experiencing such distress. Specificity, or true negative rate, was 84.8% and misclassification rate was 34.7%. Interestingly, the physicians in this study knew that the psychological status of their patients was being assessed and that they were being videotaped; thus, detection rates may actually be worse in situations where physicians are not being monitored. Finally, studies consistently show that oncologists fail to recognize major depression in their patients between 50%[50] and 87%[38] of the time. Comparisons between the diagnoses made by oncologists and liaison psychiatrists who consulted on the same patients resulted in a concordance rate of 23% for major depression, with oncologists failing to diagnose most cases.[51]

Many patients do not spontaneously bring up their distress with their oncologists.[48,52] In addition, patients may be reluctant to bring up their concerns because they believe the concerns are an inevitable part of their illness,[53] because they are embarrassed or uncomfortable, because they do not want to trouble or burden the health care professional, or because of a perceived lack of time.[52] Thus, it is essential that physicians and other health care professionals actively ask about and encourage their patients to disclose and discuss their concerns and distress.

Physicians vary in their ability to elicit their patients' psychosocial concerns.[38,54,55] Several studies have found that physicians often underidentify psychological problems in cancer patients.[48] Detmar et al,[56] for example, examined the content of the communication about QOL topics (daily activities, emotional functioning, pain, and fatigue) during outpatient visits of patients receiving palliative chemotherapy. In 20% to 45% of the visits in which patients were experiencing significant QOL problems, no time was spent discussing these problems. Specifically, emotional functioning and fatigue were unaddressed in 54% and 48% of the time, respectively.

Research suggests that physicians tend to underestimate the level of depression and severity of symptoms among cancer patients.[57,58] Psychological distress in palliative care patients tends to be underdiagnosed and undertreated.[59,60] Severe communication problems at the end of life were found among up to 40% of patients and communication problems between patients and health care professionals were associated with more spiritual problems, need for care planning, and poorer patient and family insight.[61] In another study, Sollner et al[62] examined oncology physicians' ability to identify distress in their patients. There was considerable variability between the oncologists in their ability to identify patients with significant distress. The physicians' sensitivity in recognizing moderate distress was relatively high, but their ability to detect severe distress in their patients was low. Oncologists may be uncomfortable dealing with patient emotions for a variety of reasons including lack of training, the belief that it will take too much

time, or being an emotional burden for themselves. Doctors may have difficulty responding to nonverbal cues of distress.[63]

Kennifer et al[64] examined how the type and severity of cancer patients' emotions influenced how oncologists responded through examination of 264 audio recordings between oncologists and patients with advanced cancer. In these encounters, patients were more likely to present fear than other emotions such as anger or sadness. The oncologists responded to 35% of these emotions with empathic statements and were more empathic when patients showed intense emotions. Importantly, they found that responding empathically only extended the length of consultations by an average of 21 seconds.

A recent study explored reasons why cancer patients were reluctant to disclose their emotional distress to their physicians and factors associated with these concerns among a sample of lung cancer patients in Japan.[65] Patients identified four categories of concerns about emotional disclosure to their physicians: (1) no perceived need for disclosure, (2) fear of negative impact of emotional disclosure, (3) negative attitude toward emotional disclosure, and (4) hesitation to disturb physicians with emotional disclosure. Hesitation to disturb physicians was the most prevalent reason for not disclosing distress to physicians (68% of sample). They found that men were more likely to hold this attitude than women. Older patients were more likely to report negative attitude than younger patients.

Zachariae et al[66] examined the association between oncology patients' perceived communication style with their physician and patients' satisfaction and distress. Higher scores of physician attentiveness and empathy were associated with lower levels of emotional distress following the consultation. This highlights the potential importance of the physician–patient relationship in reducing distress for cancer patients.

Other studies have found that physicians often miss opportunities to make empathic statements and responses. Pollak et al,[67] for example, found that in 398 recorded conversations between oncologists and patients with advanced disease, 37% contained at least one empathic opportunity. When the empathic opportunity occurred, physicians responded with continuers (a statement that offers empathy and allows patient to continue expressing emotion) 22% of the time. Younger oncologists and those who rated their orientation as more socioemotional than technical were more likely to respond with empathic statements. These results suggest that many opportunities to respond empathically and encourage patients to discuss their feelings and distress are missed.

One of the most frequently reported barriers to regular routine screening is lack of time. In a survey of members of the American Society of Clinical Oncology, lack of time was the most frequently cited barrier, with 76% of respondents endorsing it as an issue. Lack of time was also a significant predictor of screening, but it was not associated with using a screening instrument.[47] Interestingly, addressing patients' psychosocial needs may ultimately make oncology clinics run more efficiently. Patients with unresolved emotional needs are more likely to use community health services and to visit emergency facilities.[68] While it is true that distressed patients require more time and contact and can be frustrating for their providers, treating emotional distress can ultimately help patients and reduce the strain on their oncology team.[15]

■ CASE EXAMPLES

The following case examples demonstrate a few commonly reported barriers to addressing distress in cancer patients. These barriers are based on the common assumptions that distress in cancer is normal and that it would take too much time to address a patient's distress. Existing empirical data challenge some of the realities of these assumptions.

Case no. 1: Mrs Jones is a 50-year-old woman recently diagnosed with stage III colon cancer. She received surgery and is about to start chemotherapy. During her last visit with her oncologist, she asked questions regarding what side effects she might expect to experience with this new treatment. She appeared somewhat nervous, but was not tearful during the discussion. Her oncologist recognized this as a normal response for someone about to begin chemotherapy for the first time.

While distress may be relatively common and considered a "normal reaction" to cancer, it still requires attention. Studies of distress in cancer typically examine those meeting clinical levels of distress; however, there is benefit in identifying individuals with subthreshold distress levels. Mild-to-moderately distressed cancer patients may be at risk for developing diagnosable disorders given the stress associated with cancer and its treatment; thus, early intervention may be key. In this case example, early identification may have resulted in a referral for relaxation training, which may have assisted Mrs Smith in being able to manage the rigors of her chemotherapy regimen. Without early intervention, Mrs Smith's anxiety may have escalated to where she started having difficulties sleeping at night, thus exacerbating her fatigue during the day.

Case no. 2: If I bring up distress, it will take up too much time in my clinic. Mr Smith is a 48-year-old male recently diagnosed with non-small cell lung cancer. He is married and has two children. Mr Smith has never smoked and has led what most would consider a healthy lifestyle. The patient had difficulty holding back his tears during his consultation visit with the oncologist. The oncologist was running late in his clinic and did not want to acknowledge the distress for fear of getting even more behind.

While Mr Smith likely has a number of psychosocial issues to be discussed, the reality is that acknowledging these issues likely may have been very helpful for Mr Smith. A study published in the *Journal of Clinical Oncology* showed that just 40 seconds of compassion during a consultation can reduce patient anxiety. The oncologist could have expressed compassion and support for the patient's situation and then consulted a mental health professional to evaluate his psychological functioning. This same study demonstrated that compassion results in more positive ratings of physician characteristics.[69] Studies of physician interaction style show its role in patient satisfaction and long-term psychological adjustment.[70–74]

■ IMPROVING FOLLOW-UP TO SCREENING: SCREENING FEEDBACK AND TREATMENT RECOMMENDATIONS

The US Preventive Services Task Force[20,75–77] highlighted the critical need to link screening with adequate follow-up to screening in order to improve patient outcomes. For example, while feedback of screening results increases the recognition of depression by a factor of 2 to 3, feedback alone does not result in improvements in treatment rates for depression or in improvement of patients' depression itself. In comparison, feedback of screening results accompanied with treatment recommendations yielded consistently improved treatment rates for depression, and feedback integrated with systems of diagnostic follow-up and clinical intervention had the best chance of alleviating depression in medical patients.[21]

Studies in cancer also show that screening alone is insufficient for improving patient QOL[78] or psychosocial well-being.[79] Adequate follow-up includes tracking patterns of referral and treatment for patients, and direct intervention.[77,80,81]

KEY POINTS

■ National guidelines provide recommendations for making distress management an integral part of routine oncological care.

■ Patient distress often goes unrecognized by oncology providers.

■ Standardized assessment is important for screening and should be conducted with instruments that have good psychometric properties.

■ Screening alone is insufficient for reducing distress and improving psychosocial well-being.

■ In addition to screening, there must be feedback of screening results, diagnostic follow-up, and clinical intervention to improve patient QOL or psychosocial well-being.

REFERENCES

1. National Comprehensive Cancer Network. NCCN Clinical Practice Guidelines in Oncology™ *Distress Management V.1.2010*. 2010. http://www.nccn.org/professionals/physician-gls/PDF/distress.pdf. Accessed September 7, 2010.

2. Judd LL, Paulus MP, Wells KB, et al. Socioeconomic burden of subsyndromal depressive symptoms and major depression in a sample of the general population. *Am J Psychiatry*. 1996;153:1411–1417.

3. Maier W, Gansicke M, Weiffenbach O. The relationship between major and subthreshold variants of unipolar depression. *J Affect Disord*. 1997;45:41–51.

4. Zabora J, Brintzenhofeszoc K, Curbow B, et al. The prevalence of psychological distress by cancer site. *Psychooncology*. 2001;10:19–28.

5. Compas BE, Worsham NL, Epping-Jordan JE, et al. When mom or dad has cancer: markers of psychological distress in cancer patients, spouses, and children. *Health Psychol*. 1994;13:507–515.

6. Hagedoorn M, Sanderman R, Bolks HN, et al. Distress in couples coping with cancer: a meta-analysis and critical review of role and gender effects. *Psychol Bull*. 2008;134:1–30.

7. Ayres A, Hoon P, Franzoni J, et al. Influence of mood and adjustment to cancer on compliance with chemotherapy among breast cancer patients. *J Psychosom Res*. 1009;38:393–402.

8. Stoudemire A, Thompson T. Medication noncompliance: systematic approaches to evaluation and intervention. *Gen Hosp Psychiatry*. 1983;5:233–239.

9. Satin JR, Linden W, Phillips MJ. Depression as a predictor of disease progression and mortality in cancer patients. *Cancer*. 2009;115:5349–5361.

10. Kiecolt-Glaser JK, McGuire L, Robles T, et al. Psychoneuroimmunology: psychological influences on immune function and health. *J Consult Clin Psychol*. 2002;70:537–547.

11. Anderson B, Yang H, Farrar W, et al. Psychologic intervention improves survival for breast cancer patients. A randomized clinical trial. *Cancer*. 2008;113:3450–3458.

12. Holland J. Psychological care of patients: psychooncology's contribution. *J Clin Oncol*. 2003;21:253s–265s.

13. Jacobsen PB. Screening for psychological distress in cancer patients: challenges and opportunities. *J Clin Oncol*. 2007;25:4526–4527.

14. Institute of Medicine. *Cancer Care for the Whole Patient: Meeting Psychosocial Health Needs*. Washington, DC: The National Academies Press; 2008.

15. Holland JC, Bultz BD. The NCCN guideline for distress management: a case for making distress the sixth vital sign. *J Natl Compr Cancer Netw*. 2007;5:3–7.

16. Bultz BD, Carlson LE. Emotional distress: the sixth vital sign—future directions in cancer care. *Psychooncology*. 2006;15:93–95.

17. Thomas BC, Bultz BD. The future in psychosocial oncology: screening for emotional distress—the sixth vital sign. *Future Oncol*. 2008;4:779–784.

18. Carlson LE, Bultz BD. Cancer distress screening: needs, models, and methods. *J Psychosom Res*. 2003;55:403–409.

19. Mitchell AJ, Kaar S, Coggan C, et al. Acceptability of common screening methods used to detect distress and related mood disorders—preferences of cancer specialists and non-specialists. *Psychooncology*. 2008;17:226–236.

20. U.S. Preventive Services Task Force. Screening for depression: recommendations and rationale. *Ann Intern Med*. 2002;136:760–764.

21. Pignone M, Gaynes B, Rushton J, et al. Screening for depression in adults: a summary of the evidence for the U.S. Preventive Services Task Force. *Ann Intern Med.* 2002;136:765–776.

22. Jacobsen PB, Donovan KA, Trask PC, et al. Screening for psychologic distress in ambulatory cancer patients: a multicenter evaluation of the Distress Thermometer. *Cancer.* 2005;103:1494–1502.

23. Mitchell AJ. Accuracy of Distress Thermometer and other ultra-short methods of detecting cancer-related mood disorders: pooled results from 38 analyses. *J Clin Oncol.* 2007;25:1–12.

24. Williams J, Noel P, Cordes J, et al. Is this patient clinically depressed? *JAMA.* 2002;287:1160–1170.

25. Mahoney J, Drinka T, Abler R, et al. Screening for depression; single question versus GDS. *J Am Geriatr Soc.* 1994;42:1103–1109.

26. Chochinov H, Wilson K, Enns M, et al. "Are you depressed?" screening for depression in the terminally ill. *Am J Psychiatry.* 1997;154:674–676.

27. Mitchell AJ. Pooled results from 38 analyses of the accuracy of Distress Thermometer and other ultra-short methods of detecting cancer-related mood disorders. *J Clin Oncol.* 2007;25:4670–4681.

28. Payne D, Hoffman R, Theodoulou M, et al. Screening for anxiety and depression in women with breast cancer. Psychiatry and medical oncology gear up for managed care. *Psychosomatics.* 1999;40:64–69.

29. Coyne JC. Self-reported distress: analog or Ersatz depression? *Psychol Bull.* 1994;116:29–45.

30. Rost K, Duan N, Rubenstein L, et al. The Quality Improvement for Depression collaboration: general analytic strategies for a coordinated study of quality improvement in depression care. *Gen Hosp Psychiatry.* 2001;23:239–253.

31. Rost K, Nutting P, Smith J, et al. Improving depression outcomes in community primary care practice. *J Gen Intern Med.* 2001;16:143–149.

32. Fechner-Bates S, Coyne J, Schwenk T. The relationship of self-reported distress to depressive disorders and other psychopathology. *J Consult Clin Psychol.* 1994;62:550–559.

33. Gilbody S, House A, Sheldon T. Routinely administered questionnaires for depression and anxiety: a systematic review. *BMJ.* 2001;322:406–409.

34. Derogatis LR. *Brief Symptom 18: Administration, Scoring, and Procedures Manual.* Minneapolis, MN: NCS Pearson; 2001.

35. Zabora J, BrintzenhofeSzoc K, Jacobsen P, et al. A new psychosocial screening instrument for use with cancer patients. *Psychosomatics.* 2001;42:241–246.

36. Hall A, Hern R, Fallowfield L. Are we using appropriate self-report questionnaires for detecting anxiety and depression in women with early breast cancer? *Eur J Cancer.* 1999;35:79–85.

37. Dugan W, McDonald M, Passik S, et al. Use of the Zung self-rating depression scale in cancer patients: feasibility as a screening tool. *Psychooncology.* 1998;7:483–493.

38. Passik S, Dugan W, McDonald M, et al. Oncologists' recognition of depression in their patients with cancer. *J Clin Oncol.* 1998;16:1594–1600.

39. Visser M, Smets E. Fatigue, depression and quality of life in cancer patients: how are they related? *Support Care Cancer.* 1998;6:101–108.

40. Beck A, Steer R. *Beck Depression Inventory-II Manual.* 2nd ed. San Antonio, TX: The Psychological Corporation; 1993.

41. Hann D, Winter K, Jacobsen PJ. Measurement of depressive symptoms in cancer patients: evaluation of the Center for Epidemiological Studies Depression Scale (CES-D). *J Psychosom Res.* 1999;46:437–443.

42. Radloff LS. The CES-D scale: a self-report depression scale for research in the general population. *Appl Psychol Meas.* 1977;1:385–401.

43. Beck A. *Beck Depression Inventory.* Boston: Harcourt; 1996.

44. Beck A, Steer R. *BDI-Fast Screen for Medical Patients Manual.* San Antonio: Harcourt Assessment Company; 2000.

45. First M, Gibbon M, Spitzer R, et al. *User's Guide for the Structured Clinical Interview for DSM-IV Axis I Disorders—Research Version.* New York, NY: Biometrics Research; 1996.

46. Jacobsen PB, Ransom S. Implementation of NCCN distress management guidelines by member institutions. *J Natl Compr Cancer Netw.* 2007;5:99–103.

47. Pirl WF, Muriel A, Hwang V, et al. Screening for psychosocial distress: a national survey of oncologists. *J Support Oncol.* 2007;5:499–504.

48. Fallowfield L, Ratcliffe D, Jenkins V, et al. Psychiatric morbidity and its recognition by doctors in patients with cancer. *Br J Cancer.* 2001;84:1011–1015.

49. Newell S, Sanson-Fisher RW, Girgis A, et al. How well do medical oncologists' perceptions reflect their patients' reported physical and psychosocial prob-

lems? Data from a survey of five oncologists. *Cancer.* 1998;83:1640–1651.

50. Whooley M, Avins A, Miranda J, et al. Case-finding instruments for depression: two questions are as good as many. *J Gen Intern Med.* 1997;12:439–445.

51. Berard R, Boermeester F, Viljoen G. Depressive disorders in an out-patient oncology setting: prevalence, assessment, and management. *Psychooncology.* 1998;7:112–120.

52. Maguire P. Improving the detection of psychiatric problems in cancer patients. *Soc Sci Med.* 1985;20:819–823.

53. Arora NK. Interacting with cancer patients: the significance of physicians' communication behavior. *Soc Sci Med.* 2003;57:791–806.

54. Detmar SB, Aaronson NK, Wever LD, et al. How are you feeling? Who wants to know? Patients' and oncologists' preferences for discussing health-related quality-of-life issues. *J Clin Oncol.* 2000;18:3295–3301.

55. Gulbrandsen P, Hjortdahl P, Fugelli P. General practitioners' knowledge of their patients' psychosocial problems: multipractice questionnaire survey. *BMJ.* 1997;314:1014–1018.

56. Detmar SB, Muller MJ, Wever LD, et al. The patient–physician relationship. Patient–physician communication during outpatient palliative treatment visits: an observational study. *JAMA.* 2001;285:1351–1357.

57. Sanson-Fisher R, Girgis A, Boyes A, et al. The unmet supportive care needs of patients with cancer. Supportive Care Review Group. *Cancer.* 2000;88:226–237.

58. Sneeuw KC, Aaronson NK, Sprangers MA, et al. Evaluating the quality of life of cancer patients: assessments by patients, significant others, physicians and nurses. *Br J Cancer.* 1999;81:87–94.

59. Chochinov HM. Thinking outside the box: depression, hope, and meaning at the end of life. *J Palliat Med.* 2003;6:973–977.

60. Wilson K, Chochinov HM, de Faye B, et al. Diagnosis and management of depression in palliative care. In: Chochinov HM, Breitbart W, eds. *Handbook of Psychiatry in Palliative Medicine.* New York: Oxford University Press; 2000:25–49.

61. Higginson IJ, Costantini M. Communication in end-of-life cancer care: a comparison of team assessments in three European countries. *J Clin Oncol.* 2002;20:3674–3682.

62. Sollner W, DeVries A, Steixner E, et al. How successful are oncologists in identifying patient distress, perceived social support, and need for psychosocial counselling? *Br J Cancer.* 2001;84:179–185.

63. Butow PN, Brown RF, Cogar S, et al. Oncologists' reactions to cancer patients' verbal cues. *Psychooncology.* 2002;11:47–58.

64. Kennifer SL, Alexander SC, Pollak KI, et al. Negative emotions in cancer care: do oncologists' responses depend on severity and type of emotion? *Patient Educ Couns.* 200;76:51–56.

65. Okuyama T, Endo C, Seto T, et al. Cancer patients' reluctance to disclose their emotional distress to their physicians: a study of Japanese patients with lung cancer. *Psychooncology.* 2008;17:460–465.

66. Zachariae R, Pedersen CG, Jensen AB, et al. Association of perceived physician communication style with patient satisfaction, distress, cancer-related self-efficacy, and perceived control over the disease. *Br J Cancer.* 2003;88:658–665.

67. Pollak KI, Arnold RM, Jeffreys AS, et al. Oncologist communication about emotion during visits with patients with advanced cancer. *J Clin Oncol.* 2007;25:5748–5752.

68. Carlson LE, Bultz BD. Efficacy and medical cost offset of psychosocial interventions in cancer care: making the case for economic analyses. *Psychooncology.* 2004;13:837–849 [discussion 850–856].

69. Fogarty LA, Curbow BA, Wingard JR, et al. Can 40 seconds of compassion reduce patient anxiety? *J Clin Oncol.* 1999;17:371–379.

70. Bredart A, Bouleuc C, Dolbeault S. Doctor–patient communication and satisfaction with care in oncology. *Curr Opin Oncol.* 2005;17:351–354.

71. Brown JB, Boles M, Mullooly JP, et al. Effect of clinician communication skills training on patient satisfaction. A randomized, controlled trial. *Ann Intern Med.* 1999;131:822–829.

72. Chen JY, Tao ML, Tisnado D, et al. Impact of physician–patient discussions on patient satisfaction. *Med Care.* 2008;46:1157–1162.

73. Lienard A, Merckaert I, Libert Y, et al. Factors that influence cancer patients' anxiety following a medical consultation: impact of a communication skills training programme for physicians. *Ann Oncol.* 2006;17:1450–1458.

74. Roberts CS, Cox CE, Reintgen DS, et al. Influence of physician communication on newly diagnosed breast patients' psychologic adjustment and decision-making. *Cancer.* 1994;74:336–341.

75. Coyne J, Schwenk T, Fechner-Bates S. Nondetection of depression by primary care physicians reconsidered. *Psychiatry Prim Care.* 1995;17:3–12.

76. Coyne J. Depression in primary care: depressing news, exciting research opportunities. *Am Psychol Soc News Res*. 2001;14:1–4

77. Panel DG. *Depression in Primary Care*. Rockville, MD: Department of Health and Human Services; 1993.

78. Rosenbloom SK, Victorson DE, Hahn EA, et al. Assessment is not enough: a randomized controlled trial of the effects of HRQL assessment on quality of life and satisfaction in oncology clinical practice. *Psychooncology*. 2007;16:1069–1079.

79. Boyes A, Newell S, Girgis A, et al. Does routine assessment and real-time feedback improve cancer patients' psychosocial well-being? *Eur J Cancer Care (Engl)*. 2006;15:163–171.

80. Wells K, Sherbourne C, Schoenbaum M, et al. Impact of disseminating quality improvement programs for depression in managed care: a randomized controlled trial. *JAMA*. 2000;283:212–220.

81. Sherbourne C, Wells K, Duan N, et al. Long-term effectiveness of disseminating quality improvement for depression in primary care. *Arch Gen Psychiatry*. 2001;58:696–703.

Assessment and Management of Psychological Symptoms

Mood Disorders

• *Alan D. Valentine*

◼ INTRODUCTION

Depression in the general population is a major public health problem, its most severe form (major depression [MDD]) affecting almost 7% of American adults.[1] Depressive spectrum disorders are sufficiently common in oncology that clinicians of all specialties working in the field can expect to encounter patients with presentation of these states on a daily basis. Because of the negative emotional valence associated with cancer, depression may be overlooked or ignored as a "normal" consequence of the cancer experience, not requiring or unlikely to respond to treatment (therapeutic nihilism).[2] Depressive disorders adversely affect quality of life and appear to increase medical morbidity and symptom burden in cancer patients.[3–5] Depression predicts desire for hastened death in terminally ill patients, as does hopelessness.[6] There is increasing evidence that depression predicts early mortality from malignancy, although some studies have not found this to be the case.[7–12] Familiarity with differential diagnosis and treatment options for depressive disorders is an essential component of comprehensive care and can do much to palliate emotional distress of patients and caregivers. Diagnosis and treatment of mood disorders can be time intensive and thus potentially problematic for clinicians with busy practices or with understandable preoccupation with therapeutic decisions or focus on more acute symptoms (ie, pain, dyspnea). However, to the extent that depressive states interfere with or complicate treatment, identification and treatment of symptoms could also make care more efficient and, possibly, less stressful for clinicians.

Diagnosis of depression in oncology can be difficult. The term "depression" is nonspecific, with meanings ranging from a nonpathological emotional state common to everyday experience to so-called "reactive depressions" (adjustment disorders [AD]), to a formally defined neuropsychiatric disorder with possible organic and/or "functional" etiologies (major depressive disorder). Here we focus on the most significant depressive spectrum disorders: AD and MDD, the former being the most common presentations that clinicians will encounter.[13] Patients so affected will experience troubling persistent dysphoria or anhedonia (most likely to bring them to attention and most obviously associated with the term "depression") and may also experience thoughts of suicide and physical symptoms of consequence, including change in sleep patterns, appetite, fatigue, and cognitive function. Some symptoms of MDD are similar to those caused by malignant disease itself or its treatment. Currently there is much interest and increasing evidence to suggest that symptom clusters (ie, fatigue, anorexia, cognitive impairment, pain) common to oncology can have common biological (ie, inflammatory, neuroendocrine) etiologies.[14–16]

Patients with mood disorders may also present with mania. Present in the general population at rates of about 2.5%, patients with symptoms of mania present with elevated, expansive, or irritable mood, speech that is rapid to the point of being pressured, racing thoughts, grandiosity, decreased need for sleep, variable psychomotor agitation, and impulsivity or poor judgment resulting in risk-taking behaviors.[1,11] In settings of full-blown mania patients can be delusional. Uncontrolled primary or secondary mania can seriously compromise cancer treatment.

PREVALENCE

Clinically significant emotional distress, or criteria-defined psychiatric disorder, may be observed or detected in approximately 33% to 50% of cancer patients.[17,18] In the setting of advanced disease about 50% of patients are so affected.[19] Prevalence rates for depressive disorders in oncology vary greatly. There are several reasons for this including differences in conceptualization of depression as a disorder, assessment methodology, disease sites, and stage of disease. Massie's[20] review of almost 100 studies over the past 50 years found prevalence rates of depressive spectrum disorders from 0% to 58%, and of MDD from 0% to 38%. Taken together, studies suggest that cancer patients are affected by MDD at rates two to three times that of the general population and generally at rates equal to or higher than those encountered in other medical diseases.[20–22] The medical acuity and symptom severity of inpatients is usually greater than that of outpatients. In the setting of advanced and end-stage disease, rates of these disorders may be 35% or greater.[14]

There is some variation in rates of depression by disease site. As a generalization, tumor types with relatively poorer prognoses appear to have higher rates of significant distress.[17] The same may be true of depressive spectrum disorders. Rates of depression in pancreatic cancer range from 20% to 50%.[23–25] Similar rates have been detected in recent studies of patients with lung cancer.[26,27] Rates of depression in patients with primary brain tumors, a particularly difficult group to study, vary from 18% to 28% in ambulatory settings using defined criteria, with self-report of depressive symptoms approaching 90% soon after surgery.[28–30] High rates of depression have been associated with head and neck cancers and breast cancers, although some studies using defined diagnostic criteria or established rating instruments have found lower rates.[20,31–34]

DIAGNOSIS

Depending on setting, context, and medical status, depressed mood or affect in a cancer patient may result from one or more of several diagnostic possibilities. In most clinical settings, however, the primary considerations will be AD and MDD.

■ TABLE 5-1. Diagnostic Criteria for Adjustment Disorders

DSM-IV-TR

A. The development of emotional or behavioral symptoms in response to an identifiable stressor(s) occurring within 3 months of the onset of the stressor(s)
B. These symptoms or behaviors are clinically significant as evidenced by either of the following:
   (1) Marked distress that is in excess of what would be expected from exposure to the stressor
   (2) Significant impairment in social or occupational (academic) functioning
C. The stress-related disturbance does not meet the criteria for another specific Axis I disorder and is not merely an exacerbation of a preexisting Axis I or Axis II disorder
D. The symptoms do not represent bereavement
E. Once the stressor (or its consequences) has terminated, the symptoms do not persist for more than an additional 6 months
   Specify if:
   Acute: if the disturbance lasts less than 6 months
   Chronic: if the disturbance lasts for 6 months or longer
Adjustment disorders are coded based on the subtype, which is selected according to the predominant symptoms. The specific stressor(s) can be specified on Axis IV
With depressed mood
With anxiety
With mixed anxiety and depressed mood
With disturbance of conduct
With mixed disturbance of emotions and conduct
Unspecified

Reprinted with permission from the *Diagnostic and Statistical Manual of Mental Disorders, Text Revision*. 4th ed. American Psychiatric Association (copyright 2000).

AD are the most common psychiatric disorders in cancer patients.[18] The diagnosis as defined by the *Diagnostic and Statistical Manual of Mental Disorders—Fourth Edition, Text Revision* (DSM-IV-TR) of the American Psychiatric Association requires development of emotional distress (depression or anxiety, or both) in response to a stressor that is in excess of what would be expected or that causes significant functional impairment[10] (Table 5-1).

■ **TABLE 5-2. Criteria for Major Depressive Episode**

A. Five (or more) of the following symptoms have been present during the same 2-week period and represent a change from previous functioning; at least one of the symptoms is either (1) depressed mood or (2) loss of interest or pleasure

   Note: Do not include symptoms that are clearly due to a general medical condition, or mood-incongruent delusions or hallucinations

   (1) Depressed mood most of the day, nearly every day, as indicated by either subjective report (eg, feels sad or empty) or observation made by others (eg, appears tearful). *Note*: In children and adolescents, can be irritable mood

   (2) Markedly diminished interest or pleasure in all, or almost all, activities most of the day, nearly every day (as indicated by either subjective account or observation made by others)

   (3) Significant weight loss when not dieting or weight gain (eg, a change of more than 5% of body weight in a month), or decrease or increase in appetite nearly every day. *Note*: In children, consider failure to make expected weight gains

   (4) Insomnia or hypersomnia nearly every day

   (5) Psychomotor agitation or retardation nearly every day (observable by others, not merely subjective feelings of restlessness or being slowed down)

   (6) Fatigue or loss of energy nearly every day

   (7) Feelings of worthlessness or excessive or inappropriate guilt (which may be delusional) nearly every day (not merely self-reproach or guilt about being sick)

   (8) Diminished ability to think or concentrate, or indecisiveness, nearly every day (either by subjective account or as observed by others)

   (9) Recurrent thoughts of death (not just fear of dying), recurrent suicidal ideation without a specific plan, or a suicide attempt or a specific plan for committing suicide

B. The symptoms do not meet criteria for a mixed episode

C. The symptoms cause clinically significant distress or impairment in social, occupational, or other important areas of functioning

D. The symptoms are not due to the direct physiological effects of a substance (eg, a drug of abuse, a medication) or a general medical condition (eg, hypothyroidism)

E. The symptoms are not better accounted for by bereavement, that is, after the loss of a loved one, the symptoms persist for longer than 2 months or are characterized by marked functional impairment, morbid preoccupation with worthlessness, suicidal ideation, psychotic symptoms, or psychomotor retardation

Reprinted with permission from the *Diagnostic and Statistical Manual of Mental Disorders, Text Revision*. 4th edition. American Psychiatric Association (copyright 2000).

Both of these criteria, especially the former, are problematic as they require a subjective judgment. As a practical point it is easier to determine, from history or observation, whether symptoms interfere with ability to cope, than it is to assess what is excessive. Inquiry into the specific nature of symptoms and their precipitants is necessary.[14] No somatic or vegetative symptoms are required for diagnosis of AD, although one or more may be present. In some instances patients with such presentations may fall into the DSM-IV-TR diagnostic category of "Depression Not Otherwise Specified."[10] It is important to realize that patients with AD (sometimes referred to as "minor depression" or "reactive depression") can be in as much or more emotional distress as patients with MDD.

The accurate diagnosis of MDD in cancer patients has long been considered a significant challenge.[35] The diagnosis of MDD requires the presence of at least five symptoms that must include persistent dysphoria or anhedonia, or both, in addition to at least three to four additional symptoms[10] (Table 5-2). A particular problem is consideration of the somatic symptoms of MDD, which can be a function of the mood disorder, the malignancy, disease consequences (ie, pain), treatment side effects, or any combination of these variables. The somatic symptoms of

MDD have been considered so unreliable in the setting of cancer that numerous investigators have developed and employed substitution criteria to aid diagnosis and/or to assess severity (major vs. minor depression).[36–38] Others assert that the somatic symptoms may be reliable in the setting of cancer and should be considered.[14,39]

Diagnosis of mood disorders is accomplished by clinical interview including history and mental status examination. There are no laboratory assays or radiological imaging studies that will serve the purpose. However, review of possible contributing medical causes, including drugs and metabolic dyscrasias, should be conducted.

Clinicians often miss a diagnosis of depression, and in busy practices there may be impediments to the detailed clinical interviews that may be required. Consequently, rating scales are often used to screen for emotional distress and depression in particular. A considerable number of patient- or rater-completed instruments have been used to screen for depression in the setting of cancer. The Hospital Anxiety and Depression Scale (HADS) is possibly the instrument most often employed in clinical and research settings.[40] Currently the Patient Health Questionnaire (PHQ-9) and its companion two question screen (PHQ-2) are also widely used.[41,42] Others include the Montgomery–Asberg Depression Rating Scale (MADRS) and the Center for Epidemiological Studies Depression Scale (CES-D).[43,44]

Rating scales by themselves are probably not adequate to make a diagnosis of depression. Ideally patients with scale scores suggestive of the presence of a mood disorder would go on to clinical examination. Especially in the setting of advanced cancer and palliative care, the use of detailed screening instruments and clinical interviews may be too burdensome to be practical and it may be possible to use one- or two-question screens to assess for mood disorders.[45,46]

The differential diagnosis of patient presenting with possible depression will include AD and MDD as noted, but also mood disorders that meet some of the DSM-IV-TR criteria for MDD (depression NOS, or "minor depression"). In some instances the classification of "Depression Due to a Medical Condition" is appropriate. To the extent that depressive mood and behaviors are emotional responses "caused" by cancer or a function of biological pathology (ie, neuroendocrine or neurotransmitter dysregulation, inflammation), the term might be universally applicable. However, it is usually used in more limited settings. In oncology, pancreatic cancer and other gastrointestinal malignancies, and possibly some central nervous system cancers, are thought to present with depression in some instances.[23] Drugs that are widely recognized to have depressive side effects include corticosteroids and interferon-alpha (IFN-α).

In the setting of advanced cancer, the construct of demoralization has received clinical and research attention; these patients often present with hopelessness that appears to be a risk factor for wish for death and suicide distinct from patients with depression.[47,48] Suffering and grief reactions may also be considered.

Especially in critical care and advanced disease settings, hypoactive delirium should be considered. Such patients on close examination will have an altered level of arousal and cognitive impairment not typical of even severely depressed patients.

Disease- and Treatment-related Considerations

As noted, primary malignancies, especially pancreatic cancer, are thought to present with depression. Primary and metastatic brain tumors (and the effects of their treatment) can present with cognitive dysfunction, apathy, and psychomotor slowing suggestive of depression.[49,50]

Although central nervous system dysfunction has been associated with many cancer therapies, the list of those associated with depression is of modest length and, with exceptions, they do not routinely cause significant problems. These include vincristine and vinblastine, L-asparaginase, procarbazine, and leuprolide.[51–53] Depressive syndromes have been reported with tamoxifen, although studies indicate that the association is weak.[54]

Depressive syndromes associated with IFN-α (which may also cause mania) and interleukin-2 (IL-2) are of much greater concern.[55,56] Patients who are depressed at initiation of IFN-α therapy or during treatment should be monitored closely.[57,58] Treatment with antidepressants and/or discontinuation of IFN-α or IL-2 should be considered.

Corticosteroids, especially when employed over time (ie, management of graft vs. host disease), may cause depressive syndromes and are a common cause of mania and psychosis when present acutely or at high doses.[59,60] Central nervous system depressants, including opioid analgesics, benzodiazepines, barbiturates, and some anticonvulsants, may cause depressive syndromes in patients with idiosyncratic vulnerability, prior depression, or cognitive impairment.

Unrelieved pain is associated with increased risk of psychiatric disorders, including AD and depression in the setting of cancer, although causal relationships have not been definitely established.[14,61] The burden of other physical symptoms (ie, fatigue, cognitive impairment) may similarly predispose to mood disorders and has obvious implications for management.

Metabolic disturbances (ie, hyponatremia) and abnormalities of parathyroid and especially thyroid function are associated with depressive syndromes. Abnormalities of hepatic and renal function predispose to delirium and cognitive dysfunction that at initial assessment may mimic depression. Nutritional deficiencies (B_{12}, folate) may do the same.

Suicide

The issue of suicide, its assessment, and management (more thoroughly developed in Chapter 1) is critical to consideration of the depressed cancer patient. Suicide is associated with depression and medical illness in the general population. Cancer patients appear to experience persistent suicidal ideations or desire to die more often than patients in the community and complete suicide at rates twice that of the general population.[62,63] It is thought that many suicides in cancer patients go unreported or are attributed to other causes, and the actual rate may be higher than that found in recent studies. In addition to known risk factors for suicide (age, male gender, lack of social support), severity of depression, pain, advanced disease, and feelings of hopelessness increase risk of suicide in cancer patients.[6,48,64]

Evaluation

Patients should be assessed for mood disorders based on clinical suspicion or complaint of symptoms by patients or family members. Screening for psychosocial distress, as recommended in the guidelines of National Comprehensive Cancer Network (NCCN), takes place at diagnosis and significant disease trajectory intervals and if positive for emotional distress would then lead to specific evaluation for mood disorder.[65]

The evaluation can include use of a screening instrument (see above) and focused evaluations including history and clinical interview. Screening instruments themselves are probably not adequate to make a diagnosis of MDD. Patients with possible mood disorders must be assessed for suicide risk, including assessment of intent (passive ideations vs. active intent) and possession of a plan and its lethality. The safety of an at-risk patient must be assured, which may require admission to a primary psychiatric facility (if the patient is medically stable and meets admission criteria) or close observation in an oncology or palliative care inpatient unit.

Consistent with NCCN guidelines for assessment of mood disorders, review of contributing or comorbid symptoms (ie, pain, nausea), possible offending antineoplastic and supportive care drugs, and metabolic and endocrine (especially thyroid) status should be assessed with correction of abnormalities detected and removal or modification of pharmacological contributors if possible.[60]

■ TREATMENT

In general psychiatry, the treatment of mood disorders involves psychotherapy, pharmacotherapy, or both. Lack of randomized controlled trials is such that evidence-based support for these interventions in oncology is modest, especially for severe mood disorders. However, small studies do indicate that both forms of treatment do have some efficacy, and they are routinely employed.[16,66–68]

Psychotherapy

Supportive psychotherapy is intended to reinforce patients' coping skills, or help patients develop new ones. This is a mainstay of the treatment of AD and has a role in the management of more severe or pervasive mood disorders. It can involve elements of evidence-supported interventions including psychoeducation, supportive-expressive therapy, cognitive–behavioral therapy (CBT), and group support. The intended result is decreased isolation, increased mastery of threat, and increased ability to problem solving. While supportive psychotherapy, like any other form of psychotherapy, should be considered a formal behavioral intervention, it is likely the most common therapy used in general oncology settings, and some forms can be employed by clinicians without advanced training in the clinical behavioral sciences. *CBT* in this setting involves identification of inaccurate perceptions of variables including self, disease state, treatment outcome, and correction or modification of resultant behaviors. It may involve training in distraction or reframing techniques. CBT has application in management of AD and MDD and usually will require referral to a qualified psychotherapist. *Group psychotherapy* is routinely employed in supportive therapy for patients and caregivers. It has possible application in treatment of formal mood disorders but also requires formal training.

Pharmacotherapy

Results of limited clinical trials, consensus clinical guidelines, and general practice trends all support the use of antidepressants to treat depressive disorders in cancer (see Table 5-3). Evidence to support use of antidepressants for AD in cancer is extremely limited but as a practical point this is likely often done, especially by nonpsychiatrists, as is use of the same medications for palliation of affective distress in subsyndrome depressive states.[69,70] There is no "gold standard" antidepressant in the setting of cancer. Choice of antidepressant is usually a function of a drug's side effect and tolerance, cost, and, increasingly, drug–drug interactions.

Some generalizations are applicable to the various classes of antidepressants:

1. The drugs are usually well tolerated. In ambulatory settings and over time, weight gain, sexual dysfunction, and nausea can be problematic, but this is variable.
2. The drugs for the most part do not work quickly, taking anywhere from 1 to 4 weeks to achieve some effect. Dose escalation may be necessary. However, caution is required in seriously ill and elderly patients, who generally should be started at low doses with careful escalation if tolerated.
3. There are no effective parenteral formulations available for routine clinical use.
4. It is prudent to follow recommendations for antidepressant therapy in the general population: 4 to 6 months of treatment efficacy before consideration of discontinuation.[71] Patients should not come off these drugs too early. They also need not be maintained on antidepressants indefinitely. Regular follow-up to monitor response is required.

Selective Serotonin Reuptake Inhibitors (SSRIs)

These drugs are mainstays of antidepressant therapy in primary care and general psychiatry settings and quite possibly in oncology as well. Many of the drugs in this class have indications for management of anxiety disorders and several have been used off-label for management of disease- or treatment-related hot flashes.

SSRIs have been associated with hyponatremia/SIADH, bleeding syndromes thought due to decreased platelet aggregation, and possibly thrombocytopenia. Used alone, but especially in combination with other antidepressants, antipsychotics, and monoamine oxidase inhibitors (eg, linezolid, procarbazine), and, possibly, in the setting of hormone-secreting tumors (pheochromocytomas), these drugs can induce serotonin toxicity (serotonin syndrome) characterized by headache, autonomic instability, tremor or frank myoclonus, and altered mental status.

SSRIs are variable inhibitors of the 2D6 isoenzyme of the hepatic cytochrome P450 metabolic pathway. There is increasing evidence that potent 2D6 inhibitors (including paroxetine and fluoxetine) have serious adverse effects on the antineoplastic efficacy of tamoxifen, which is thought to be 2D6-mediated.[72,73] The adverse effects in this setting of SSRIs that are moderate (sertraline) or weak 2D6 inhibitors (citalopram, escitalopram) are less clear.

Serotonin–Norepinephrine Reuptake Inhibitors (SNRIs)

SNRIs include venlafaxine, desvenlafaxine, and duloxetine. Venlafaxine is among several drugs (including SSRIs) used to treat hot flashes. In addition to its indication for depression, duloxetine is approved for management of diabetic neuropathic pain. This has led to fairly common use against chemotherapy-induced neuropathy, and it may be an attractive consideration in the treatment of depressed patients with persistent pain.

The side-effect profile of the SNRIs is quite similar to that of the SSRIs. Toxicity can include serotonin syndrome, and abrupt discontinuation can lead to unpleasant withdrawal symptoms that actually are similar to mild–moderate serotonin toxicity.

At time of this writing, venlafaxine's modest 2D6 inhibition is such that it is one of the few antidepressants (with citalopram and escitalopram) thought to be reliably safe to use with tamoxifen. The same assumption may be applicable to desvenlafaxine.

"Atypical" Antidepressants

The side-effect profiles of these drugs make them attractive considerations in certain settings.

Bupropion is thought to be a dopamine/norepinephrine reuptake inhibitor. It is an "activating" antidepressant that may be useful in the setting of fatigue or mild cognitive slowing. Compared with other antidepressants, its use is associated with minimal risk of sexual dysfunction and it is weight neutral. Bupropion's separate indication for adjunctive treatment of nicotine dependence has potential advantages in management of depressed

■ TABLE 5-3. Selected Antidepressants Used in Cancer Patients

Drug	Starting Dose	Maintenance Dose	Comments
Selective serotonin reuptake inhibitors			
• Citalopram	10 mg/day	20–40 mg/day	Possible nausea, weight gain, sexual dysfunction
• Escitalopram	5–10 mg/day	10–20 mg/day	Possible nausea, weight gain, sexual dysfunction
• Fluoxetine	10–20 mg/day	20–60 mg/day	Long half-life; possible nausea, sexual dysfunction; variable effects on weight; strong 2D6 inhibition
• Paroxetine	20 mg/day	20–60 mg/day	Possible nausea, sedation, weight gain; sexual dysfunction; strong 2D6 inhibition
• Sertraline	25–50 mg/day	50–150 mg/day	Possible nausea, weight gain
Serotonin–norepinephrine reuptake inhibitors			
• Venlafaxine	37.5 mg/day	75–225 mg/day	Possible nausea; may be useful for hot flashes, neuropathic pain; should be tapered to discontinuation
• Desvenlafaxine	50 mg/day	50 mg/day	Possible nausea
• Duloxetine	30 mg/day	30–60 mg/day	Possible nausea, sedation; possible adjunct for neuropathic pain
Tricyclic antidepressants			
• Amitriptyline	25–50 mg qhs	50–200 mg/day	Significant sedation; anticholinergic effects; adjunct for neuropathic pain
• Nortriptyline	25–50 mg qhs	50–200 mg/day	Moderate sedation; adjunct for neuropathic pain
Atypical antidepressants			
• Bupropion	75 mg/day	150–450 mg/day	Activating; usually no sexual dysfunction; risk of seizures in predisposed patients; adjunct for smoking cessation
• Mirtazapine	15 mg qhs	15–45 mg qhs	Sedating, variable appetite stimulant, antiemetic effects; available as sol-tab
Psychostimulants			
Methylphenidate	2.5 mg q AM, noon 2.5 mg q AM, noon	10–60 mg/day	Activating rapid effect possible; possible insomnia, anxiety, variable blood pressure
Dextroamphetamine		10–60 mg/day	Activating rapid effect possible; possible insomnia, anxiety, variable blood pressure

smokers. The drug is associated with risk of seizures in at-risk patients including those with prior histories of seizures and brain tumors, and in the setting of alcohol withdrawal or at doses >450 mg per day. The drug is thought to be a moderate CYP2D6 inhibitor.

Mirtazapine is a noradrenergic/specific serotonin/H1 histamine receptor antagonist. This leads to side effects including appetite stimulation/weight gain and drowsiness. These effects are common causes for discontinuation in the general population but can be helpful in symptom control of selected cancer patients. Mirtazapine also appears to have mild anxiolytic and antiemetic effects. The drug is available in a rapidly dissolving sol-tab formulation. Mirtazapine is a weak CYP1A2 and CYP3A4 inhibitor. It has been associated with neutropenia.

Trazodone is a specific serotonin reuptake inhibitor/receptor antagonist with potent antihistaminic and alpha-adrenergic receptor blockade effects. At high doses (450–600 mg per day) it has efficacy as an antidepressant in the general population, but its side effects (sedation, orthostasis, priapism) make its use for this purpose problematic in cancer patients. Trazodone is more often used as a hypnotic at doses of 50 to 150 mg.

Tricyclic Antidepressants

First-line antidepressants before introduction of SSRIs, tricyclic antidepressants (TCAs), are norepinephrine/serotonin reuptake inhibitors with variable alpha-adrenergic blockade effects. While effective antidepressants, their side effects (orthostasis, weight gain, sexual dysfunction, constipation) make them somewhat difficult to use at therapeutic doses in cancer patients. They are associated with cardiac conduction delays and are potentially lethal in overdose. In oncology, TCAs are more often used at low doses as adjunctive therapies against neuropathic pain.

Psychostimulants

Although not formally approved for the purpose, psychostimulants including methylphenidate and D-amphetamine are often used effectively to treat depressed cancer patients, especially in the setting of advanced disease, comorbid fatigue, or "failure to thrive" syndromes.[16,74–77] The drugs, which are direct and indirect dopamine agonists, tend to work fairly quickly. Monitored appropriately, they can be used to "jump start" a coadministered standard antidepressant. In contrast to side effects when used in other settings, appetite often improves. Psychostimulants should be administered cautiously in patients with unstable blood pressures or cardiac dysrhythmias. Insomnia and anxiety are common side effects, but can be minimized by use of short-acting formulations (taken in the morning and early afternoon) and gradual dose escalation to effect.

Antimania Drugs

These include lithium, some anticonvulsants/mood stabilizers, and the atypical antipsychotics. Lithium is quite effective in treatment of bipolar disorder, but there are often compliance issues and the drug's many side effects (including alterations of thyroid, renal, and cardiac function, and alteration of hematological indices) make it difficult to use in oncology.[78] Consequently, patients on or considered for lithium therapy probably should be followed by psychiatrists.

Anticonvulsants/mood stabilizers can be used to treat primary mania or steroid-induced mania and may have application to treatment of neuropathic pain. They include valproic acid, lamotrigine, and carbamazepine. They are associated with significant drug–drug interactions, sedation, and rare hematological reactions including agranulocytosis.[79]

The atypical antipsychotics including olanzapine, risperidone, ziprasidone, and quetiapine are probably easier to use in primary oncology settings. They are associated with variable sedation, weight gain, cardiac conduction delays, and metabolic syndrome, requiring careful monitoring during treatment.

■ SUMMARY

Depressive disorders are common (mania less so), but should not be considered normal, in the setting of cancer. General consensus and a growing evidence-based literature support aggressive assessment and multimodal management of depressive symptoms in cancer patients. Oncologists and other clinicians who are not mental health specialists can make significant contributions to this basic component of supportive oncology and comprehensive cancer care.

KEY POINTS

- Depressive mood disorders, especially AD and MDD, are "common," but should not be considered "normal" in the setting of cancer. Primary and secondary mania will also be encountered.

- Diagnosis of depressive disorders in oncology can be difficult because symptoms may also be a function of disease or treatment side effects. Validated rating scales are useful for screening purposes.

- Evaluation of pain control and suicide risk is critical in assessment of depressed patients.

- A few primary antineoplastic agents and several supportive care drugs can cause secondary depressive syndromes. Drug side effects, metabolic disturbances, and central nervous system dysfunction (ie, hypoactive delirium) can cause or mimic depression.

- Treatment of mood disorders in cancer patients includes psychotherapy, antidepressant therapy, or both. There is no "gold standard" antidepressant for use in oncology.

REFERENCES

1. Kessler RC, Chiu WT, Demler O, et al. Prevalence, severity, and comorbidity of 12-month DSM-IV disorders in the National Comorbidity Survey Replication. *Arch Gen Psychiatry*. 2005;62:617–627.

2. Chochinov HM. Depression in cancer patients. *Lancet Oncol*. 2001;2:499–505.

3. Weitzner MA, Meyers CA, Stuebing KK, Saleeba AK. Relationship between quality of life and mood in long-term survivors of breast cancer treated with mastectomy. *Support Care Cancer*. 1997;5:241–248.

4. van den Beuken-van Everdingen MH, de Rijke JM, Kessels AG, et al. Quality of life and non-pain symptoms in patients with cancer. *J Pain Symptom Manage*. 2009;38:216–233.

5. Delgado-Guay M, Parsons HA, Li Z, et al. Symptom distress in advanced cancer patients with anxiety and depression in the palliative care setting. *Support Care Cancer*. 2009;17:573–579.

6. Breitbart W, Rosenfeld B, Pessin H, et al. Depression, hopelessness, and desire for hastened death in terminally ill patients with cancer. *JAMA*. 2000;284: 2907–2911.

7. Hjerl K, Andersen EW, Keiding N, et al. Depression as a prognostic factor for breast cancer mortality. *Psychosomatics*. 2003;44:24–30.

8. Prieto JM, Atala J, Blanch J, et al. Role of depression as a predictor of mortality among cancer patients after stem-cell transplantation. *J Clin Oncol*. 2005;23:6063–6071.

9. Satin JR, Linden W, Phillips MJ. Depression as a predictor of disease progression and mortality in cancer patients: a meta-analysis. *Cancer*. 2009;115:5349–5361.

10. Nakaya N, Saito-Nakaya K, Akizuki N, et al. Depression and survival in patients with non-small cell lung cancer after curative resection: a preliminary study. *Cancer Sci*. 2006;97:199–205.

11. Nakaya N, Saito-Nakaya K, Akechi T, et al. Negative psychological aspects and survival in lung cancer patients. *Psychooncology*. 2008;17:466–473.

12. Zonderman AB, Costa PT Jr, McCrae RR, Costa PTJ. Depression as a risk for cancer morbidity and mortality in a nationally representative sample. *JAMA*. 1989;262: 1191–1195.

13. American Psychiatric Association. *Diagnostic and Statistical Manual of Mental Disorders, Text Revision*. Washington, DC: American Psychiatric Association; 2000.

14. Cleeland CS, Bennett GJ, Dantzer R, et al. Are the symptoms of cancer and cancer treatment due to a shared biologic mechanism? A cytokine-immunologic model of cancer symptoms. *Cancer*. 2003;97:2919–2925.

15. Miller AH, Ancoli-Israel S, Bower JE, et al. Neuroendocrine-immune mechanisms of behavioral comorbidities in patients with cancer. *J Clin Oncol*. 2008;26:971–982.

16. Seruga B, Zhang H, Bernstein LJ, et al. Cytokines and their relationship to the symptoms and outcome of cancer. *Nat Rev Cancer*. 2008;8:887–899.

17. Zabora J, BrintzenhofeSzoc K, Curbow B, Hooker C, Piantadosi S. The prevalence of psychological distress by cancer site. *Psychooncology*. 2001;10:19–28.

18. Derogatis LR, Morrow GR, Fetting J. The prevalence of psychiatric disorders among cancer patients. *JAMA*. 1983;249:751–757.

19. Miovic M, Block S. Psychiatric disorders in advanced cancer. *Cancer*. 2007;110:1665–1676.

20. Massie MJ. Prevalence of depression in patients with cancer. *J Natl Cancer Inst Monogr*. 2004;32:57–71.

21. Pirl WF. Evidence report on the occurrence, assessment, and treatment of depression in cancer patients. *J Natl Cancer Inst Monogr*. 2004;32:32–39.

22. Hotopf M, Chidgey J, Addington-Hall J, Ly KL. Depression in advanced disease: a systematic review Part 1. Prevalence and case finding. *Palliat Med*. 2002;16: 81–97.

23. Joffe RT, Rubinow DR, Denicoff KD, Maher M, Sindelar WF. Depression and carcinoma of the pancreas. *Gen Hosp Psychiatry*. 1986;8:241–245.

24. Jacobsson L, Ottosson JO. Initial mental disorders in carcinoma of pancreas and stomach. *Acta Psychiatr Scand Suppl*. 1971;221:120–127.

25. Fras I, Litin EM. Comparison of psychiatric manifestations in carcinoma of the pancreas, retroperitoneal malignant lymphoma, and lymphoma in other locations. *Psychosomatics*. 1967;8:275–277.

26. Neron S, Correa JA, Dajczman E, Kasymjanova G, Kreisman H, Small D. Screening for depressive symptoms in patients with unresectable lung cancer. *Support Care Cancer*. 2007;15:1207–1212.

27. Pirl WF, Temel JS, Billings A, et al. Depression after diagnosis of advanced non-small cell lung cancer and survival: a pilot study. *Psychosomatics*. 2008;49:218–224.

28. Pringle AM, Taylor R, Whittle IR. Anxiety and depression in patients with an intracranial neoplasm before and after tumour surgery. *Br J Neurosurg*. 1999;13:46–51.

29. Wellisch DK, Kaleita TA, Freeman D, Cloughesy T, Goldman J. Predicting major depression in brain tumor patients. *Psychooncology*. 2002;11:230–238.

30. Litofsky NS, Farace E, Anderson F Jr, et al. Depression in patients with high-grade glioma: results of the Glioma Outcomes Project. *Neurosurgery.* 2004;54: 358–366 [discussion 66–67].

31. Archer J, Hutchison I, Korszun A. Mood and malignancy: head and neck cancer and depression. *J Oral Pathol Med.* 2008;37:255–270.

32. Fulton C. The prevalence and detection of psychiatric morbidity in patients with metastatic breast cancer. *Eur J Cancer Care.* 1998;7:232–239.

33. Osborne RH, Elsworth GR, Hopper JL. Age-specific norms and determinants of anxiety and depression in 731 women with breast cancer recruited through a population-based cancer registry. *Eur J Cancer.* 2003;39:755–762.

34. Kissane DW, Grabsch B, Love A, Clarke DM, Bloch S, Smith GC. Psychiatric disorder in women with early stage and advanced breast cancer: a comparative analysis. *Aust N Z J Psychiatry.* 2004;38:320–326.

35. McDaniel JS, Musselman DL, Porter MR, Reed DA, Nemeroff CB. Depression in patients with cancer. Diagnosis, biology, and treatment. *Arch Gen Psychiatry.* 1995;52:89–99.

36. Endicott J. Measurement of depression in patients with cancer. *Cancer.* 1984;53:2243–2249.

37. Akechi T, Ietsugu T, Sukigara M, et al. Symptom indicator of severity of depression in cancer patients: a comparison of the DSM-IV criteria with alternative diagnostic criteria. *Gen Hosp Psychiatry.* 2009;31:225–232 [see comment].

38. Cavanaugh S. Depression in the medically ill. *Psychosomatics.* 1995;36:48–59.

39. Akechi T, Nakano T, Akizuki N, et al. Somatic symptoms for diagnosing major depression in cancer patients. *Psychosomatics.* 2003;44:244–248.

40. Zigmond AS, Snaith RP. The hospital anxiety and depression scale. *Acta Psychiatr Scand.* 1983;67:361–370.

41. Kroenke K, Spitzer RL, Williams JB. The PHQ-9: validity of a brief depression severity measure. *J Gen Intern Med.* 2001;16:606–613.

42. Kroenke K, Spitzer RL, Williams JB. The Patient Health Questionnaire-2: validity of a two-item depression screener. *Med Care.* 2003;41:1284–1292.

43. Montgomery SA, Asberg M. A new depression scale designed to be sensitive to change. *Br J Psychiatry.* 1979;134:382–389.

44. Radloff LS. The CES-D scale: a self report depression scale for research in the general population. *Appl Psychol Meas.* 1973;1:385–401.

45. Chochinov HM, Wilson KG, Enns M, Lander S. "Are you depressed?" Screening for depression in the terminally ill. *Am J Psychiatry.* 1997;154:674–676.

46. Whooley MA, Avins AL, Miranda J, Browner WS. Case-finding instruments for depression. Two questions are as good as many. *J Gen Intern Med.* 1997;12:439–445.

47. Clarke DM, Kissane DW. Demoralization: its phenomenology and importance. *Aust N Z J Psychiatry.* 2002;36:733–742.

48. Chochinov HM, Wilson KG, Enns M, Lander S. Depression, hopelessness, and suicidal ideation in the terminally ill. *Psychosomatics.* 1998;39:366–370.

49. Weitzner MA. Psychosocial and neuropsychiatric aspects of patients with primary brain tumors. *Cancer Invest.* 1999;17:285–291.

50. Taphoorn MJ, Klein M. Cognitive deficits in adult patients with brain tumours. *Lancet Neurol.* 2004;3: 159–168 [review].

51. Holland J, Fasanello S, Onuma T. Psychiatric symptoms associated with L-asparaginase administration. *J Psychiatr Res.* 1974;10:105–113.

52. Massie MJ, Holland JC. Diagnosis and treatment of depression in the cancer patient. *J Clin Psychiatry.* 1984;45:25–29.

53. Pirl WF, Greer JA, Goode M, et al. Prospective study of depression and fatigue in men with advanced prostate cancer receiving hormone therapy. *Psychooncology.* 2008;17:148–153.

54. Day R, Ganz PA, Costantino JP. Tamoxifen and depression: more evidence from the National Surgical Adjuvant Breast and Bowel Project's Breast Cancer Prevention (P-1) Randomized Study. *J Natl Cancer Inst.* 2001;93: 1615–1623.

55. Meyers CA, Valentine AD. Neurological and psychiatric adverse effects of immunological therapy. *CNS Drugs.* 1995;3:56–68.

56. Greenberg DB, Jonasch E, Gadd MA, et al. Adjuvant therapy of melanoma with interferon-alpha-2b is associated with mania and bipolar syndromes. *Cancer.* 2000;89:356–362.

57. Capuron L, Ravaud A, Dantzer R. Early depressive symptoms in cancer patients receiving interleukin 2 and/or interferon alfa-2b therapy. *J Clin Oncol.* 2000;18: 2143–2151.

58. Trask PC, Esper P, Riba M, Redman B. Psychiatric side effects of interferon therapy: prevalence, proposed mechanisms, and future directions. *J Clin Oncol.* 2000;18:2316–2326.

59. Stiefel FC, Breitbart WS, Holland JC. Corticosteroids in cancer: neuropsychiatric complications. *Cancer Invest.* 1989;7:479–491.

60. Patten SB, Barbui C. Drug-induced depression: a systematic review to inform clinical practice. *Psychother Psychosom.* 2004;73:207–215.

61. Laird BJ, Boyd AC, Colvin LA, et al. Are cancer pain and depression interdependent? A systematic review. *Psychooncology.* 2009;18:459–464.

62. Walker J, Waters RA, Murray G, et al. Better off dead: suicidal thoughts in cancer patients. *J Clin Oncol.* 2008;26:4725–4730.

63. Misono S, Weiss NS, Fann JR, et al. Incidence of suicide in persons with cancer. *J Clin Oncol.* 2008;26:4731–4738.

64. Akechi T, Okamura H, Yamawaki S, Uchitomi Y. Why do some cancer patients with depression desire an early death and others do not? *Psychosomatics.* 2001;42:141–145.

65. NCCN practice guidelines for the management of psychosocial distress. National Comprehensive Cancer Network. *Oncology (Huntingt).* 1999;13:113–147.

66. Rodin G, Lloyd N, Katz M, et al. The treatment of depression in cancer patients: a systematic review. *Support Care Cancer.* 2007;15:123–136.

67. Williams S, Dale J. The effectiveness of treatment for depression/depressive symptoms in adults with cancer: a systematic review. *Br J Cancer.* 2006;94:372–390.

68. Fulcher CD, Badger T, Gunter AK, et al. Putting evidence into practice: interventions for depression. *Clin J Oncol Nurs.* 2008;12:131–140.

69. Razavi D, Kormoss N, Collard A, Farvacques C, Delvaux N. Comparative study of the efficacy and safety of trazodone versus clorazepate in the treatment of adjustment disorders in cancer patients: a pilot study. *J Int Med Res.* 1999;27:264–272.

70. Fisch M. Treatment of depression in cancer. *J Natl Cancer Inst Monogr.* 2004;32:105–111.

71. Practice guideline for the treatment of patients with major depressive disorder (revision). *Am J Psychiatry.* 2000;157:1–45.

72. Jin Y, Desta Z, Stearns V, et al. CYP2D6 genotype, antidepressant use, and tamoxifen metabolism during adjuvant breast cancer treatment. *J Natl Cancer Inst.* 2005;97:30–39.

73. Kelly CM, Juurlink DN, Gomes T, et al. Selective serotonin reuptake inhibitors and breast cancer mortality in women receiving tamoxifen: a population based cohort study. *BMJ.* 2010;340:c693.

74. Sood A, Barton DL, Loprinzi CL. Use of methylphenidate in patients with cancer. *Am J Hospice Palliat Care.* 2006;23:35–40.

75. Price A, Hotopf M. The treatment of depression in patients with advanced cancer undergoing palliative care. *Curr Opin Support Palliat Care.* 2009;3:61–66.

76. Olin J, Masand P. Psychostimulants for depression in hospitalized cancer patients. *Psychosomatics.* 1996;37:57–62.

77. Orr K, Taylor D. Psychostimulants in the treatment of depression: a review of the evidence. *CNS Drugs.* 2007;21:239–257.

78. Greenberg DB, Younger J, Kaufman SD. Management of lithium in patients with cancer. *Psychosomatics.* 1993;34:388–394.

79. Yap KY, Chui WK, Chan A. Drug interactions between chemotherapeutic regimens and antiepileptics. *Clin Ther.* 2008;30:1385–1407.

Anxiety in Cancer Patients

• *Anis Rashid*

■ INTRODUCTION

Anxiety is the most common and a very stressful condition in patients with cancer diagnoses. High level of anxiety is seen in up to 50% of newly diagnosed cancer patients.[1] It has also been noticed that a large number of patients with a principal anxiety disorder have one or more coexisting diagnoses at the time of initial evaluation. Anxiety is more common in younger age groups, single females, with low level of education and poor social support, and those of lower economic status.[2] The reason for this is that with maturity and more experience, the ability to mobilize resources, and adaptability, patients develop skills to cope better with illness. It has also been reported that patients with advanced disease and lower performance status endorse a higher level of stress.[3]

The level of anxiety may fluctuate during the course of the illness, but the symptoms persist throughout the initial consultation, workup, follow-up visits, and treatment. Patients may become more anxious before the first consultation, and reassurance usually does not bring the anxiety level down.[4] Anxiety level increases during treatment in anticipation of side effects, relapse, or spread of the disease. Patients with preexisting anxiety disorders are more likely to develop severe anxiety when faced with a cancer diagnosis.[5]

Increased anxiety may interfere with patients' understanding of the disease, decision making, treatment compliance, and response to treatment. It may impair normal functioning and alter their quality of life. Reducing anxiety may play a big role in the overall treatment outcome.

A better understanding of different anxiety states, their pathophysiological and psychological responses, and a measure of the strength and coping skills of patients is essential. It will help determine a treatment plan and strategies most effective and meaningful for patients.

Anxiety may be state anxiety, which is situational anxiety in response to the current threat, or trait anxiety, which is baseline anxiety prevailing over a period of many years.[1] The response to any threat or challenge is much more pronounced in patients with baseline anxiety.

Anxiety may occur at different times during the course of the illness as the patient undergoes different stages from diagnosis to survivorship. The impact of being diagnosed with cancer is very stressful. At the same time the patient receives a lot of information regarding further workups, including blood tests, scans, and information about treatment options, chemotherapy versus surgery or radiation, side effects of the chemotherapeutic agents, the possibility of prolonged hospital stay, and short- and long-term follow-up plans. He or she feels overwhelmed and flooded with information. The patient sees himself or herself caged in a situation from which escape is impossible or life threatening. He or she is not able to absorb all the information and starts having psychological and physiological responses. The patient loses sleep and appetite, develops anxiety, feels helpless, and loses interest in other activities. From the biological perspective this can be referred to as "overstimulation anxiety."[6]

The level of anxiety may vary from one individual to another with cancer diagnosis. Patients who do not have preexisting anxiety disorder and who focus on learning about the specific cancer diagnosis and treatment options experience less anxiety. These patients may be categorized as "repressors."[6] They avoid thinking about the consequences of the cancer diagnosis and side effects of treatment, and divert their mental energy to looking for solutions. They focus on treatment options and positive outcome. Patients with preexisting anxiety disorder and those with brain metastases and lung cancers have physiological responses leading to severe anxiety.[5] Intense anxiety is more prevalent in patients with severe pain, disability, no response to treatment, and poor social support systems.

Levels of anxiety also depend to some degree on the stage of cancer and related complications.[5] Patients with advanced-stage cancers usually do not fear death; they have increased anxiety, fearing uncontrolled or poorly controlled pain, dependency on others, and abandonment by the family members.[5]

Preexisting anxiety disorders and phobias must also be taken into account while treating cancer patients. Some patients have preexisting anxiety disorders such as needle phobia, claustrophobia, or phobias about taking medications.

Needle phobia, which affects 10% of the population, may have dramatic impact on day-to-day life.[7] Simple blood draw for a patient with needle phobia becomes an ordeal and needs a lot of preparation including pre-medications and precautions. Similar is the situation for patients going for MRIs or other scans if they are claustrophobic. In some cases levels of anxiety are so high that these tests cannot be performed without sedation.

■ CASE REPORT

Miss C was a 42-year-old Caucasian lady with mild mental retardation, needle phobia, and a diagnosis of melanoma, who was seen on an urgent basis due to "out-of-control behavior." She was sent to the laboratory for a blood draw. On referral Miss C was screaming, very anxious, and aggressive. She clearly said she would not get a needle stick under any circumstances. No one was able to console her and convince her for the need of blood work. She preferred to die of cancer but would not let anybody put a needle into her body. She was sent back from the laboratory. Days passed by and Miss C did not show up in the clinic. One late afternoon she showed up in the clinic escorted by a patient advocate and asked for full treatment of her cancer but would not agree for blood work. Cancer diagnosis on top of the existing fear for

needle made the situation worse. Miss C was referred to the psychiatry clinic for evaluation and management of needle phobia. Reassurance, use of topical anesthetic before needle stick, fast-acting antianxiety medications, education of the patient, and the medical staff helped her go through blood work and further management.

■ PREVALENCE

Anxiety is a common symptom affecting cancer patients. The prevalence of anxiety disorder in cancer patients ranges between 13% and 16%.[8] In a study with breast cancer patients the prevalence of posttraumatic stress disorder (PTSD) was 3% to 19%.[8] A higher prevalence of anxiety is seen in patients with chronic pain, ranging between 20% and 40%. More than 50% of patients with cancer diagnoses suffer with pain, and exhibit increased anxiety and distress. Increased anxiety has been reported in ovarian cancer patients due to significant pain.[8]

Cancer pain may not only cause anxiety, but also trigger the memories of past emotional traumas and exacerbate symptoms of anxiety and distress. It has been shown that adequate pain control with medication and cognitive–behavioral approaches to enhance adjustment and capability to cope will remarkably reduce anxiety in patients.[8] Patients being diagnosed with gynecological cancers express more distress because the body parts involved are emotionally charged and are associated with sexuality, femininity, and childbearing.[9]

Anxiety levels in men who are at risk for prostate cancer range from 10% to 15%.[10] However, a higher anxiety level in the range of 50% or more is seen in patients who present for screening. This level falls after a negative biopsy or negative screening result.[10] Lung cancer, known as the leading cause of cancer death in both men and women and responsible for 30% of all cancer-related deaths in the United States, evokes extreme anxiety and depression in patients when diagnosed.[11] This is seen in all types of lung cancer, especially non-small cell lung cancer, due to disease burden, major psychosocial impact, metastasis at the time of diagnosis, and poor prognosis. In a study in Scotland it was shown that only 10% of patients endorsed severe anxiety and 6% showed borderline anxiety at their first presentation.[12] Primary brain tumor patients suffer from many neuropsychiatric problems associated with their diagnosis and treatment, which affects their quality of life. The initial analysis in a study sample designed to see the psychiatric illnesses in brain tumor patients demonstrated that 48% patients endorsed generalized anxiety disorder (GAD), with only 5% having preexisting psychiatric illnesses.[13]

Cancer patients of all age groups experience symptoms of anxiety, but it has been reported in a study conducted in the Norwegian Radium Hospital that patients under 30 years of age and over 70 years of age express less anxiety as compared with others.[14] The Psychosocial Collaborative Oncology Group has found that preexisting anxiety disorder is present in 4% of patients diagnosed with cancer.[8] This trait anxiety makes patients more vulnerable to any stress and reduces the ability to cope. The diagnosis of cancer, cancer pain, and side effects of the treatment can reactivate this existing condition and lead to sense of loss of control and tax patients' ability to cope with the situation.

■ PATHOPHYSIOLOGY

There is a strong genetic component in the development of major psychiatric disorders. Stressful life events in early childhood play a major role leading to anxiety and depression later in life. In a well-documented study of 2000 women it was shown that women with a history of childhood sexual or physical abuse develop more symptoms of anxiety and depression and had more frequently attempted suicide as compared with women without a history of childhood sexual or physical abuse.[15] These women are more prone to develop severe anxiety disorder including panic disorder and GAD. It seems that persistent changes in central nervous system (CNS) corticotrophin-releasing factor (CRF) due to early life trauma are responsible for these psychiatric disorders and are the main mediator between stressful experiences and development of mood disorders.[15]

The stress response is characterized by the activation of the hypothalamic–pituitary–adrenal axis (HPA). It results in both the synthesis and the secretion of CRF. Hypersecretion of CRF is the main element in the chain responsible for autonomic and behavioral responses seen in anxiety. Cell bodies of CRF are found in high density in the hypothalamic *paraventricular* nucleus, while the neurons project to the median eminence. In anxiety, CRF is secreted from nerve terminals into the hypothalamo-hypophyseal portal circulation connecting hypothalamus and the pituitary. The CRF then stimulates the production of proopiomelanocortin (POMC) and adrenocorticotropic hormone (ACTH). ACTH then stimulates the

synthesis and secretion of glucocorticoids, which maintains the homeostasis in stress. Glucocorticoids also control the activity of HPA axis by negative feedback inhibition system. In negative feedback system glucocorticoids dampen HPA axis.[15]

In a positive feedforward cascade, glucocorticoids are responsible for behavioral responses seen in stress. CRF-releasing neurons are also found in the amygdala and cortical regions. CRF presence in amygdala suggests its role in the modulation of affective stress response. Originating from amygdale these neurons project into the locus ceruleus and increase tyrosine hydrooxylase activity, which further increases the synthesis and release of norepinephrine. Due to its action on locus ceruleus, CRF is responsible for vigilance-, arousal-, and anxietylike behavioral responses. Extensive evidence has shown that CRF is responsible for autonomic, immune, and behavioral stress response. Laboratory animals have shown stress responses when CRF is directly administered into the CNS. Centrally administered CRF also shows the behavioral responses seen in acute anxiety and stress. Increased activity of the HPA axis is seen in psychological stress only and not after physical stress such as hemorrhage. This suggests the involvement of corticolimbic pathways in stress and anxiety.[15] In contrast, it has been shown that patients with PTSD have low adrenocortical activity. In a study with Vietnam veterans it was shown that these patients have low nadir and increased peak of cortisol release as compared with controls.[15] The release of increased cortisol at the time of stress is damaging to hippocampal neurons and may persist for years. This results in lower hippocampal volumes in patients with PTSD.

Release of glucocorticoids and/or catacholamines at the time of stress also interferes and may modulate the encoding of memories. Hence, the memories of acute stress, initial panic attack, or anxiety remain unforgettable and come to surface with any trivial stimulus or cue.[15]

Another theory suggests that dysfunctional γ-aminobutyric acid (GABA) system may be responsible for autonomic and behavioral changes in stress and anxiety. This theory is based on the clinical experiences gained with the use of benzodiazepines and its efficacy in the treatment of anxiety disorders.[16] Another neurotransmitter involved in the pathogenesis of anxiety is serotonin. In acute stress and threatening situations synaptic serotonin is increased, and limbic and cortical regions receive this signal and prepare the individual to adapt and respond to the situation.

■ PSYCHODYNAMIC CONCEPTS OF ANXIETY

Different psychodynamic aspects of anxiety have been described in the literature. Freud described two types of anxiety influencing the ego system, which is the conscious control of the personality and is responsible for perception, defenses, cognition, and mood. Signal anxiety generates smaller doses of anxiety and alerts the ego defense mechanism to deal with it. This type of anxiety may be labeled as positive anxiety, as it helps the person to deal with the situation. Traumatic anxiety is seen in panic attacks, when the ego defense mechanism is overwhelmed and is unable to deal with the fears and dangers posited in the situation. Freud also described developmental anxiety due to fears and dangers faced in childhood. He believed that meaningful internal dangers faced in young life may lead to eruption of anxiety later in life. These fears may be the fear of loss of an object, such as loss of a parent, loss of an object's love, or fear of castration.[17]

■ TYPES OF ANXIETY DISORDERS

Generalized Anxiety Disorder

In the cancer setting the criterion of GAD is modified from 6 months' duration to 2 weeks of symptoms.[18] Patients have preexisting anxiety disorder, for an average 5 to 10 years before being formally diagnosed with the disorder. Cancer patients have increased anxiety about their prognosis, treatment side effects, prolonged hospital stay, recurrence, loss of income, dependency, pain, disability, and untimely death.[18] If in proportion, anxiety may influence patients positively, enforcing them to change their behavior, avoiding risky behavior and being compliant with the treatment plan.

Panic Disorder with or without Agoraphobia

Panic disorder results in a discrete period of intense fear or discomfort, in which four or more of the following symptoms develop abruptly and reach a peak within 10 minutes. The symptoms include palpitations, pounding heart or accelerated heart rate, sweating, trembling or shaking, and sensation of shortness of breath or smothering. Patients may feel chest pain or discomfort, nausea, or abdominal distress. They may feel dizzy or lightheaded and fear losing control or going crazy. Patients may develop paresthesias, chills, or hot flashes or may endorse symptoms of derealization or depersonalization. They may fear dying.[19]

When panic attacks become more frequent, patients worry excessively about additional attacks and their implications. Panic disorder may be misinterpreted in cancer patients due to disease-related physical symptoms, such as shortness of breath due to pleural effusion, pneumonia, or atelectasis. Patients with cancer-related uncontrolled pain, or just wanting to go home after a prolonged hospital stay, may be diagnosed as having a panic attack. A careful evaluation is necessary to rule out an organic etiology.

Adjustment Disorder with Anxiety

The important criterion for adjustment disorder with anxiety is the presence of a stressor leading to the development of symptoms within a 3-month period. The symptoms should resolve within the next 6 months. If symptoms persist longer than 6 months, then the diagnosis changes to any one of the anxiety disorder spectrum diagnoses. Usually the symptoms are out of proportion to the degree of the stressor. This classification is indicative of chances of recovery rather than a chronic illness.[18] In practice almost all patients endorse symptoms of anxiety after being diagnosed with cancer. *Diagnostic and Statistical Manual IV* (DSM-IV) does not classify adjustment disorder with anxiety under anxiety disorder spectrum, but as an independent class.

Anxiety due to General Medical Conditions

The symptoms of anxiety in this category are due to the direct physiological consequences of a general medical condition, and there is a temporal association between the onset of general medical condition and the anxiety symptoms.[18] Certain medical conditions are closely associated with mood disorder. Cancer diagnoses, especially brain tumors, and cardiovascular disorders such as myocardial infarction are good examples. Among brain tumor patients, those with temporal lobe tumors are more vulnerable to developing anxiety. Post-myocardial infarction patients develop anxiety mostly as a part of widely described post-stroke syndrome.[21]

Other diseases that may cause or contribute to anxiety include thyroid diseases, Parkinson's disease, pulmonary diseases such as asthma or COPD, and seizures. Rare causes include pheochromocytoma, hyperparathyroidism, hypocalcemia, and hypomagnesemia.[21]

Substance-induced Anxiety Disorder

Substance-induced anxiety is the direct physiological effect of a substance or medication on mood. A long list of medications commonly used in medical practice are known to cause anxious mood. Steroids used very frequently in cancer patients may induce anxiety and emotional lability. Proinflammatory cytokines such as interferon may cause anxiety or a panic attack. Thyrotropic drugs, sympathomimetic drugs, or stimulants used to treat cancer-induced fatigue may cause anxiety and agitation. Antinausea medication such as metoclopamide and prochlorperazine may cause restlessness, anxiety, and akathesia.[18] Caffeine used widely may cause anxiety and restlessness. It is present in coffee, tea, caffeinated drinks, coffee ice cream, weight-loss medications, and headache medications.[21] Over-the-counter decongestants containing pseudoephedrine may cause tachyphylaxis and anxiety.[21] While substance may cause anxiety, at times withdrawal of the medication may also produce acute anxiety.[21] Benzodiazepine, nicotine, or alcohol withdrawal may cause symptoms of intense anxiety and restlessness.

Illicit drugs that may cause anxiety include hallucinogen or phencyclidine when used in excessive amounts (Table 6-1).

■ POSTTRAUMATIC STRESS DISORDER

Approximately 3% to 5% cancer survivors develop symptoms of PTSD while the prevalence of PTSD in general population is 7.8%.[19] The etiology of PTSD is different in cancer patients in two ways:

1. The trauma leading to PTSD arises from within the person's own body as opposed to outside threat.
2. The ongoing stress is not the past experience but mainly the fear of having a relapse of the disease.

Some clinicians believe that the trauma of being diagnosed with a life-threatening illness is sufficient to cause these symptoms. The prolonged hospitalization and the severe side effects of the chemotherapeutic agents play a major role in the development of the symptoms of PTSD. Other contributory factors include intensive care unit experiences, poor pain control, and increased physical symptoms in the immediate postoperative period. Patients with previous psychiatric disorders, poor social support system, and recent stressors are more vulnerable to develop symptoms of PTSD. The location and the severity of cancer are not directly related to the development of PTSD.

DSM-IV criteria of PTSD are as follows:

1. **Criteria A:**
   - The person experienced, witnessed, or was confronted with an event that involved or threatened actual death or serious injury or a threat to physical integrity of self or others.
   - The person's response involved intense fear, helplessness, or horror.
2. **Criteria B:**
   - The traumatic event is persistently re-experienced by one or more of the following:
     (a) recurrent and intrusive distressing recollections of the events;
     (b) recurrent distressing dreams of the event;
     (c) reliving the experience, illusions, hallucinations, and dissociative flashback episodes;
     (d) intense psychological distress at exposure to internal and external cues;
     (e) physiological reactivity on exposure to internal or external cues.
3. **Criteria C:**
   - Persistent avoidance of stimuli associated with the trauma and numbing of general responsiveness as indicated by three or more of the following:
     (a) efforts to avoid thoughts, feelings, or conversations associated with the trauma;
     (b) efforts to avoid activities, places, or people that arouse recollections of the trauma;
     (c) inability to recall an important aspect of the trauma;
     (d) markedly diminished interest or participation in significant activities;
     (e) feelings of detachment or estrangements from others;
     (f) restricted range of affect;
     (g) sense of foreshortened future.
4. **Criteria D:**
   - Persistent symptoms of increased arousal as indicated by two or more of the following:
     (a) difficulty falling or staying asleep;
     (b) irritability or outbursts of anger;
     (c) difficulty concentrating;
     (d) hypervigilance;
     (e) exaggerated startle response.
5. **Criteria E:**
   - Duration of the disturbance is more than 1 month.
6. **Criteria F:**
   - The disturbance causes significant stress or impairment in social occupational or other important areas of functioning.

PTSD may be classified as following:

- Acute: if duration of symptoms is less than 3 months.

■ **TABLE 6-1. Substances that may cause Anxiety**

Class	Examples	Notes
Androgens	Nandrolone	Most problems occur when abused
	Methyltestosterone	
Angiotensin-converting enzyme inhibitors	Captopril	Often stimulating
	Lisinopril	
Anticholinergics	Atropine	
	Benztropine	
	Dicyclomine	
	Hyoscyamine	
Antidepressants	Serotonin reuptake inhibitors	
	Bupropion	
	Tricyclic agents	
Antiemetics	Prochlorperazine	Anxiety may actually be akathisia
	Promethazine	
Antimigraine agents	Sumatriptan	
	Naratriptan	
Antimycobacterial agents	Isoniazid	
Antineoplastic agents	Vinblastine	
	Ifosfamide	
Antipsychotics	Thiothixene	Anxiety may actually be akathisia
	Haloperidol	
Antiviral agents	Acyclovir	
	Didanosine	
	Foscarnet	
	Ganciclovir	
	Efavirenz	
Beta-adrenergic agonists	Albuterol	
	Metaproterenol	
Cannabinoids	Dronabinol	
Class I antiarrhythmics	Lidocaine	
	Procainamide	
	Quinidine	
Corticosteroids	Prednisone	
	Methylprednisolone	
Dopaminergic agents	Carbidopa–levodopa	
	Amantadine	
	Pergolide	
Estrogens	Conjugated estrogens	May cause panic attacks and depression
	Ethinyl estradiol	
	Levonorgestrel implant	
Gonadotropin-releasing hormone active agents	Leuprolide	
Histamine H2 receptor antagonists	Cimetidine	
	Famotidine	
	Nizatidine	
Interferons	Interferon-alpha	
	Interferon-beta	

Continued

■ TABLE 6-1. Substances that may cause Anxiety (continued)

Class	Examples	Notes
Methylxanthines	Caffeine	
	Theophylline	
Sympathomimetics	Ephedrine	
	Epinephrine	
	Phenylephrine nasal	
	Pseudoephedrine	
Nonsteroidal anti-inflammatory drugs	Indomethacin	
	Naproxen	
	Salicylates	
Opiates	Meperidine	Owing to drug withdrawal, meperidine may directly cause anxiety with progression to delirium.[20]
Opioid antagonists	Naltrexone	Observe for opiate withdrawal
Progestins	Medroxyprogesterone acetate	
	Norethindrone	
Prokinetic agents	Metoclopramide	Anxiety may be due to akathisia
Psychostimulants	Methylphenidate	
	Dextroamphetamine	
Sedative-hypnotics	Benzodiazepines	Anxiety due to drug withdrawal
	Barbiturates	
	Alcohol	

Reprinted with permission from the *Diagnostic and Statistical Manual of Mental Disorders, Text Revision*. 4th ed. American Psychiatric Association (copyright 2000).[21]

- Chronic: if duration of symptoms is 3 months or more.
- With delayed onset: if onset of symptoms is at least 6 months after the stressor.[22]

■ DIAGNOSIS

When evaluating anxiety in cancer patients, it is important for the clinician to consider the full range of the potential causes of anxiety and to separate the organic anxiety from functional anxiety, as the treatment varies. Physicians should not only keep in mind the possibility of preexisting anxiety disorder, but also look into other possibilities. Is this anxiety the direct psychological reaction to the medical illness? Is this reaction due to the direct result of the treatment or medication, or is this anxiety directly due to the biological effects of the medical illness?[21] The clinician has to keep in mind common medical conditions that present with symptoms of acute stress and anxiety.

Hypoxia is one of the most common medical conditions seen in our patient population that results in anxiety. Medical comorbidities involving lungs and pleura such as pneumonia, pleural effusion, and atelectasis cause difficulty in breathing and shortness of breath and subsequently result in anxiety. Reassurance with treatment of the underlying etiology would be the right approach. Many chemotherapeutic regimens, especially the ones that include high-dose steroids in the protocol, may produce anxiety and agitation in cancer patients.

Side effects of chemotherapeutic agents, especially nausea and vomiting, add to the problem, making the picture more complicated. Anticipatory anxiety on top of organic cause may further contribute and exacerbate the condition.

Once the organic cause is ruled out, the diagnostic interview using DSM-IV-TR criteria is the gold standard.[21]

When approaching an anxious patient, the clinician should consider all the possible factors leading to anxiety. The often unavoidable uncertainty associated with the cancer diagnosis, its treatment, and prognosis leads to extreme anxiety and distress. Patients with predisposition to anxiety or patients with preexisting anxiety disorders are more vulnerable to develop anxiety during the course of illness. Some patients worry excessively that they might have a serious illness. For example, patients who have a family history of breast cancer become anxious going for a routine mammogram.[21]

Severe anxiety is frequently seen during the period when patients are waiting for test results. Prolonged uncertainty about the prognosis or efficacy of the treatment is also anxiety provoking and very stressful for cancer patients. Many cancer patients experience ongoing fears of recurrence, resulting in continued anxiety. While approaching these patients, the clinician should look for the underlying fear resulting in anxiety and address this accordingly.

Many patients worry about the impact of the cancer diagnosis and treatment on their body image. Head and neck cancer patients are apprehensive about the changes in their facial appearance, while breast cancer patients fear losing their femininity and body shape after breast surgery. Similarly, men fear becoming impotent after prostate surgery or ablation treatments. Fear of being dependent on others or fear of uncontrolled pain is another related area that needs to be explored and addressed.

Fear of death is another area of concern. When evaluating patients with death anxiety, the clinician should explore the specific reasons for fear of death in both patients and their families. Assessment of death anxiety should also include the discussion with patients regarding the existential thoughts about dying, and reflections about the meaning of one's life. In some cases patients are actually at peace with dying but fear that their family will not be able to survive without them. In that case bringing the family members into discussion and reassurance will reduce anxiety in these patients and lead to a peaceful dying process.

Last but not least, some patients develop anxiety due to the fear of negative response from the treating physician. These are patients who do not follow instructions about medication compliance, blood sugar checkups, or instructions to quit smoking or stop drinking alcohol. These patients may cancel their appointments to avoid an unpleasant interaction with the physician. Some of these patients may fear to disclose important medical information to the treating physician and become responsible for aggravating their own illness. They may develop guilt and feel disconnected from their treating physicians. Just to make a phone call to make an appointment raises their anxiety level and they try to avoid it as long as possible. Clinicians should look for these cues and explore the reasons for excessive anxiety in these patients. Awareness of the negative countertransference is essential.[21]

Screening for anxiety can be performed utilizing three different approaches. The simplest approach is when the clinician would ask the patient if he or she is anxious or worried. This single-symptom assessment is quick and easy, but not very reliable.

The more reliable and valid approach is to use standard screening measures. These include the Hospital Anxiety and Depression Questionnaire, the State Trait Anxiety Inventory, and the Anxiety Subscale of Brief Symptom Inventory. GAD scale, GAD-7, has the advantage to match more closely with the DSM-IV criteria and has recently been used effectively in medical practice. The third approach describes clinical syndromes, such as panic disorder, GAD, and social phobia, that comply with the criteria matching with the DSM-IV classification. The advantage of this approach is in the diagnosis and management of these patients (Tables 6-2 to 6-4).

■ MANAGEMENT

Treatment of anxiety disorders in cancer patients may be different from the treatment of anxiety in any other medical illness. Anxiety in cancer patients could be a normal response to cancer diagnosis, or the symptoms may persist to become pathological anxiety. These patients frequently have other comorbid psychiatric illnesses, usually major depression, and their symptoms fluctuate during the course of their illness. Anxiety is a normal response to cancer diagnosis that may resolve in days or weeks. This short-term anxiety motivates the patient to seek medical and psychological help and to apply coping strategies. Maladaptive and pathological anxiety seen in cancer patients leads to persistent social and occupational functional impairment.[8]

The most important initial step in the treatment of anxiety is empathic listening.[21] It helps the clinician to understand the patient's main concerns and fears and address these issues accordingly.

■ TABLE 6-2. Hospital Anxiety and Depression Scale

This questionnaire will help your physician to know how you are feeling. Ready every sentence. Place an "X" on the answer that best describes how you have been feeling during the last week. You do not have to think too much to answer. In this questionnaire, spontaneous answers are more important

A 1) I feel tense or wound up
   3 ( ) Most of the time
   2 ( ) A lot of the time
   1 ( ) From time to time
   0 ( ) Not at all

D 2) I still enjoy the things I used to enjoy
   0 ( ) Definitely and quite badly
   1 ( ) Not quite so much
   2 ( ) Only a little
   3 ( ) Hardly at all

A 3) I get a sort of frightened feeling as if something is about to happen
   3 ( ) Very definitely and quite badly
   2 ( ) Yes, but not too badly
   1 ( ) A little, but it does not worry me
   0 ( ) Not at all

D 4) I can laugh and see the funny side of things
   0 ( ) As much as I always could
   1 ( ) Not quite as much now
   2 ( ) Definitely not so much now
   3 ( ) Not at all

A 5) Worrying thought goes through my head
   3 ( ) A great deal of the time
   2 ( ) A lot of the time
   1 ( ) From time to time but not too often
   0 ( ) Only occasionally

D 6) I feel cheerful
   3 ( ) Not at all
   2 ( ) Not often
   1 ( ) Sometimes
   0 ( ) Most of the time

A 7) I can sit at ease and feel relaxed
   0 ( ) Definitely
   1 ( ) Usually
   2 ( ) Not often
   3 ( ) Not at all

D 8) I feel as I am slowed down
   3 ( ) Nearly all the time
   2 ( ) Very often
   1 ( ) Sometimes
   0 ( ) Not at all

A 9) I get a sort of frightened feeling like butterflies in the stomach
   0 ( ) Not at all
   1 ( ) Occasionally
   2 ( ) Quite often
   3 ( ) Very often

D 10) I have lost interest in my appearance
   3 ( ) Definitely
   2 ( ) I do not take so much care as I should
   1 ( ) I may not take quite as much care
   0 ( ) I take just as much care as ever

A 11) I feel restless, as if I had to be on the move
   3 ( ) Very much indeed
   2 ( ) Quite a lot
   1 ( ) Not very much
   0 ( ) Not at all

D 12) I look forward with enjoyment to things
   0 ( ) As much as I ever did
   1 ( ) Rather less than I used to
   2 ( ) Definitely less than I used to
   3 ( ) Hardly at all

A 13) I get sudden feeling of panic
   3 ( ) Very often indeed
   2 ( ) Quite often
   1 ( ) Not very often
   0 ( ) Not at all

D 14) I can enjoy a good TV or radio program or book
   0 ( ) Often
   1 ( ) Sometimes
   2 ( ) Not often
   3 ( ) Very seldom

■ **TABLE 6-3. Hamilton Rating Scale for Anxiety**

Instructions: This checklist is to assist the physician or psychiatrist in evaluating each patient as to his degree of anxiety and pathological condition. Please fill in the appropriate rating:
None = 0; mild = 1; moderate = 3; severe, grossly disabling = 4

Item	Rating	Item	Rating
Anxious: worries, anticipation of the worst, fearful anticipation, irritability		Somatic (sensory): tinnitus, blurring of vision, hot and cold flushes, feelings of weakness, pricking sensation	
Tension: feelings of tension, fatigability, startle response, moved to tears easily, trembling, feelings of restlessness, inability to relax		Cardiovascular symptoms: tachycardia, palpitations, pain in chest, throbbing of vessels, fainting feelings, missing beat	
Fears: of dark, of strangers, of being left alone, of animals, of traffic, of crowds		Respiratory symptoms: pressure of constriction in chest, choking feelings, sighing, dyspnea	
Insomnia: difficulty in falling asleep, broken sleep, unsatisfying sleep and fatigue on walking, dreams, nightmares, night terrors		Gastrointestinal symptoms: difficulty in swallowing, wind, abdominal pain, burning sensations, abdominal fullness, nausea, vomiting, borborygmi, looseness of bowels, loss of weight, constipation	
Intellectual (cognitive): difficulty in concentration, poor memory		Genitourinary symptoms: frequency of micturition, urgency of micturition, amenorrhea, menorrhagia, development of frigidity, premature ejaculation, loss of libido, impotence	
Depressed mood: loss of interest, lack of pleasure in hobbies, depression, early waking, diurnal swing		Autonomic symptoms: dry mouth, flushing, pallor, tendency to sweat, giddiness, tension headache, raising hair	
Somatic (muscular): pains and aches, twitching, stiffness, myoclonic jerks, grinding of teeth, unsteady voice, increased muscular tone		Behavior at interview: fidgeting, restlessness or pacing, tremor of hands, furrowed brow, strained face, sighing or rapid respiration, facial pallor, swallowing, belching, brisk tendon jerks, dilated pupils, exophthalmos	

Adapted from Hedlund JL, Vieweg BW. The Hamilton rating scale for depression. *J Operational Psychiatry*. 1979;10(2):149–165.

■ TABLE 6-4. GAD 7

Over the past 2 weeks, How Often have You been Bothered by the Following Problems?	Not At All	Several Days	More than Half the Days	Nearly Every Day
1. Feeling nervous, anxious, or on edge	0	1	2	3
2. Not being able to stop or control worrying	0	1	2	3
3. Worrying too much about different things	0	1	2	3
4. Trouble relaxing	0	1	2	3
5. Being so restless that it is hard to sit still	0	1	2	3
6. Becoming easily annoyed or irritable	0	1	2	3
7. Feeling afraid as if something awful might happen	0	1	2	3

Total score _____ = add columns _____ + _____ + _____

If you checked off any problems, how difficult have these problems made it for you to do you work, take care of things at home, or get along with other people?	Not difficult at all ☐	Somewhat difficult ☐	Very difficult ☐	Extremely difficult ☐

Treatment of anxiety in cancer patients begins by providing adequate information regarding their illness, concerning available treatment options and resources and giving support.[25] Poor or incomplete information may generate mistrust of the health care providers. Three different treatment approaches are available, which include pharmacotherapy, psychotherapy, and a combination approach.

The overemphasis on psychopharmacology may ignore the beneficial role of psychotherapy in these patients.[21] Different psychotherapeutic approaches include supportive, cognitive–behavioral, group, and psychodynamic therapies. Hypnosis, guided imagery, and relaxation techniques have been used successfully in many cancer centers.

Supportive Psychotherapy

Supportive therapy involves empathic listening for fears and misperceptions, educating the patient about the medical illness, and providing sympathy and support. Effective communication skills are essential while providing information. Workshops with open questioning sessions, discussion about psychological problems, and discouraging reassurance have led to more disclosure of psychosocial issues. Anxious patients are hypersensitive to threatening stimuli. Even in the absence of progression of the disease, simple bodily symptoms increase their anxiety. Seeking medical advice for the newly developed symptoms is understandable, while reassurance-seeking behavior is maladaptive. Sometimes well-meaning reassurance for cancer-related symptoms may worsen anxiety.[25] Making a definite plan to differentiate minor symptoms from those that need medical attention will reduce anxiety.

An important aspect of the supportive therapy is to mobilize the patient's support system including family and friends. In addition, resources available at the treatment centers such as nurses, social workers, chaplains, and other allied health care workers can provide support to the medically ill patients.[21] Patients who have strong religious beliefs may get relief and reduce their stress from pastoral counseling.

In terminally ill patients relieving physical symptoms such as pain and dyspnea may reduce anxiety. While facing death maintaining hope and changing the plan from full recovery to having time to accomplish certain short-term goals may help patients reduce their stress. Therapists can help patients find meaning in their lives despite their illness and reduce emotional distress.

Cognitive–Behavioral Therapy

Cognitive–behavioral therapy developed and refined by Beck in 1960 is based on an ever-evolving formulation of patients and their problems in cognitive terms. It requires strong therapeutic alliance and teaches patients to identify, evaluate, and respond to their dysfunctional thoughts and beliefs.[26] It has been proven to be very effective in treating anxiety disorders. Cognitive techniques are used to uncover and correct the distorted or dysfunctional thoughts and beliefs that lead to emotional and behavioral changes. Behavioral techniques such as systemic desensitization and therapies about self-regulation and bodily functions have been very successful in reducing anxiety in cancer patients. These therapies include biofeedback and relaxation techniques, such as breathing exercises, self-hypnosis, and meditation. Guided imagery has also been used successfully to reduce anxiety. Meditation reduces the frequency of panic attacks, and biofeedback helps wean patients from the ventilator. Relaxation techniques have been used to decrease the need of medications in certain conditions and to overall reduce anxiety.

Psychodynamic Therapy

This approach is used in patients who are not very ill, can be engaged easily, and are emotionally resilient. This type of therapy focuses on conscious and unconscious meaning of illness to the patient. It involves an understanding of the patient's developmental history, psychodynamics aspects of his or her social and personal life, and his or her defense mechanisms. The clinician can help the patient develop strategies to cope better if the clinician understands what strategies had helped him in the past. Psychodynamic psychotherapy may uncover some aspects of the patient's life that may lead to further distress and anxiety. This includes imagined or real guilt and recollection of past unhealthy relationships that may be repeated in the new patient–doctor relationship. Full understanding of the psychodynamic aspect of a patient's life will help the

clinician to identify the conflicts with the treating physicians and resolve the issues that may be interfering with recovery.

Countertransference reactions also cause problems for the treating physician as they may lead to frustration due to progression of the disease or treatment failure. The clinician may overcompensate by providing excessive reassurance or may overlook a symptom in an unconscious attempt to reduce his or her own anxiety. Psychiatrists may play an important role here identifying these conflicts and defenses so that they do not interfere with the optimal patient care. Psychotherapy may be continued later as an outpatient to help the patient cope with continued illness and to improve functioning.

Group Therapy

Support groups are very helpful for medically ill patients. These groups provide emotional support, education about stress management, and coping strategies. Sharing their life experiences and emotions help patients to deal with the stress better, resulting in improved functioning.

Pharmacotherapy

Once a decision is made to start pharmacological treatment, a broad range of medication class and types are available that can be used safely in this patient population. The choices are based on patient's personal and family history of response to the medication. The medications can be used on an as-needed basis or on a schedule at a regular interval.

Benzodiazepines

Benzodiazepines are the most effective drugs and are used most frequently in the treatment of anxiety. Diazepam and chlordiazepoxide were among the first of these to be used. Alprazolam works quickly to bring the anxiety level down; hence, it is the most desired drug in patients with anxiety. Alprazolam has a short half-life and its effect is short-lived; hence, rebound anxiety and withdrawal symptoms are common. Lorazepam is the drug that can be given in intravenous, intramuscular, and oral forms and does not have an active metabolite; hence, it is the most popular drug in hospitalized patients. Like lorazepam, temazepam and oxazepam are directly glucorinated by uridine 5′-diphosphate glucuronosyltransferases (UGTs). Since UGTs are less affected than cytochrome

P450 system by chronic liver disease, these three are the preferred drugs for use in patients with liver disease.[27] For patients who need long-term use of benzodiazepine, the drug of choice would be clonazepam. Sedatives and hypnotics are also used for patients who are kept awake due to anxiety. These are best used on a short-term basis to avoid side effects and to maintain the effectiveness. The most commonly used drug in this class is zolpidem, a nonbenzodiazepine drug that acts on benzodiazepine receptors. Benzodiazepines can cause excessive sedation and may cause cognitive disturbances, especially in elderly patients with impaired brain functioning such as a history of dementia, head injury, or a history of excessive alcohol intake. Benzodiazepines serve as respiratory depressant and should be used with caution in patients with respiratory problems or sleep apnea. All benzodiazepines lead to tolerance and dependence, and should be avoided especially in patients with history of substance abuse. In some patients who are reliable and do not have a history of chemical dependency, these drugs can be used safely for a longer period of time without causing any problem.

Antidepressants

Another class of drugs commonly used to control symptoms of anxiety is selective serotonin reuptake inhibitors (SSRIs). This group includes fluoxetine, sertraline, paroxetine, citalopram, escitalopram, and fluvoxamine. These medications are relatively safe and do not cause cardiac conduction problems, orthostatic hypotension, and physical dependence. These drugs have few side effects and therefore can be used safely in medically ill patients. Since these drugs may take 4 to 6 weeks to act, initial treatment of anxiety may include the use of benzodiazepines. Once the patient is stable and starts responding to SSRIs, benzodiazepines can be withdrawn easily. One of the main side effects of these medications is a sexual side effect, which could be a concern especially in younger patients. SSRIs may cause gastrointestinal disturbances including nausea and vomiting; hence, they are given with food. These side effects are transient and usually last for few days only.

Another side effect of some concern may be SSRI-associated syndrome of inappropriate secretion of antidiuretic hormone. An uncommon side effect is the increase in parkinsonian symptoms in patients with Parkinson's disease. All SSRIs are equally effective and choice of medication is based on side-effect profile. Sedating drugs such as paroxetine are used in highly anxious patients and the stimulating SSRI, fluoxetine, is used in patients with symptoms of fatigue. In cancer setting medications with fewer drug interactions such as citalopram and escitalopram are preferred.

Serotonin–norepinephrine reuptake inhibitors (SNRIs) are also used to treat anxiety. In a small number of patients this drug may cause an elevation in diastolic blood pressure, which is dose dependent. Clinicians need to monitor blood pressure readings when starting this medication. If there is a sustained increase in the blood pressure, either the dose needs to be reduced or medication should be stopped.

Mirtazapine is a unique drug that is used very often to control anxiety. It is an alpha-adrenoreceptor antagonist, and antagonist at 5-HT_{2A}, 5-HT_{2C}, and 5-HT_3 receptors. It is a highly sedating drug that controls nausea and promotes appetite; hence, it is commonly used in cancer patients who have anxiety, insomnia, weight loss, and chemotherapy-induced nausea. It is also a very potent antihistamine and this property is useful in certain skin conditions to control itching.

Antipsychotics

Antipsychotics are not approved to treat anxiety but have shown their efficacy in the management of anxiety, especially when benzodiazepines are contraindicated. Patients who do not respond to benzodiazepines or have cognitive impairment or agitation respond best to haloperidol. Thioridazine (Mellaril) in low doses or second-generation antipsychotics such as olanzapine (Zyprexa) or quetiapine (Seroquel) in low doses have been very effective in the treatment of anxiety. FDA has labeled neuroleptics with a black box warning especially with thioridazine. Newer-generation antipsychotics have a more favorable side-effect profile and are used more commonly.

Antihistamines

Antihistamines are sometimes used to treat anxiety and insomnia in cancer patients. Hydroxyzine and diphenhydramine are more commonly used antihistamines. Diphenhydramine being over the counter is considered benign, but it may cause dizziness, excessive sedation, and confusion. These medications are used when benzodiazepines cannot be prescribed due to respiratory depressant side effects or in patients with a history of chemical dependency.

Beta-blockers

This group of drugs is highly useful to treat anxiety associated with drug-induced akathisia. While treating chemotherapy-induced nausea, high doses of antiemetic drugs are prescribed, the most commonly used being metoclopramide. The major side effect of this drug is akathisia. The feeling of extreme restlessness and anxiety keeps the patient awake and on his or her toes. He or she does not find a comfortable position and is not able to rest. The first-line treatment of this condition is beta-blockers. These drugs control anxiety symptoms by blocking autonomic hyperarousal and calming the patient down. Beta-blockers are contraindicated in patients with asthma and diabetes.

Anticonvulsants

Anticonvulsants are prescribed to control anxiety and panic attacks especially in patients with temporal lobe abnormalities. Divalproic acid and carbamazepine have been used successfully to treat anxiety in patients with head injury.

■ SUMMARY

Anxiety is the most common initial psychiatric diagnosis in cancer patients. The burden of anxiety can add difficulties when discussing treatment options; hence, early detection of pathological anxiety and differentiating it from the normal response to cancer diagnosis is essential. Different rating scales have shown efficacy and are used regularly in many centers. Once the diagnosis of anxiety disorder is made, the choice of therapy is based on patients' personal and family history. Combination therapies that include psychotherapy and medication have shown better results. The choice of medication should be based on medical history, past experiences with the medication, and side-effect profile. Spiritual support may lessen anxiety in highly spiritual patients regardless of influence of gender, age, diagnosis, and marital status.[28] Complete elimination of the symptoms may not be possible, and reassurance may worsen anxiety. Compassionate listening, thorough assessment, and skillful intervention and support by the clinician will reduce anxiety and suffering in cancer patients and improve quality of life.[29]

KEY POINTS

- Anxiety is the most common psychological disorder in cancer patients.
- Anxiety in cancer is more common in patients with preexisting anxiety disorders.
- Etiology and prevalence of anxiety among different age groups, socioeconomic conditions, and different types of cancers are identified.
- Pathophysiology and psychodynamic concepts of anxiety are discussed.
- Anxiety can be managed by pharmacological and nonpharmacological methods of treatment.

REFERENCES

1. Sheldon LK, Swanson S, Dolce A, Marsh K, Summers J. Putting evidence into practice: evidence-based interventions for anxiety. *Clin J Oncol Nurs.* 2008;12(5):789–797.

2. Mirza I, Jenkins R. Risk factors, prevalence, and treatment of anxiety and depressive disorders in Pakistan: systematic review. *BMJ.* 2004;328:794.

3. Hammerlid E, Ahlner-Elmqvist M, Bjordal K, et al. A prospective multicentre study in Sweden and Norway of mental distress and psychiatric morbidity in head and neck cancer patients. *Br J Cancer.* 1999;80(5–6):766–774.

4. Miovic M, Block S. Psychiatry disorders in advanced cancer. *Cancer.* 2007 Oct 15;110(8):1665–1676.

5. Anxiety and cancer patients. July 7, 2004. Available at: MedicineNet.com. Accessed March 25, 2010.

6. Kelvens C. Fear and anxiety. Spring 1997. Available at: CSUN.edu. Accessed March 25, 2010.

7. Cox L. Needle phobia more common than many believe. January 2008. Available at: Abcnews.go.com/health. Accessed April 13, 2010.

8. Steinman RH. The cancer patient with anxiety and chronic pain. *Int Assoc Study of Pain.* 2009;17:1–6.

9. Hersch J, Juraskova I, Price M, Mullan B. Psychosocial interventions and quality of life in gynaecological cancer patients: a systematic review. *Psychooncology.* 2009;18(8):795–810.

10. Dale W, Bilir P, Han M, Meltzer D. The role of anxiety in prostate carcinoma: a structured review of the literature. *Cancer.* 2005 1;104(3):467–478.

11. Statistics of lung cancer. 2009. Available at: Beverlyfund. org. Accessed March 25, 2010.

12. Montazeri A, Milroy R, Hole D, McEwen J, Gillis CR. Anxiety and depression in patient with lung cancer before and after diagnosis: findings from a population in Glasgow, Scotland. *J Epidemiol Community Health.* 1998;52(3):203–204.

13. Arnold SD, Forman LM, Brigidi BD, et al. Evaluation and characterization of generalized anxiety and depression in patients with primary brain tumors. *Neuro-oncol.* 2008;10(2):171–181.

14. Aass N, Fosså SD, Dahl AA, Moe TJ. Prevalence of anxiety and depression in cancer patients seen at the Norwegian Radium Hospital. *Eur J Cancer.* 1997;33(10): 1597–1604.

15. Heim C, Nemeroff CB. The impact of early adverse experiences on brain systems involved in the pathophysiology of anxiety and affective disorders. *Biol Psychiatry.* 1999;16(11):1509–1522.

16. Nemeroff CB. The role of GABA in the pathophysiology and treatment of anxiety disorders. *Psychopharmacol Bull.* 2003;37(4):133–146.

17. Milrod B, Cooper AM, Shear MK. Psychodynamic concepts of anxiety. In: Stein DJ, Hollander E, eds. *Textbook of Anxiety Disorders.* 1st ed. Washington, DC: American Psychiatric Publishing; 2001:81–92.

18. Levin TT, Alici Y. Anxiety disorders. In: Holland JC, Breltbart WS, Jacobsen PB, Lederberg ML, Loscalzo MJ, McCorkle R, eds. *Psycho-Oncology.* 2nd ed. New York, NY: Oxford University Press Publishing; 2010: 324–330.

19. Diagnostic and Statistical Manual of Mental Disorders IV Text Revision. *Anxiety Disorders.* 4th ed. Washington, DC: American Psychiatric Association Publishing; 2000:467–468.

20. Kaiko RF, Foley KM, Grabinski PY, et al. Central nervous system excitatory effects of meperidine in cancer patients. *Ann Neurol.* 1983;13:180–185.

21. Epstein SA, Hicks D. Anxiety disorders. In: Levenson JL, ed. *Textbook of Psychosomatic Medicine.* 1st ed. Arllngron, VA: American Psychiatric Publishing; 2005:251–270.

22. Holland JC, Greenberg DB, Hughes MK. Screening instruments: Hospital Anxiety and Depression Scale. In: *Quick Reference for Oncology Clinicians: The Psychiatric and Psychological Dimensions of Cancer Symptom Management.* 2004:6–18.

23. Blacker D. Hamilton Rating Scale for Anxiety. (From Hamilton M. The assessment of anxiety states by rating. *Br J Psychiatry.* 1959;32:50, with permission) Psychiatric Rating Scales. Textbook of Psychiatry. 8th ed. 2005:946.

24. Spitzer RL, Kroenke K, Williams JB, Löwe B. A brief measure for assessing generalized anxiety disorder: *The GAD-7.* (Reprinted from ARCH INTERN MED/ VOL 166). American Medical Association Publishing; 2006;1092–1097.

25. Stark DP, House, A. Anxiety in cancer patients. *Br J Cancer.* 2000;83(10):1261–1267.

26. Beck JS. Cognitive therapy: basics and beyond. *Introduction.* New York, NY: The Guilford Press Publishing; 1995:1–12.

27. Cozza KL, Armstrong SC, Oesterheld JR. *Concise Guide to Drug Interaction Principles for Medical Practice: Cytochrome P450s, UGTs, P-Glycoproteins: Metabolism in Depth: Phase II.* 2003;(3): 27–43.

28. Kaczorowski JM. Spiritual well-being and anxiety in adults diagnosed with cancer. *Hospice J.* 1990;5(3–4): 105–116.

29. Block SD. Psychological issues in end-of-life care. *J Palliat Med.* 2006;9(3):751–772.

Delirium

• *James D. Duffy and Alan D. Valentine*

■ INTRODUCTION

Every clinician should be able to recognize delirium. As the most common behavioral complication of cancer treatment, delirium is often a harbinger of a serious medical disorder and is associated with increased morbidity and mortality, and increased length and cost of hospital stay.[1–5] In addition to its physical implications, delirium typically is a terrifying experience that has a lasting psychological impact on patients and their families. The experience of delirium is remembered by the majority of patients and may result in long-term psychological morbidity for patients and their families.[6] Delirium interferes with the patient's ability to communicate and hinders the clinician's attempts to evaluate physical symptoms and to perform a detailed physical examination. Delirious patients are more likely to have an accidental fall or other injury during their hospital stay.[7] A diagnosis of delirium is a predictor of longer hospital stay and is also associated with more difficulty in identifying posthospital placement options for the patient.

Many terms have been used to describe the syndrome subsumed under the DSM-IV-TR syndrome of delirium (Table 7-1). Terms such as acute confusional state, acute brain failure, organic brain syndrome, and encephalopathy are still used by different clinicians to describe patients who meet criteria for delirium. This nosologic imprecision inevitably results in confusion among clinicians and families, and hampers the development of standardized approaches to assessment and management.[8] Because

delirium occurs so frequently in intensive care settings, it is still sometimes referred to as "ICU psychosis" and, unfortunately, may be regarded almost as a natural consequence of intensive care (the so-called "ICU psychosis").[9–11]

Lipowski[12] defined delirium as "a transient organic syndrome characterized by acute onset, global impairment of cognitive function, altered level of consciousness, inability to attend, psychomotor agitation or retardation, and disruption of sleep–wake cycle." This definition takes into account criteria not required by the *Diagnostic and Statistical Manual* of the American Psychiatric Association (Table 7-1).[13] Several important points are relevant to both definitions of delirium:

1. *Delirium is essentially a disorder of attention.* This is because the ability to focus, sustain, and redirect attention is the bedrock of all cognition and behavior. As a disorder of attention, delirium will produce impairments in virtually all areas of behavior.

2. *Delirium is a syndrome.* It is critical to realize that delirium is not a disease but is the syndromic manifestation of one or more underlying pathophysiological processes.

3. *Delirium is not caused by a preexisting psychological condition and is NOT a "functional" reaction to stress.* The prominent affective changes seen in delirium frequently lead clinicians to misinterpret behavioral change as being driven by emotional or psychodynamic factors.

4. *Delirium is a very dynamic syndrome.* Changes in attentional capacity in delirious patients will result in

■ **TABLE 7-1.** Evaluation of the Delirious Patient

History and chart review; attention to medications
Clinical interview and mental status examination
Physical examination; attention to neurological status
Laboratory assessment: complete blood count with differential and platelets, electrolytes, creatinine, BUN, calcium, magnesium, albumin, liver function tests, thyroid, glucose, RPR function tests, O2 saturation/ arterial blood gases
Chest x-ray, EKG
Urine, blood cultures, cerebral spinal fluid studies, if indicated
Serum/urine drug and alcohol screens, serum drug levels
As indicated: B_{12} and folate levels, serum drug levels, EEF brain CT/MRI

fluctuating levels of arousal, degrees of cognitive impairment, and psychomotor behavior. Patients may experience "lucid intervals" in which they appear completely intact and appear to be recovering, only to lapse back into an impaired state.

5. *Delirium is the "great psychiatric masquerader."* The myriad signs and symptoms of delirium are often misinterpreted as another psychiatric disorder. Unless the clinician maintains a high index of suspicion for delirium in all medically ill patients, the risk of misdiagnosis is high—leading to inappropriate management and a failure to recognize the precipitating physical etiology of the patient's behavioral change. Delirium is often the first sign of physical illness in the elderly and cognitively impaired patient, and its recognition can alert the astute clinician to the necessity for a thorough medical workup. The failure to detect delirium is associated with increased mortality, while earlier detection leads to lower mortality and shorter length of stays.[14,15]

■ PREVALENCE

Delirium is the most common behavioral disorder experienced by cancer patients and occurs in 26% to 44% of patients with advanced cancer admitted to an acute hospital, and as many as 80% of patients with advanced cancer will exhibit delirium in the days preceding their death.[15,16] Approximately 50% of stem cell transplant patients will experience a delirium in the first postoperative month.[17]

Most of the data relating to the prevalence of delirium have been generated from general medical populations. Prevalence rates for delirium in perioperative and critical care settings vary greatly. Most of the surgical literature involves assessment of delirium after orthopedic and cardiac surgery. In postoperative patient populations, delirium rates of 7% to 52% have been reported, with differences attributed to factors including study methodology, setting, disease site, and age of population.[18,19] Rates of greater than 40% have been detected in patients taken to surgery for hip fracture.[20,21]

■ RISK FACTORS FOR DELIRIUM

Certain patient populations are at a greater risk for becoming delirious. In the general medical population, almost two thirds of delirium occurs in the context of comorbid cognitive impairment. Delirium is 2.0 to 3.5 times more common in patients with dementia compared with nondemented controls.[22,23] In most patients, several factors act together to determine their risk for manifesting delirium. In this regard, Inouye and Charpentier have developed a predictive model that includes four predisposing factors (ie, cognitive impairment, severe illness, visual impairment, and high blood urea) and five precipitating factors (ie, more than three prescribed medications, restraints, malnutrition, catheterization, and any iatrogenic event). These factors predicted a 17-fold variation in the related risk for developing delirium.[24]

There are some data to suggest a genetic vulnerability to delirium with a reported association between polymorphisms of both the dopamine transporter gene and the neuropeptide Y gene and the risk of developing alcohol withdrawal–related delirium.[25,26] Many cancer patients are malnourished and have low serum albumin levels. This results in greater bioavailability of many drugs and a greater risk of developing their neuropsychiatric side effects such as delirium.[27]

The reversibility and prognosis of delirium is determined by the interaction between patients' premorbid vulnerability and the etiology of their delirium. Given this, younger and healthier patients with an adverse drug reaction are far more likely to have a favorable outcome compared with older, frail cancer patients with a metabolic or major organ failure etiology for their delirium.

Delirium is a potent predictor of death. Mortality rates during the index hospitalization during which delirium occurred range from 4% to 65%.[28] Agitated delirium is associated with the lowest mortality (10%) compared to 38% mortality in hypoactive delirium and 30% in mixed delirium.[29]

CLINICAL FEATURES OF DELIRIUM

Clinical manifestations of delirium can vary greatly from patient to patient. Delirium typically develops over a period of hours or a few days. The earlier stages of delirium may include irritability, anxiety, or illogical thinking that may be misdiagnosed as willful, maladaptive behavior by the patient.

Subtypes of delirium including hyperactive, hypoactive, and mixed forms have been described.[30] The *hyperactive* form of delirium includes behaviors that are likely most consistent with what clinicians routinely associate with delirium. These signs include increased psychomotor activity, often to the point of agitation or combativeness, rapid or pressured speech that is often (not always) illogical, hyperalertness or hypervigilance, hallucinations and delusions, impulsive and/or disinhibited behavior, and fluctuations of mood and affect over a range of emotional states including irritability and hostility, paroxysmal sadness, and euphoria. In the intensive care setting such presentations can constitute an active emergency, the patient being at risk to remove intravenous lines, oxygen desaturate, or self-extubate, fall, or injure bystanders. It is also this form of delirium that is most frightening to family members, because it is unexpected and often so uncharacteristic of the patient's baseline personality.

Hypoactive (apathetic) delirium produces behavioral changes that are often unrecognized, or misinterpreted as depression or amotivation. Hypoactive delirium is more likely to occur in older patients and in a palliative care setting.[31,32] The patient with hypoactive delirium demonstrates decreased motor activity, slow speech and thought processes (to the point of being blocked) though often as illogical as in the hyperactive form, a decreased level of arousal and indifference or lack of attention to external stimuli, and a flat, unreactive affect. Hypoactive delirium is associated with a higher mortality than hyperactive delirium.[33]

Mixed delirium is characterized by fluctuating features of both the hyperactive and hypoactive delirium. This fluctuation in outward behavioral signs is not surprising when one considers that waxing and waning attention is the hallmark of delirium. The behavior of a patient in a mixed delirium may vary from day to day or within a day, often without warning and without any predictability in the variability. Lucid intervals are characterized by periods in which the patient appears cognitively and behaviorally intact. It may appear that the delirium has resolved only to once again exhibit features of delirium—making therapeutic decisions difficult. Close monitoring of the patient's attentional status (as measured by bedside measures of attention such as digit span), and not simply the patient's overt behavior, is therefore important to the diagnosis and treatment of delirium.

Patients vulnerable for delirium will often experience symptoms at night or in the early morning (so-called "*sundowning*").[34] Nighttime agitation places the delirious patient at risk for gradual disruption of sleep–wake cycle, further exacerbating delirium. In intensive care settings where there may be considerable activity and sensory stimulation at all hours, a frank diurnal variation in onset or intensity of delirium may be less noticeable. In this setting it may also be more difficult to approximate a normal sleep–wake cycle, and control of the variable may be more easily obtained if/when the patient is moved out of the ICU. It is important to recognize that any increase in environmental stimuli (such as turning on a noisy television in the patient's room) will likely cause an exacerbation in the agitation of the delirious patient. The clinician should also recognize that their questioning may overwhelm the patient's limited attentional resources and precipitate escalating agitation.

ETIOLOGY OF DELIRIUM

There are numerous causes of delirium. Many of these etiologies are life threatening, but potentially reversible. A diagnosis of delirium therefore signals a medical emergency that dictates an immediate and extensive workup to determine the etiology. Although the etiology of delirium in terminally ill patients may be difficult, it can often be determined in such patients[35] (Fig. 7-1).

Medications

Medication effects may be the most common precipitants of delirium in hospitalized patients, and the list of drugs with any potential to cause altered mental status is extensive[37,38] (Table 7-2). Since an altered mental status thought secondary to effects of anesthesia is common, some investigators choose not to include the initial 24 postoperative hours in studies of delirium.[39,40] Route of delivery of anesthesia does not appear to influence development of delirium.[41] Other medications that are routinely associated

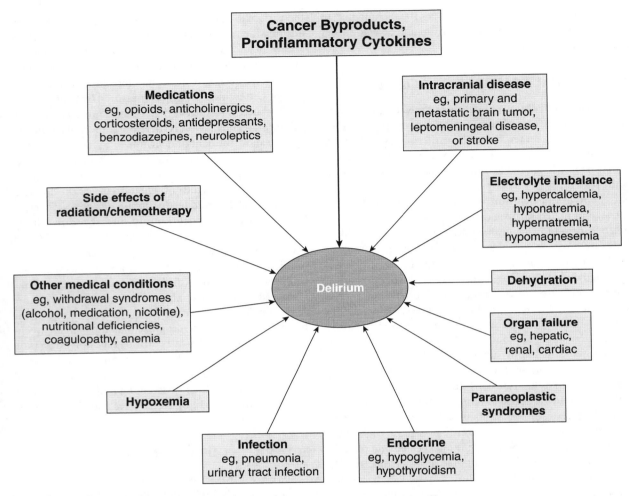

FIGURE 7-1. Factors contributing to the development of delirium in cancer patients.[36]

with altered mental status in this setting include opioid analgesics, benzodiazepine sedative-hypnotics, corticosteroids, antiarrhythmics, and sympathomimetics.[42] Anticholinergic drugs have long been associated with a characteristic hyperactive delirium and anticholinergic processes are the best studied causes of delirium.[43–45] It is important to note that geriatric patients are at a potentially higher risk for drug-induced delirium because of altered (slowed) drug metabolism and because of the higher rate of baseline cognitive impairment.

Although there are multiple causes of delirium, the clinical features are stereotypical. This suggests that delirium is produced by dysregulation in a common

pathway involving cholinergic, dopaminergic, and serotonergic neural systems.[46] In particular, any medication with anticholinergic activity is particularly likely to have delirium as a side effect. In this regard, when assessing a patient for delirium, it is important to look for other anticholinergic effects (ie, mydriasis, hyperthermia, fever without sweating, dry skin, and urinary retention).

Among cancer patients, opioids are the most common cause of delirium and more than 75% of advanced cancer patients receiving opiates exhibit altered mental status.[47] The risk for delirium doubles if the daily dose equivalent of subcutaneous morphine is above 90 mg per day.[48] Clinical features of opioid-induced neurotoxicity (OIN)

■ TABLE 7-2. Drugs Associated with Delirium (Partial List)

Anesthetics
  General: halothane, enflurane
Anticholinergics
  Atropine, scopolamine, benztropine
Anticonvulsants
  Phenytoin, carbamazepine
Antiarrhythmics
  Lidocaine, mexiletine, procainamide, amiodarone, quinidine, digoxin
Antihypertensives
  β-Blockers, clonidine, methyldopa
Antiviral agents
  Acyclovir, ganciclovir, foscarnet, interferon
Antifungal agents
  Amphotericin
Antibiotics
  Cephalosporins, chloramphenicol, tetracyclines, sulfonamides
Corticosteroids
Immunosuppressants
  Cyclosporine, FK-506
H_1-receptor antagonists
  Diphenhydramine
H_2-receptor antagonists
  Cimetidine, ranitidine
Prokinetic drugs
  Metoclopramide
Respiratory agents
  Albuterol, theophylline
Narcotic analgesics
Nonsteroidal anti-inflammatory drugs
Sedative-hypnotic drugs
  Barbiturates, benzodiazepines
Antineoplastic agents
  Cytosine arabinoside, ifosfamide, methotrexate, interleukin

include delirium, sedation, visual and tactile hallucinations, myoclonus, seizures, hyperalgesia, and allodynia. Although the pathogenesis of OIN remains uncertain, it is thought to be caused by the accumulation of toxins that produce anticholinergic effects, the endocytosis of opioid receptors, and the activation of *N*-methyl-d-aspartate receptors.[49] Meperidine is no longer recommended to treat pain because of the high rate of neurotoxicity associated with its metabolite normeperidine.

Numerous antineoplastic therapies have been associated with delirium. These include methotrexate, bleomycin, *cis*-platinum, asparginase, vinblastine, bis-chloronitrosourea, procarbazine, cytosine arabinoside, ifosfamide, tacrolimus, and cyclophosphamide.[50] Biological response modifiers, especially interleukin-2 and interferon-alpha, are, especially if used in combination, associated with delirium and sometimes with a prolonged encephalopathic state.[51]

Metabolic Disturbances

Electrolyte and metabolic abnormalities are common causes of postoperative delirium, with hypoxia (often related to respiratory failure, anemia, or both) the most frequent precipitant.[8]

Sepsis

Altered mental status can be the first sign of evolving infection. Since immunocompromised cancer patients may not mobilize any overt clinical signs of infection, the clinician should rule out sepsis as an etiology of delirium in all such patients.

Direct and Indirect CNS Effects of Cancer

These include the local CNS of primary and metastatic brain lesions, as well as paraneoplastic syndromes and leptomeningeal carcinomatosis.[51]

Substance Abuse and Withdrawal

The clinician should always be alert to the presence of alcohol withdrawal delirium and/or substance abuse. A detailed substance use history should be obtained from the patient (and the family). Alcohol withdrawal is most likely to produce an agitated delirium with florid evidence for autonomic instability. In addition to alcohol, the clinician should also be alert to the possibility of prescription benzodiazepine abuse. Opiate withdrawal should not produce delirium. The possibility of intentional overdose should always be entertained, particularly in the presence of a past psychiatric history or severe undertreated pain.

■ ASSESSMENT OF DELIRIUM

The diagnosis of delirium is clinical and based on history and observation of the patient, physical examination, and laboratory studies. As noted above, presentations

■ **TABLE 7-3.** Differential Diagnosis of Delirium

Dementia
Major depression
Substance intoxication, withdrawal
Schizophrenia/schizophreniform disorder
Bipolar mania
Brief psychotic disorder
Nonspecific agitation
    Unrelieved pain
    Hypoxia
    Anxiety, fear
    Akathisia

of delirium can closely resemble other neuropsychiatric disorders and conditions in which there is no global impairment of central nervous system function (Tables 7-3 and 7-4).

Screening Instruments

Several screening instruments are available to assist in the assessment of delirious patients. However, even the most reliable and frequently used instruments have a significant associated error rate, and all patients who score above threshold levels on these scales should go on to careful clinical evaluation. Furthermore, the clinician should not rely entirely on these instruments and should always closely evaluate the mental status of any patient who exhibits behavioral change of any kind.

The Mini-Mental State Examination (MMSE) may be the most frequently used screen of cognitive function and is often employed to assess delirious patients. However, it does not distinguish delirium from dementia and patients may score poorly on the test for a number of reasons not directly related to delirium.[52] The MMSE is therefore not a suitable instrument for assessing delirium.

The Confusion Assessment Method (CAM) developed by Inouye et al[53] is frequently used and is designed to allow nonpsychiatric clinicians to screen for presence of delirium. It has been modified for use in ICU settings with patients who are intubated or otherwise unable to communicate.[54,55] Other instruments including the Delirium Rating Scale (DRS) and the Memorial Delirium Assessment Scale (MDAS) are used more frequently to assess severity of delirium and can be used to follow patients over time and assess response to therapy, and also as research instruments.[56,57]

Clinical Evaluation and Mental Status Examination

The clinical evaluation of a patient thought to be delirious will include elements of history, observation and interview of the patient, and mental status examination.[8] The patient is likely to be unreliable or unavailable (eg, an intubated patient) as a historian, so it is often necessary to rely on family members, nursing staff, and others for information on the time course and characteristics (including diurnal variation with symptoms worse at night) of changes in behavior, arousal, and cognitive function. History of use of medications, use or discontinuation of alcohol and illicit drugs, baseline cognitive function, and other events (eg, falls) are critical in consideration of possible evolving delirium.

Observation and clinical interview of the patient includes assessment of level of arousal, psychomotor agitation or retardation, affective stability, distractibility, impersistence, and assessment for presence of illusions, hallucination, and delusions. It is important to keep in mind that the patient in the early or prodromal stages of a delirium may show little evidence of abnormality to observation.[8]

Depending on the patient's behavioral status, it may or may not be possible to complete a detailed mental status examination. Since delirium is essentially a disorder of attention, the most important part of the mental status exam is an assessment of the patient's attentional status. Simple tasks of attention include days, months, and digit span forwards and backwards. The delirious patient will

■ **TABLE 7-4.** Behavioral Aids to Management of Delirium

Maintain background light and sound
    Music or television
    Lights dimmed at night
Reorient patient frequently
    Calendars, message boards
Minimize sensory deprivation
    Replace glasses or hearing aides
Facilitate patient contact with family and other support symptoms
Maintain communication with family, caregivers
Use physical restraints only if absolutely necessary
    Check patient and release restrains frequently
    Consider one-on-one attendant as alternative

perform poorly on these tasks, and in such cases, there is nothing to be gained from further detailed cognitive testing. It is helpful to obtain a quantitative determination of the patient's attention (eg, digits forwards and backwards) that can be used as a baseline against which to measure his or her progress.

Physical Examination

A thorough physical examination is a vital part of the clinical assessment of the delirious patient. Clinical evidence of anticholinergic toxicity should be assessed. Stigmata for chronic alcohol use may provide important clues on etiology. The neurological examination should identify any localizing signs or evidence for intracranial sepsis or raised intracranial pressure.

Laboratory Assessment and Other Tests

All laboratory and/or neurodiagnostic workup should be directed by a reasoned diagnostic hypothesis. Having said this, particularly in severely obtunded patients, the workup of the delirious patient is often empirical and includes a wide range of tests. This includes serum chemistries: electrolytes, creatinine, blood urea nitrogen, calcium, magnesium, liver function assays, thyroid functions, as well as urinalysis and complete blood count with differential and platelet count. Chest x-ray and EKG should be reviewed or obtained. Serum drug levels should be checked in patients on some medications including immunosuppressants (eg, cyclosporine, tacrolimus), anticonvulsants, cardiac drugs (eg, digoxin), and psychotropics (eg, lithium, tricyclic antidepressants), and in patients known or suspected of use of illicit drugs. Vitamin B_{12} and serum folate levels should be checked in patients known or suspected to be alcohol-dependent.

Other tests should be considered in certain settings, but are probably not routinely necessary. Neuroimaging (CT, MRI) may be helpful if physical exam reveals focal neurological signs, and in the absence of other obvious causes of delirium, or when delirium persists despite appropriate treatment. The electroencephalogram (EEG) will almost always reveal diffuse, nonspecific slowing in the delirious patient. While EEG evaluation is probably not routinely necessary, it should be obtained in cases of suspected seizures. The EEG may also be useful in attempts to distinguish delirium from other causes of similar behavior (eg, dementia, severe depression, "functional" psychiatric disorders).[58]

■ MANAGEMENT

Prevention

The potential consequences of delirium are such that it should be prevented or detected and treated as early as possible. Patients who might be expected to develop delirium (eg, geriatrics, known cognitive impairment, alcohol dependence) should be monitored closely and evaluated frequently. Preoperative assessment that predicts and allows for early intervention has potential to significantly impact morbidity and costs associated with intensive treatment.[59]

Although repeated formal attempts have been made to prevent delirium, a recent Cochrane review concluded that the evidence on the efficacy of interventions to prevent delirium is sparse. However, Inouye et al[60,61] reported that an environmental intervention program was effective in reducing the incidence of delirium in elderly hospitalized patients.

Behavioral and Environmental Management

As described above, the physical environment will have a powerful influence on the clinical manifestations of delirium. In particular, the typical ICU environment is likely to exacerbate the agitation of a delirious patient. Every effort should be made to reduce sensory stimulation, normalize the sleep–wake cycle, and provide environmental cues that will orient patients to their location and the date. Family members are likely to be very comforting for the patient but should be instructed to avoid becoming too emotionally demonstrative or intrusive. The patient should be treated in a room that is sheltered from other activities in the ICU. Physical restraints should be avoided and are considered a last resort for behavioral management. In most cases, the delirious patient (particularly if agitated) will require constant observation so that fall injuries or other potentially self-injurious behaviors can be avoided. It is important to recognize delirium early in its course and not to defer treatment until the patient exhibits florid symptoms.

Pharmacotherapy

Until reversible causes for delirium have been identified and treated, pharmacotherapy remains the mainstay of treatment. Unfortunately, because of the very practical limitations imposed by the ethical constraints inherent to any study of the delirious patient, the scientific database for assessing the most effective and safest strategy for treating delirium remains sparse. In this regard, a 2007 Cochrane review reported only three studies that meet criteria for review.[62]

The aim of psychopharmacological treatment of delirium is to optimize the patient's behaviors and cognitive function without causing excess sedation. Neuroleptics remain the first-line treatment of choice with haloperidol, a potent D2 receptor antagonist with little anticholinergic activity, the most commonly used agent.[62] Although not approved for intravenous administration, haloperidol is routinely and effectively given by this route, facilitating rapid delivery, and usually produces minimal anticholinergic toxicity, extrapyramidal effects, or effects on cardiac, respiratory, and hepatic function.[63–66]

Although the dosage requirements vary, mild agitation can typically be managed with 0.5 to 2.0 mg haloperidol slowly intravenously and moderate to severe agitation with 2.0 to 5.0 haloperidol. Rather than utilizing escalating doses, the authors recommend more frequent dosing (up to every 30 minutes if necessary). Once the patient's agitation is stabilized, a scheduled dose of haloperidol every 4 to 6 hours (with hourly prn doses available) is usually effective. Once the etiology of the patient's delirium has been identified and reversed, it is usually possible to taper the haloperidol scheduled dose over the next 1 or 2 days. The rate of dose taper will be dependent on the patient's comorbid risk factors. The American Psychiatric Association[66] guidelines for the treatment of delirium recommend low-dose haloperidol (ie, 1–2 mg PO every 4 hours as needed or 0.25–0.50 mg PO every 4 hours in elderly patients).

Benzodiazepines are not a first-line treatment for delirium and may actually exacerbate cognitive dysfunction and may increase psychomotor agitation in the delirious patient.[68] However, if control of severe agitation is not achieved with two to three doses of haloperidol, it is often necessary to add an intravenous benzodiazepine (ie, lorazepam, midazolam) or propofol with the goal of sedating the patient until haloperidol is effective and/or the etiology of the patient's delirium has been identified. Such patients require close observation and should be managed in the intensive care unit. It is important to identify patients who are in alcohol withdrawal since they will require both a benzodiazepine (for management of alcohol withdrawal) and a neuroleptic (for management of psychosis and agitation).

Although intravenous haloperidol is usually well tolerated, it has been associated with Q-Tc interval prolongation and ventricular arrhythmia (torsades de pointes). In 2007, the FDA[69] recommended electrocardiogram monitoring for all patients receiving intravenous haloperidol. Risk factors for developing torsades de pointes include congenital prolonged Q-T syndrome, underlying heart disease, bradycardia, ischemic heart disease, female sex, liver disease, electrolyte imbalances, concomitant use of other medications that may prolong the Q-T interval, and rapid and high dose of haloperidol.[70] Correction of reversible risk factors and cardiac monitoring with measurement of Q-Tc intervals is therefore recommended in all patients receiving intravenous haloperidol, with reduction or discontinuation of haloperidol if the Q-Tc interval is above 450 milliseconds or increases 25% over baseline.[71,72] Akathisia should be suspected if motor agitation increases with escalation of haloperidol doses.

The atypical antipsychotics (eg, risperidone, olanzapine, quetiapine, ziprasidone, aripiprazole) are increasingly being used to treat delirium. The 2007 Cochrane review concluded that haloperidol (at a dose of 3.5 mg per day), olanzapine, and risperidone were equally effective in the treatment of delirium.[69] In a study of delirium in elderly hospitalized patients,[73] olanzapine was found to be effective in 76% of patients. Patients with hypoactive delirium, over age 70, and/or dementia were less likely to demonstrate therapeutic benefit from olanzapine. The starting dose of olanzapine in this study was 2.5 to 5 mg with up to a total daily dose of 20 mg. In a study of oncology patients, oral risperidol (mean dose 1.02 mg daily) was reported to be equally effective as oral haloperidol (mean dose 1.71 mg daily) for the treatment of delirium.[74] Haloperidol doses above 4.5 mg are more likely to produce EPS when compared with atypical antipsychotics. However, lower-dose haloperidol (ie, below 3.5 mg daily) does not appear to have a high incidence of EPS.[62,74] Although the atypical antipsychotics are attractive because they are less likely to produce Q-Tc interval prolongation and extrapyramidal effects, the lack of available IV preparations limits their utility in ICU settings. Given its beneficial side-effect profile (ie, more sedation and less effect on the Q-T interval), quetiapine is being prescribed with increasing frequency to treat delirium. A double-blind study reported that quetiapine, when dose-escalated to desired effect, may be associated with faster resolution of delirium, reduced time of delirium and agitation, and a more favorable disposition at hospital discharge than patients who receive as-needed intravenous haloperidol therapy alone.[75]

Although cholinesterase inhibitors have been described in case reports to help some delirious patients, a Cochrane review does not support their routine use for this indication.[76]

As described above, opiates are a frequent cause of delirium in cancer patients. In such situations, lowering the dose of the offending opiate and/or switching to another opiate usually results in rapid resolution of the patient's delirium.

■ SUMMARY

Delirium is the most common behavioral disorder encountered in cancer patients. It is often a harbinger of a serious, often life-threatening medical condition. All clinicians should therefore be able to recognize the signs of delirium and recognize that it represents a medical, and not simply a psychiatric, emergency.

KEY POINTS

- Delirium is essentially a disorder of attention.
- Delirium represents a medical emergency.
- Delirium may often be misdiagnosed as another psychiatric disorder.
- Delirium is more common in patients with cognitive deficits.
- The agitation associated with delirium can be effectively treated with psychopharmacological agents.

REFERENCES

1. Tuma R, DeAngelis LM. Altered mental status in patients with cancer. *Arch Neurol.* 2000;57(12):1727–1731.

2. Tune L, Carr S, Cooper T, Klug B, Golinger RC. Association of anticholinergic activity of prescribed medications with postoperative delirium. *J Neuropsychiatry Clin Neurosci.* 1993;5(2):208–210.

3. Ely EW, Gautam S, Margolin R, et al. The impact of delirium in the intensive care unit on hospital length of stay. *Intensive Care Med.* 2001;27(12):1892–1900.

4. Caraceni A, Nanni O, Maltoni M, et al. Impact of delirium on the short term prognosis of advanced cancer patients. Italian Multicenter Study Group on Palliative Care. *Cancer.* 2000;89(5):1145–1149.

5. Franco K, Litaker D, Locala J, Bronson D. The cost of delirium in the surgical patient. *Psychosomatics.* 2001;42(1):68–73.

6. Breitbart W, Gibson C, Tremblay A. The delirium experience: delirium recall and delirium-related distress in hospitalized patients with cancer, their spouses/caregivers, and their nurses. *Psychosomatics.* 2002;43(3):183–194.

7. Pautex S, Hermann FR, Zulian GB. Factors associated with falls in patients with cancer hospitalized for palliative care. *J Palliat Med.* 2008;11:878–884.

8. Lipowski ZJ. Update on delirium. *Psychiatr Clin North Am.* 1992;15(2):335–346.

9. Curtis T. 'Climbing the walls' ICU psychosis: myth or reality? *Nurs Crit Care.* 1999;4(1):18–21.

10. Fricchione G. What is an ICU psychosis? *Harv Ment Health Lett.* 1999;16(6):7.

11. McGuire BE, Basten CJ, Ryan CJ, Gallagher J. Intensive care unit syndrome: a dangerous misnomer. *Arch Intern Med.* 2000;160(7):906–909.

12. Lipowski ZJ. *Delirium: Acute Confusional States.* New York, NY: Oxford University Press; 1990.

13. American Psychiatric Association. *Diagnostic and Statistical Manual of Mental Disorders.* 4th ed. Washington, DC: American Psychiatric Association; 1994.

14. Kakuma R, du Fort GG, Arsenault L. Delirium in older emergency department patients discharged home: effect on survival. *J Am Geriatr Soc.* 2003;51:443–450.

15. Rockwood K, Cosway S, Stolee P. Increasing the recognition of delirium in elderly patients. *J Am Geriatr Soc.* 1994;42:252–256.

16. Liptzin B, Levkoff SE. An empirical study of delirium subtypes. *Br J Psychiatry.* 1992;161:843–845.

17. Fann JR, Roth-Rowmer S, Burington BE. Delirium in patients undergoing hematopoetic stem cell transplantation. *Cancer.* 2002;95:1971–1981.

18. Bucht G, Gustafson Y, Sandberg O. Epidemiology of delirium. *Dement Geriatr Cogn Disord.* 1999;10(5):315–318.

19. van der Mast RC. Postoperative delirium. *Dement Geriatr Cogn Disord.* 1999;10(5):401–405.

20. Galanakis P, Bickel H, Gradinger R, Von Gumppenberg S, Forstl H. Acute confusional state in the elderly following hip surgery: incidence, risk factors and complications. *Int J Geriatr Psychiatry.* 2001;16(4):349–355.

21. Holmes JD, House AO. Psychiatric illness in hip fracture. *Age Ageing.* 2000;29(6):537–546.

22. Wahlund L, Bjorlin GA. Delirium in clinical practice: experience from a specialized delirium ward. *Dement Geriatr Cogn Disord.* 1999;10:389–392.

23. Erkinjuntti T, Wokstrom J, Parlo J. Dementia among medical inpatients: evaluation of 2000 consecutive admissions. *Arch Intern Med.* 1986;146:1923–1926.

24. Inouye SK, Charpentier PA. Precipitating factors for delirium in hospitalized elderly patients: predictive model and interrelationships with baseline variability. *JAMA.* 1996;275:852–857.

25. Gorwood P, Limosin F, Batel P. The A9 allele of the dopamine transporter gene is associated with delirium tremens and alcohol-withdrawal seizure. *Biol Psychiatry.* 2003;53:85–92.

26. Koehnke MD, Schick S, Lutz U. Severity of alcohol withdrawal symptoms and the T1128C polymorphism of the neuropeptide Y gene. *J Neural Transm.* 2002;109:1423–1429.

27. Dickson LR. Hypoalbuminemia in delirium. *Psychosomatics.* 1991;32:317–323.

28. Cameron DJ, Thomas RI, Mulvihill M. Delirium: a test of DSM-III criteria on medical patients. *J Am Geriatr Soc.* 1987;35:1007–1010.

29. Oloffson SM, Weitzner MA, Valentine AD. A retrospective study of the psychiatric management and outcome of delirium in the cancer patient. *Support Care Cancer.* 1996;4:351–357.

30. Lipowski ZJ. Delirium (acute confusional states). *JAMA.* 1987;258(13):1789–1792.

31. Peterson JF, Bun BT, Dittus RS, et al. Delirium and its motoric subtypes: a study of 614 critically ill patients. *J Am Geriatr Soc.* 2006;54(3):479–484.

32. Spiller JA, Keen JC. Hypoactive delirium: assessing the extent of the problem for inpatient specialist palliative care. *Palliat Med.* 2006;20(1):17–23.

33. Leonard M, Raju B, Conroy M, et al. Reversibility of delirium in terminally ill patients and predictors of mortality. *Palliat Med.* 2008;22(7):848–854.

34. Burney-Puckett M. Sundown syndrome: etiology and management. *J Psychosoc Nurs Ment Health Serv.* 1996;34(5):40–43.

35. Bruera E, Miller L, McCallion J, Macmillan K, Krefting L, Hanson J. Cognitive failure in patients with terminal cancer: a prospective study. *J Pain Symptom Manage.* 1992;7(4):192–195.

36. Bush SH, Bruera E. The assessment and management of delirium in cancer patients. *Oncologist.* 2009;14:1039–1049.

37. Brown TM, Stoudemire A. *Psychiatric Side Effects of Prescription and Over-the-counter Medications.* Washington, DC: American Psychiatric Press Inc; 1998.

38. Brown TM. Drug-induced delirium. *Semin Clin Neuropsychiatry.* 2000;5(2):113–124.

39. Rasmussen LS, Moller JT. Central nervous system dysfunction after anesthesia in the geriatric patient. *Anesthesiol Clin North Am.* 2000;18(1):59–70.

40. Boucher BA, Witt WO, Foster TS. The postoperative adverse effects of inhalational anesthetics. *Heart Lung J Acute Crit Care.* 1986;15(1):63–69.

41. Parikh SS, Chung F. Postoperative delirium in the elderly. *Anesth Analg.* 1995;80(6):1223–1232.

42. Marcantonio ER, Juarez G, Goldman L, et al. The relationship of postoperative delirium with psychoactive medications. *JAMA.* 1994;272(19):1518–1522.

43. Tune LE, Damlouji NF, Holland A, Gardner TJ, Folstein MF, Coyle JT. Association of postoperative delirium with raised serum levels of anticholinergic drugs. *Lancet.* 1981;2(8248):651–653.

44. Tune LE. Post-operative delirium. *Int Psychogeriatr.* 1991;3:325–332.

45. Trzepacz PT. Delirium. Advances in diagnosis, pathophysiology, and treatment. *Psychiatr Clin North Am.* 1996;19(3):429–448.

46. Trepacz PT. Is there a final common pathway in delirium? Focus on acetylcholine and dopamine. *Semin Clin Neuropsychiatry.* 2000;5(2):132–148.

47. Leipzig RM, Goodman H, Gray G. Reversible narcotic-associated mental status impairment in patients with metastatic cancer. *Pharmacology.* 1987;35:47–54.

48. Gaudreau JD, Gagnon P, Harel F, et al. Psychoactive medications and risk of delirium in hospitalized cancer patients. *J Clin Oncol.* 2005;23:6712–6718.

49. Vella-Brincat J, MacLeod AD. Adverse effects of opioids on the central nervous systems of palliative care patients. *J Pain Palliat Care Pharmacother.* 2007;62:521–525.

50. Breitbart W, Friedlander M. Confusion/delirium. In: Bruera E, Higginson I, Ripamonti C, von Gunten C, eds. *Palliative Medicine.* London, UK: London Hodder Press; 2006:688–700.

51. Meyers CA, Valentine AD. Neurological and psychiatric adverse effects of immunological therapy. *CNS Drugs.* 1995;3:56–58.

52. Folstein MF, Folstein SE, McHugh PR. "Mini-mental state". A practical method for grading the cognitive state of patients for the clinician. *J Psychiatr Res.* 1975;12(3):189–198.

53. Inouye SK, van Dyck CH, Alessi CA, Balkin S, Siegal AP, Horwitz RI. Clarifying confusion: the confusion assessment method. A new method for detection of delirium. *Ann Intern Med.* 1990;113(12):941–948.

54. Bergeron N, Dubois MJ, Dumont M, Dial S, Skrobik Y. Intensive Care Delirium Screening Checklist: evaluation of a new screening tool. *Intensive Care Med.* 2001;27(5):859–864.

55. Bergeron N, Skrobik Y, Dubois MJ. Delirium in critically ill patients. *Crit Care (Lond).* 2002;6(3):181–182.

56. Trzepacz PT, Baker RW, Greenhouse J. A symptom rating scale for delirium. *Psychiatry Res.* 1988;23(1):89–97.

57. Breitbart W, Rosenfeld B, Roth A, Smith MJ, Cohen K, Passik S. The Memorial Delirium Assessment Scale. *J Pain Symptom Manage.* 1997;13(3):128–137 [comment].

58. Jacobson SA, Leuchter AF, Walter DO. Conventional and quantitative EEG in the diagnosis of delirium among the elderly. *J Neurol Neurosurg Psychiatry.* 1993;56(2):153–158.

59. Inouye SK. Prevention of delirium in hospitalized older patients: risk factors and targeted intervention strategies. *Ann Med.* 2000;32(4):257–263.

60. Siddiqi N, Stockdale R, Britton AM, Holmes J. Interventions for preventing delirium in hospitalized patients. *Cochrane Database Syst Rev.* 2007;(2):CD005563.

61. Inouye SK, Bogardus ST, Charpentier PA. A multicomponent intervention to prevent delirium in hospitalized older patients. *N Engl J Med.* 1999;340(9):669–766.

62. Lonergan E, Britton AM, Luxenberg J. Antipsychotics for delirium. *Cochrane Database Syst Rev.* 2007;(2):CD005594.

63. Adams F. Emergency intravenous sedation of the delirious, medically ill patient. *J Clin Psychiatry.* 1988;49(suppl):22–27.

64. Akechi T, Uchitomi Y, Okamura H, et al. Usage of haloperidol for delirium in cancer patients. *Support Care Cancer.* 1996;4(5):390–392.

65. Crippen DW. Pharmacologic treatment of brain failure and delirium. *Crit Care Clin.* 1994;10(4):733–766.

66. Fish DN. Treatment of delirium in the critically ill patient. *Clin Pharm.* 1991;10(6):456–466.

67. American Psychiatric Press Association. Practice guidelines for the treatment of delirium. *Am J Psychiatry.* 199;156:S1–S20.

68. Breitbart W, Marotta R, Platt MM, et al. A double-blind trial of haloperidol, chlorpromazine, and lorazepam in the treatment of delirium in hospitalized AIDS patients. *Am J Psychiatry.* 1996;153(2):231–237.

69. U.S. Food and Drug Administration. *Haloperidol (Marketed as Haldol, Haldol Decanoate and Haldol Lactate).* Silver Spring, MD: U.S. Food and Drug Administration; 2007.

70. Zemrak WR, Kenna GA. Association of antipsychotic and antidepressant drugs with Q-T interval prolongation. *Am J Health Syst Pharm.* 2008;65:1029–1038.

71. Metzger E, Friedman R. Prolongation of the corrected QT and torsades de pointes cardiac arrhythmia associated with intravenous haloperidol in the medically ill. *J Clin Psychopharmacol.* 1993;13(2):128–132.

72. Lawrence KR, Nasraway SA. Conduction disturbances associated with administration of butyrophenone antipsychotics in the critically ill: a review of the literature. *Pharmacotherapy.* 1997;17(3):531–537.

73. Breitbart W, Tremblay A, Gibson C. An open trial of olanzapine for the treatment of delirium in hospitalized cancer patients. *Psychosomatics.* 2002;43(3):175–182.

74. Han CS, Kim Y. A double-blind trial of risperidone and haloperidol for the treatment of delirium. *Psychosomatics.* 2004;45(4):297–301.

75. Devlin, JW, Roberts, RJ, Fong, JJ, et al. Efficacy and safety of quetiapine in critically ill patients with delirium: a prospective, multicenter, randomized, double-blind, placebo-controlled pilot study. *Crit Care Med.* 2010;38(2):419–427.

76. Overshott R, Karim S, Burns A. Cholinesterase inhibitors for delirium. *Cochrane Database Syst Rev.* 2008;(1):CD005317.

Nicotine Dependence

• Maher Karam-Hage and Paul Cinciripini

In the United States approximately 443,000 deaths in 2007 were attributable to cigarette smoking, according to the Centers for Disease Control and Prevention (CDC). This number makes cigarette smoking the principal cause of premature death and disability in the country.[1] In addition, the average annual smoking-attributable health care expenditures nationwide were approximately $96 billion during 2001–2004. Then when combined with productivity losses of $97 billion, the total economic burden of smoking was approximately $193 billion per year.[2] Furthermore, the International Agency for Research on Cancer has reported that tobacco smoking is causally linked to 13 types of neoplastic disease.[3] Unfortunately, despite tobacco control efforts, including public education about the health hazards of smoking, many smokers continue to encounter extreme difficulty quitting and maintaining long-term abstinence from tobacco.

According to the 2007 National Health Interview Survey, one fifth of the US population consisted of current smokers, smoking rates were substantially higher among those with less than a high school education than those with more education, and 40% of the current smokers had made at least one quit attempt of at least 24 hours in the previous year.[1] According to the National Survey on Drug Use and Health performed that same year, nearly 42% of adults 18 to 25 years old reported using cigarettes in the previous month, whereas only 8% reported using an illicit drug and 7% were classified as heavy alcohol users.[4] Finally, in the most recent Monitoring the Future (MTF) survey conducted in 2009, 20%, 33%, and 43% of 8th-, 10th-, and 12th-grade students, respectively,

reported that they had smoked cigarettes in their lifetime, as well as 9%, 15%, and 16%, respectively, reported they have used smokeless tobacco in their lifetime.[5]

Although most smokers (~70%) report an interest in quitting, if not receiving assistance in smoking cessation, fewer than 6% are abstinent at 1 month after their quit date and fewer than 2% are abstinent at 1 year.[6] Difficulty in maintaining abstinence is strongly related to affective and cognitive dysfunction, which may persist for some time after the initial cessation in addition to postcessation cigarette cravings.[7]

The health consequences associated with smoking tobacco are substantial and life-threatening. Smoking is the primary causal factor for 30% of deaths due to cancer and 80% of deaths related to chronic obstructive pulmonary disease.[8] The three leading causes of smoking-attributable deaths are lung cancer, ischemic heart disease, and chronic obstructive pulmonary disease. In the last half century the number of smoking-related deaths has remained relatively unchanged even though cigarette use has declined substantially.[2]

■ BIOLOGICAL, BEHAVIORAL, AND COGNITIVE ASPECTS OF NICOTINE DEPENDENCE

The Reward Pathway

Like most drugs associated with abuse and dependence, nicotine stimulates a rapid increase in dopamine release in the nucleus accumbens and the ventral tegmental area. The stimulation typically occurs within 10 seconds

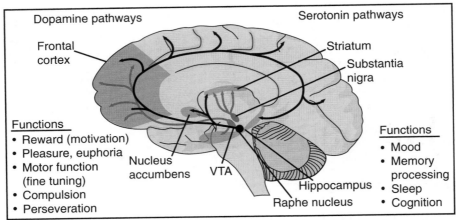

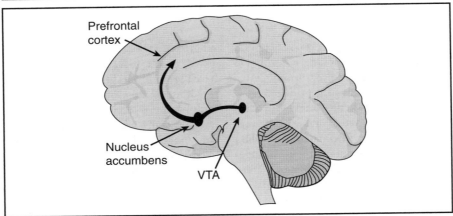

FIGURE 8-1. The dopamine and serotonin pathways with their respective functions, contrasted to the reward pathway consisting of the nucleus accumbens and ventral tegmental area (VTA) with projections to the frontal and prefrontal cortex.[12]

of smoking a cigarette.[9–11] Under normal circumstances, these two areas of the brain are activated by the consumption of food, social affiliation, and sexual activity, which are all activities linked to survival of the individual or species. The key component of the reward pathway within the mesocorticolimbic system is the neurotransmitter dopamine. The reward pathway projects from the nucleus accumbens and ventral tegmental area to the prefrontal cortex, the amygdala, and the olfactory tubercle (Fig. 8-1). Several other brain systems (neurotransmitters and pathways) are thought to be involved in the process of addiction to a substance, while dopamine appears to be the final common neurotransmitter in the reward pathway. The γ-aminobutyric acid, glutamate, and cholinergic systems have been shown to be involved

in the process of neuroadaptation that in the long term leads to addiction.[13]

Nicotine stimulates the reward pathway via nicotinic receptors that trigger several neurotransmitter systems. Nicotinic receptors, which are a subtype of cholinergic receptors, are present throughout the central nervous system, and they exert various effects (excitatory, inhibitory, or modulatory) depending on their location in the brain, which impacts the level of activity of several neurotransmitters, including dopamine, norepinephrine, serotonin, glutamate, and γ-aminobutyric acid. In addition, the endogenous opioid and the cannabinoid-1 (CB-1) receptors are thought to modulate nucleus accumbens activity that results from nicotinic receptor activation.[14] In summary, in the last several decades research on nicotine addiction has focused primarily on dopamine, which is believed to be the main determinant of nicotine and other drug addictions.[3,9,15,16] However, the neurotransmitter systems involved in addiction probably include most, if not all, of the other major systems in the brain in a dynamic interplay. This interaction is thought to result in the neuroadaptations necessary to form and maintain substance addiction.[17]

Neuronal Adaptation

Some individuals are more vulnerable than others to substance abuse or dependence. This vulnerability is mediated by genetic, environmental, and cultural factors. The pleasurable sensation produced by activation of the reward pathway is associated with the acute use of a substance such as nicotine. Repeated administration of nicotine over months or years is likely to lead to increased tolerance, and then to withdrawal in the absence of nicotine. Tolerance and withdrawal are the physiologic hallmarks of dependence and are thought to be related to neuroadaptive effects occurring within the brain.[18] Interestingly, the chronic use of drugs of abuse and dependence (including nicotine) appears to result in a generalized decrease in dopaminergic neurotransmission. This decrease is likely to be as a *homeostatic* response to the intermittent yet repetitive increases in dopamine induced by the frequent and sustained use of such drugs.[19] Another implication of neuroadaptation is the increase in levels of corticotropin-releasing factor induced by substance use or abuse; this increase is associated with the activation of central stress pathways. Sensitization and counteradaptation are the two major neuroadaptive models that have been proposed. That is to explain how changes in reward pathway may result in the development of substance dependence. Sensitization can be thought of as an increase in "wanting" a drug after intermittent but repeated use; this can facilitate the transition from occasional use to chronic use and tolerance.[20] The counteradaptation model postulates that the initial positive feelings of reward (resulting from the use of a drug) are followed by an opposing rather than synchronous development of tolerance. Finally, tolerance is often manifested by the appearance of withdrawal symptoms associated with the lack of the substance.[21]

Other models of nicotine addiction are based on mechanisms associated with cognitive control and reinforcement learning,[22] in particular the negative reinforcement associated with withdrawal from nicotine, which is usually followed by reduction in negative affect when smoking a cigarette.[23]

Cognitive Impairment

While much of the focus of earlier research on nicotine addiction has been related to its effects on reward processes and mesolimbic dopamine neurotransmission,[3,9,11,15,16] a growing body of literature has accumulated on nicotine's noradrenergic and dopaminergic effects on attention, information processing, and affective regulation. These effects may be of considerable importance in understanding the maintenance of dependence. Neurologic deficits common to attention deficit and substance use disorders, such as impaired performance, lack of motivation, decreased working memory, and impaired executive function, have been well documented[24] for both children and adults.[25–29] Overlapping and interrelated brain areas may be responsible for the attentional and executive impairments common to the two disorders.[30,31] The involvement of the prefrontal cortex and anterior cingulate cortex in both drug dependence and attentional/cognitive disorders, including nicotine and neurophysiologic deficits related to cognitive dysfunction, highlights such commonalities.

Drug-addicted individuals, including smokers, continue to use drugs even when faced with negative consequences and diminished reward, which suggests loss of control.[20] The failure to regulate (ie, inhibit) this drive points to a dysfunction within the prefrontal cortex,[17] the anterior cingulate, and orbitofrontal cortices.[32]

Nicotine and Negative Affect

One of the most fundamental aspects of nicotine dependence involves its neuroregulatory function on mood. The relationship between negative affect and the maintenance and cessation of smoking behavior plays a prominent role in theories of nicotine dependence.[23] In this model of negative affect it is theorized that individuals addicted to a substance learn to detect internal cues. Those internal cues signal that negative affect is approaching as drug levels fall within the body. To prevent the onset of these negative feelings, the addicted person would self-administer the drug. This process often proceeds without conscious awareness, but the longer an individual is without the drug, the more likely these negative feelings will enter the person's conscious awareness, thus providing direct reinforcement that taking the drug does relieve his or her negative affect. This relationship has driven the development of new pharmacologic[33–35] and behavioral[36,37] approaches to the treatment of addiction.

The experience of negative affect is a significant contributor to the risk of relapse, and many smokers cite reducing negative affect as an important reason to smoke. The term "negative affect" refers to a composite index of many negative mood states, including feelings of depression, dysphoria, irritability, and nervousness. Negative affect is usually measured by Likert-type scales such as the Positive and Negative Affect Schedule (PANAS),[38] the Profile of Mood States (POMS),[39] and similar checklists of adjectives.[40]

Finally, negative affect that follows a quit attempt has been related to treatment failure and relapse across a variety of treatment modalities.[7,41,42] Indeed, the presence of negative affect following cessation has been found to characterize more than half of all smoking lapses, and one fifth of lapses occur under conditions of extreme negative mood.[40]

Genetics

Heritability
Recent family, twin, and molecular genetic studies have provided compelling evidence of a role of genetic factors in governing smoking initiation, continuation, and cessation. Estimated heritability rates are in a range of 47% to 76% for initiation and 62% for persistence.[43–48] The concordance rates for smoking, not smoking, and quitting are higher for monozygotic than for dizygotic twins, and the concordance rate for smoking in 82 pairs of identical twins reared apart was 79%.[44] A meta-analysis of data from eight studies revealed an estimated heritability rate of 60% for smoking; for the maintenance of dependent smoking behavior, the percent genetic contribution is about 70%.[49] Three linkage studies of smoking behavior have suggested that the alleles that influence smoking behavior occur in only a small proportion of families.[50–52]

Genome-wide Association Studies of Nicotine Dependence and Treatment Outcome
The following genome-wide association studies related to nicotine dependence have recently been published. Uhl et al[53] used 520,000 single-nucleotide polymorphisms and the DNA pooling approach. They prepared pools of DNA from nicotine-dependent European–American participants in a smoking cessation trial and control individuals and then analyzed the results between smokers and nonsmokers and between successful and unsuccessful quitters to identify several genes of interest. Uhl and colleagues[54] also conducted a genome-wide association study to examine successful versus unsuccessful quitters across three clinical trials. One trial used nicotine replacement (results from this sample were also previously published by this group[53]) and two trials used bupropion in mixed racial samples. The combined sample for all three trials totaled 540 individuals (124 in the nicotine replacement therapy [NRT] trials and 266 and 150, respectively, in the two bupropion trials). Altogether, several thousand single-nucleotide polymorphisms with nominal significance and covering more than 100 genes were noted. Clearly, much more information is needed, taking a more traditional approach than genome-wide association techniques. That is to examine both the predictors of abstinence and the pharmacogenetic effects of smoking cessation medications.

Candidate Gene Studies for Nicotine Dependence and Treatment Outcome
More than 60 unique genes have been noted in candidate gene studies of nicotine dependence. Several reviews have been published in this area,[55–60] mostly concluding that small sample size and replicability pose significant issues in interpreting the study results. The limited characterization of the phenotype (ie, simple classification as a smoker or nonsmoker) may further restrict the information that can be obtained from these studies. Most of the assessed candidate genes involve nicotine metabolism or the function of central nervous system receptors or neuron transmitters. These genes include all the major single-nucleotide polymorphisms that have been researched in the literature related to smoking and to dopamine pathways and nicotinic receptors (eg, DRD2, DOPA, ANKK1, DAT, COMT, CHRNA4, and CHRNB2).[61–65] A handful of candidate studies have examined genetic predictors of response to treatment such as NRT and bupropion.[66] Like the candidate gene studies on nicotine dependence, most of these studies have focused on markers in the dopamine pathway because of the importance of dopaminergic neurotransmission in nicotine reinforcement.

■ DIAGNOSIS

According to the *Diagnostic and Statistical Manual of Mental Disorders*, fourth edition (DSM-IV),[67] the presence of three or more of seven criteria for at least a year satisfies the definition of "dependence" (classically known as "addiction"). After prolonged smoking, the user develops nicotine tolerance and exhibits withdrawal symptoms when nicotine is absent. Nicotine may also be responsible for three other criteria for dependence: loss of control over smoking (eg, not being able to reduce or stop smoking, or smoking more than intended), compulsive use (eg, spending more time using the substance or giving up important events to use the substance), and continued smoking despite adverse consequences (eg, heart attack, emphysema, or cancer).

Another widely used scale to assess for nicotine dependence is the Fagerström Test for Nicotine Dependence (FTND) (Table 8-1). This tool, and its first item in particular ("How soon after you wake up do you smoke your first cigarette?"), measures physiologic dependence (ie, tolerance and withdrawal) reliably well. However, it does not reliably measure some of the other dimensions of nicotine dependence, especially the behavioral dimensions. Four points or more out of a possible maximum of 10 are customarily used to diagnose physiologic dependence on nicotine.[69,70]

The Wisconsin Inventory of Smoking Dependence Motives (WISDM)[71] is a more recently developed multidimensional scale of nicotine dependence. This comprehensive scale includes measures of cognitive enhancement, negative reinforcement, positive reinforcement, automaticity, affiliative attachment, loss of control, behavioral choice/amelioration, craving, cue exposure/associative processes, social/environmental goals, taste/sensory processes, weight control, and tolerance. The WISDM has been validated and found to be reliable in measuring nicotine dependence; it is reported to have internal consistency along a 13-factor model.[72]

Smoking and Psychiatric Comorbidities

There is substantial evidence that smoking is closely linked with several psychiatric comorbidities, suggesting shared biological pathways between nicotine dependence and these psychiatric conditions. For example, the current smoking rate among individuals with no mental illness, past-month mental illness, and lifetime mental illness has been reported to be 22%, 34%, and 41%, respectively. Remarkably, smokers with a mental disorder in the past month reportedly consumed 44% of all cigarettes smoked in the same nationally representative sample.[73] Several studies have demonstrated a positive relationship between alcohol use, abuse, or dependence, substance abuse, and other psychiatric disorders and

■ **TABLE 8-1. Items and Scoring for Fagerström Test for Nicotine Dependence (FTND)** [68]

Questions	Answers	Points
(1) How soon after you wake up do you smoke your first cigarette?	Within 5 min	3
	6–30 min	2
	31–60 min	1
	After 60 min	0
(2) Do you find it difficult to refrain from smoking in places where it is forbidden (eg, in church, at the library, in a cinema)?	Yes	1
	No	0
(3) Which cigarette would you hate most to give up?	The first one in the morning	1
	All others	0
(4) How many cigarettes per day do you smoke?	10 or less	0
	11–20	1
	21–30	2
	31 or more	3
(5) Do you smoke more frequently during the first hours after waking than during the rest of the day?	Yes	1
	No	0
(6) Do you smoke if you are so ill that you are in bed most of the day?	Yes	1
	No	0

Reproduced with permission from Ref.68

smoking.[73–80] For example, the lifetime prevalence rate of alcohol dependence or drug abuse is an estimated 23% to 30% among adult smokers.[81,82] Among tobacco-dependent and nondependent current smokers, lifetime rates of mood and anxiety disorders have been reported to range from 33% to 46% and from 12% to 26%, respectively.[81] Similarly, among tobacco-dependent smokers, the 12-month prevalence of any mood or anxiety disorder was 22%.[83] Smokers also have an elevated risk of a first onset of major depression, panic disorder, or generalized anxiety disorder.[84,85,86] Regarding cognitive dysfunction, the odds ratio (OR) comparing ever smokers with never smokers was positively related to the number of attention-deficit hyperactivity disorder symptoms. In addition, lifetime regular smoking had an inverse relationship between the number of attention-deficit hyperactivity disorder symptoms and the age of onset. Further, a positive relationship between the number of symptoms and the number of cigarettes smoked has also been observed.[87]

■ TREATMENT

The US Department of Health and Human Services[88] updated the Clinical Practice Guidelines for Treating Tobacco Use and Dependence (CPG-TTUD) in 2008. These guidelines are evidence based and they are considered as the standard of practice in providing smoking cessation treatment; they revolve around 10 key recommendations (Table 8-2).

Recovery from nicotine dependence is maximized when a comprehensive biological, psychological, and social (ie, biopsychosocial) assessment is performed. Such assessments, which should account for the smoker's motivation for change, can guide both psychosocial therapy and pharmacologic treatment. Pharmacologic treatments are used as an adjunct to psychosocial therapy. When psychosocial and medical treatments are provided in concert, the odds of a patient quitting smoking are usually doubled. However, medication alone can alleviate some of the effects of nicotine withdrawal, decrease cravings for tobacco use, and decrease the risk of relapse.

Nicotine replacement products and non-nicotine-based medications such as sustained-release bupropion (bupropion SR) (Zyban or Wellbutrin SR) and varenicline (Chantix) have a big impact on tobacco cessation, reduction of cravings, and mitigation of nicotine withdrawal symptoms. While bupropion SR and varenicline are first-line therapies for tobacco dependence, nortriptyline (Pamelor) and clonidine (Catapres) are considered second-line therapies (Table 8-3).

Pharmacologic agents for nicotine dependence can be grouped based on their mode of action on nicotinic receptors: nicotinic receptor agonists (ie, NRTs), nicotinic receptor antagonists (bupropion and mecamylamine), nicotinic receptor partial agonists (cytisine and varenicline), and medications with no known action on nicotinic receptors (eg, nortriptyline and clonidine).

Nicotinic Receptor Agonists

NRTs were the first pharmacologic treatments to be offered for smoking cessation. In general, the quit rate among smokers who take an NRT is double that of non-NRT users.[89] The US Food and Drug Administration (FDA) has approved the following NRTs for smoking cessation: 16- or 24-hour prescription or over-the-counter (OTC) patches, prescription nasal spray or buccal inhaler, and OTC polacrilex gum, flavored gum, or flavored lozenges (Table 8-3).

In a recent review, Silagy et al[90] identified 103 trials that compared smoking abstinence rates achieved with an NRT compared with a control (placebo or a non-NRT drug). The overall OR for abstinence with NRTs compared with placebo was 1.77 (95% confidence interval [CI], 1.66–1.88). In addition, combinations of NRTs were more effective than any NRT alone. Silagy and colleagues concluded that (1) 8 weeks of patch therapy are as effective as longer courses of patch therapy, and there is no evidence that tapering off patch therapy is better than ending patch therapy abruptly, (2) wearing a patch only during waking hours (for 16 hours per day) is as effective as wearing a patch for 24 hours per day, (3) gum may be offered on a fixed-dose or as-needed basis, (4) highly dependent smokers (eg, those who need to smoke within 30 minutes of waking) and those who have been unable to quit with 2-mg gum would need a 4-mg gum, and (5) the effectiveness of NRTs appears to be largely independent of the intensity of psychosocial therapeutic support provided to the smoker.

If someone has had prior success quitting with one type of NRT, using the same product again may have some advantage over trying another NRT. NRTs can be safely combined, leading to improved abstinence rate compared with a single NRT.[91] A particularly useful combination is using the patch plus one of the episodic NRTs (lozenge, buccal inhaler, gum, or nasal spray). Two considerations in deciding to offer combined NRTs are patient's previous success with an NRT and higher level of nicotine dependence. Patient's education and management of expectations are key aspects of the clinical visit before treatment begins. This is especially true for combination approaches, such as the simultaneous use of two NRTs or of the nicotinic receptor antagonist bupropion plus an NRT. The use of NRTs such as gums, inhalers, and patches has also been deemed safe even if a patient continues to smoke.[97] The use of NRTs while

■ TABLE 8-2. Ten Key Guideline Recommendations from the Clinical Practice Guidelines on Treating Tobacco Use and Dependence

The overarching goal of these recommendations is that clinicians strongly recommend the use of effective tobacco dependence counseling and medication treatments to their patients who use tobacco, and that health systems, insurers, and purchasers assist clinicians in making such effective treatment available

1. Tobacco dependence is a chronic disease that often requires repeated intervention and multiple attempts to quit. Effective treatments exist, however, that can significantly increase rates of long-term abstinence

2. It is essential that clinicians and health care delivery systems consistently identify and document tobacco use status and treat every tobacco user seen in a health care setting

3. Tobacco dependence treatments are effective across a broad range of populations. Clinicians should encourage every patient willing to make a quit attempt to use the counseling treatments and medications recommended in this guideline

4. Brief tobacco dependence treatment is effective. Clinicians should offer every patient who uses tobacco at least the brief treatments shown to be effective in this guideline

5. Individual, group, and telephone counseling are effective, and their effectiveness increases with treatment intensity. Two components of counseling are especially effective, and clinicians should use these when counseling patients making a quit attempt:
   • Practical counseling (problem solving/skills training)
   • Social support delivered as part of treatment

6. Numerous effective medications are available for tobacco dependence, and clinicians should encourage their use by all patients attempting to quit smoking—except when medically contraindicated or with specific populations for which there is insufficient evidence of effectiveness (ie, pregnant women, smokeless tobacco users, light smokers, and adolescents):
   • Seven first-line medications (5 nicotine and 2 non-nicotine) reliably increase long-term smoking abstinence rates: bupropion SR, nicotine gum, nicotine inhaler, nicotine lozenge, nicotine nasal spray, nicotine patch, varenicline
   • Clinicians also should consider the use of certain combinations of medications identified as effective in this guideline

7. Counseling and medication are effective when used by themselves for treating tobacco dependence. The combination of counseling and medication, however, is more effective than either alone. Thus, clinicians should encourage all individuals making a quit attempt to use both counseling and medication

8. Telephone quitline counseling is effective with diverse populations and has a broad reach. Therefore, both clinicians and health care delivery systems should both ensure patient access to quitlines and promote quitline use

9. If a tobacco user currently is unwilling to make a quit attempt, clinicians should use the motivational treatments shown in this guideline to be effective in increasing future quit attempts

10. Tobacco dependence treatments are both clinically effective and highly cost-effective relative to interventions for other clinical disorders. Providing coverage for these treatments increases quit rates. Insurers and purchasers should ensure that all insurance plans include the counseling and medication identified as effective in this guideline as covered benefits

Reprinted with permission from *Treating Tobacco Use and Dependence: 2008 Update*.[88]

continuing to smoke has helped reduce the number of cigarettes smoked each day by as much as 50% among participants who were not motivated to quit. Those studies noted a lack of significant nicotine toxicity or major adverse events.[93–95]

A recent large and well-designed placebo-controlled trial was conducted among volunteers recruited from the community. Three monotherapies (bupropion, patch, and lozenge) and two combination therapies (bupropion plus lozenge and patch plus lozenge) were compared; the patch

■ **TABLE 8-3. Meta-analysis (2008): Effectiveness and Abstinence Rates for Various Medications and Medication Combinations Compared with Placebo at 6 Months' Postquit (n = 83 Studies)**

Medication	Number of Arms	Estimated Odds Ratio (95% CI)	Estimated Abstinence Rate (95% CI)
Placebo	80	1.0	13.8
Monotherapies			
Varenicline (2 mg/day)	5	3.1 (2.5–3.8)	33.2 (28.9–37.8)
Nicotine nasal spray	4	2.3 (1.7–3.0)	26.7 (21.5–32.7)
High-dose nicotine patch (>25 mg) (this included both standard and long-term duration)	4	2.3 (1.7–3.0)	26.5 (21.3–32.5)
Long-term nicotine gum (>14 weeks)	6	2.2 (1.5–3.2)	26.1 (19.7–33.6)
Varenicline (1 mg/day)	3	2.1 (1.5–3.0)	25.4 (19.6–32.2)
Nicotine inhaler	6	2.1 (1.5–2.9)	24.8 (19.1–31.6)
Clonidine	3	2.1 (1.2–3.7)	25.0 (15.7–37.3)
Bupropion SR	26	2.0 (1.8–2.2)	24.2 (22.2–26.4)
Nicotine patch (6–14 weeks)	32	1.9 (1.7–2.2)	23.4 (21.3–25.8)
Long-term nicotine patch (>14 weeks)	10	1.9 (1.7–2.3)	23.7 (21.0–26.6)
Nortriptyline	5	1.8 (1.3–2.6)	22.5 (16.8–29.4)
Nicotine gum (6–14 weeks)	15	1.5 (1.2–1.7)	19.0 (16.5–21.9)
Combination therapies			
Patch (long-term; >14 weeks) + ad lib NRT (gum or spray)	3	3.6 (2.5–5.2)	36.5 (28.6–45.3)
Patch + bupropion SR	3	2.5 (1.9–3.4)	28.9 (23.5–35.1)
Patch + nortriptyline	2	2.3 (1.3–4.2)	27.3 (17.2–40.4)
Patch + inhaler	2	2.2 (1.3–3.6)	25.8 (17.4–36.5)
Patch + second-generation antidepressants (paroxetine, venlafaxine)	3	2.0 (1.2–3.4)	24.3 (16.1–35.0)
Medications not shown to be effective	3	1.0 (0.7–1.4)	13.7 (10.2–18.0)
Selective serotonin reuptake inhibitors (SSRIs)	2	0.5 (0.2–1.2)	7.3 (3.1–16.2)
Naltrexone			

Refer www.surgeongeneral.gov/tobacco/gdlnrefs.htm for the articles used in this meta-analysis.

and lozenge combination produced the greatest benefit relative to placebo for smoking cessation. Treatment with lozenge alone or bupropion alone produced comparable effects as their combination.[96] An effectiveness trial by the same research group using the same therapies was conducted among primary care patients.[108] At 6-month follow-up bupropion SR plus lozenge resulted in an abstinence rate of 30%. This combination was superior to each monotherapy tested. In addition, the combination

of the patch and lozenge was superior to either medication alone.[108]

Nicotinic Receptor Antagonists

Bupropion

The FDA originally approved bupropion SR (chemical name: amfebutamone) as an antidepressant. It is considered an atypical antidepressant because it does not have a clearly known mechanism of action. However, its pharmacodynamic properties include inhibition of norepinephrine reuptake and to some extent dopamine reuptake. These inhibitory properties may be its mechanisms of action as an antidepressant and possibly as an antismoking medication as well.[98] In addition, bupropion was found to have some activity as a noncompetitive antagonist on high-affinity α4β2 subnicotinic acethlcholinergic receptors.[99] One of the drug's metabolites, (2S,3S)-hydroxybupropion, could have even more powerful antagonist activity against α4β2 receptors than bupropion itself. This metabolite may also reduce nicotine reward, withdrawal symptoms, and cravings.[100] In 1991 bupropion was approved under the name Zyban for the treatment of tobacco dependence. Bupropion SR therapy is typically started 1 to 2 weeks before the planned quit date at a dosage of 150 mg per day for 3 to 7 days; then it is increased to 150 mg twice daily.

Unfortunately bupropion SR use is limited by its contraindication for patients with a family or personal history of seizure, a personal history of head trauma, or a history of bulimia and anorexia nervosa. The most commonly reported adverse events with bupropion's use are anxiety, insomnia, dry mouth, or tremors; therefore, bupropion need to be used cautiously in patients who may already have these symptoms. Finally, bupropion SR is relatively contraindicated with patients who have elevated liver enzyme levels since its metabolites may accumulate and lead to toxic effects.

A recent meta-analysis, based on 31 clinical trials including more than 10,000 smokers, showed bupropion SR to be twice as effective as placebo in achieving long-term (6–12 months) tobacco abstinence (OR = 1.94; 95% CI, 1.72–2.19).[101] Bupropion SR also has been shown to be effective in primary care settings[102] and in several special clinical populations, such as schizophrenic patients,[103] depressed patients,[104] veterans,[105] and smokers with posttraumatic stress disorder.[106] The addition of an NRT to bupropion SR therapy is believed to help relieve nicotine withdrawal, at least in the immediate postcessation period. A large controlled trial showed that the combination of bupropion SR and one form of NRT, the patch, was more effective than either alone at the end of active treatment of 8 weeks but not at 6- or 12-month follow-up.[107] As mentioned above, a more recent effectiveness trial was conducted with patients seeking treatment at primary care clinics; it compared head to head three monotherapies (bupropion, patch, and lozenge) and two combination therapies (bupropion plus lozenge and patch plus lozenge). In that trial the combination of bupropion SR and lozenge was superior to all of the monotherapies (OR = 0.46–0.56). Furthermore, the patch plus lozenge combination was superior to the patch alone or bupropion alone (OR = 0.56 and 0.54, respectively[108]).

Bupropion SR offers unique advantages for smokers who have comorbid depression or attention-deficit hyperactivity disorder; it may alleviate the comorbid symptoms in addition to helping them quit smoking. Another advantage may be its attenuating the weight gain associated with smoking cessation, an important issue for those smokers who are obese, overweight, or afraid of gaining weight after quitting.[109] Finally, bupropion has a subtle positive effect on sexual dysfunction (mechanism not known); this is an important advantage since smoking is known to cause sexual dysfunction.[110]

Although other antidepressants and anxiolytics have not generally been found to be efficacious for smoking cessation,[101] bupropion's antidepressant actions may make it a particularly attractive choice for smokers vulnerable to negative affect or among those with some level of affective or cognitive impairment. For example, bupropion tripled the 1-year smoking cessation rates in women who had history of depression, compared with placebo.[111] However, the absolute cessation rates may not differ significantly among smokers with and without a history of depression.[101] Apart from smoking cessation, bupropion has long been indicated for the treatment of depression; the paucity of data on depressed smokers is mostly because these individuals are typically excluded from smoking cessation pharmaceutical trials. More recently bupropion has also been shown to prevent the recurrence of smoking among people with history of depression.[112] Direct controlled trials of bupropion with actively depressed smokers have yet to be performed; nevertheless, open, small, or noncontrolled trials have shown promising results.[111]

Mecamylamine

Mecamylamine, a classic nicotinic receptor antagonist, is used in research settings for smoking cessation. In preclinical and clinical studies, it was shown to increase the efficacy of nicotine patch therapy. In a review paper on the topic, Lancaster et al.[113] reported that: (a) one study compared mecamylamine alone to placebo with no effectiveness. (b) Another early study compared a combination of mecamylamine and the nicotine patch with placebo and found a significant effect for this combination. (c) A more recent study comparing nicotine patch alone to nicotine patch plus mecamylamine found no significant differences. Also, mecamylamine produces unpleasant side effects, such as postganglionic effects (eg, orthostatic hypotension) and strong anticholinergic effects (eg, dry mouth and constipation), which have limited its use to research in either clinical or laboratory settings.[113]

Nicotinic Receptor Partial Agonists

Varenicline

Varenicline (Chantix in the United States, Champix in other countries) is the first pharmaceutically designed compound with partial agonist effects on nicotinic receptors to become available in the market. It is a selective partial agonist that stimulates $\alpha4\beta2$ nicotinic cholinergic receptors; consequently, it stimulates dopamine release in the nucleus accumbens, though to a lesser extent (40–60% less) than nicotine itself. By binding to nicotinic receptors throughout its relatively long half-life of 24 hours, varenicline displays antagonistic properties as well. It prevents the full stimulation of those receptors that ensues when nicotine is coadministered.[114] Because of these properties, varenicline may provide relief from withdrawal symptoms (via its agonist effect) while blocking the rewarding effects of nicotine (via its antagonist effect).[115] Studies with animals have demonstrated that varenicline also acts as a full agonist of the $\alpha7$ nicotinic cholinergic receptor. Although this property has no clear benefit for smoking cessation,[116] it may provide benefits for smokers with chronic mental disorders such as schizophrenia.

Two randomized, double-blind clinical trials[117,118] have demonstrated varenicline to be more effective for smoking cessation than placebo (OR $\approx$ 3) and bupropion-SR (OR $\approx$ 2). Those studies compared varenicline (2 mg per day), bupropion-SR (300 mg per day), and placebo. The overall continuous abstinence rates from the end of treatment (12 weeks) to 1 year were 21%, 16%, and 8%, respectively, for one study[117] and 23%, 14%, and 10%, respectively, for the other study.[118] In a combined analysis of the two trials, varenicline resulted in significantly higher continuous abstinence

rates at 1 year than placebo alone or bupropion alone ($P < .05$ for both comparisons).[119] In this pooled analysis, compared with placebo, varenicline nearly tripled the odds of a smoker quitting even when continued abstinence was used as the outcome measure during the last 4 weeks of medication treatment (OR = 3.09; 95% CI, 1.95–4.91; $P < .001$). In a continuation of treatment study an additional 12 weeks of varenicline therapy (for a total of 24 weeks) was given to patients who had abstained from smoking at some point during the first 3 months of varenicline therapy.[120] In that double-blind continuation trial, successful quitters were randomly assigned to receive varenicline or placebo. Those on varenicline reported significantly less cravings and diminished withdrawal symptoms throughout the trial, and 70% remained abstinent at the end of the extension. In contrast, only 50% remained abstinent if they had received a placebo extension. Furthermore, the 1-year follow-up abstinence rate (after medication treatment) was doubled if patients had received a 3-month extension of varenicline rather than placebo (25% and 12%, respectively).[121]

The most common adverse effect of varenicline is nausea, occurring in up to 30% of patients (approximately twice the rate of nausea as for patients taking a placebo); however, in the majority of cases the nausea was mild to moderate. The other commonly reported adverse events are flatulence and abnormal dreams. Recently, the FDA has received a large amount of reports indicating increased depressive symptoms, occurrence or increase in suicidal ideation, and difficulty with motor coordination. As a result, the agency mandated the inclusion of specific warnings about these symptoms to the medication label; it also recommended that patients stop the medication immediately and report to their health care providers. The FDA[122] has commissioned further analysis of existing data, and to start prospective studies to clarify the relationship of these adverse effects to varenicline and the magnitude of such occurrences. For many patients, the prospect of using a new option, varenicline, could possibly motivate them to quit smoking, especially those who have not succeeded with more established smoking cessation medications. Finally a combination strategy such as adding bupropion SR to varenicline may increase the efficacy of smoking cessation.[123] The combination may also mitigate the emergence of depression, and other neuropsychiatric symptoms.[124] Two double-blind, controlled trials are under way to investigate the efficacy of such combination.[125,126]

Cytisine

Cytisine (Tabex) is a nicotinelike alkaloid derived from the plant *Laburnum anagyroides*. Although cytisine was used for smoking cessation in the Soviet Union (SU) for many years, little was known in the United States about this compound until the fall of the SU in the 1990s. Studies of cytisine for smoking cessation were mostly from SU countries; some are open-label trials, and those that were controlled were not designed rigorously. More recently, a review paper reported a meta-analysis of two double-blind, placebo-controlled studies of cytisine with pooled OR for smoking cessation of 1.83 (95% CI, 1.12–2.99) at 3 and 6 months. Another study reported in the same review paper was a double-blind, placebo-controlled trial; that study also resulted in a similar OR of 1.77 (95% CI, 1.29–2.43) but at the 2-year follow-up.[127]

Other Medications

Clonidine, a second-line pharmacotherapy for smoking cessation, has exhibited significant efficacy in clinical trials. Its superiority to placebo has been reported in two meta-analyses that included a total of 13 placebo-controlled clinical trials, with respective ORs of quitting smoking of 2.4 (95% CI, 1.70–3.28) and 2.0 (95% CI, 1.30–3.00).[128] However, its three times per day dosing and undesirable side-effect profile (eg, dry mouth, dizziness, somnolence, and orthostatic hypotension) have limited its use and therefore its role as a second-line medication.

Nortriptyline might facilitate smoking cessation by itself or with behavioral treatment. There are six well-designed controlled studies showing the drug's significant effects on smoking cessation, with an OR of 2.1 compared with placebo.[129] However, nortriptyline has significant disadvantages, including anticholinergic and cardiac side effects, as well as potential for lethality if overdose occurs. These issues resulted in classifying it as a second-line medication for smoking cessation.

Other potentially useful medications for smoking cessation that are not approved by the FDA at this time include rimonabant, a CB-1 receptor blocker, Quit Pack, which is a combination of mecamylamine and bupropion

SR, topiramate (an ion channel anticonvulsant), and a nicotine vaccine. The vaccine is a unique concept as it is proposed to develop active immunization to help the immune system recognize nicotine as a foreign substance and develop antibodies against it.[130] Establishing the efficacy and effectiveness of these treatments will require further study.

Nonpharmacologic Treatments

Behavioral treatment delivered by physicians, psychologists, nurses, pharmacists, dentists, and other clinicians increases their patients' smoking abstinence rates when "the five A's" are applied: ask patients if they smoke, advise them to quit, assess motivation for change, assist if they are willing to change, and arrange for follow-up.[88]

Sixty-four studies met selection criteria for meta-analyses performed for the Clinical Practice Guidelines for Treating Tobacco Use and Dependence (CPG-TTUD) in 2000; these meta-analyses were needed to examine the effectiveness of interventions using various types of counseling and behavioral therapies. The results revealed that four specific types of counseling and behavioral therapy categories yield statistically significant increases in abstinence rates relative to no contact (ie, untreated control conditions). These categories are: (1) providing practical counseling such as problem solving/skills training/stress management; (2) providing support during a smoker's direct contact with a clinician (intratreatment social support); (3) intervening to increase social support in the smoker's environment (extratreatment social support); and (4) using aversive smoking procedures (rapid smoking, rapid puffing, other smoking exposure).[88] These recommendations remained the same for the updated CPG-TTUD in 2008, since there were no newer studies or therapies to warrant additional analysis.

Finally, more intensive behavioral treatments usually translate into higher abstinence rates, but not every smoker requires the same amount of behavioral intervention. In a meta-analysis for the CPG-TTUD of 2008, an incremental improvement in abstinence rates was observed and categorized in intervals. Those intervals based on the number of sessions were: [1] abstinence of 22% (OR = 1), [2 and 3] abstinence of 28% (OR = 1.4), [4–8] abstinence of 27% (OR = 1.3), and >[8] abstinence of 33% (OR = 1.7). On the other hand, the vast majority of pharmacologic trials provide only minimal behavioral therapy of around 10 minutes of duration.[88]

REFERENCES

1. CDC. Cigarette smoking among adults, United States, 2007. *MMWR Morb Mortal Wkly Rep.* 2007;56(44): 1157–1161.

2. CDC. Smoking-attributable mortality, years of potential life lost, and productivity losses—United States, 2000–2004. *MMWR Morb Mortal Wkly Rep.* 2008;57(45): 1226–1228.

3. International Agency for Research on Cancer. Tobacco smoking. IARC Monographs on the Evaluation of Carcinogenic Risk of Chemicals to Man. 1986;38:312–314.

4. Substance Abuse and Mental Health Services Administration. *Results from the 2007 National Survey on Drug Use and Health: National Findings.* Rockville, MD: DHHS; 2008. DHHS Publication No. SMA 08-4343.

5. Johnston LD, O'Malley PM, Bachman JG, Schulenberg J. *Smoking Continues Gradual Decline Among U.S. Teens, Smokeless Tobacco Threatens a Comeback.* Ann Arbor, MI: University of Michigan News Service; 2009.

6. USDHHS. *Reducing Tobacco Use: A Report of the Surgeon General.* Atlanta, GA: U.S. Department of Health and Human Services, Public Health Service, Centers for Disease Control, Centers for Chronic Disease Prevention and Health Promotion, Office on Smoking and Health; 2000.

7. Kenford SL, Smith SS, Wetter DW, Jorenby DE, Fiore MC, Baker TB. Predicting relapse back to smoking: contrasting affective and physical models of dependence. *J Consult Clin Psychol.* 2002;70:216–227.

8. CDC. Annual smoking-attributable mortality, years of potential life lost, and productivity losses—United States, 1997–2001. *MMWR Morb Mortal Wkly Rep.* 2005;54(25):625–628.

9. Nisell M, Marcus M, Nomikos GG, Svensson TH. Differential effects of acute and chronic nicotine on dopamine output in the core and shell of the rat nucleus accumbens. *J Neural Transm.* 1997;104:1–10.

10. Nomikos GG, Damsma G, Wenkstern D, Fibiger HC. Acute effects of bupropion on extracellular dopamine concentrations in rat striatum and nucleus accumbens studied by in vivo microdialysis. *Neuropsychopharmacology.* 1989;2:273–279.

11. Pidoplichko vI, DeBiasi M, Williams JT, Dani JA. Nicotine activates and desensitizes midbrain dopamine neurons. *Nature.* 1997;390:401–404.

12. NIDA. The neurobiology of drug addiction. *NIDA Notes.* Available at: http://www.nida.nih.gov/pubs/teaching/Teaching2/Teaching.html. Accessed 9-9-2010.

13. Lowinson JH, Ruiz P, Millman RB, Langrod JG. *Substance Abuse: A Comprehensive Textbook.* New York, NY: Lippincott Williams & Wilkins; 2005.

14. Le FB, Forget B, Aubin HJ, Goldberg SR. Blocking cannabinoid CB1 receptors for the treatment of nicotine

dependence: insights from pre-clinical and clinical studies. *Addict Biol.* 2008;13(2):239–252.

15. Carr LA, Basham JK, York BK, Rowell PP. Inhibition of uptake of 1-methyl-4-phenylpyridinium ion and dopamine in striatal synaptosomes by tobacco smoke components. *Eur J Pharmacol.* 1992;215:285–287.

16. Pontieri FE, Tanda G, Orzi F, Di Chiara G. Effects of nicotine on the nucleus accumbens and similarity to those of addictive drugs. *Nature.* 1996;382:255–257.

17. Volkow ND, Fowler JS, Wang GJ. The addicted human brain viewed in the light of imaging studies: brain circuits and treatment strategies. *Neuropharmacology.* 2004;47(suppl 1):3–13.

18. Benowitz NL. Neurobiology of nicotine addiction: implications for smoking cessation treatment. *Am J Med.* 2008;121(4 suppl 1):S3–S10.

19. Volkow ND, Fowler J, Wang G-J. Role of dopamine in drug reinforcement and addiction in humans: results from imaging studies. *Behav Pharmacol.* 2002;13:355–366.

20. Robinson TE, Berridge KC. Incentive-sensitization and addiction. *Addiction.* 2001;96(1):103–114.

21. Ueda H. Anti-opioid systems in morphine tolerance and addiction—locus-specific involvement of nociceptin and the NMDA receptor. *Novartis Found Symp.* 2004;261:155–162.

22. Curtin JJ, McCarthy DE, Piper ME, Baker TB. Implicit and explicit drug motivational processes: a model of boundary conditions. In: Reinout R, Stacy A, eds. *Handbook of Implicit Cognition and Addiction.* Thousand Oaks, CA: Sage Publications; 2006:233–250.

23. Baker TB, Piper ME, McCarthy DE, Majeskie MR, Fiore MC. Addiction motivation reformulated: an affective processing model of negative reinforcement. *Psychol Rev.* 2004;111(1):33–51.

24. Wilens TE, Biederman J. Alcohol, drugs, and attention-deficit/hyperactivity disorder: a model for the study of addictions in youth. *J Psychopharmacol.* 2006;20(4):580–588. Epub 2005 September.

25. Epstein JN, Conners CK, Erhardt D, March JS, Swanson JM. Asymmetrical hemispheric control of visual–spatial attention in adults with attention deficit hyperactivity disorder. *Neuropsychology.* 1997;11(4):467–473.

26. Barkley RA. Behavioral inhibition, sustained attention, and executive functions: constructing a unifying theory of ADHD. *Psychol Bull.* 1997;121(1):65–94.

27. Seidman LJ, Biederman J, Faraone SV, Weber W, Ouellette C. Toward defining a neuropsychology of attention deficit-hyperactivity disorder: performance of children

and adolescents from a large clinically referred sample. *J Consult Clin Psychol.* 1997;65(1):150–160.

28. Beitchman JH, Douglas L, Wilson B, et al. Adolescent substance use disorders: findings from a 14-year follow-up of speech/language-impaired and control children. *J Clin Child Psychol.* 1999;28(3):312–321.

29. Tapert SF, Baratta MV, Abrantes AM, Brown SA. Attention dysfunction predicts substance involvement in community youths. *J Am Acad Child Adolesc Psychiatry.* 2002;41(6):680–686.

30. Faraone SV, Biederman J. Efficacy of Adderall for attention-deficit/hyperactivity disorder: a meta-analysis. *J Atten Disord.* 2002;6(2):69–75.

31. Chambers RA, Taylor JR, Potenza MN. Developmental neurocircuitry of motivation in adolescence: a critical period of addiction vulnerability. *Am J Psychiatry.* 2003;160(6):1041–1052.

32. Lubman DI, Yucel M, Pantelis C. Addiction, a condition of compulsive behaviour? Neuroimaging and neuropsychological evidence of inhibitory dysregulation. *Addiction.* 2004;99(12):1491–1502.

33. Hall SM, Humfleet GL, Reus VI, Munoz RF, Hartz DT, Maude-Griffin R. Psychological intervention and antidepressant treatment in smoking cessation. *Arch Gen Psychiatry.* 2002;59:930–936.

34. Hurt RD, Sachs DPL, Glover ED, et al. A comparison of sustained-release bupropion and placebo for smoking cessation. *N Engl J Med.* 1997;337:1195–1202.

35. Cinciripini PM, Tsoh JT, Wetter DW, et al. Combined effects of venlafaxine, nicotine replacement & brief counseling on smoking cessation. *Exp Clin Psychopharmacol.* 2005;13(4):282–292.

36. Hall SM, Sees KL, Munoz RF, et al. Mood management and nicotine gum in smoking treatment: a therapeutic contact and placebo-controlled study. *J Consult Clin Psychol.* 1996;64(5):1003–1009.

37. Brown RA, Kahler CW, Niaura R, et al. Cognitive–behavioral treatment for depression in smoking cessation. *J Consult Clin Psychol.* 2001;69(3):471–480.

38. Watson D, Clark LA, Tellegen A. Development and validation of brief measures of positive and negative affect: the PANAS scales. *J Pers Soc Psychol.* 1988;54:1063–1070.

39. McNair DM, Lorr M, Droppleman LF. *Profile of Mood States Manual.* San Diego, CA: Education and Industrial Testing Service; 1992.

40. Shiffman S, Paty J, Gnys M, Kassel J, Hickcox M. First lapses to smoking: within-subjects analysis of real-time reports. *J Consult Clin Psychol.* 1996;64(2):366–379.

41. Borrelli B, Niaura R, Keuthen NJ, et al. Development of major depressive disorder during smoking-cessation treatment. *J Clin Psychiatry.* 1996;57(11):534–538.

42. Burgess ES, Kahler CW, Niaura R, Abrams DB, Goldstein MG, Miller IW. Patterns of change in depressive symptoms during smoking cessation: who's at risk for relapse? *J Consult Clin Psychol.* 2002;70(2):356–361.

43. Spitz MR, Shi H, Hudmon KS, et al. A case–control study of the dopamine D2 receptor gene and smoking status in lung cancer. *J Natl Cancer Inst.* 1998;90(5):358–363.

44. Carmelli D, Swan GE, Robinette D, Fabsitz R. Genetic influence on smoking—a study of male twins. *N Engl J Med.* 1992;327:829–833.

45. Lerman C, Shields PG, Audrain J, et al. The role of the serotonin transporter gene in cigarette smoking. *Cancer Epidemiol Biomarkers Prev.* 1998;7:253–255.

46. Picciotto MR, Zoli M, Rimondini R, et al. Acetylcholine receptors containing the beta2 subunit are involved in the reinforcing properties of nicotine. *Nature.* 1998;391:173–177.

47. Lerman C, Caporaso NE, Audrain J, et al. Evidence suggesting the role of specific genetic factors in cigarette smoking. *Health Psychol.* 1999;18(1):14–20.

48. Sabol SZ, Nelson ML, Fisher C, et al. A genetic association for cigarette smoking behavior. *Health Psychol.* 1999;18(1):7–13.

49. True WR, Heath AC, Scherrer JF, et al. Genetic and environmental contributions to smoking. *Addiction.* 1997;92(10):1277–1287.

50. Bergen AW, Korczak JF, Weissbecker KA, Goldstein AM. A genome-wide search for loci contributing to smoking and alcoholism. *Genet Epidemiol.* 1999;17(suppl 1):S55–S60.

51. Duggirala R, Almasy L, Blangero J. Smoking behavior is under the influence of a major quantitative trait locus on human chromosome 5q. *Genet Epidemiol.* 1999;17(suppl 1):S139–S144.

52. Straub RE, Sullivan PF, Ma Y, et al. Susceptibility genes for nicotine dependence: a genome scan and followup in an independent sample suggest that regions on chromosomes 2, 4, 10, 16, 17, and 18 merit further study. *Mol Psychiatry.* 1999;4:129–144.

53. Uhl GR, Liu QR, Drgon T, Johnson C, Walther D, Rose JE. Molecular genetics of nicotine dependence and abstinence: whole genome association using 520,000 SNPs. *BMC Genet.* 2007;8:10.

54. Uhl GR, Liu QR, Drgon T, et al. Molecular genetics of successful smoking cessation: convergent genome-wide association study results. *Arch Gen Psychiatry.* 2008;65(6):683–693.

55. Carter BL, Long TY, Cinciripini PM. A meta-analytic review of the CYP2A6 genotype and smoking behavior. *Nicotine Tob Res.* 2004;6(2):221–227.

56. Lessov-Schlaggar CN, Pergadia ML, Khroyan TV, Swan GE. Genetics of nicotine dependence and pharmacotherapy. *Biochem Pharmacol.* 2008;75(1):178–195.

57. Li MD. Identifying susceptibility loci for nicotine dependence: 2008 update based on recent genome-wide linkage analyses. *Hum Genet.* 2008;123(2):119–131.

58. Munafo M, Clark T, Johnstone E, Murphy M, Walton R. The genetic basis for smoking behavior: a systematic review and meta-analysis. *Nicotine Tob Res.* 2004;6(4):583–597.

59. Munafo MR, Flint J. Meta-analysis of genetic association studies. *Trends Genet.* 2004;20(9):439–444.

60. Munafo MR, Johnstone EC. Genes and cigarette smoking. *Addiction.* 2008;103(6):893–904.

61. Gelernter J, Yu Y, Weiss R, et al. Haplotype spanning TTC12 and ANKK1, flanked by the DRD2 and NCAM1 loci, is strongly associated to nicotine dependence in two distinct American populations. *Hum Mol Genet.* 2006;15(24):3498–3507.

62. Huang W, Payne TJ, Ma JZ, et al. Significant association of ANKK1 and detection of a functional polymorphism with nicotine dependence in an African-American sample. *Neuropsychopharmacology.* 2009;34(2):319–330. Epub 2008 Mar 19.

63. Saccone SF, Hinrichs AL, Saccone NL, et al. Cholinergic nicotinic receptor genes implicated in a nicotine dependence association study targeting 348 candidate genes with 3,713 SNPs. *Hum Mol Genet.* 2007;16(1):36–49.

64. Hutchison KE, Allen DL, Filbey FM, et al. CHRNA4 and tobacco dependence: from gene regulation to treatment outcome. *Arch Gen Psychiatry.* 2007;64(9):1078–1086.

65. Zhang H, Ye Y, Wang X, Gelernter J, Ma JZ, Li MD. DOPA decarboxylase gene is associated with nicotine dependence. *Pharmacogenomics.* 2006;7(8):1159–1166.

66. David SP, Brown RA, Papandonatos G, et al. Pharmacogenetic clinical trial of sustained-release bupropion for smoking cessation. *Nicotine Tob Res.* 2007;9(8):821-833. Erratum in: *Nicotine Tob Res.* 2007;9(11):1243.

67. American Psychiatric Association. *Diagnostic and Statistical Manual of Mental Disorders.* 4th revised ed. Washington, DC: American Psychiatric Association; 2000.

68. Heatherton TF, Kozlowski LT, Frecker RC, Fagerström KO. The Fagerström Test for Nicotine Dependence: a revision of the Fagerström Tolerance Questionnaire. *Br J Addict.* 1991;86:1119–1127.

69. Payne TJ, Smith PO, McCracken LM, McSherry WC, Anthony MM. Assessing nicotine dependence: a comparison of the Fagerstrom Tolerance Questionnaire (FTQ) with the Fagerstrom Test for Nicotine Dependence (FTND) in a clinical sample. *Addict Behav*. 1994;19:307–374.

70. Pomerleau CS, Pomerleau OF, Majchrzak MJ, Kloska DD, Malakuti R. Relationship between Fagerstrom Tolerance Questionnaire scores and plasma cotinine. *Addict Behav*. 1990;15:73–80.

71. Piper ME, Piasecki TM, Federman EB, et al. A multiple motives approach to tobacco dependence: the Wisconsin Inventory of Smoking Dependence Motives (WISDM-68). *J Consult Clin Psychol*. 2004;72(2):139–154.

72. Shenassa E, Graham A, Burdzovic J, Buka S. Psychometric properties of the Wisconsin Inventory of Smoking Dependence Motives (WISDM-68): a replication extension. *Nicotine Tob Res*. 2010;11(8):1002–1010.

73. Lasser K, Boyd JW, Woolhandler S, Himmelstein DU, McCormick D, Bor DH. Smoking and mental illness: a population-based prevalence study. *JAMA*. 2000;284(20):2606–2610.

74. Breslau N, Johnson EO, Hiripi E, Kessler R. Nicotine dependence in the United States: prevalence, trends, and smoking persistence. *Arch Gen Psychiatry*. 2001;58(9):810–816.

75. Covey LS, Hughes DC, Glassman AH, Blazer DG, George LK. Ever-smoking, quitting, and psychiatric disorders: evidence from the Durham, North Carolina, epidemiologic catchment area. *Tob Control*. 1994;3:222–227.

76. Glassman AH, Helzer JE, Covey LS, et al. Smoking, smoking cessation, and major depression. *JAMA*. 1990;264(12):1546–1549.

77. Williams JM, Ziedonis D. Addressing tobacco among individuals with a mental illness or an addiction. *Addict Behav*. 2004;29(6):1067–1083.

78. Barkley RA, Fischer M, Edelbrock CS, Smallish L. The adolescent outcome of hyperactive children diagnosed by research criteria: I. An 8-year prospective follow-up study. *J Am Acad Child Adolesc Psychiatry*. 1990;29(4):546–557.

79. Borland BL, Heckman HK. Hyperactive boys and their brothers. A 25-year follow-up study. *Arch Gen Psychiatry*. 1976;33(6):669–675.

80. Hartsough CS, Lambert NM. Pattern and progression of drug use among hyperactives and controls: a prospective short-term longitudinal study. *J Child Psychol Psychiatry*. 1987;28(4):543–553.

81. Breslau N. Psychiatric comorbidity of smoking and nicotine dependence. *Behav Genet*. 1995;25(2):95–101.

82. Batel P, Pessione F, Maitre C, Rueff B. Relationship between alcohol and tobacco dependencies among alcoholics who smoke. *Addiction*. 1995;90(7):977–980.

83. Grant BF, Hasin DS, Chou SP, Stinson FS, Dawson DA. Nicotine dependence and psychiatric disorders in the United States: results from the national epidemiologic survey on alcohol and related conditions. *Arch Gen Psychiatry*. 2004;61(11):1107–1115.

84. Breslau N, Klein DF. Smoking and panic attacks: an epidemiologic investigation. *Arch Gen Psychiatry*. 1999;56(12):1141–1147.

85. Breslau N, Peterson EL, Schultz LR, Chilcoat HD, Andreski P. Major depression and stages of smoking: a longitudinal investigation. *Arch Gen Psychiatry*. 1998;55:161–166.

86. Kendler KS, Neale MC, MacLean CJ, Heath AC, Eaves LJ, Kessler RC. Smoking and major depression: a casual analysis. *Arch Gen Psychiatry*. 1993;50(1):36–43.

87. Kollins SH, McClernon FJ, Fuemmeler BF. Association between smoking and attention-deficit/hyperactivity disorder symptoms in a population-based sample of young adults. *Arch Gen Psychiatry*. 2005;62(10):1142–1147.

88. Fiore MC, Jaen CR, Baker TB, et al. *Treating Tobacco Use and Dependence: 2008 Update, Clinical Practice Guideline*. Rockville, MD: U.S. Department of Health and Human Services Public Health Service; 2008.

89. Karam-Hage M, Cinciripini PM. Pharmacotherapy for tobacco cessation: nicotine agonists, antagonists, and partial agonists. *Curr Oncol Rep*. 2007;9(6):509–516.

90. Silagy C, Lancaster T, Stead L, Mant D, Fowler G. *Nicotine Replacement Therapy for Smoking Cessation*. Chichester, UK: John Wiley & Sons Ltd; 2004. Report No. 3.

91. Fagerström KO, Tejding LR, Ake W, Lunell E. Aiding reduction of smoking with nicotine replacement medications. A strategy for the hopeless? *Tob Control*. 1997;6(4):311–316.

92. Piper ME, Smith SS, Schlam TR, et al. A randomized placebo controlled clinical trial of 5 smoking cessation pharmacotherapies. *Arch Gen Psychiatry*. 2009;66(11):1253–1262.

93. Bolliger CT, Zellweger JP, Danielsson T, et al. Smoking reduction with oral nicotine inhalers: double blind, randomised clinical trial of efficacy and safety. *BMJ*. 2000;321(7257):329–333.

94. Etter JF, Laszlo E, Zellweger JP, Perrot C, Perneger TV. Nicotine replacement to reduce cigarette consumption in smokers who are unwilling to quit: a randomized trial. *J Clin Psychopharmacol*. 2002;22(5):487–495.

95. Wennike P, Danielsson T, Landfeldt B, Westin A, Tonnesen P. Smoking reduction promotes smoking cessation: results from a double blind, randomized, placebo-controlled trial of nicotine gum with 2-year follow-up. *Addiction.* 2003;98(10):1395–1402.

96. Piper ME, Smith SS, Schlam TR, et al. A randomized placebo-controlled clinical trial of 5 smoking cessation pharmacotherapies. *Gen Psychiatry.* 2009;66(11):1253–1262.

97. Kozlowski LT, Giovino GA, Edwards B, et al. Advice on using over-the-counter nicotine replacement therapy-patch, gum or lozenge-to quit smoking. *Addict Behav.* 2007;32(10):2140–2150.

98. Ascher JA, Cole JO, Colin JN, et al. Bupropion: a review of its mechanism of antidepressant activity. *J Clin Psychiatry.* 1995;56:395–401.

99. Slemmer JE, Martin BP, Damaj I. Bupropion is a nicotine antagonist. *J Pharmacol Exp Ther.* 2000;295:321–327.

100. Damaj MI, Carroll FI, Eaton JB, et al. Enantioselective effects of hydroxy metabolites of bupropion on behavior and on function of monoamine transporters and nicotinic receptors. *Mol Pharmacol.* 2004;66(3):675–682.

101. Hughes JR, Stead LF, Lancaster T. Antidepressants for smoking cessation. *Cochrane Database Syst Rev.* 2007;(1):CD000031.

102. Murray RL, Coleman T, Antoniak M, et al. The effect of proactively identifying smokers and offering smoking cessation support in primary care populations: a cluster-randomized trial. *Addiction.* 2008;103(6):998–1006.

103. Evins AE, Cather C, Deckersbach T, et al. A double-blind placebo-controlled trial of bupropion sustained-release for smoking cessation in schizophrenia. *J Clin Psychopharmacol.* 2005;25(3):218–225.

104. Brown RA, Niaura R, Lloyd-Richardson EE, et al. Bupropion and cognitive–behavioral treatment for depression in smoking cessation. *Nicotine Tob Res.* 2007;9(7):721–730.

105. Beckham JC. Smoking and anxiety in combat veterans with chronic posttraumatic stress disorder: a review. *J Psychoactive Drugs.* 1999;31(2):103–110.

106. Hertzberg MA, Moore SD, Feldman ME, Beckham JC. A preliminary study of bupropion sustained-release for smoking cessation in patients with chronic posttraumatic stress disorder. *J Clin Psychopharmacol.* 2001;21(1):94–98.

107. Jorenby DE, Leischow SJ, Nides MA, et al. A controlled trial of sustained-release bupropion, a nicotine patch, or both for smoking cessation. *N Engl J Med.* 1999;340(9):685–691.

108. Smith SS, McCarthy DE, Janovitch S, et al. Comparative effectiveness of 5 smoking cessation pharmacotherapies in primary care clinics. *Arch Intern Med.* 2009;169(22):2148–2155.

109. Mooney ME, Sofuoglu M. Bupropion for the treatment of nicotine withdrawal and craving. *Expert Rev Neurother.* 2006;6(7):965–981.

110. Clayton AH, Pradko JF, Croft HA, et al. Prevalence of sexual dysfunction among newer antidepressants. *J Clin Psychiatry.* 2002;63(4):357–366.

111. Smith SS, Jorenby DE, Leischow SJ, et al. Targeting smokers at increased risk for relapse: treating women and those with a history of depression. *Nicotine Tob Res.* 2003;5:99–109.

112. Clayton AH. Extended-release bupropion: an antidepressant with a broad spectrum of therapeutic activity? *Expert Opin Pharmacother.* 2007;8(4):457–466.

113. Lancaster T, Stead LF. Mecamylamine (a nicotine antagonist) for smoking cessation. *Cochrane Database Syst Rev.* 2000;(2):CD001009.

114. Coe JW, Brooks PR, Vetelino MG, et al. Varenicline: an alpha4beta2 nicotinic receptor partial agonist for smoking cessation. *J Med Chem.* 2005;48(10):3474–3477.

115. Tonstad S. Varenicline for smoking cessation. *Expert Rev Neurother.* 2007;7(2):121–127. Review.

116. Mihalak KB, Carroll FI, Luetje CW. Varenicline is a partial agonist at alpha4beta2 and a full agonist at alpha7 neuronal nicotinic receptors. *Mol Pharmacol.* 2006;70(3):801–805.

117. Gonzales D, Rennard SI, Nides M, et al. Varenicline, an alpha4beta2 nicotinic acetylcholine receptor partial agonist, vs sustained-release bupropion and placebo for smoking cessation: a randomized controlled trial. *JAMA.* 2006;296(1):47–55.

118. Jorenby DE, Hays JT, Rigotti NA, et al. Efficacy of varenicline, an alpha4beta2 nicotinic acetylcholine receptor partial agonist, vs placebo or sustained-release bupropion for smoking cessation: a randomized controlled trial. *JAMA.* 2006;296(1):56–63.

119. Nides M, Glover ED, Reus VI, et al. Varenicline versus bupropion SR or placebo for smoking cessation: a pooled analysis. *Am J Health Behav.* 2008;32(6):664–675.

120. Tonstad S, Tonnesen P, Hajek P, Williams KE, Billing CB, Reeves KR. Effect of maintenance therapy with varenicline on smoking cessation: a randomized controlled trial. *JAMA.* 2006;296(1):64–71.

121. West R, Baker CL, Cappelleri et al. Effect of varenicline and bupropion on craving, nicotine withdrawal symptoms, and rewarding effects of smoking during a smok-

ing. *Psychopharmacology (Berl)*. 2008;197(3):371–377. Epub 2007.

122. US Food and Drug Administration. *Public Health Advisory, Important Information on Chantix (Varenicline)*. Rockville, MD: Department of Health and Human Services; February 1, 2008.

123. Ebbert JO, Croghan IT, Sood A, Schroeder DR, Hays JT, Hurt RD. Vareniclin and bupropion sustained release combination therapy for smoking cessation. *Nicotine Tob Res*. 2009;11(3):234–239.

124. Karam-Hage M, Shah K, Cinciripini PM. Adding bupropion-SR to vareniciline helps with depression and suicidal ideation. *Prim Care Companion J Clin Psychiatry*. 2010;12(2):PCC.09l00800.

125. Croghan IT. Varenicline and bupropion for smoking cessation (CHANBAN). *ClinicalTrials.gov*; 2010. Available at: http://www.clinicaltrials.gov/ct2/show/NCT0093581 8?term=bupropion+and+varenicline&rank=5. Accessed 9-9-2010.

126. Cinciripini PM. Combining varenicline and bupropion for smoking cessation. *ClinicalTrials.gov*; 2010. Available at: http://www.clinicaltrials.gov/ct2/show/NCT0094361 8?term=bupropion+and+varenicline&rank=9. Accessed 9-9-2010.

127. Etter JF. Cytisine for smoking cessation: a literature review and a meta-analysis. *Arch Intern Med*. 2006;166(15):1553–1559.

128. Gourlay SG, Stead LF, Benowitz NL. Clonidine for smoking cessation. *Cochrane Database Syst Rev*. 2004;(3):CD000058.

129. Hughes JR, Stead LF, Lancaster T. Nortriptyline for smoking cessation: a review. *Nicotine Tob Res*. 2005;7(4): 491–499.

130. Wagena EJ, de Vos A, Horwith G, van Schayck C. The immunogenicity and safety of a nicotine vaccine in smokers and nonsmokers: results of a randomized, placebo-controlled phase 1/2 trial. *Nicotine Tob Res*. 2008;10(1): 213–218.

Substance Abuse and Cancer

• *Kathie Rickman*

THE SUBSTANCE ALCOHOL

Alcohol is widely used in our society. Most individuals who use alcohol drink in ways that do not increase risk of alcohol use problems. Some, however, drink in ways or at times during their life course that increase risk to themselves or others. Still others who use alcohol may derive a health benefit from its use.[1]

According to Nels Ericson at the US Department of Justice,[2] "research has long shown that the abuse of alcohol, tobacco, and illicit drugs is the single most serious health problem in the United States, straining the health care system, burdening the economy, and contributing to the health problems and death of millions of Americans every year. Today, substance abuse causes more deaths, illnesses, and disabilities than any other preventable health condition." He states that substance abuse is the nation's number one preventable health problem. The economic costs of drug and alcohol abuse in the United States are estimated to exceed $275 billion per year; this includes lost productivity, medical expenses, crime, and other costs. More than 22 million people are in need of addiction treatment according to the *Robert Woods Johnson Foundation Knowledge Asset Policy Brief*[3] dated September 2008.

Alcohol's causal link to cancer has been known for decades.[4,5] The continued use of substances has a known adverse effect on human immune function. Alcohol is the favorite mood-altering drug in the United States. Its effects, both pleasant and unpleasant, are well known. What is not as well known is that alcohol is a toxic drug that produces pathological changes in tissue and organs and can cause death. A recent report from the Substance Abuse and Mental Health Services Administration shows a small percentage of people are kicking smoking while alcohol- and illicit drug–use levels remain steady. Alcohol still leads tobacco as the most commonly used substance. Marijuana is the most commonly used illicit drug. The rate of illicit drug use in 2007 among persons aged 12 or older was 8% to 10% in the general population in the United States. The illicit drugs include hallucinogens (including Ecstasy), cocaine, methamphetamines, and prescription drugs. More information on distribution of drug and alcohol use by state can be found at www.nida.nig.gov.

ALCOHOL LINKS TO CERTAIN CANCERS

In 2000, the *National Toxicology Program Report* to the US Department of Health and Human Services[1] listed ethyl alcohol as a human carcinogen for the first time. Consumption of alcoholic beverages is *causally* related to cancers of the mouth, pharynx, larynx, and esophagus. Cohort and case–control studies consistently find moderate to strong associations between alcohol consumption and those cancers. Evidence also supports a weaker but possibly causal relationship between alcohol consumption and increased risk of cancers of the breast and liver. Epidemiologic research has demonstrated a dose-dependent association between alcohol consumption and certain types of cancer; as alcohol consumption increases, so does the risk of developing certain cancers.[7]

Irigaray et al[8] looked at lifestyle factors and reported that drinking alcohol contributes to the formation of some types of cancer in men who drink more than two alcoholic drinks per day and in women who drink more than one alcoholic drink per day. Their research reported that strong associations between alcohol use and cancer are found in the mouth, esophagus, larynx, pharynx, breast, and liver. Those who drink heavily and smoke cigarettes or use other kinds of tobacco are at an even greater risk for most of these cancers. Multiple other factors were listed as well.

Breast Cancer

The *type* of alcohol a woman drinks makes no difference; the *amount* of alcohol consumed is linked to the risk of developing breast cancer according to a study of 70,033 women in Spain.[8] A study of 150,000 women worldwide by British researchers concluded that drinking as little as one drink per day increases the risk of breast cancer.[9] *Any* kind of alcohol consumed changes the levels of female hormones, thus causing more estrogen receptor–positive breast cancer. Since there is convincing scientific evidence that alcohol is a cause of breast and other cancers, the American Institute of Cancer Research recommends that women keep to one drink per day, if they drink at all.[10]

From the massive "Million Women Study" in England conducted between 1996 and 2001, 1,280,296 women who attended breast cancer screening completed questionnaires asking about quantity of wine, beer, and spirits consumed on average each week. Light-to-moderate drinking predicted a statistically significant increased risk of rectal, liver, and breast cancers. Researchers reported that the equivalent of a glass of wine or one beer per day increased a woman's risk of developing breast cancer by 12%, the risk of liver cancer by 25%, and the risk of rectal cancer by 10%. Each additional alcoholic drink regularly consumed per day was associated with 11 additional breast cancers per 1000 women up to age 75, one additional cancer of the oral cavity and pharynx, one additional cancer of the rectum, and an increase of 0.7 each for esophageal, laryngeal, and liver cancers. For these cancers combined, there was an excess of about 15 cancers per 1000 women per drink per day. Women in the study who drank alcohol consumed, on average, one drink per day, which is typical in most high-income countries such as the United Kingdom and the United States. Very few drank three or more drinks per day.

With an average follow-up time of more than 7 years, 68,775 women were diagnosed with cancer.[11]

"Although the magnitude of the excess absolute risk associated with one additional drink per day may appear small for some cancer sites, the high prevalence of moderate alcohol drinking among women in many populations means that the proportion of cancers attributable to alcohol is an important public health issue," the authors write. In an accompanying editorial, Lauer and Sorlie,[12] of the National Heart, Lung, and Blood Institute, in Bethesda, Maryland, emphasize that these new results derived from such a large study population should give readers a pause.

The news is not all bad, however. Researchers at the Centre for Addiction and Mental Health (CAMH)[13] in Canada have clarified the link between alcohol consumption and the risk of head and neck cancers, showing that people who stop drinking can significantly reduce their cancer risk. According to CAMH principal investigator Dr Jürgen Rehm, existing research consistently shows a relationship between alcohol consumption and an increased risk for cancer of the esophagus, larynx, and oral cavity. Dr Rehm and his team analyzed epidemiologic literature from 1966 to 2006 to further investigate this association and their results were published in the September 2008 issue of the *International Journal of Cancer*. Risk of head and neck cancer only reduced significantly after 10 years of cessation. After more than 20 years of alcohol cessation, the risks for both cancers were similar to those seen in people who never drank alcohol.

Seniors and Alcohol

A large percentage of certain cancers occurs in populations aged >50.[14] Of note, alcohol and substance abuse is statistically at epidemic proportions among the elderly and remains mostly unreported. Therefore, it is prudent to assess older adults for substance use as part of the initial overall intake assessment for cancer. Representatives of the American Medical Association[15,16] speculate that hospital admissions of elderly patients with alcohol-related problems range from 22% to 35%. They point out that the real numbers of elderly alcohol abusers are not known because so many physicians fail to ask their older patients if they drink, how much they drink, and how long they have been drinking. Older women with a history of alcohol use are significantly more likely to be diagnosed with hormonally sensitive forms of breast cancer than nondrinkers. Women who are undergoing hormone replacement therapy and who drink just *one drink* per day *double* their chances of developing breast cancer, according to a study published in the *Annals of Internal Medicine*.[17] Women and seniors in general should be educated by health care providers about the risk of drinking on a regular basis, especially when taking certain types of medication as advised in the *Alcoholism Alert*, July 2006.[18]

Colorectal Cancers

Colorectal cancer is the second leading cause of cancer death in the United States and seems to develop years earlier in males who drink alcohol and smoke cigarettes according to research conducted at Evanston Northwestern Healthcare.[19] Wakai et al[20] report, in a study by a Japanese cancer center of 58,000 men and women, that men who drank alcohol regularly were *twice as likely* to develop colon cancer than men who do not drink at all.

Cho et al[21] reviewed the findings of eight cohort studies consisting of 489,979 people. They found that 4687 people developed colorectal cancer. Compared with people who reported drinking no alcohol, people who reported drinking more than 30 g of alcohol per day (the equivalent of two average-sized drinks) had a small increase in risk for colorectal cancer. The increase in risk was highest in people who drank more than 45 g of alcohol per day, which is slightly more than three average-sized drinks.

■ SUBSTANCE USE DISORDERS (SUDS) IN CANCER PATIENTS

Substance use and abuse is just *one* of the many comorbidities found in cancer patients. "It is the time to assess for substance use or abuse and address the issue of how it will interfere with cancer treatment," says the National Cancer Institute[22] in its January 2008 report. Substance abuse in cancer patients without previous history is rare. Substance users often present with comorbidities that are treated while undergoing cancer care. Patients abusing alcohol, prescription drugs, or illicit drugs present with problems, which if *not* addressed may significantly affect treatment outcomes. If SUDS were thought of and treated like other medical illnesses, substance users might not be considered bad people who need to get good, but rather sick people who need to get well. This attitude appears to be more in keeping with compassionate health care practice rather than one of criticism or judgment.

■ IMPORTANCE OF SCREENING

According to the *American Family Physician*,[23] 10% of the population in the United States abuses drugs or alcohol, and 20% of patients seen by family physicians have substance abuse problems, excluding tobacco use. These patients can be identified by relying on regular screening or a high index of suspicion based on "red flags" obtained in various clinical situations. The modified CAGE questionnaire is one example, but several alternatives are available. The best screening test is one that the physician will routinely use as screening tools have proven to be effective in identifying patients who abuse substances.[23]

Routine screening for problems with alcohol is a relatively recent practice, but has a solid base of support. In 1990, the Institute of Medicine's[25] landmark report on broadening the base of alcohol and other drug abuse treatment recommended that patients in all medical settings be screened for the full spectrum of problems that can accompany alcohol use and, when necessary, be offered brief intervention or referral to treatment services. The level of screening used by a clinician typically depends on the patient's characteristics, whether he or she has other medical or psychiatric problems, the physician's skills and interest, and the amount of time available.[26]

Clinicians under strict time constraints may have time to ask a patient only one screening question about his or her alcohol consumption. One study has demonstrated that a positive response to the question "On any single occasion during the past 3 months, have you had more than 5 drinks containing alcohol?" accurately identifies patients who meet either NIAAA's criteria for at-risk drinking or the criteria for alcohol abuse or dependence specified in DSM-IV.[27]

The best known screening instrument for alcohol use is the CAGE questionnaire,[28] developed decades ago to be used in primary care settings. It consists of four questions asked by a health care provider to identify issues related to DSM-IV criteria diagnostic for alcoholism. When two questions are answered in the affirmative, there is a 72% reliability factor for a probable problem with alcohol. Three or four positive answers indicate a diagnosis of alcohol dependence (see Table 9-1).

Other useful screen tools for assessing substance use include the following:

1. Alcohol Use Disorders Identification Test (AUDIT)[29];
2. Michigan Alcohol Screening Test (MAST)[30];

■ **TABLE 9-1. CAGE Questionnaire**

(1) Have you ever felt you should *cut* down on your drinking?

(2) Have people *annoyed* you by criticizing your drinking?

(3) Have you ever felt bad or *guilty* about your drinking?

(4) Have you ever had a drink first thing in the morning to steady your nerves or get rid of a hangover (*eye opener*)?

3. Drug Abuse Screening Test (DAST)[31];
4. Substance Abuse Screening and Severity Instrument (SASSI).[32]

■ **LABORATORY TESTS**

Laboratory tests can be useful to determine current or recent use of alcohol and other substances, but they are not diagnostic. The most useful laboratory tests to confirm alcohol-abuse problems are gamma-glutamyl transpeptidase (GGT, a hepatic enzyme that is elevated in persons who use alcohol excessively), mean corpuscular volume (MCV) also elevated in heavy drinkers, and carbohydrate-deficient transferring (CDT). A urine toxicology screen is the best test to confirm problems with other drugs.[33]

■ **COMMON INDICATORS OF PROBLEMS (RED FLAGS):**

Common complaints in patients abusing alcohol may include the following:

- sleep disorders;
- history of frequent trauma or accidental injuries;
- depression and/or anxiety;
- labile hypertension and other elevated vital signs;
- GI symptoms such as epigastric distress, diarrhea, and weight changes;
- sexual dysfunction.

The symptoms are listed on the American Society of Addiction Medicine (ASAM) Alcohol Screening Card. These and other symptoms of substance use can be found at www.asam.org/publ. These symptoms are often red flags that should cause the health care provider to ask more in-depth questions about substance use. Additional physical findings that suggest alcohol and other drug problems include mild tremor, alcohol on breath, aftershave, mouthwash, mints, gum, enlarged, tender liver, nasal or conjunctiva irritation, hepatitis B or C, and HIV (see Table 9-2).

When faced with the crisis of being diagnosed with cancer, a patient may turn to the use of substances that have proven to be effective in calming anxiety or inducing sleep such as alcohol, nicotine, or prescription drugs. Because cancer treatment often includes the use of toxic chemicals and medications, the risk of overburdening the liver becomes a clinical reality. The ideal and safest course for the patient is to stop the intake of alcohol, tobacco, and nonessential chemicals during cancer treatment. Detoxification from substances offers safety to patients undergoing surgery, chemotherapy, and radiation treatments for their cancer.[34]

■ **DETOXIFICATION PRINCIPLES**

Detoxification from large amounts of alcohol over long periods should be managed under the direct supervision of a physician to reduce or eliminate the possibility of alcohol withdrawal syndrome (AWS). The Clinical Institute Withdrawal Assessment of Alcohol (CIWA) scale has been used successfully to assess symptoms of severity of withdrawal and to recommend doses of benzodiazepine medication administration. Alcohol withdrawal symptoms include agitation, anxiety, auditory disturbances, clouding of sensorium, headache, nausea/vomiting, paroxysmal sweats, tactile disturbances, tremor, and visual disturbances.[35] A similar assessment scale for use in patients using opioids is the Clinical Opiate Withdrawal Scale (COWS).[36] This scale includes assessment of the following symptoms: elevated vital signs, sweats, restlessness, pupil size, bone/joint aches, runny nose or tearing, GI upset, tremor, yawning,

■ **TABLE 9-2. Signs and Symptoms: Alcohol Withdrawal**

Anxiety	Agitation
Headache	Seizures
Nausea	Vomiting
Disorientation	Seizures
Tactile disturbances	Tremor
Visual disturbances	Elevated V/S

■ **TABLE 9-3. Opioid Withdrawal Signs and Symptoms**

Abdominal cramps	Irritability
Agitation	Insomnia
Anorexia	Lacrimation
Anxiety	Muscle spasms
Arthralgias	Myalgias
Diarrhea	Rhinorrhea
Dilated pupils	Goose bumps
Yawning	Elevated V/S
Diaphoresis	

anxiety or irritability, and gooseflesh. It is useful for determining severity of withdrawal symptoms and corresponding medication dosages (see Table 9-3).

Pharmacologic treatment of AWS involves the use of medications that are cross-tolerant with alcohol. Benzodiazepines have been shown to be safe and effective, particularly for preventing or treating seizures and delirium, and are the preferred agents for treating the symptoms of AWS.[37] The choice of agent is based on pharmacokinetics, presenting symptoms, location, and availability of patient to provider. For patients who have been drinking large quantities of alcohol for a long period of time, inpatient and supervised detoxification is preferred. Unsupervised withdrawal from alcohol or benzodiazepines can be life threatening and requires medical oversight. Treatment with these agents may be preferable in patients who metabolize medications less effectively, particularly the elderly and those with liver failure.

■ WITHDRAWAL CASE STUDY

Mr W is a 45-year-old Caucasian male who was diagnosed with lymphoma 2 months prior to admission. He came into the hospital 3 days ago to begin induction chemotherapy before receiving an autologous bone marrow transplant. He had been smoking one pack of cigarettes per day up to this point. Before admission, he had been prescribed oxycontin 90 mg BID along with oxycodone 10 mg every 4 to 6 hours for breakthrough pain. I was called to see the patient on Monday when it was discovered by the APN on the service that Mr W had a history of alcoholism and opioid dependence and was appearing increasingly anxious and agitated. He had poor appetite and had not slept well since admission.

I interviewed Mr W and recognized that he was in both acute nicotine and opiate withdrawal. He admitted abusing opiates and was taking up to 480 mg of combined oxycontin and oxycodone a day. He had smoked on the day of admission, 3 days ago. History revealed two previous treatments for alcohol dependence as well as a brief period of heroin addiction. Physical symptoms at the time of interview included sweats and chills for 24 hours, nausea without vomiting, abdominal cramping with intermittent diarrhea, muscle pain, insomnia, agitation, anxiety, and goose bumps. The nurses on the unit were unfamiliar with these classic opiate withdrawal symptoms compounded by abrupt cessation of nicotine use, which were causing Mr W's discomfort and irritability.

Treatment included 21-mg transdermal nicotine patch daily while hospitalized to minimize his wanting to leave the floor to go outside to smoke. In addition, he was prescribed clonazepam 0.5 mg every 12 hours and methadone 10 mg TID for 3 days, which was then titrated down to 5 mg BID over the next 4 days. He was followed closely for additional symptoms of anxiety, insomnia, and agitation.

Although anxiety in patients with cancer appearing for treatment is not unusual, when accompanied by the physical symptoms listed above, more questions must be asked. Epidemiologic studies show that between 30% and 60% of patients with anxiety disorders have comorbid conditions such as depression or an SUD.[38] Whenever acute anxiety or history of benzodiazepine use is found, additional inquiry is indicated.[39]

■ NICOTINE AND CANCER

Cigarette smoking is a risk factor for various types of cancer. Nicotine, a major alkaloid in tobacco, is responsible for different aspects in the pathogenesis of smoking-related malignancies. Nicotine not only perpetuates smoking behavior in smokers, which results in further intake of tobacco-derived carcinogens, but also directly increases cellular mutagenic events. Current evidence also supports that nicotine can be metabolized into highly carcinogenic nitrosamines. In addition, nicotine by itself stimulates cancer cell proliferation through multiple mitogenic signaling pathways. Nicotinic stimulation also provides prosurvival signals to cancer cells such that they are more resistant to apoptosis induced by chemotherapeutic agents or ionizing radiation. Moreover, there is evolving evidence suggesting that nicotine can stimulate tumor-associated angiogenesis, a biological process essential for tumor growth and metastasis.[40] It has also been reported that nicotine enhances cancer cell invasiveness and weakens host cancer-killing immunity.[40] Taken together, nicotine seems to play an important role in the initiation, promotion, and progression of smoking-related cancers. A controlled surveillance study on cancer risk of current nicotine users, especially those on nicotine replacement therapy, is therefore justified.[40]

KEY POINTS

- SUDS are common in cancer patients.
- Continued use of alcohol, tobacco, and illicit substances as well as abuse of prescription medication may interfere with successful outcomes of cancer treatment.
- Substance abuse screening tools work when used.
- Detoxification from alcohol and other substances should be accomplished before beginning cancer treatment.
- Nicotine replacement interventions are useful during cancer treatment.

REFERENCES

1. US Department of Health and Human Services. *Tenth Special Report to the US Congress on Alcohol and Health.* Rockville, Md: US DHHS; 2000.

2. US Department of Justice Fact Sheet. September 2001. No. 17.

3. McCarty D. *Substance Abuse Treatment: Benefits and Cost. Knowledge Asset Policy Brief.* Greensboro, NC: Robert Woods Johnson Foundation; September 2008. Substance Abuse Policy Research Program.

4. Tuyns AJ. Epidemiology of alcohol and cancer. *Cancer Res.* 1979;39:2820.

5. Benedetti A, Parent ME, Siemiatycki J. Lifetime consumption of alcoholic beverages and risk of 13 types of cancer in men: results from a case–control study in Montreal. *Cancer Detect Prev.* 2009;32(5–6):352–362.

6. Substance Abuse and Mental Health Services Administration, Office of Applied Studies. *Results from the 2007 National Survey on Drug Use and Health: National Findings.* NSDUH Series H-34, DHHS Publication No. SMA 08-4343). Rockville, MD; 2008.

7. Bagnardi V, Blangiardo M, La Vecchia C, Corrao G. Alcohol Consumption and the Risk of Cancer: A Meta-Analysis. *Alcohol Res Health.* 2001;25.

8. Irigaray P, Newby JA, Clapp R, et al. Lifestyle-related factors and environmental agents causing cancer: an overview. *Biomed Pharmacother.* 2007;61(10):640–658.

9. Klatsky A. Wine, women and … spirits, beer, & breast cancer risk. In: European Cancer Conference 14; September 2007; Barcelona.

10. Allen NE, Beral V, Casabonne D, et al. Moderate alcohol intake and cancer incidence in women. *J Natl Cancer Inst.* 2009;101:296–305.

11. Reeves GK, Pirie K, Green J, Bull D, Beral V, Million Women Study Collaborators. Reproductive factors and specific histological types of breast cancer: prospective study and meta-analysis. *Br J Cancer.* 2009;100(3):538–544.

12. Lauer M, Sorlie P. Alcohol, cardiovascular disease, and cancer: treat with caution. *J Natl Cancer Inst.* 2009;101:282–283.

13. Centre for Addiction and Mental Health. Alcohol and cancer: is drinking the new smoking? *Science Daily.* Available at: http://www.sciencedaily.com. Retrieved June 24, 2009.

14. Li CI, Malone KE, Porter PL, Weiss NS, Tang MT, Daling JR. The relationship between alcohol use and risk of breast cancer by histology and hormone receptor status among women 65–79 years of age. *Cancer Epidemiol Biomarkers Prev.* 2003;12(10):1061–1066.

15. Medical Review Board. Ignoring the problem of senior substance abuse; doctors reluctant to make diagnosis. *Alcoholism Newsletter.* July 2006. Available at: www.about.com. Accessed June 2010.

16. O'Connell H, Chin AV, Cunningham C, Lawlor B. Alcohol use disorders in elderly people—redefining an age old problem in old age. *BMJ.* 2003;327:664.

17. Cher WY, Colditz GA, Rosner B, et al. Use of postmenopausal hormones, alcohol and risk for invasive breast cancer. *Ann Intern Med.* 2002;137:798–804.

18. National Institute on Alcohol Abuse and Alcoholism. *NIH Alcohol Alert, No. 74: Alcohol Research: A Lifespan Perspective*; 2008. NIAAA Publication Center, Rockville, MD; 2008.

19 Zismca A. Nickolov A. et al. Associations between the age at diagnosis and location of colorectal cancer and

the use of alcohol and tobacco. *Arch Int Med.* 2006;166: 629–634.

20. Wakai K, Kojima M, Tamakoshi K, et al. Alcohol consumption and colorectal cancer risk. *J Epidemiol.* 2005;15(suppl II):S173–S179.

21. Cho E, Smith-Warner S, Ritz J, et al. Alcohol intake and colorectal cancer: a pooled analysis of 8 cohort studies. *Ann Intern Med.* 2004;140(8):603–613.

22. National Cancer Institute. *Substance Abuse Issues in Cancer;* 2008.

23. Mersy DJ. Recognition of alcohol and substance abuse. *Am Fam Physician.* 2003;67(7):1529–1532.

24. Committee on Treatment of Alcohol Problems, Institute of Medicine. *Broadening the Base of Treatment for Alcohol Problems.* Report of a Study by a Committee of the Institute of Medicine, Division of Mental Health and Behavioral Medicine. (BOOK: ISBN: 10:0-309-04038-8). Washington, DC: National Academy Press; 1990.

25. National Institute of Alcohol Abuse and Alcoholism Alert #65, April, 2005. Screening for Alcohol Use and Alcohol Related Problems.

26. Taj N, Devera-Sales A, Vinson DC. Screening for problem drinking: does a single question work? *J Fam Pract.* 1998;46(4):328–335.

27. Diagnostic and Statistical Manual of Mental Disorders, 4th ed. Arlington, VA: American Psychiatric Association; 2000.

28. Ewing JA. Detecting alcoholism: the CAGE questionnaire. *JAMA.* 1984;252(14):1905–1907.

29. Saunders, JB, Aasland, OF, Babor, TF, De La Fuente, JR, Grant, M. Development of the Alcohol Use Disorders Identification Test (AUDIT): WHO collaborative project on early detection of persons with harmful alcohol consumption-II. *Addiction.* 1993;88(6):791–804.

30. Selzer ML. The Michigan Alcoholism Screening Test: the quest for a new diagnostic instrument. *Am J Psychiatry.* 1971;127:1653–1658.

31. Gavin DR, Ross HE, Skinner HA. Diagnostic validity of the Drug Abuse Screening Test in the assessment of DSM-III drug disorders. *Br J Addict.* 1989;84(3): 301–307.

32. Miller GA. *The Substance Abuse Subtle Screening Inventory (SASSI) Manual.* 2nd ed. Springville, Ind: The SASSI Institute; 1999.

33. Mersy DJ. Recognition of alcohol and substance abuse. *Am Fam Physician.* 2003;Apr 1;67(7):1529–1532.

34. Watson RR, ed. *Alcohol and Cancer.* Florida: CRC Press; 1992.

35. Sullivan JT, Sykora K, Schneiderman J, Naranjo CA, Sellers EM. Assessment of alcohol withdrawal: the revised Clinical Institute Withdrawal Instrument for Alcohol Scale (CIWA-Ar). *Br J Addict.* 1989; 84:1353–1357.

36. Wesson DR, Ling W. The Clinical Opiate Withdrawal Scale (COWS). *J Psychoactive Drugs.* 2003;35(2):253–259.

37. Mayo-Smith FF. Pharmacologic management of alcohol withdrawal. A meta-analysis and evidence based practice guidelines. American Society of Addiction Medicine Working Group on Pharmacologic Management of Alcohol Withdrawal. *JAMA.* 1997;278:144–151.

38 Comorbid Drug Abuse and Mental Illness: A Research Update from the National Institute on Drug Abuse. October 2007.

39. Regier DA, Farmer ME, Rae DS, et al. Comorbidity of mental disorders with alcohol and other drug abuse, results from the Epidemiological Catchment Area (ECA) Study. *JAMA.* 1990;264:2511–2518.

40. Karger B. Tobacco use and cancer: an epidemiological perspective. In: Wu W, Wong H, Yu L, Cho CH, Purohit V, eds. Alcohol, Tobacco and Cancer. 2006:253–267.

Sexuality and Cancer

• *Mary K. Hughes*

While living with cancer, a person experiences numerous assaults on his or her quality of life. One of these is to a person's sexuality. It is important to remember that the sexual dysfunction is not limited to treatment changes in organs associated with sexual response.[1] Treatments and/or the disease itself can cause changes in sexuality, but health care providers rarely ask about sexuality issues because of concepts about the importance of sexuality in the context of the disease.[2] This causes patients to think they are the only ones with sexuality issues since they are asked about other intimate issues such as bowel and bladder habits, but not sexuality issues.

All cancers can impact sexuality and intimacy.[1] Unlike other side effects of cancer and its treatment, sexual problems do not tend to resolve after several years of disease-free survival.[3] Schover et al[4] report sexuality to be one of the first elements of daily living disrupted by a cancer diagnosis. Sexual relationships make a significant contribution to the quality of life for almost everyone.[5] According to Leiblum et al,[6] all patients regardless of age, sexual orientation, marital status, or life circumstances should have the opportunity to discuss sexual matters with their health care professional. But it is not easy to talk about despite living in a culture that is saturated with overtly sexual images, graphic lyrics, and explicit advertising.[7] Bruner and Boyd[8] assert that the promotion of sexual health is vital for preserving quality of life and is an integral part of total or holistic cancer management.

The benefits of discussing sexuality with the patient are numerous, and are listed as follows:

- it demonstrates a desire by the clinician to treat the entire patient, not just the diseased body part;
- it legitimizes the topic for discussion;
- it emphasizes the importance of maintaining normal activities and relationships during and after treatment;
- it may identify patients at risk for sexual dysfunction after treatment.[9–12]

In order for providers to begin assessing sexuality in people with cancer, they must first understand what sexuality encompasses. It is a broad term including social, emotional, and physical components.[13] It is not just genitals or gender, but includes body image, love of self and others, relating to others, and pleasure.[13] It is genetically endowed (whether a person has XX or XY chromosomes), phenotypically embodied (how masculine or feminine a person is), hormonally nurtured, not age related, but matured by experience, and cannot be bought, sold, or destroyed despite what is done to a person.[14,15] Sexuality includes affection, sexual orientation, sexual activity, eroticism, reproduction, intimacy, and gender roles, and encompasses feelings of trust.[16–18] It also includes:

- the belief that one is capable of attracting the attention and affection of another;
- giving and receiving sexual pleasure;
- feeling of belonging;

- being accepted by another;
- the conviction that we are worthy to live and enjoy life.[19,20]

According to Dibble et al,[21] sexuality is only limited by imagination and physical challenges.

Sexual expression is influenced by cultural norms, past experiences, and the developmental stage of the individual.[10,18,22] Expressions of sexuality include style of dress, values, and attitudes as well as hugging, touching, kissing, acting out scenarios/fantasies, sex toys, masturbation, sexual intercourse, and oral genital stimulation, either alone or with others.[16,18,21,23] Sexual behaviors may involve oral, vaginal, and/or anal penetration.[21] They are influenced by:

- religious beliefs;
- age;
- education;
- level of comfort with one's body and physical functioning;
- experiences of sexual abuse and trauma;
- one's partner's wishes;
- comfort level with one's own sexual orientation and gender identity.[24,25]

Maslow[26] described sexual activity to be a basic need in his hierarchy of needs while love and connection to others was at a higher level. Everyone has a lifelong need for touch and emotional connection to others regardless of current relationship status.[23] Sexual intercourse is not the defining characteristic of a person's sexuality; a sexual relationship includes the need to be touched and held along with closeness and tenderness.[19,27]

In a meta-analysis of studies of women's sexual intercourse frequency, Schneidewind-Skibbe et al[28] report that in women in Europe, the United States, and Asia, sexual activity diminished with age, but in Africa and South America, age did not change frequency. In a study of sexual problems and distress in women in the United States, Shifren et al[29] found that although 44% report a sexual problem, only 22% felt this caused personal distress. Sexual concerns must be associated with distress to be considered a medical problem. Malcarne et al[30] report that the quality of a couple's relationship can be altered even by successful treatment because of the changes in the person with cancer, both emotional and physical.

Masters and Johnson[31] described the human sexual response cycle that begins with libido, which Freud described as instinctual because without it, people would not want to have sex and procreate. Gregoire[32] reports that men are more attracted to visual sexual stimuli, whereas women are more attracted to auditory and written material, particularly stimuli associated within the context of a loving and positive relationship. Women are not linear in their sexual response, but more circular.[33] They may experience sexual excitement before they have a desire for sexual activity. Sexual excitement is the phase where the penis becomes rigid enough to use and the vagina lubricates and enlarges in depth and width, and the clitoris enlarges.[22,34,35] Erection is the male counterpart to vaginal secretions from the sexual physiology perspective.[36] Orgasm is the height of sexual pleasure and the release of sexual tension. The penis emits semen through muscular spasms and there are rhythmic contractions of the vagina and the cervix lifts up out of the vaginal vault. The last phase of the cycle is the resolution phase where the genitals return to their normal, nonexcited state. There is an evaluation of the sexual experience as well as relaxation and contentment during this phase.[37,38] In this phase is the refractory period where the genitals are resistant to sexual stimulation. In males, this period can be a matter of minutes in youth, but take days in older men or with certain medications or medical conditions.

Sexual dysfunction is failure of any aspect of the sexual response cycle to function properly.[39] Goldstein et al[40] report that sexual dysfunction is 90% psychological and 75% physiological. But when a person with cancer has sexual dysfunction, it is mostly physiological. Rothschild[41] describes many causes of sexual dysfunction:

- psychosocial/interpersonal stressors;
- medical illness;
- depressive illness;
- medication;
- sexual disorder (DSM-IV).

The following constitute a sexual problem:

- physiological dysfunction;
- altered experiences;
- own perceptions and beliefs;
- partner's perceptions and expectations;
- altered circumstances;
- past experiences.[32]

Thaler-DeMers[1] reports that treatment decisions made at the time of diagnosis impact the interpersonal relationships, sexuality, and reproductive capacity of all cancer survivors. What are possible causes of sexual dysfunction in a person with cancer? Most often they are treatment related due to the changes in physiological, psychological, and social dimensions of sexuality and disruption in one or more phases of the sexual response cycle.[23,42] As early as 1981, Derogatis and Kourlesis[43] reported that the majority of patients have sexual problems after cancer treatment. Treatments can cause both acute and chronic side effects that affect sexuality.

Determinants of sexual dysfunction with chemotherapy or biologics include:

* type of drug;
* dose of drug;
* cumulative dose;
* length of treatment;
* age of individual;
* sex of individual;
* drug combinations;
* methods to manage side effects;
* length of time after treatment.[20,44,45]

Types of chemotherapeutic agents associated with sexual or reproductive dysfunction include:

* alkylating agents;
* antimetabolites;
* natural products;
* hormonal agents or antagonists;
* biologic agents.[46–53]

Side effects of radiation therapy depend on what part of the body is involved. With cranial or total body irradiation, there is an endocrine axis disruption that can cause ovarian failure. Any radiation to the pelvis, abdomen, or testes can cause oligospermia, uterine damage, and decreased elasticity, volume, and blood supply, and sexuality changes can be experienced months to years after radiation is completed.[54,55]

Hormonal therapy includes steroids, aromatase inhibitors, antiandrogens, and antiestrogen. Indirectly, hormones affect mood, self-image, sexual perception, and energy.[56]

Side effects of surgery depend on:

* location of surgery;
* rate of healing;
* meaning of lost/altered body part to individual.

Side effects of surgery can be extensive and long-lasting and include:

* erectile dysfunction (ED);
* change in ejaculation;
* poor body image;
* scarring;
* loss of tactile sensation in reconstructed breast;
* limited range of motion;
* body asymmetry;
* alibido;
* anorgasmia;
* bowel and/or bladder incontinence;
* infertility;
* stoma;
* ostomy;
* amputation;
* change in female genitalia;
* premature menopause;
* lymphedema;
* increased oral secretions;
* dry mouth.[1,25,57–66]

The nononcologic problems confronting patients after therapy, many of which are the direct result of treatment, need to be considered and addressed.[67]

Besides chemotherapy, biologic agents, and hormones, there are numerous medications that can have sexual side effects that range from decreased desire to difficulty reaching orgasm. These include:

* neurotransmitters;
* stimulants;
* hallucinogens;
* sedatives;
* narcotics;
* anxiolytics;
* anticholinergics;
* antipsychotics;
* lipid-lowering drugs;
* H_2 antagonists;
* many antidepressants;
* phenothiazines;
* antihypertensives;
* recreational drugs;
* alcohol;
* herbals and vitamins;
* anticonvulsants.[32,55,68–70,143,144]

In a study by Montejo-Gonzalez et al,[146] selective serotonin reuptake inhibitors (SSRI) increased the incidence of sexual dysfunction in men, but the dysfunction was more intense in women. Piazza et al[147] found no association between improvement in depression and improvement in sexual functioning after SSRI treatment in women.

Menopausal symptoms can be very distressing to women and interfere with sexuality because of the changes in their bodies.[46] These changes happen gradually in women without cancer and they have time to adjust and enjoy sexual activity 5 to 10 years longer with fewer sexual problems than women with cancer who rapidly experience menopause.[73,74,148]

Wilmoth[69] reports that women with breast cancer identified an altered sexual self that included loss of:

- body parts;
- bleeding (becoming old);
- sexual sensations;
- womanhood.

One should note that while dyspareunia assumes pain with penile–vaginal intercourse, it may be a source of distress as well for women with same-sexed partners, where touch and/or finger or object penetration is uncomfortable.[76] Katz[71] found that physical appearance was important in gay culture and having a partner show acceptance of treatment- or disease-related physical changes was comforting. Chronic graft-versus-host disease (GVHD) after a hematopoietic stem cell transplant can contribute to vaginal introital stenosis and mucosal changes that contribute to dyspareunia, vaginal irritation, and increased sensitivity of genital tissues.[78] Vaginal dryness and concomitant decrease in vulval blood flow can contribute to genital discomfort, dyspareunia, and a decrease in urethral blood flow, which is thought to be a significant factor in urgency incontinence.[36] Sarrel[36] asserts that dyspareunia caused by vaginal dryness can lead to fear of penetration and associated vaginismus, which can affect the woman's partner. Table 10-1 describes types of female sexual dysfunction as defined by DSM-IV.[84]

Sexual dysfunction in men is not as complex as in women and is usually associated with age and illness. Ideally male testosterone levels should be tested before beginning cancer treatment as a baseline indicator of a man's normal level.[85] Types of male sexual dysfunction and possible causes include:

- ED;
- low libido;
- age-related factors:
  - loss of willing partner, opportunity, and privacy;
  - decreased frequency of activity;
  - decreased arousal in response to psychological stimuli;
  - decreased tactile sensitivity of penis;
  - increased refractory period after orgasm;
  - increased rates of ED with age;
  - physical disease:
    - peripheral vascular;
    - diabetic neuropathy;
    - cancer;
  - psychiatric illness:
    - dementia;
    - depression;
  - lifestyle factors:
    - physical inactivity;
    - boredom;
    - loneliness;
    - smoking;
    - alcohol consumption;
- ejaculation problems:
  - retrograde;
  - dry;
  - premature.[32,79,86]

It should be remembered that sexual dysfunctions are not all-or-nothing phenomena, but occur on a continuum—in terms of frequency and severity. Comorbidity of sexual dysfunctions is common. Gregoire[32] reports that almost half the men with low libido also have another sexual dysfunction, and 20% of men with ED have low libido. The patient's partner and their relationship probably have a more profound effect on sexual health than on any other aspect of health.

An estimated 30 million men in the United States experience some degree of ED at any given time.[87] It is more common in men who are obese, smokers, and physically inactive or have been treated for diabetes, heart disease, or hypertension.[88,89] Kupelian et al[81] reported that ED is predictive of metabolic syndrome in men with a body mass index higher than 25. It is important to get a medical history of patients to see whether they have factors other than cancer treatment history that could contribute to ED.

Knight and Latini[82] concluded that for many men, next to survival, sexuality is one of the most important considerations in prostate cancer treatment decision making. Men with colorectal cancer report more problems with sexual function related to their surgeries than women with similar treatment for similar diagnoses.[59,60] Some studies show that partners of patients with cancer experience more psychological distress than their cancer-affected mate.[92–96] Neese et al[89] note that less than half of men with sexual dysfunction believed that their partners supported them in their efforts to find help.

■ **TABLE 10-1. American Psychiatric Association Categories of Sexual Dysfunction**[79–83]

Type of Female Sexual Dysfunction	Description
Persistent or recurrent disorders of interest/desire (hypoactive sexual desire disorder [HSDD])	An absence of desire at any time during the sexual experience designates disorder
Disorders of subjective and genital arousal	If subjective, no response to any type of sexual stimulation, but may have genital arousal
	If genital arousal disorder, subjective arousal to nongenital stimulation (usually postmenopausal women), but impaired or absent genital sexual arousal
	Combined—absence or very diminished feelings of sexual arousal from any type of sexual stimulation as well as absence of genital sexual arousal
Persistent sexual arousal disorder	In the absence of sexual interest and desire, spontaneous, intrusive, unwanted genital throbbing unrelieved by orgasm
Orgasmic disorder (female orgasmic disorder [FOD])	Lack of, markedly diminished, or delay of orgasms despite sexual arousal regardless of stimulation
Sexual pain disorders	
Vaginismus	Reflexive tightening around the vagina when vaginal entry is attempted despite woman's desire for penetration. No physical abnormalities present. Often associated with fear, anticipation, or pain
Dyspareunia	Pain with attempted or completed vaginal entry
Sexual aversion disorder involving dysfunctions of sexual desire (FSAD)	Extreme anxiety and/or disgust at the anticipation of or attempt to have any sexual activity
Sexual dysfunction secondary to a general medical condition or substance induced	Medications, chronic or acute illnesses, fatigue, pain

Treatment decisions made at the time of diagnosis impact interpersonal relationships, sexuality, and reproductive capacity of all survivors.[1] Schover[98] reports that one of the greatest concerns of cancer survivors of childbearing age is the effect of treatment on fertility. Reproductive concerns that emerge within the cancer experience are negatively associated with quality of life.[99] Studies show that most young survivors are interested in having children, especially if they were childless at the time of their cancer diagnosis.[98,100] Difficulties with fertility increase with age and are much more common for women greater than 40 years.[84,101] Pregnancy does not appear to increase the risk of cancer recurrence.[102] The ability to preserve fertility depends on:

- age;
- type of cancer;
- combination of treatments;
- type of treatment.[103–106]

The American Society of Clinical Oncologists recommends that:

- Oncologists address the possibility of infertility with patients in their reproductive years.
- Fertility preservation should be considered as early as possible during treatment.
- Standard fertility preservation practice is:
  ○ sperm cryopreservation for men;
  ○ embryo cryopreservation for women;
  ○ other methods considered investigational.[107,108]

Unfortunately, fertility preservation takes time, is expensive, and can delay treatment, and many cancers need to be treated promptly.[46] One study showed significant depression, grief, and sexual difficulties in women whose cancer treatment caused infertility.[109] Psychological responses to infertility may include:

- grief;
- anger;
- depression;
- sadness;
- loss of femininity/masculinity;
- changes in self-image.[1,23]

Body image is a key aspect of sexuality and includes one's feelings and attitudes about one's body.[17,110] Body image changes can profoundly alter feelings of attractiveness, which is an important aspect of sexuality.[1] External changes that are visible to others as well as internal changes affect body image.[17,111] Body image changes can be temporary or permanent and include:

- alopecia;
- change in facial hair;
- weight changes;
- scarring;
- ostomies;
- stomas;
- placement of drains and venous access lines;
- amputations;
- skin changes (texture/color);
- incontinence of bowel and/or bladder;
- gynecomastia;
- change in penis/testicle size;
- change in shape of breast.[23,149]

Mood can affect sexual functioning in a negative or positive way.[112] Psychological issues that can alter sexual functioning include:

- frustration;
- stigma;
- embarrassment;
- anxiety;
- anger;
- irritability;
- depression;
- loneliness;
- despair;
- grief;
- interference of age-appropriate goals;
- performance anxiety;
- changes in personality;
- mood swings;
- misinformation;

- guilt and shame;
- disappointment;
- fear of:
  - death,
  - rejection,
  - never feeling better,
  - abandonment,
  - how cancer will affect others,
  - social role change,
  - how attractiveness changes,
  - never finishing treatment,
  - pain,
  - recurrence with sexual activity,
  - cancer spread with sexual activity,
  - loss of control,
  - dependency.[150,113–120,142,145]

It is important to get depression and anxiety treated (see Chapters 5 and 6).

The culture in which one grew up as well as the culture in which one currently lives not only affects how one copes with cancer, but also influences one's sexuality.[46] Katz's study[71] found that homophobia does not affect current cancer care experiences of gay and lesbian patients, and health care providers accepted the support of the patient's same-sexed partners. Often health care practitioners do not know the sexual orientation or gender identity of their patients.[21] Dibble et al[21] further state that because of heterosexism, those who do not share a heterosexual orientation may have difficult lives especially when they are ill. Heterosexism is the belief that heterosexuality is the only "normal" option for relationships.[21] Most of the research on the effects of cancer and its treatment on sexuality has been limited to heterosexual women or women assumed to be heterosexual.[121]

People in isolated, rural areas may feel a lack of support and resources to address sexuality changes. Someone with cancer may mistakenly feel they are contagious. Partners of women with cancer often are fearful of hurting or infecting them because of lack of information or misinformation from the practitioner about resuming sexual activity.[122] Cancer is expensive to treat, and often financial and insurance concerns interfere with sexuality because of being distracted. The stress of cancer and its treatments can exacerbate underlying marital tension and likewise affect the sexual relationship.[46] Other sociocultural influences on sexual changes include:

- marital status;
- race;

- education;
- attitude toward cancer/treatment;
- gender preference;
- family traditions;
- religion;
- change in touch/intimacy;
- lack of partner;
- significance of body part;
- role change;
- job loss/pressures;
- end-of-life issues;
- relationship inequalities.[4, 113,116,122–125]

One of the most important factors in adjusting sexually after surviving cancer is a woman's feelings about sexuality before cancer. Many people have adopted a pattern of sexual behavior before their diagnosis and attempt to return to it after treatment. If they experience discomfort or failure to function as before, they will stop trying and feel they cannot enjoy sexual activity.[126] Some couples who are cancer survivors and are in a stressful relationship with an unsupportive partner tend to have more distress, which can lead to avoidant coping behaviors.[127] They avoid talking about difficult issues including sexuality. Conversely, during the time of treatment, the cancer experience encourages a more intimate and intense interpersonal relationship.[1] There are few studies that have attempted any type of psychosocial intervention to assist survivors in integrating the cancer experience into their personal life.[1] If one is not partnered, there is the question of when to reveal one's cancer history: at the beginning of a relationship or wait until the relationship develops.

According to Tomlinson,[118] the main difference between taking a history about a sexual problem and an ordinary medical history is the level of embarrassment and discomfort of the patient and the health care provider. A discussion of sexual changes can begin by acknowledging the sexual changes brought about by the cancer or the treatment of the cancer.[1] Sexual changes after treatment are routinely unaddressed or only barely touched on despite patients having significant needs for education, support, and practical help with managing them. Regardless of our role in providing care to the patient, most of us do not have experience talking about sexuality and intimacy in a frank, direct, and authentic manner.[7] Annon's PLISSIT model[119] has four components: P, permission; LI, limited information; SS, specific suggestions; and IT, intensive therapy. The practitioner gives the patient permission (P) to think about cancer and sexuality at the same time by asking, "What sexuality changes have you noticed since your cancer?," which lets them know that they are not the only ones to experience sexuality changes. By asking open-ended questions, the health care provider is better able to get a thoughtful response from the patient.[113] Giving patients time to answer is important. Try to remain relaxed with good eye contact to let them know that you are interested in this area of their lives. Addressing sexuality issues early on in the assessment and treatment of the patient allows the nurse to open up a line of communication with the patient so that these issues can be addressed as they come up in the future.[113]

Providing patients with limited information (LI) about side effects from treatments by saying, "Sometimes people notice sexuality changes when they get this treatment," lets them know that you are comfortable talking about sexuality issues. One of the first steps toward sexual rehabilitation is sex education.[120]

Describing specific suggestions (SS) such as books to read and positions to use can offer them help with the problem. Other suggestions can include:

- vaginal lubricants and moisturizers;
- videos;
- contraceptive options;
- planning for sexual activity;
- communicating more openly about sexual needs;
- exploring one's own body;
- safer sexual practices;
- different means of sexual expression;
- better symptom control;
- using erotic devices;
- using erotica;
- sensate focus.[121–124]

Some patients are in difficult relationships, which only get worse with cancer treatment and need intensive therapy (IT) from a marital or a sex therapist. Having a list of those resources in the community can be helpful to the patient. But Schover[125] reports that patients often prefer to receive information from a member of the health care team instead of being sent to a sex specialist.

Giving referrals depends on patients who may benefit from specialized assistance if they need:

- PDE5 inhibitors;
- penile implants;
- penile injections;
- penile suppositories;
- vacuum erection device;

- fertility specialists;
- EROS-CT for women;
- physical therapist for pelvic floor exercises;
- reconstructive surgery;
- breast implants;
- hormone therapy;
- psychosexual therapy.[4,22,46,126–128]

The patient usually does not voluntarily ask sex-related questions, so it is up to the health care provider to integrate sexuality into the routine care of all oncology patients.[113] Sexual morbidities after breast cancer diagnosis include an immediate reduction in sexual activity and responsiveness.[129–132] Andersen[112] found that women diagnosed with breast cancer recurrence were less sexually active initially, but increased their activity to pre-recurrence rates unless they had distance metastasis. Even when patients are dealing with end-of-life issues, it is important to be aware of their sexuality concerns and address these.[133]

Interventions for sexual dysfunction resulting from cancer treatment can be limited because of the hormone status of the tumor. Women with estrogen receptive positive breast cancer are often unable to use any estrogen products, while some oncologists give them the go-ahead to use an estrogen vaginal ring, vaginal creams, or tablets. A study reported that use of vaginal estradiol tablet was associated with a rise in systemic estradiol levels, which reverses estrogen suppression achieved by aromatase inhibitors and should be avoided.[107] Greenwald and McCorkle[132] reported that women with cervical cancer had their sexual desire and enjoyment rebound 6 years after treatment, but they struggled with sexuality issues until then, whereas most of the symptoms of sexual dysfunction in patients with breast cancer are related to estrogen deprivation due to premature menopause caused by chemotherapy and antiestrogen hormonal therapy. Furthermore, there are some oncologists who will allow the use of off-label androgen gel for those women to improve libido. Studies have demonstrated that testosterone has positive effects on women's sexuality and that higher doses show greater effects.[134] It is controversial and should be left up to the discretion of the medical oncologist. Women with other types of cancer can use oral estrogen replacement if they are comfortable with that and their oncologist has approved use. Maintenance of vaginal health through hormonal and nonhormonal methods is important not only for overall well-being of the postmenopausal female, but also for the elimination of sexual dysfunctions that occur because of atrophic vaginitis.[135]

Levine[136] asserts that it is important to preserve motivation for women to have sex and that there are common enemies to accomplishing this:

- anger and disappointment with partner;
- insufficient psychological intimacy;
- fatigue;
- disappointment with self for:
  - too much to do,
  - too little time to accomplish tasks,
  - depressing character trait (do not like an aspect of themselves).

Levine[136] further describes sexual activity as a rebonding mechanism:

- serves as an eraser for ordinary annoyances;
- prevents hostility between partners;
- decreases extramarital temptations;
- provides psychological intimacy.

Men with prostate cancer do not have the option to take testosterone replacements for low libido for fear of stimulating the tumor. However, men with other types of cancer can take testosterone replacements without fear of increasing their risk of prostate cancer.[137] Asking about desire includes inquiring about sexual fantasies and dreams that have to do with testosterone levels.

According to Ritchie,[138] the most important factor in improving care of sexual problems in cancer is to ask about them. In most published studies, patients have stated that they would like more information about sex than they received from their physician.

Ways to incorporate assessment of sexuality concerns into clinical practice include addressing sexuality through patients' perceptions of:

- body image;
- family roles and functions;
- relationships;
- sexual function.[139]

The Institute of Medicine report,[140] *From Cancer Patient to Cancer Survivor: Lost in Transition*, recommends intervention for consequences of cancer and its treatment including sexual side effects. By legitimizing the topic of sexuality from the onset of patient assessment, health care providers support patients who then find it easier to raise issues of sexuality as they evolve. Recognizing the pleasure that sexual activity brings and the pain its absence can create can prompt the health care provider to include a sexual assessment on all patients.[113] Kaplan[141] points out that a strong therapeutic alliance is formed with the cancer patient and also with his or her partner when the health care practitioner expresses concern about the couple's sexual well-being and when the practitioner sees to it that everything possible has been done to restore their sexual relationship.

KEY POINTS

- Sexuality has been defined.
- Human sexual response has been discussed.
- Comparison has been made between sexual dysfunction and sexual problems.
- Causes of sexual dysfunction have been listed.
- Interventions for sexual dysfunction have been discussed.

REFERENCES

1. Thaler-DeMers D. Intimacy issues: sexuality, fertility, and relationships. *Semin Oncol Nurs.* 2001;17:255–262.

2. Bitzer J, Platano G, Tschudin S, Alder J. Sexual counseling for women in the context of physical diseases: a teaching model for physicians. *J Sex Med.* 2007;4:29–37.

3. Schover LR. Premature ovarian failure and its consequences: vasomotor symptoms, sexuality, and fertility. *J Clin Oncol.* 2008;26:753–758.

4. Schover L, Montague D, Lakin M. Sexual problems. In: Devita VT, Hellman S, Rosenberg SA, eds. *Cancer: Principles and Practices of Oncology.* 5th ed. Philadelphia, Pa: Lippincott-Raven; 1997:2857–2871.

5. Filiberti A, Audisio RA, Gangeri L, et al. Prevalence of sexual dysfunction in male cancer patients treated with rectal excision and coloanal anastomosis. *Eur J Cancer.* 1994;20:43–46.

6. Leiblum SR, Baume RM, Croog SH. The sexual functioning of elderly hypertensive women. *J Sex Marital Ther.* 1994;20:259–270.

7. Bober SL. From the guest editor: out in the open: addressing sexual health after cancer. *Cancer J.* 2009;15:13–14.

8. Bruner DW, Boyd CP. Assessing women's sexuality after cancer therapy: checking assumptions with the focus group technique. *Cancer Nurs.* 1999;22:438–447.

9. McKee AL Jr, Schover LR. Sexuality rehabilitation. *Cancer.* 2001;92:1008–1012.

10. Pelusi J. Sexuality and body image. Research on breast cancer survivors documents altered body image and sexuality. *Am J Nurs.* 2006;106:32–38.

11. Speer JJ, Hillenberg B, Sugrue DP, et al. Study of sexual functioning determinants in breast cancer survivors. *Breast J.* 2005;11:440–447.

12. Rogers MP. Breast cancer program: tools to help deliver enhanced outcomes. In: ONS 9th Annual IOL & APN Conference; 2008; Seattle, Wash:6–48.

13. Southard NZ, Keller J. The importance of assessing sexuality: a patient perspective. *Clin J Oncol Nurs.* 2009;13:213–217.

14. Smith DB. Sexuality and the patient with cancer: what nurses need to know. *Oncol Patient Care Pract Guidel Specialized Nurse.* 1994;4:1–3.

15. Winze JP, Carey MP. *Sexual Dysfunction: A Guide for Assessment and Treatment.* New York, NY: Guilford Press; 1991.

16. Sexual Health. World Health Organization. 2002. Available at: http://www.who.int/reproductive-health/gender/sexualhealth.htm. Accessed June 8, 2010.

17. Krebs L. What should I say? Talking with patients about sexuality issues. *Clin J Oncol Nurs.* 2006;10:313–315.

18. Wilmoth MC. Life after cancer: what does sexuality have to do with it? 2006 Mara Mogensen Flaherty Memorial Lectureship. *Oncol Nurs Forum.* 2006;33:905–910.

19. Shell JA. Sexuality. In: Carroll-Johnson R, Gorman L, Bush N, eds. *Oncology Nursing.* St Louis, Mo: Mosby; 2007:546–564.

20. Krebs LU. Sexuality and reproductive issues. In: Yasko JM, ed. *Nursing Management of Symptoms associated with Chemotherapy.* 5th ed. West Conshohocken, Pa: Meniscus Health Care Communications; 2001: 205–214.

21. Dibble S, Eliason MJ, Dejoseph JF, Chinn P. Sexual issues in special populations: lesbian and gay individuals. *Semin Oncol Nurs.* 2008;24:127–130.

22. Katz A. *Breaking the Silence on Cancer and Sexuality.* Pittsburgh, Pa: Oncology Nursing Society; 2007.

23. Tierney DK. Sexuality: a quality-of-life issue for cancer survivors. *Semin Oncol Nurs.* 2008;24:71–79.

24. Dibble SL, Eliason MJ, Christiansen MA. Chronic illness care for lesbian, gay, & bisexual individuals. *Nurs Clin North Am.* 2007;42:655–674; viii.

25. Bruner DW. Quality of life: sexuality issues for cancer patients. Paper presented at: NCCN Conference; Nurses' session, February 2005.

26. Maslow A. A theory of human motivation. *Psychol Rev.* 1943;50:370–396.

27. Stausmire JM. Sexuality at the end of life. *Am J Hosp Palliat Care.* 2004;21:33–39.

28. Schneidewind-Skibbe A, Hayes RD, Koochaki PE, Meyer J, Dennerstein L. The frequency of sexual intercourse reported by women: a review of community-based studies and factors limiting their conclusions. *J Sex Med.* 2008;5:301–335.

29. Shifren JL, Monz BU, Russo PA, Segreti A, Johannes CB. Sexual problems and distress in United States women: prevalence and correlates. *Obstet Gynecol.* 2008;112:970–978.

30. Malcarne VL, Banthia R, Varni JW, Sadler GR, Greenbergs HL, Ko CM. Problem-solving skills and emotional distress in spouses of men with prostate cancer. *J Cancer Educ.* 2002;17:150–154.

31. Masters WH, Johnson VE. *Human Sexual Response.* 1st ed. Boston, Mass: Little Brown; 1966.

32. Gregoire A. Male sexual problems. In: Tomlinson JM, ed. *ABC of Sexual Health.* 2nd ed. Malden, Mass: Blackwell Publishing Inc; 2005:37–39.

33. Basson R. Human sex–response cycles. *J Sex Marital Ther.* 2001;27:33–43.

34. Kandeel FR, Koussa VK, Swerdloff RS. Male sexual function and its disorders: physiology, pathophysiology, clinical investigation, and treatment. *Endocr Rev.* 2001;22:342–388.

35. Schiavi RC, Segraves RT. The biology of sexual function. *Psychiatr Clin North Am.* 1995;18:7–23.

36. Sarrel P. Genital blood flow and ovarian secretions. *Obstet Gynecol*; 75(suppl4):265–305.

37. Zilbergeld B, Ellison C. Desire discrepancies and arousal problems in sex therapy. In: Leiblum S, Pervin L, eds. *Principles and Practice of Sex Therapy.* New York, NY: Guilford Press; 1980.

38. Gallo-Silver L. The sexual rehabilitation of persons with cancer. *Cancer Pract.* 2000;8:10–15.

39. Maurice WL. *Sexual Medicine in Primary Care.* St Louis, Mo: Mosby; 1999.

40. Goldstein I, Meston CM, Traish AM, et al. Future directions. In: *Women's Sexual Function and Dysfunction: Study, Diagnosis, and Treatment.* London: Taylor & Francis; 2007:745–748.

41. Rothschild AJ. Assessing for sexual side effects of medications. Paper presented at: CME Conference; lunch lecture, November 1998.

42. Schover L. Reproductive complications and sexual dysfunction in cancer survivors. In: Ganz PA, ed. *Cancer Survivorship; Today and Tomorrow.* New York, NY: Springer; 2007:251–271.

43. Derogatis LR, Kourlesis SM. An approach to evaluation of sexual problems in the cancer patient. *CA Cancer J Clin.* 1981;31:46–50.

44. Knobf MT. The influence of endocrine effects of adjuvant therapy on quality of life outcomes in younger breast cancer survivors. *Oncologist.* 2006;11:96–110.

45. Averette HE, Boike GM, Jarrell MA. Effects of cancer chemotherapy on gonadal function and reproductive capacity. *CA Cancer J Clin.* 1990;40:199–209.

46. Krebs LU. Sexual and reproductive dysfunction. In: Yarbro C, Frogge MH, Goodman M, Groenwald S, eds. *Cancer Nursing: Principles and Practice.* 5th ed. Sudbury, Mass: Jones & Bartlett Publishers; 2000:831–885.

47. Guy JL, Ingram BA. Medical oncology: the agents. In: McCorkle R, Grant M, Frank-Stromborg M, Baird S, eds. *Cancer Nursing: A Comprehensive Textbook.* 2nd ed. Philadelphia, Pa: WB Saunders; 1996:359–394.

48. Langhorne M. Chemotherapy. In: Otto S, ed. *Oncology Nursing.* 3rd ed. St Louis, Mo: Mosby-Year Book; 1997:530–572.

49. Martin V, Walker FE, Goodman M. Delivery of cancer chemotherapy. In: McCorkle R, Grant M, Frank-Stromborg M, Baird S, eds. *Cancer Nursing: A Comprehensive Textbook.* 2nd ed. Philadelphia, Pa: WB Saunders; 1996:395–433.

50. Perry MC, Anderson CM, Dorr VJ, Wilkes JD. *Companion Handbook to the Chemotherapy Sourcebook.* Baltimore, Md: Lippincott Williams & Wilkins; 1999.

51. Reiger PT. *Clinical Handbook for Biotherapy.* Sudbury, Mass: Jones & Bartlett Publishers; 1999.

52. Skeel RT. *Handbook of Cancer Chemotherapy.* 5th ed. Philadelphia, Pa: Lippincott Williams & Wilkins; 1999.

53. Wilkes GM. *1999 Oncology Nursing Drug Handbook.* Sudbury, Mass: Jones & Bartlett Publishers; 1999.

54. Kelly D. Changed men: the embodied impact of prostate cancer. *Qual Health Res.* 2009;19:151–163.

55. Galbraith ME, Crighton F. Alterations of sexual function in men with cancer. *Semin Oncol Nurs.* 2008;24:102–114.

56. Barton D. The significance of serum testosterone concentrations for female cancer survivors. In: 9th National Conference on Cancer Nursing Research; 2007; Hollywood, Calif. *Oncol Nurs Forum.* 2007:170.

57. Lamb MA. Psychosexual issues: the woman with gynecologic cancer. *Semin Oncol Nurs.* 1990;6:237–243.

58. Hendren SK, O'Connor BI, Liu M, et al. Prevalence of male and female sexual dysfunction is high following surgery for rectal cancer. *Ann Surg.* 2005;242:212–223.

59. Maurer CA, Z'Graggen K, Renzulli P, Schilling MK, Netzer P, Buchler MW. Total mesorectal excision preserves male genital function compared with conventional rectal cancer surgery. *Br J Surg.* 2001;88:1501–1505.

60. Schmidt CE, Bestmann B, Kuchler T, Kremer B. Factors influencing sexual function in patients with rectal cancer. *Int J Impot Res.* 2005;17:231–238.

61. Salem HK. Radical cystectomy with preservation of sexual function and fertility in patients with transitional cell carcinoma of the bladder: new technique. *Int J Urol.* 2007;14:294–298 [discussion 9].

62. Katz A. Sexuality after hysterectomy. *J Obstet Gynecol Neonatal Nurs.* 2002;31:256–262.

63. Stanford JL, Feng Z, Hamilton AS, et al. Urinary and sexual function after radical prostatectomy for clinically localized prostate cancer: the Prostate Cancer Outcomes Study. *JAMA.* 2000;283:354–360.

64. Bruner DW, Berk L. Altered body image and sexual health. In: Yarbro CH, Frogge MH, Goodman M, eds. *Cancer Symptom Management.* Sudbury, Mass: Jones and Bartlett Publishers; 2004:141–156.

65. Bakewell RT, Volker DL. Sexual dysfunction related to the treatment of young women with breast cancer. *Clin J Oncol Nurs.* 2005;9:697–702.

66. Jung BF, Ahrendt GM, Oaklander AL, Dworkin RH. Neuropathic pain following breast cancer surgery: proposed classification and research update. *Pain.* 2003;104:1–13.

67. Auchincloss SS, Holland J, Hughes M. Gynecological. In: Holland J, Greenberg D, Hughes M, eds. *Quick Reference for Oncology Clinicians: The Psychiatric and Psychological Dimensions of Cancer Symptom Management.* Charlottesville, Va: IPOS Press; 2006.

68. Hughes M. Sexual dysfunction. In: Holland J, Greenberg D, Hughes M, eds. *Quick Reference for Oncology Clinicians: The Psychiatric and Psychological Dimensions of Cancer Symptom Management.* Charlottesville, Va: IPOS Press; 2006.

69. Wilmoth MC. The aftermath of breast cancer: an altered sexual self. *Cancer Nurs.* 2001;24:278–286.

70. Rosenbaum TY. Managing postmenopausal dyspareunia: beyond hormone therapy. *Female Patient.* 2006;31:1–5.

71. Katz A. Gay and lesbian patients with cancer. *Oncol Nurs Forum.* 2009;36:203–207.

72. Schubert MA, Sullivan KM, Schubert MM, et al. Gynecological abnormalities following allogeneic bone marrow transplantation. *Bone Marrow Transplant.* 1990;5:425–430.

73. American Psychiatric Association. *Diagnostic and Statistical Manual of Mental Disorders: DSM-IV-TR.* Washington, DC: Author; 2000.

74. Basson R, Leiblum S, Brotto L, et al. Revised definitions of women's sexual dysfunction. *J Sex Med.* 2004;1:40–48.

75. Basson R, Althof S, Davis S, et al. Summary of the recommendations on sexual dysfunctions in women. *J Sex Med.* 2004;1:24–34.

76. Yi JC, Syrjala KL. Sexuality after hematopoietic stem cell transplantation. *Cancer J.* 2009;15:57–64.

77. Feldman HA, Goldstein I, Hatzichristou DG, Krane RJ, McKinlay JB. Impotence and its medical and psychosocial correlates: results of the Massachusetts Male Aging Study. *J Urol.* 1994;151:54–61.

78. Esposito K, Giugliano F, Di Palo C, et al. Effect of lifestyle changes on erectile dysfunction in obese men: a randomized controlled trial. *JAMA.* 2004;291:2978–2984.

79. Lue T. Physiology of penile erection and pathophysiology of erectile dysfunction and priapism. In: Walsh C, Retik A, eds. *Campbell's Urology.* 8th ed. Philadelphia, PA: WB Saunders; 2002:1591–1618.

80. Seftel AD. Erectile dysfunction a decade later: another paradigm shift. *J Urol.* 2006;176:10–11.

81. Kupelian V, Shabsigh R, Araujo AB, O'Donnell AB, McKinlay JB. Erectile dysfunction as a predictor of the metabolic syndrome in aging men: results from the Massachusetts Male Aging Study. *J Urol.* 2006;176:222–226.

82. Knight SJ, Latini DM. Sexual side effects and prostate cancer treatment decisions: patient information needs and preferences. *Cancer J.* 2009;15:41–44.

83. Harden J. Developmental life stage and couples' experiences with prostate cancer: a review of the literature. *Cancer Nurs.* 2005;28:85–98.

84. Oktay K, Sonmezer M. Ovarian tissue banking for cancer patients: fertility preservation, not just ovarian cryopreservation. *Hum Reprod.* 2004;19:477–480.

85. Carlson LE, Bultz BD, Speca M, St. Pierre M. Partners of cancer patients—part I. Impact, adjustment, and coping across the illness trajectory. *J Psychosoc Oncol.* 2000;18:39–63.

86. Kiss A, Meryn S. Effect of sex and gender on psychosocial aspects of prostate and breast cancer. *BMJ.* 2001;323:1055–1058.

87. Perez MA, Skinner EC, Meyerowitz BE. Sexuality and intimacy following radical prostatectomy: patient and partner perspectives. *Health Psychol.* 2002;21:288–293.

88. Sestini AJ, Pakenham KI. Cancer of the prostate—a biopsychosocial review. *J Psychosoc Oncol.* 2000;18:17–38.

89. Neese LE, Schover LR, Klein EA, Zippe C, Kupelian PA. Finding help for sexual problems after prostate cancer treatment: a phone survey of men's and women's perspectives. *Psychooncology.* 2003;12:463–473.

90. Wenzel L, Dogan-Ates A, Habbal R, et al. Defining and measuring reproductive concerns of female cancer survivors. *J Natl Cancer Inst Monogr.* 2005;34:94–98.

91. Schover LR. Psychosocial aspects of infertility and decisions about reproduction in young cancer survivors: a review. *Med Pediatr Oncol.* 1999;33:53–59.

92. Simon B, Lee SJ, Partridge AH, Runowicz CD. Preserving fertility after cancer. *CA Cancer J Clin.* 2005;55:211–228 [quiz 63–64].

93. Partridge AH, Burstein HJ, Winer EP. Side effects of chemotherapy and combined chemohormonal therapy in women with early-stage breast cancer. *J Natl Cancer Inst Monogr.* 2001;30:135–142.

94. Fossa SD, Dahl AA. Fertility and sexuality in young cancer survivors who have adult-onset malignancies. *Hematol Oncol Clin North Am.* 2008;22:291–303, vii.

95. Dow KH, Kuhn D. Fertility options in young breast cancer survivors: a review of the literature. *Oncol Nurs Forum.* 2004;31:E46–E53.

96. Leonard M, Hammelef K, Smith GD. Fertility considerations, counseling, and semen cryopreservation for males prior to the initiation of cancer therapy. *Clin J Oncol Nurs.* 2004;8:127–131, 45.

97. Wallace WH, Anderson RA, Irvine DS. Fertility preservation for young patients with cancer: who is at risk and what can be offered? *Lancet Oncol.* 2005;6:209–218.

98. Schover LR. Sexuality and fertility after cancer. *Hematology (Am Soc Hematol Educ Program).* 2005;523–527.

99. Lamb MA. Effects of cancer on the sexuality and fertility of women. *Semin Oncol Nurs.* 1995;11:120–127.

100. American Society of Clinical Oncology. ASCO recommendations on fertility preservation in cancer patients: guideline summary. *J Oncol Pract.* 2006;2:143–146.

101. Carter J. Cancer-related infertility. *Gynecol Oncol.* 2005;99:S122–S123.

102. DeFrank JT, Mehta CC, Stein KD, Baker F. Body image dissatisfaction in cancer survivors. *Oncol Nurs Forum.* 2007;34:E36–E41.

103. Butler L, Banfield V, Sveinson T, Allen K. Conceptualizing sexual health in cancer care. *West J Nurs Res.* 1998;20:683–699 [discussion 700–705].

104. Mitchell WB, DiBartolo PM, Brown TA, Barlow DH. Effects of positive and negative mood on sexual arousal in sexually functional males. *Arch Sex Behav.* 1998;27:197–207.

105. Massie M. Breast. In: Holland J, Greenberg D, Hughes M, eds. *Quick Reference for Oncology Clinicians: The Psychiatric and Psychological Dimensions of Cancer Symptom Management.* Charlottesville, Va: IPOS Press; 2006.

106. Fisher SG. The psychosexual effects of cancer and cancer treatment. *Oncol Nurs Forum.* 1983;10:63–68.

107. Cull A, Cowie VJ, Farquharson DI, Livingstone JR, Smart GE, Elton RA. Early stage cervical cancer: psychosocial and sexual outcomes of treatment. *Br J Cancer.* 1993;68:1216–1220.

108. Kritcharoen S, Suwan K, Jirojwong S. Perceptions of gender roles, gender power relationships, and sexuality in Thai women following diagnosis and treatment for cervical cancer. *Oncol Nurs Forum.* 2005;32:682–688.

109. Boehmer U, Potter J, Bowen DJ. Sexual functioning after cancer in sexual minority women. *Cancer J.* 2009;15:65–69.

110. Ferrell BR, Dow KH, Leigh S, Ly J, Gulasekaram P. Quality of life in long-term cancer survivors. *Oncol Nurs Forum.* 1995;22:915–922.

111. Dobkin PL, Bradley I. Assessment of sexual dysfunction in oncology patients: review, critique, and suggestions. *J Psychosoc Oncol.* 1991;9:43–75.

112. Andersen BL. In sickness and in health: maintaining intimacy after breast cancer recurrence. *Cancer J.* 2009;15:70–73.

113. Hughes MK. Sexuality and the cancer survivor: a silent coexistence. *Cancer Nurs.* 2000;23:477–482.

114. Hughes MK. Alterations of sexual function in women with cancer. *Semin Oncol Nurs.* 2008;24:91–101.

115. Humphreys CT, Tallman B, Altmaier EM, Barnette V. Sexual functioning in patients undergoing bone marrow transplantation: a longitudinal study. *Bone Marrow Transplant.* 2007;39:491–496.

116. Basson R. Women's sexual dysfunction: revised and expanded definitions. *CMAJ.* 2005;172:1327–1333.

117. Manne SL, Ostroff J, Winkel G, Grana G, Fox K. Partner unsupportive responses, avoidant coping, and distress among women with early stage breast cancer: patient and partner perspectives. *Health Psychol.* 2005;24:635–641.

118. Tomlinson JM. Talking a sexual history. In: Tomlinson JM, ed. *ABC of Sexual Health.* 2nd ed. Malden, Mass: Blackwell Publishing Inc; 2005:13–16.

119. Annon JS. The PLISSIT model: a proposed conceptual scheme for the behavioral treatment of sexual problems. *J Sex Educ Ther.* 1976;2:1–15.

120. Smith DB, Babaian RJ. The effects of treatment for cancer on male fertility and sexuality. *Cancer Nurs.* 1992;15:271–275.

121. Masters WH, Johnson VE, Kolodny RC. *Human Sexuality.* New York, NY: HarperCollins; 1992.

122. Clayton AH. Sexual function and dysfunction in women. *Psychiatr Clin North Am.* 2003;26:673–682.

123. Hughes MK. Sexuality changes in the cancer patient: MD Anderson case reports and review. *Nurs Interv Oncol.* 1996;8:15–18.

124. Notelovitz M. Management of the changing vagina. *J Clin Pract Sex.* 1990:16–21.

125. Schover LR. Sexual rehabilitation after treatment for prostate cancer. *Cancer.* 1993;71:1024–1030.

126. Guirguis WR. Oral treatment of erectile dysfunction: from herbal remedies to designer drugs. *J Sex Marital Ther.* 1998;24:69–73.

127. Padma-Nathan H, Hellstrom WJ, Kaiser FE, et al. Treatment of men with erectile dysfunction with transurethral alprostadil. Medicated Urethral System for Erection (MUSE) Study Group. *N Engl J Med.* 1997;336:1–7.

128. Albaugh JA. Intracavernosal injection algorithm. *Urol Nurs.* 2006;26:449–453.

129. Yurek D, Farrar W, Andersen BL. Breast cancer surgery: comparing surgical groups and determining individual differences in postoperative sexuality and body change stress. *J Consult Clin Psychol.* 2000;68:697–709.

130. Ganz PA, Rowland JH, Desmond K, Meyerowitz BE, Wyatt GE. Life after breast cancer: understanding women's health-related quality of life and sexual functioning. *J Clin Oncol.* 1998;16:501–514.

131. Henson HK. Breast cancer and sexuality. *Sex Disabil.* 2002;20:261–275.

132. Greenwald HP, McCorkle R. Sexuality and sexual function in long-term survivors of cervical cancer. *J Womens Health.* 2008;17:955–963.

133. Shell JA, Carolan M, Zhang Y, Meneses KD. The longitudinal effects of cancer treatment on sexuality in individuals with lung cancer. *Oncol Nurs Forum.* 2008;35:73–79.

134. Heiman JR. Treating low sexual desire—new findings for testosterone in women. *N Engl J Med.* 2008;359:2047–2049.

135. Bachmann GA. Sexual issues at menopause. *Ann N Y Acad Sci.* 1990;592:87–94 [discussion 123–133].

136. Levine SB. *Demystifying Love: Plain Talk for the Mental Health Professional.* New York, NY: Routledge-Taylor & Francis Group; 2007.

137. Slater S, Oliver RT. Testosterone: its role in development of prostate cancer and potential risk from use as hormone replacement therapy. *Drugs Aging.* 2000;17:431–439.

138. Ritchie K. Sexual issues in gynecologic cancer. *Clin Consult Obstet Gynecol.* 1997;3:118–121.

139. Mick JM. Sexuality assessment: 10 strategies for improvement. *Clin J Oncol Nurs.* 2007;11:671–675.

140. Institute of Medicine. *From Cancer Patient to Cancer Survivor: Lost in Transition.* Washington, DC: National Academies Press; 2005.

141. Kaplan HS. A neglected issue: the sexual side effects of current treatments for breast cancer. *J Sex Marital Ther.* 1992;18:3–19.

142. Auchincloss S. Sexual dysfunction after cancer treatment. *J Psychosoc Oncol.* 1991;9:23–41.

143. Crenshaw TL, Goldberg JP, eds. *Sexual Pharmacology: Drugs that effect Sexual Functioning.* New York, NY: WW Norton; 1996.

144. Sadock V. Psychotropic drugs and sexual dysfunction. *Prim Psychiatry.* 1995;4:16–17.

145. Ofman US. Psychosocial aspects of sexuality in the patient with cancer. *Oncol Patient Care Pract Guidel Specialized Nurse.* 1994;4:14–15.

146. Montejo-Gonzalez AL, Llorca G, Izquierdo JA, et al. SSRI-induced sexual dysfunction: fluoxetine, paroxetine, sertraline, and fluvoxamine in a prospective, multicenter, and descriptive clinical study of 344 patients. *J Sex Marital Ther.* 1997;23:176–194.

147. Piazza LA, Markowitz JC, Kocsis JH, et al. Sexual functioning in chronically depressed patients treated with SSRI antidepressants: a pilot study. *Am J Psychiatry.* 1997;154:1757–1759.

148. Conde DM, Pinto-Neto AM, Cabello C, Sa DS, Costa-Paiva L, Martinez EZ. Menopause symptoms and quality of life in women aged 45 to 65 years with and without breast cancer. *Menopause.* 2005;12:436–443.

149. Fobair P, Stewart SL, Chang S, D'Onofrio C, Banks PJ, Bloom JR. Body image and sexual problems in young women with breast cancer. *Psychooncology.* 2006;15:579–594.

150. Kendall A, Dowsett M, Folkerd E, Smith I. Caution: vaginal estradiol appears to be contraindicated in postmenopausal women on adjuvant aromatase inhibitors. *Ann Oncol.* 2006;17:584–587.

CHAPTER 11

Cancer-related Fatigue

• *Carmen P. Escalante and Ellen F. Manzullo*

■ INTRODUCTION

Fatigue is the most common symptom among cancer patients and a common symptom among cancer survivors. Cancer-related fatigue (CRF) is defined as a distressing, persistent, subjective sense of tiredness or exhaustion related to cancer or cancer treatment that is not proportional to recent activity and interferes with usual functioning.[1] In comparison to the fatigue experienced by healthy individuals, CRF is more severe, more distressing,[2,3] and less likely to be relieved by rest.[4] The International Classification of Diseases, 10th revision (ICD-10), describes the CRF diagnostic criteria as follows[5–7]:

1. Six or more of 11 possible fatigue symptoms, with 1 being "significant fatigue," have been present every day or nearly every day during the same 2-week period in the past month.
2. The symptoms cause clinically significant distress or impairment in important aspects of functioning.
3. The symptoms are the result of cancer or cancer treatment.
4. The symptoms are not primarily due to a comorbid psychiatric disorder.

Fatigue is a symptom with multiple dimensions that includes physical, emotional, and mental aspects. It can be experienced anywhere along the spectrum of cancer care, from diagnosis to treatment to long-term follow-up. This symptom affects 70% to 100% of cancer patients.[8] Fatigue is also experienced by cancer survivors, and when strict ICD-10 diagnostic criteria are used, the prevalence of fatigue among survivors ranges from 17% to 21%.[6]

■ CAUSES AND PATHOPHYSIOLOGY OF CRF

Fatigue can be due to the patient's malignancy, cancer treatment, or any of a multitude of comorbid conditions. In some patients, fatigue is the presenting symptom of the malignancy. For example, a patient with a hematologic malignancy might have significant anemia resulting in the sensation of fatigue. In other patients, fatigue is related to the cancer treatment. For example, patients receiving high-dose chemotherapy can experience fluctuations in fatigue, with worsening of the fatigue as their blood counts reach their nadir and subsequent improvement as the counts recover.[9] Patients receiving radiotherapy may experience worsening fatigue as their treatment progresses.[10] As for the effects of surgery on fatigue, there are limited data available at this time. Patients receiving biologic response modifiers can experience severe fatigue, and it can affect their treatment regimen.[11] Finally, fatigue can be related to the presence of comorbid conditions. The list of medical conditions that are associated with fatigue is quite long and includes endocrine disorders such as hypothyroidism, sleep disorders, coronary artery disease, metabolic abnormalities, depression, and anxiety, to name a few. Fatigue can also be caused by medical therapy, and thus it is important to review patients' medication lists.

Research into the pathophysiology of CRF is in its infancy. There are currently several proposed mechanisms for this symptom. The theory of serotonin dysregulation proposes that CRF is caused by an increase in brain serotonin levels in localized regions of the brain and an upregulation of certain 5-HT receptors, which results in decreases in somatomotor drive, modified hypothalamic–pituitary axis function, and a perceived decreased ability to perform physical activity.[12,13] The theory of hypothalamic–pituitary axis dysfunction suggests that cancer or its treatment directly or indirectly causes change in the hypothalamic–pituitary axis function, resulting in endocrine changes that are related to fatigue.[14,15] The vagal afferent hypothesis postulates that cancer or cancer treatment results in a release of neuroactive agents that activate vagal afferents, thus decreasing somatic motor output and causing sustained changes in particular areas of the brain associated with fatigue.[16–18] Finally, the muscle metabolism hypothesis suggests that cancer or cancer treatment results in a defect in adenosine triphosphate regeneration in skeletal muscle, which decreases a person's ability to perform work and results in fatigue.[19,20]

SCREENING FOR CRF

Clinicians need to inquire about fatigue since it can have a profound effect on a cancer patient's life. The degree of fatigue can vary, and in its most severe form, fatigue can result in patients not being able to engage in routine activities of daily living. Some patients are even faced with disability issues since they are not able to perform their normal job duties. Fatigue can result in significant levels of stress for both the patient and caregivers. However, there are several barriers that can contribute to inadequate assessment of this symptom. Patients might not mention fatigue because of concern that they might not receive usual treatment or that they might be viewed as complainers. Some patients fear that fatigue is indicative of recurrent disease, and some think it is an expected result of their cancer treatment. On the other hand, clinicians are often faced with time constraints, limiting their ability to inquire about fatigue. Also, clinicians might be hesitant to inquire about fatigue because of lack of knowledge regarding its evaluation and treatment.

CLINICAL EVALUATION OF CRF

Cancer patients should be screened during active treatment, during transition from active treatment to surveillance, and at appropriate intervals as clinically indicated in long-term follow-up by either their primary care physician or their oncologist. Patients in long-term follow-up with symptoms of fatigue will require more frequent monitoring of this symptom than those not experiencing fatigue. Several survey tools for assessing fatigue are available.[21–24] An effective tool must be reproducible and practical. In a busy clinical practice, a simple one-question screen for fatigue, "How would you rate your fatigue on a scale of 0–10 over the past week?," may be most helpful. The National Comprehensive Cancer Network has published a practice guideline for CRF that may be helpful to clinicians.[25]

MANAGEMENT OF CRF

All patients and families should be educated regarding the pattern and severity of fatigue they may experience. CRF varies depending on many factors, such as type of malignancy, modality of treatment, anemia, other comorbidities, and emotional disturbances (Table 11-1).

Approach to Mild Fatigue

Patients with mild fatigue (rated 1–3 on a scale of 0–10) and without interference in daily activities should be given information about fatigue and general CRF management strategies. These strategies encompass energy conservation and distraction.[26,27] Energy conservation includes prioritizing and pacing activities and delegating less important activities to others. A diary may help patients identify periods of high and low energy, which may allow them to plan routines during periods of peak energy and postpone less essential tasks. Other energy conservation strategies are use of labor-saving devices, limiting naps, performing one activity at a time, and devising a daily schedule. Distraction may also aid patients with fatigue and may be accomplished through games, music, reading, or social pastimes.

Approach to Moderate and Severe Fatigue

Patients with moderate fatigue (rated 4–6 on a scale of 1–10) or severe fatigue (7–10 on a scale of 1–10), especially patients having difficulty with daily tasks, should be given information about fatigue and general CRF management strategies and should receive a detailed medical evaluation. A comprehensive history of the specifics of the fatigue is necessary and should cover fatigue onset, duration, intensity, and changes over time; other related

■ **TABLE 11-1. Factors contributing to CRF**

Symptom burden
　Pain
　Anxiety
　Depression
Sleep dysfunction
　Obstructive sleep apnea
　Restless leg syndrome
　Narcolepsy
　Insomnia
Nutritional imbalances
　Weight changes
　Changes in caloric intake
　Fluid and electrolyte imbalances
　Motility disorders
Physical function changes
　Physical inactivity
　Physical deconditioning
Medical issues
　Anemia (various etiologies)
　Other comorbidities
　　Infection
　　Cardiac dysfunction
　　Connective tissue diseases
　　Pulmonary dysfunction
　　Renal dysfunction
　　Hepatic dysfunction
　　Neurologic dysfunction
　　Endocrine dysfunction
　　　Hypothyroidism
　　　Hypogonadism
　　　Diabetes mellitus
　　　Adrenal insufficiency
Medications
　Sedating agents (hypnotics, narcotics, neuropathic
　　agents, etc)
　Beta-blockers
　Supplements (homeopathic agents)
　Other (drug interactions and other medication side
　　effects)
Cancer treatment effects
　Chemotherapy
　Radiotherapy
　Surgery
　Bone marrow transplantation
　Biologic response modifiers
　Hormonal treatment
Direct effects of the malignancy

symptoms; and factors linked to fatigue improvement or decline. In addition, history of cancer treatment, extent of disease and response to treatment, other existing comorbidities and their status, and Eastern Cooperative Oncology Group performance status should be elicited. Because medication interactions or side effects, such as sedation and anxiety, commonly contribute to fatigue, a thorough review of medications should be performed, including prescribed medications, over-the-counter medications, and herbal, vitamin, and mineral supplements. Smoking, use of alcohol and illicit drugs, work history, exercise tolerance, and family history should also be reviewed with the patient. For patients with other symptoms in addition to fatigue (depression, anxiety, pain, sleep disturbances, or nutritional problems), other survey tools may be helpful in determining the burden of these symptoms and are frequently useful in tracking symptom trends over time.

The physical examination should be comprehensive. It may focus on particular organ systems guided by a thorough review of systems.

Frequently, a diagnostic workup is necessary, especially in a patient not recently evaluated. A review of measurements of the hemoglobin and hematocrit, electrolytes (ie, sodium, potassium, chloride, and bicarbonate), creatinine, blood urea nitrogen, glucose, magnesium, calcium, phosphorus, total bilirubin, serum transaminase, alkaline phosphatase, lactic dehydrogenase, albumin, and total protein obtained within an appropriate time frame prior to the assessment should be considered. A thyroid-stimulating hormone test will aid in assessing hypothyroidism. Other more specific testing (for testosterone, antinuclear antibody, or creatinine kinase) should be ordered on the basis of the specific findings of the history and physical examination.

Often patients believe that fatigue is a symptom of recurrence or progression of the malignancy, which contributes to increased anxiety and worry. Once it is clear that recurrence or progression is not the source of the fatigue, reassurance may help to allay patients' fears and anxiety.

Treatment may involve further consultation with other services, such as physical medicine and rehabilitation, physical and occupational therapy, psychiatry and neuropsychology, and social and nutritional services, depending on the findings of the general evaluation.

Interventions for treatment of CRF include both nonpharmacologic and pharmacologic interventions.

■ **TABLE 11-2. CRF Treatment Interventions**

Nonpharmacologic interventions
Psychosocial (category 1 evidence)
    Education
    Support groups
    Individual counseling
    Coping strategies
    Stress management training
    Individualized behavioral intervention
Exercise (category 1 evidence)
Attention-restoring therapy
Dietary management
Sleep therapy
    Cognitive behavioral therapy (stimulus control, sleep
        restriction, sleep hygiene)
Pharmacologic interventions
Stimulants
    Methylphenidate
    Modafinil
Antidepressants
    Selective serotonin reuptake inhibitors (paroxetine,
        sertraline)
    Bupropion
Steroids
Hematopoietic growth factors
    Erythropoietin
    Darbopoetin

Frequently, a combination of interventions is necessary (Table 11-2).

■ NONPHARMACOLOGIC INTERVENTIONS

Nonpharmacologic interventions for CRF include psychosocial interventions, exercise, attention-restoring therapy, dietary management, and sleep therapy. Psychosocial interventions and exercise have the strongest supporting evidence (category 1).

Psychosocial Interventions

Various interventions have been utilized to reduce stress and increase psychosocial support, thereby reducing fatigue. These interventions have included education,[28] support groups,[29] individual counseling,[30] comprehensive coping strategies,[31] stress management training,[32] and individualized behavioral interventions.[33] Although fatigue was a secondary endpoint in many studies of psychosocial interventions, there is sufficient evidence to support psychosocial interventions in managing this symptom, and that evidence is rated category 1. A recent meta-analysis of psychological and activity-based interventions for CRF included 30 randomized clinical trials.[34] Of the psychological trials, half were rated as fair or better in quality and demonstrated significant findings favoring the intervention. Some of the interventions utilized included listening to a guided imagery tape daily, prioritizing daily activities, and discussing how fatigue had affected lifestyle and emotional well-being.

Exercise

Among nonpharmacologic interventions for managing CRF, exercise is the intervention with the strongest evidence supporting its effectiveness.[35-38] Physical exercise training programs may increase functional capacity, leading to decreased effort in performing usual activities and decreased fatigue.[39,40] There have been a diverse array of studies utilizing exercise as an intervention for CRF, encompassing patients on active treatment as well as patients who have completed treatment.[41,42,43] Limitations of these studies include small sample sizes, a multitude of study designs, study population limited to women with breast cancer in many cases, and variations in length of exercise interventions, ranging from 6 weeks to 6 months. Some exercise types that have been utilized are bed cycle ergometer, home-based walking programs, and stationary cycling; some studies allowed participants to choose their preferred aerobic exercise. In addition, strength and resistance training, flexibility training, routine stretching, yoga, and seated exercise have been studied.

The effects of exercise for management of CRF were reported in a 2008 *Cochrane* analysis[44] based on 28 randomized controlled trials. The majority of the trials included breast cancer patients, and 16 studies were in supervised, institutional programs. The interventions ranged in duration from 3 to 32 weeks, with an average of 12 weeks. Exercise was shown to be statistically more effective than the control both during and after treatment.

Exercise programs should be individualized to meet the requirements of each patient and take into account the patient's overall medical status, the patient's level of physical conditioning, and the specifics of cancer treatment. Age and gender may influence the decision making, but their significance varies from patient to patient. Patients with substantial deconditioning may benefit from a rehabilitation or physical therapy program.

Attention-restoring Therapy

Attentional fatigue has been defined as a decreased capacity to concentrate or to direct attention during stressful or demanding situations.[45] Activities that have been shown to have a restorative influence on cancer patients' attention include bird watching and sitting in the park.

Dietary Management

Frequently, cancer patients have alterations in nutrition. Patients may experience nausea, vomiting, diarrhea, constipation, anorexia, or cachexia due to the treatment of the malignancy or the malignancy itself. Patients may also have volume status changes. Assessment of hydration and electrolyte balance is important in addressing fatigue.

Sleep Therapy

Sleep abnormalities are often present in cancer patients and frequently difficult to manage. Patients may present with difficulties ranging from hypersomnia to insomnia. Commonly, issues involve sleep quality rather than sleep quantity. Many factors may affect sleep, including daytime napping, anxiety and depression, medication side effects, dietary issues, and nocturnal waking due to hot flashes and bathroom usage. These sleep abnormalities may contribute to the burden of fatigue. Nonpharmacologic interventions aimed at improving sleep quality include cognitive behavioral interventions, complementary therapies, psychoeducational and informational interventions, and exercise therapies.[46]

Cognitive behavioral interventions utilized for sleep improvement include stimulus control, sleep restriction, and sleep hygiene. With stimulus control, patients are requested to go to bed when sleepy, have a routine bedtime and rising time, and get out of bed following 20 minutes of wakefulness after first going to bed and after nighttime awakening. Sleep restriction involves avoidance of long or late day naps and limiting total time in bed. Sleep hygiene advice includes avoiding caffeine and exercise near bedtime, comfortable sleep surroundings (dark, cool, peaceful, and relaxing), and soothing activities near bedtime (reading or listening to tranquil music). Several studies have demonstrated the benefit of cognitive behavioral interventions for sleep improvement and consequently fatigue reduction.[47,48,49]

Cognitive behavioral interventions may be combined with complementary treatments to promote relaxation. Techniques studied have included breathing control, progressive muscle relaxation, guided imagery, massage therapy, yoga, muscle relaxation, and mindfulness-based stress reduction. Preliminary studies of these techniques are suggestive of fatigue reductions.[50,51]

■ PHARMACOLOGIC INTERVENTIONS

Occasionally, pharmacologic interventions are needed to address CRF. Some side effects of these agents may include prolonged daytime sleepiness, fatigue, withdrawal symptoms and dependency issues, rebound insomnia, sleep maintenance issues, and memory disturbances; these potential side effects should be considered when pharmacologic interventions are contemplated.

The classes of pharmacologic interventions that have been most studied in managing CRF include stimulants and antidepressants. In addition, steroids, the cholinesterase inhibitor donepezil, multivitamins, and l-carnitine have been investigated. However, there is a paucity of prospective, randomized clinical trials using these agents.

Stimulants

The stimulants most frequently utilized in treatment of CRF are methylphenidate and modafinil.

Methylphenidate is a central nervous system stimulant similar to amphetamine that has a short plasma half-life (2 hours), a rapid onset of action, and a duration of action of 3 to 6 hours.[52] The initial starting dose is usually 5 mg in the morning and at noon with titration as necessary to a maximum dosage of 1 mg/kg per day. A long-acting preparation is also available that allows once-daily dosing. The most frequent side effects are tachycardia, nervousness, insomnia, and anorexia, usually experienced at higher doses. Open-label studies have suggested an improvement in fatigue with methylphenidate.[53,54] In a recent study, Bruera et al[55] randomized 112 patients to 5 mg of methylphenidate or placebo. Patients were able to repeat doses every 2 hours as needed up to 20 mg daily. Significant improvement of fatigue compared with baseline was shown in both groups at 1 week. These observed benefits may be due to daily contact with the study nurse or a placebo effect. A *Cochrane* analysis of two trials utilizing methylphenidate with a total of 264 patients was recently completed.[56] Findings showed a significant advantage of methylphenidate over placebo for treatment of CRF. Larger prospective clinical trials are necessary to verify these results.

Modafinil is a nonamphetamine central nervous system stimulant approved for treatment of narcolepsy. It reaches peak plasma concentration at 2 to 4 hours, has a half-life of 15 hours, and reaches steady state at 2 to 4 days.[57] In limited studies for treatment of CRF, modafinil has been well tolerated.[58,59] The starting dose is 100 to 200 mg in the morning, with a second dose at noon or shortly thereafter, up to a maximum dose of 400 mg per day. In a study in multiple sclerosis patients with fatigue, modafinil at 200 mg daily produced improvement in fatigue.[60] A pilot study utilizing modafinil for fatigue noted improvement across cognitive, mood, and fatigue outcome measures, with a maximum benefit at 8 weeks after initiation of treatment.[61] Another larger, randomized trial suggested a benefit with modafinil compared with placebo; however, this benefit was limited to patients with severe fatigue.[62]

In a recent placebo-controlled trial utilizing dextroamphetamine (10 mg twice daily) in 50 patients with advanced cancer and fatigue who were receiving palliative care, no benefit was noted.[63] It is not known whether the short duration of treatment (8 days), poor performance status, and spectrum of medications utilized may have influenced the results. Further study of dextroamphetamine is necessary before any definitive conclusions can be drawn.

Antidepressants

Fatigue and depression are commonly associated. There have been three placebo-controlled, randomized trials of selective serotonin reuptake inhibitors (paroxetine, sertraline) in cancer patients, and these did not show any improvement in fatigue, although improvement was seen in depressive symptoms.[64–66] Although fatigue and depression are viewed as commonly overlapping symptoms, the findings from these three trials reinforce the concept that fatigue is a distinct entity, different from depression.

In patients with sleep dysfunction and depression, antidepressants such as nortriptyline and amitriptyline may be beneficial owing to their sedative aspects. In a small, preliminary, open-label study of bupropion in cancer patients with fatigue and with or without moderate to severe depression,[67] both groups had improvement in fatigue and depressive symptoms. These results suggest that bupropion may have potential in aiding patients with CRF; however, larger, randomized clinical trials are necessary for confirmation. The different findings in trials utilizing antidepressants for CRF may be related to differing classes and mechanisms of action of the agents.

Other Pharmacologic Treatments

Steroids

Steroids have been most helpful in patients with CRF in the end stage of cancer.[68] Side effects of steroids limit their routine use. In trials utilizing steroids for CRF, other outcome measures, such as strength, weakness, or activity level, were substituted for fatigue; however, there is no consensus that these measures accurately reflect fatigue.[69,70,71]

Donepezil

Donepezil is a selective acetylcholinesterase inhibitor. Bruera et al[72] evaluated the effectiveness of donepezil in 142 patients randomly assigned to receive donepezil 5 mg or placebo daily for 1 week. All patients were offered open-label donepezil at week 2. Donepezil did not show a benefit compared with placebo for treatment of CRF.

Multivitamins

Multivitamins were studied in a double-blind, randomized crossover trial compared with placebo as an intervention for fatigue.[73] Forty breast cancer patients undergoing radiotherapy were given either placebo or Centrum Silver multivitamins and then switched at the midpoint of radiotherapy. No significant changes were noted with multivitamin administration. Lower rates of fatigue were seen in patients who finished the placebo intervention than in those who completed multivitamin treatment.

l-Carnitine

Cruciani et al[74] utilized l-carnitine for treatment of CRF in 29 patients with cancer and carnitine deficiency. The study had a double-blind phase followed by an open-label phase. All patients received l-carnitine for 2 weeks. The findings did not show improvement of CRF with l-carnitine supplementation.

Hematopoietic Growth Factors

Both erythropoietin and darbopoetin have been utilized in treating chemotherapy-induced anemia in patients with cancer. Some studies have reported improvements in fatigue with these drugs when they produce correction of anemia.[75,76] Most recently, however, these agents have become controversial due to findings related to thromboembolic events, increased mortality rates, and other adverse cancer outcomes. There are several guidelines available regarding use of these agents for chemotherapy-related anemia along with specific recommendations based on tumor diagnosis and hemoglobin levels.[77]

■ COMPLEMENTARY AND ALTERNATIVE MEDICINE

There is much interest in utilizing complementary and alternative medicine for managing CRF. Therapies investigated have included acupuncture, aromatherapy, adenosine triphosphate infusions, energy conservation and activity management, healing touch, hypnosis, lectin-standardized mistletoe extract, levocarnitine, massage, mindfulness-based stress reduction, polarity therapy, relaxation, sleep promotion, support groups, and Tibetan yoga. A recent review of complementary therapies for CRF concluded that there are insufficient data to recommend any specific CAM intervention for CRF and that large, randomized clinic trials are needed.[78]

There have been two small trials suggesting a benefit from acupuncture against CRF. In a phase 2 trial, Vickers et al[79] utilized acupuncture in 37 patients who had completed chemotherapy more than 2 years previously. These patients did not have severe depression or anemia. Outpatient acupuncture was administered twice weekly for 4 weeks or once weekly for 6 weeks. The mean improvement in Brief Fatigue Inventory score between baseline and follow-up was 31%. Twelve patients improved by 40% or more, and three patients had greater than 75% improvement in fatigue. In another trial[80] 47 cancer patients with moderate to severe fatigue were randomly assigned to acupuncture ($n = 15$) for six 20-minute sessions over 2 weeks, acupressure ($n = 16$) and self-administered massage/pressure on acupuncture points daily for 2 weeks, or sham acupressure (control) ($n = 16$). At study conclusion, 36% of the acupuncture group, 19% of the acupressure group, and 0.6% of the sham acupressure group had fatigue improvement. Further study of acupuncture is necessary to determine whether there is benefit.

■ SUMMARY

CRF is often an extremely challenging symptom to manage both during and after active cancer treatment. Other conditions that may contribute to the burden of fatigue should be identified and assessed. Both nonpharmacologic and pharmacologic interventions are available, and often multiple interventions are necessary. The nonpharmacologic therapies, including psychosocial interventions and exercise, have the strongest supporting evidence. There is less supporting evidence for the other interventions, but they still may be effective for some patients. An evidence-based clinical guideline for treatment of CRF is available for clinicians through the National Comprehensive Cancer Network.[25]

KEY POINTS

- CRF is the most common symptom in cancer patients and is often associated with other symptoms (pain, depression, anxiety, and sleep dysfunction).
- Patients should be routinely screened for CRF and provided with appropriate information regarding the expected intensity and duration of fatigue with the treatments administered.
- Patients with mild fatigue should be given information about fatigue and general CRF management strategies.
- Patients with moderate to severe fatigue require a detailed medical evaluation, including a comprehensive history exploring specific aspects of fatigue and a thorough physical examination. They should also receive information about fatigue and general CRF management strategies similar to that given to patients with mild fatigue.
- Nonpharmacologic interventions include psychosocial interventions, exercise, attention-restoring therapy, dietary management, and sleep therapy.
- Psychosocial interventions and exercise have the strongest supporting evidence (category 1).
- Pharmacologic treatment interventions include stimulants, antidepressants, and steroids.
- Antidepressants have not been effective for CRF in patients without depressive symptoms.
- Because of their side effects, steroids are most frequently used in patients with CRF at the end of life.
- Continued research to identify pathophysiologic mechanisms and more effective treatment strategies for CRF is imperative.

REFERENCES

1. Mock V, Atkinson A, Baresvick A, et al. NCCN practice guidelines for cancer related fatigue. *Oncology (Huntington)*. 2000;14:151–161.

2. Andrykowski MA, Curran SL, Lightner R. Off-treatment fatigue in most cancer survivors: a controlled comparison. *J Behav Med.* 1998;21:1–18.

3. Stone P, Hardy J, Broadley K, Tookman AJ, Kuroska A, A'Hern R. Fatigue in advance cancer: a prospective controlled cross-sectional study. *Br J Cancer.* 1999;79:1479–1486.

4. Glaus A, Craw R, Hammond S. A qualification study to explore the concept of fatigue/tiredness in cancer patients and in healthy individuals. *Eur J Cancer Care (Engl).* 1996;5:8–23.

5. Portenoy RK, Itri LM. Cancer-related fatigue: guidelines for evaluation and management. *Oncologist.* 1999;4:1–10.

6. Cella D, Davis K, Breitbart W, Curt G, Fatigue Coalition ancer-related fatigue: prevalence of proposed diagnostic criteria in a United States sample of cancer survivors. *J Clin Oncol.* 2001;19:385–391.

7. Sadler IJ, Jacobson PB, Booth-Jones M, et al. Preliminary evaluation of a clinical syndrome approach to assessing cancer-related-fatigue. *J Pain Symptom Manage.* 2002;23:406–416.

8. Hofman M, Ryas JL, Figueroa-Moseley CP, Jean-Pierre P, Morrow GR. Cancer-related-fatigue: the scale of the problem. *Oncologist.* 2007;12(suppl 1):4–10.

9. Knobel H, Loge JH, Norday T, et al. High level of fatigue in lymphoma patients treated with high does therapy. *J Pain Symptom Manage.* 2000:19:446–456.

10. Wang XS, Janjan NA, Guo H, et al. Fatigue during preoperative chemoradiation for respectable rectal cancer. *Cancer.* 2001;92:1725–1732.

11. Brophy LR, Sharp EJ. Physical Symptoms of combination biotherapy: a quality-of-life issue. *Oncol Nurs Forum.* 1991 18:25–30

12. Newsholme EA, Blomstrand E. Tryptohan, 5-hydroxytryptamine and a possible explanation for central fatigue. *Adv Exp Med Biol.* 1995;384:315–320.

13. Gandevia SC, Allen GM, McKenzie DK. Central fatigue. Critical issues, quantification and practical implications. *Adv Exp Med Biol.* 1995;384:281–294.

14. Swain MG, Maric M. Defective corticotropin-releasing hormone medicated neuroendocrine and behavioral responses in cholestatic rats: implications for cholestatic liver disease-related sickness behaviors. *Hepatology.* 1995;22:1560–1564.

15. Bakheit AM, Behan PO, Dinan TG, et al. Possible up-regulation of hypothalamic 5-hydroxytryptamine receptors in patients with postviral fatigue syndrome. *BMJ.* 1992;304:1010–1012.

16. Opp MR, Toth LA. Somnogenic and pyrogenic effects of interleukin-1beta and lipopolysaccharide in intact and vagotomized rats. *Life Sci.* 1998:62:923–936.

17. Hansen MK, Krueger JM. Subdiaphragmatic vagotomy blocks the sleep-and-fever-promoting effects of interleukin-1beta. *Am J Physiol.* 1997;273:R1246–R1253.

18. Kapas L, Hansen MK, Chang HY, Krueger JM. Vagotomy attenuates but does not prevent the somnogenic and febrile effects of lipopolysaccharide in rats. *Am J Physiol.* 1998;274:R406–R411.

19. Dimeo F, Stieglitz RD, Novelli-Fischer U, et al. Correlation between physical performance and fatigue in cancer patients. *Ann Oncol.* 1997;8:1251–1255.

20. Akechi T, Kugaya A, Okamura H, et al. Fatigue and its associated factors in ambulatory cancer patients: a preliminary study. *J Pain Symptom Manage.* 1999;17:42–48.

21. Mendoza TR, Wang XS, Cleeland CS, et al. The rapid assessment of fatigue severity in cancer patients; use of the Brief Fatigue Inventory. *Cancer.* 1999;85:1186–1196.

22. Schwartz AL. The Schwartz Cancer Fatigue Scale: testing reliability and validity. *Oncol Nurs Forum.* 1998;25:711–717.

23. Hann DM, Denniston MM, Baker F. Measurement of fatigue in cancer patients: further validation of the Fatigue Symptom Inventory. *Qual Life Res.* 2000;9:847–854.

24. Smets EM, Garssen B, Bonke B, et al. The Multidimensional Fatigue Inventory (MFI) psychometric qualities of an instrument to assess fatigue. *J Psychosom Res.* 1995;39:315–325.

25. Mock V, Atkinson A, Barsevick AM, et al. Cancer-related fatigue. Clinical practice guidelines in oncology. *J Natl Compr Cancer Netw.* 2007;5:1054–1078.

26. Barsevick AM, Dudley W, Beck S, et al. A randomized clinical trial of energy conservation for patients with cancer-related fatigue. *Cancer.* 2004;100:1302–1310.

27. Richardson A, Ream EK. Self-care behaviours initiated by chemotherapy patients in response to fatigue. *Int J Nurs Stud.* 1997;34:35–43.

28. Yates P, Aranda S, Hargraves M, et al. Randomized controlled trial of an educational intervention for managing fatigue in women receiving adjuvant chemotherapy for early-stage breast cancer. *J Clin Oncol.* 2005; 23:6027–6036.

29. Fawzy FI, Cousins N, Fawzy NW, et al. A structured psychiatric intervention for cancer patients. I. Changes over time in methods of coping and affective disturbance. *Arch Gen Psychiatry.* 1990;47:720–725.

30. Fawzy NW. A psychoeducational nursing intervention to enhance coping and affective state in newly

diagnosed malignant melanoma patients. *Cancer Nurs.* 1995;18:427–438.

31. Gaston-Johansson F, Fall-Dickson JM, Nanda J, et al. The effectiveness of the comprehensive coping strategy program on clinical outcomes in breast cancer autologous bone marrow transplantation. *Cancer Nurs.* 2000;23:277–285.

32. Jacobsen PB, Meade CD, Stein KD, et al. Efficacy and costs of two forms of stress management training for cancer patients undergoing chemotherapy. *J Clin Oncol.* 2002;20:2851–2862.

33. Given B, Given CW, McCorkle R, et al. Pain and fatigue management: results of a nursing randomized clinical trial. *Oncol Nurs Forum.* 2002;29:949–956.

34. Jacobsen PB, Donovan KA, Vadaparampil ST, et al. Systematic review and meta-analysis of psychological and activity-based interventions for cancer-related fatigue. *Health Psychol.* 2007;26:660–667.

35. Galvao DA, Newton RU. Review of exercise intervention studies in cancer patients. *J Clin Oncol.* 2005;23:899–909.

36. McNeely ML, Campbell KL, Rowe BH, et al. Effects of exercise on breast cancer patients and survivors: a systematic review and meta-analysis. *CMAJ.* 2006;175:34–41.

37. Kangas M, Bovbjerg DH, Montgomery GH. Cancer-related fatigue: a systematic and meta-analytic review of non-pharmacological therapies for cancer patients. *Psychol Bull.* 2008;134:700–741.

38. Dimeo F, Schwartz S, Wesel N, et al. Effects of an endurance and resistance exercise program on persistent cancer-related fatigue after treatment. *Ann Oncol.* 2008;19:1495–1499.

39. Segal R, Evans W, Johnson D, et al. Structured exercise improves physical functioning in women with stages I and II breast cancer: results of a randomized controlled trial. *J Clin Oncol.* 2001;19:657–665.

40. Windsor PM, Nicol KF, Potter J. A randomized, controlled trial of aerobic exercise for treatment-related fatigue in men receiving radical external beam radiotherapy for localized prostate carcinoma. *Cancer.* 2004;101:550–557.

41. Courneya KS, MacKey JR, Bell GS, et al. Randomized controlled trial of exercise training in postmenopausal breast cancer survivors: cardiopulmonary and quality of life outcomes. *J Clin Oncol.* 2003;21:1660–1668.

42. Segal RJ, Reid RD, Courneya KS, et al. Resistance exercise in men receiving and rogen deprivation therapy for prostate cancer. *J Clin Oncol.* 2003;21:1653–1659.

43. Courneya KS, Friedenreich CM. Physical exercise and quality of life following cancer diagnosis: a literature review. *Ann Behav Med.* 1999;21:171–179.

44. Cramp F, Daniel J. Exercise for the management of cancer-related fatigue in adults. *Cochrane Database Syst Rev.* 2008:CD006145.

45. Cimprich B. Attentional fatigue following breast cancer surgery. *Res Nurs Health.* 1992;15:199–207.

46. Page MS, Berger AM, Johnson LB. Putting evidence into practice: evidence-based interventions for sleep–wake disturbances. *Clin J Oncol Nurs.* 2006;10:753–767.

47. Berger AM, Kuhn BR, Farr LA, Von Essen SG, Chamberlain J, Lynch JC, Agrawal S. One-year outcomes of a behavioral therapy intervention trial on sleep quality and cancer-related fatigue. *J Clin Oncol.* 2009;27(35):6033–6040.

48. Berger AM, Kuhn BR, Farr LA, Lynch JC, Agrawal S, Chamberlain J, Von Essen SG. Behavioral therapy intervention trial to improve sleep quality and cancer-related fatigue. *Psychooncology.* 2009;18(6):634–646.

49. Espie CA, Fleming L, Cassidy J, Samuel L, Taylor LM, White CA, Douglas NJ, Engleman HM, Kelly HL, Paul J. Randomized controlled clinical effectiveness trial of cognitive behavior therapy compared with treatment as usual for persistent insomnia in patients with cancer. *J Clin Oncol.* 2008;26(28):4651–4658.

50. Cohen L, Warneke C, Fouladi RT, et al. Psychological adjustment and sleep quality in a randomized trial of the effects of a Tibetan yoga intervention in patients with lymphoma. *Cancer.* 2004;100:2253–2260.

51. Carlson LE, Garland SN. Impact of mindfulness-based stress reduction (MBSR) on sleep, mood, stress and fatigue symptoms in cancer outpatients. *Int J Behav Med.* 2005;12:278–285.

52. Wargin W, Patrick K, Kilts C, et al. Pharmacokinetics of methylphenidate in man, rat and monkey. *J Pharmacol Exp Ther.* 1983;226:382–386.

53. Bruera E, Driver L, Barnes EA, et al. Patient-controlled methylphenidate for the management of fatigue in patients with advanced cancer: a preliminary report. *J Clin Oncol.* 2003;21:4439–4443.

54. Sarhill N, Walsh D, Nelson KA, et al. Methylphenidate for fatigue in advanced cancer: a prospective open-label pilot study. *Am J Hosp Palliat Care.* 2001;18:187–192.

55. Bruera E, Valero V, Driver L, et al. Patient controlled methylphenidate for cancer fatigue: a double-blind, randomized, placebo-controlled trial. *J Clin Oncol.* 2006;24:2073–2078.

56. Minton O, Richardson A, Sharpe M, et al. Drug therapy for the management of cancer related fatigue. *Cochrane Database Syst Rev.* 2008;(1):CD006704. DOI: 10.1002/14651858.CD—6704.pub2.

57. Wong YN. Single-dose pharmacokinetics of modafinil and methylphenidate given alone or in combination in healthy male volunteers. *J Clin Pharmacol.* 1998;38(3):276–282.

58. Jean-Pierre P, Morrow ER, Roscoe JA, et al. A Phase 3 randomized, placebo-controlled, double-blind, clinical trial of the effect of modafinil on cancer related fatigue among 631 patients receiving chemotherapy: a University of Bochestes Cancer Center Community Clinical Oncology Research base study. *Cancer.* 2010;116(14):3513–3520.

59. Blackhall L, Petroni G, Shu J, et al. A Pilot study evaluating the safety and efficacy of modafinil for cancer-related fatigue. *J Palliat Med.* 2009;12(5):433–439.

60. Rammohan KW, Rosenberg JH, Lynn DJ, et al. Efficacy and safety of modafinil (Provigil) for the treatment of fatigue in multiple sclerosis: a two centre phase 2 study. *J Neurol Neurosurg Psychiatry.* 2002;72(2):179–183.

61. Kaleita TA, Wellisch DK, Graham CA, et al. Pilot study of modafinil for treatment of neurobehavioral dysfunction and fatigue in adult patients with brain tumors [abstract]. *J Clin Oncol.* 2006;24:58s.

62. Morrow GR, Jean-Pierre P, Roscoe JA, et al. A phase III randomized, placebo-controlled, double-blind trial of a eugeroic agent in 642 cancer patients reporting fatigue during chemotherapy: a URCC CCOP study [abstract]. *J Clin Oncol.* 2008;26:504s.

63. Auret KA, Schug SA, Bremner AP, Bulsara M. A randomized, double-blind, placebo-controlled trial assessing the impact of dexamphetamine on fatigue in patients with advanced cancer. *J Pain Symptom Manage.* 2009;37:613.

64. Morrow GR, Hickok JT, Roscoe JA, et al. Differential effects of paroxetine on fatigue and depression: a randomized, double-blind trial from the University of Rochester Cancer Center Community Clinical Oncology Program. *J Clin Oncol.* 2003;21:4635–4641.

65. Stockler MR, O'Connell R, Nowak AK, et al. Effect of sertraline on symptoms and survival in patients with advanced cancer, but without major depression: a placebo-controlled double blind randomized trial. *Lancet Oncol.* 2007;8:603–612.

66. Palesh O, Mustian KM, Roscoe JA, et al. Effect of paroxetine on depression and insomnia in 547 fatigued cancer patients undergoing chemotherapy [abstract]. *J Clin Oncol.* 2008;26:502s.

67. Moss EL, Simpson JS, Pelletier G, et al. An open-label study of the effects of bupropion SR on fatigue, depression and quality of life of mixed-site cancer patients and their partners. *Psychooncology.* 2006;15:259–267.

68. Bruera E, Roca E, Cedaro L, et al. Action of oral methylprednisolone in terminal cancer patients: a prospective randomized double-blind study. *Cancer Treat Rep.* 1985;69:751–754.

69. Moertel CG, Schutt AJ, Reitemeier RJ, Hahn RG. Corticosteroid therapy of preterminal gastrointestinal cancer. *Cancer.* 1974;33(6):1607–1609.

70. Bruera E, Roca E, Cedaro L, Carraro S, Chacon R. Action of oral methylprednisolone in terminal cancer patients: a prospective randomized double-blind study. *Cancer Treat Rep.* 1985;69(7-8):751–754.

71. Della Cuna GR, Pellegrini A, Piazzi M. Effect of methylprednisolone sodium succinate on quality of life in preterminal cancer patients: a placebo-controlled, multicenter study. The Methylprednisolone Preterminal Cancer Study Group. *Eur J Cancer Clin Oncol.* 1989;25(12):1817–1821.

72. Bruera E, El Osta B, Valero V, et al. Donepezil for cancer fatigue: a double-blind, randomized, placebo-controlled trial. *J Clin Oncol.* 2007;25:3475–3481.

73. De Souza F, Bensi CG, Trufelli DC, et al. Multivitamins do not improve radiation therapy-related fatigue: results of a double-blind randomized crossover trial. *Am J Clin Oncol.* 2007;30:432–436.

74. Cruciani RA, Dvorkin E, Homel P, et al. l-Carnitine supplementation in patients with advanced cancer and carnitine deficiency: a double-blind, placebo-controlled study. *J Pain Symptom Manage.* 2009;37:622–631.

75. Lyman GH, Glaspy J. Are there clinical benefits with early erythropoietic intervention for chemotherapy-induced anemia? A systematic review. *Cancer.* 2006;106(1):223–233.

76. Gabrilove JL, Perez EA, Tomita DK, et al. Assessing symptom burden using the MD Anderson symptom inventory in patients with chemotherapy-induced anemia: results of a multicenter, open-label study (SURPASS) of patients treated with darbepoetin-alpha at a dose of 200 microg every 2 weeks. *Cancer.* 2007;110(7):1629–1640.

77. Rizzo JD, Lichtin AE, Woolf SH, et al. Use of epoetin in patients with cancer: evidence-based clinical practice guidelines of the American Society of Clinical Oncology and the American Society of Hematology. *J Clin Oncol.* 2002;20(19):4083–4107.

78. Sood A, Barton DL, Bauer BA, et al. A critical review of complementary therapies for cancer-related fatigue. *Integr Cancer Ther.* 2007;6:8–13.

79. Vickers AJ, Straus DJ, Fearon B, et al. Acupuncture for postchemotherapy fatigue: a phase II study. *J Clin Oncol.* 2004;22:1731–1735.

80. Molassiotis A, Sylt P, Diggins H. The management of cancer-related fatigue after chemotherapy with acupuncture and acupressure: a randomized controlled trial. *Complement Ther Med.* 2007;15:228–237.

CHAPTER 12

Interface between Psychiatry, Sleep, and Cancer

• *Mary Rose and Rhonda Robert*

Overwhelmingly, cancer patients report sleepiness as well as fatigue as among the most disabling side effects they experienced following cancer and its treatment. Approximately 30% to 60% of all cancer patients report sleep disturbance as a significant problem,[1,2] with long-term cancer survivors being 40% more likely than the normative population to experience distress.[3] At time of treatment, distress is even more significant; of those sampled with the Hamilton Anxiety Depression Scale in a general oncology waiting room in Argentina, 74.9% surpassed the cutoff score for anxiety, depression, or both.[4] In another study of US patients awaiting chemotherapy, depression and anxiety were prevalent, with 45% of those sampled endorsing sleep disturbance.[5]

Sleep is exquisitely sensitive to psychosocial challenge and medical compromise. Those with cancer are vulnerable to sleep disturbance from several forces. Cancer patients come into their illnesses with a level of psychiatric and medical comorbidities that are at least equivalent to those represented in the general population (and possibly more given the increased incidences of cancer associated with some lifestyle habits). It therefore stands to reason that manifestation of psychiatric illness, psychological vulnerabilities, and maladaptive coping would intensify with the added compromise of cancer and its treatments.

There is evidence that some patients grow with regard to psychosocial sophistication following cancer, a process termed *benefit finding*.[3,6,7] However, patients who grow through adverse experience are likely not newly developing this capacity as a consequence of their cancer experience, but rather they are individuals who already have the disposition to turn adversity around and to use the challenge of the cancer experience to develop broader coping and perspective on the world and themselves.

Our task, then, in understanding the interface between cancer, psychiatric disturbance, and sleep is to break down each and develop possible directions for future strategies in treating sleep disturbance based on psychiatric issues faced by cancer patients. An additional task is to guide patients to feel more enabled and more realistically optimistic about their ability to modify symptoms.

The interface between cancer, psychiatry, and sleep is a tridirectional one. Each may adversely or beneficially affect the other. The two major sleep-related compromises that patients face in cancer are insomnia and airway-related sleep disorders. The latter, although less significantly associated with psychological causes than the former, has been shown to affect mood substantially. Another area of frequent sleep disturbance that deserves attention is circadian rhythm disturbance, which has recently been gaining investigative interest. Movement disorders such as periodic limb movement disorders (PLMD) and restless legs syndrome (RLS) are additional areas that affect cancer patients.

A major focus of this chapter is primary insomnia related to the diagnosis of cancer and its treatments. The International Classification of Sleep Disorders (ICSD-9)[8] differentiates several forms of insomnia, the principal ones of which for our purposes include: psychophysiological insomnia, insomnia caused by a medical disorder, and insomnia caused by psychiatric disorder. Pediatric insomnia is coded as *insomnia of childhood*, notably a V code, which has fallen under much debate. The adult cancer patient is most often challenged with one of the first three of these diagnostic categories. We will also discuss airway-related sleep disorders and circadian rhythm disorders. The most commonly used diagnostic categories in recent years have been coded 307.42—a sort of catch-all for a persistent disorder of initiating or maintaining sleep. This is described in the ICD-9 as hyposomnia, insomnia, or sleeplessness associated with: anxiety, conditioned arousal, depression, psychosis, idiopathic insomnia, paradoxical insomnia, primary insomnia, or psychophysiological insomnia. These three are probably the most fitting diagnostic concepts for cancer patients. The practitioner interested in a more in-depth diagnostic classification of sleep disorders should use the ICSD.[9]

Insomnia may be *primary* or *secondary*. This distinguishing issue is important when it comes to decision making with regard to pharmacological management as well as capacity for insight-oriented cognitive–behavioral management of symptoms.

Specific identification and weighing of the degree to which a medical condition (eg, cancer, anemia, thyroid dysfunction, limb movement disorder, chemotherapy toxicity, possible airway-related disturbance), psychological adjustment and stressors (eg, fears about change in one's identity, partner stress, fertility fears, disfigurement, existential focus), night sweats/hot flashes, GI and GU upset, and pain contribute to a sleep disorder is a challenge; often, causes of insomnia are multifactorial, synergistic, and not readily attributable to a single etiology.

Thus, a patient complaint of insomnia requires that one reviews several critical issues that will differentiate how the patient should be treated. Possibly one of the most critical symptoms to clarify is that of fatigue versus insomnia. It is critical to determine whether the insomnia is related to sleep onset difficulty (hyperarousal and poor sleep habits), early morning spontaneous wakings (typical of depression), or middle awakenings (possible nocturia, periodic limb movement, apneas, pain, hot flashes, medication elimination). If an airway-related problem or movement disorder may be present, then a nocturnal polysomnography (NPSG) is indicated. If those problems are not present, then it has to be determined whether the patient is in the midst of medical and physiological transitions that may be significantly contributing to symptoms. In such a case, the full range of insomnia- or hypersomnia-related causes, such as psychological stress, hypervigilance and anxiety, depression,

pharmacological habits, alcohol use, activity change, and medications, must be evaluated.

Research indicates that circadian changes are less frequently the culprit, but significant changes to the timing of sleep and energy levels may be a marker that a phase change is at the source of the problem. Circadian rhythm disorders have been reported in some subgroups of cancer patients, which makes considerable sense with regard to the multitude of hormonal changes that occur with cancer treatments. Circadian disruption has been linked to fatigue and depression during chemotherapy and early recovery in breast cancer patients.[10]

■ INSOMNIA AND MOOD DISTURBANCE IN THE GENERAL POPULATION

Depression and anxiety with regard to sleep disturbance are typically interwoven. Insomnia is a significant predictor of depression. In a major population study of 14,915 subjects sampled from the general population in the United Kingdom, Germany, Italy, and Portugal, extensive interviews were conducted to assess mental health and sleep parameters.[11] Investigators found that 28% of those with insomnia had a current diagnosis of a mental disorder, and 25.6% had a psychiatric history. Presence of severe insomnia, diagnosis of primary insomnia, insomnia related to a medical condition, and insomnia that lasted more than 1 year were predictors of a psychiatric history. In most cases of mood disorders, insomnia appeared prior to (>40%) or concurrently with (>22%) mood disorder symptoms. When anxiety disorders were involved, insomnia appeared mostly in the same time frame as (>38%) or after (>34%) the anxiety disorder started.[11]

In another study, 17% to 50% of subjects with insomnia that lasted 2 weeks or longer had developed a major depressive episode at the time of later interview.[12] In a review of more than 250 journal articles, Tsuno et al[13] reported that the comorbidity of insomnia with depression occurs in about 90% of patients with depression.

The above mentioned studies suggest that insomnia may be a prequel to depression, especially for persons who are undergoing stressful life circumstances. When managing the cancer patient with insomnia, we should be mindful that at the time of diagnosis, the patient is likely undergoing significant existential crisis, life change adjustments, and stressors. Changes consequent to radiation, chemotherapy, and surgery add additional but not well-understood challenges to the biochemistry that may affect sleep onset, sleep maintenance, early morning awakenings, and overall restfulness.

The diathesis–stress model is of particular importance in understanding the interface between insomnia, cancer, and adjustment to illness. This model suggests that stable individual differences present prior to a trauma may function as vulnerability factors in the development of symptoms. Fragile sleep, or sleep that is vulnerable to noise, light, or temperature variations, may be more at play in an already hypervigilant patient and should be considered with regard to not only behavioral interventions, but also pharmacological options. Presence of vulnerability risk factors such as anxious personality, poor coping, lack of social support, and depression will most certainly worsen insomnia. This model loops back to earlier-noted studies on benefits finding that suggest that the presence of resilience and perhaps realistic optimism may lead some to actually thrive or grow through their adversity.

A vast majority of insomnia patients who do not have significant iatrogenic causes of their insomnia are likely to have difficulty with generalized anxiety and hypervigilance related to treatment and the cancer diagnosis itself. Although many patients may deny generalized anxiety, examination of phobias, habits, and ruminations will often bring out more clinical evidence of anxious symptoms. Many patients guard these habits; thus, a careful interview, involvement of family, and rapport are critical to uncovering underlying symptoms. Certainly, for patients vulnerable to mood disturbance, insomnia is a significant risk factor when they are faced with the consequences of a cancer diagnosis, chemotherapy, social upheaval, physical changes, loss of income, job security, and other medical treatments.

One challenge for sleep researchers working with cancer patients is to determine why certain types of cancers are associated with a greater risk of subjective sleep disorders such as insomnia. Cancer patients with the most serious risk for sleep disorders include those with cancers of the head and neck, breast, and lung. Head and neck and lung cancer patients are afflicted with a high incidence of airway-related sleep disturbance.[14] However, breast cancer patients have one of the highest rates of insomnia among all cancer patients.[15] Importantly, many cancer patients report significant sleep disturbance, both insomnia and apparent circadian disruption, surfacing months prior to their cancer diagnosis.[16,17] Thus, the combination of various cancer treatments and hormonal changes may lead patients even more heavily toward both difficulty initiating sleep and hormone-related fragmentation of sleep. Research on insomnia and hot flashes suggests one possible reason why this population may be at particular risk for sleep disturbance. The prevalence of symptoms of chronic insomnia increases with the severity of hot flashes and reached more than 80% in perimenopausal women and postmenopausal women who endorsed severe hot flashes.[18]

HOSPITALIZATION AND SLEEP QUALITY

During hospitalization, patients often face extreme sleep disturbance from roommates, staff entering the room throughout the night, noise in the hallway, light, change in diet, pain and general discomfort, and change in sleep environment. One study found that morphine alone (without fentanyl) caused less disturbance to sleep.[19] Management of ancillary disruptors to sleep such as pain is essential.[20,21] Again, the underlying cause of the insomnia, and not simply the insomnia as an isolated disease, should be treated.

POLYSOMNOGRAPHY, PHYSIOLOGICAL MARKERS, AND INSOMNIA

Over the past decade, we have learned considerably more about the pathophysiology of primary insomnia. Polysomnography suggests that the sleep of those with primary insomnia differs from that of good sleepers in several ways. Feige et al[22] showed overall impairment of sleep architecture, including increased arousal during REM. Beta activity is defined as EEG activity greater than 13 Hz and commonly 18 to 25 Hz and associated with lighter stages of sleep. High-frequency activity is associated with central nervous system arousal in that beta/gamma activity occurs maximally during shallow stages of sleep. Beta activity has been found to be more prominent in those with primary insomnia compared with those with insomnia secondary to major depression and with good sleepers.[23] Perlis et al[23,24] have also found that beta activity increased in non-REM and at sleep onset in patients with insomnia compared with good sleepers. This high-frequency activity tends to be correlated with discrepancies between objective and subjective total sleep time and sleep latency. These studies provide some objective weight to the common report from insomniacs of subjectively experiencing wakefulness even with the finding of objective sleep.

An additional area or pathophysiological difference is that patients with primary insomnia tend to be hypermetabolic, running at a slightly higher metabolic rate than age-matched controls.[25] Bonnet and Arand[26] found elevated whole body metabolic rate as demonstrated by elevated VO2 in both primary insomnia and sleep state misperception compared with good sleepers.

■ SLEEP AS A PREDICTOR OF FATIGUE

Fatigue and sleepiness are often erroneously used interchangeably. [27] A PubMed search of publications using the keywords "sleep" and "cancer" suggests that researchers often refer to sleepiness when fatigue is intended. Typically, fatigue is defined as a mental and/or physical weariness, while sleep is defined as a propensity to fall asleep and difficulty maintaining wakefulness. How fatigue is defined in various clinical populations as a symptom and not a disease entity in itself remains variable and is still debated by cancer specialists.

Sleep quality and daytime sleepiness have been found to be good predictors of fatigue in multiple regression analysis.[28] Insomnia tends to be routinely associated with fatigue, although it is infrequently associated with sleepiness. In fact, most insomniacs indicate low sleepiness on the Epworth Sleepiness Scale (a well-normed self-report measure of daytime sleepiness).[29] Greater inactivity (a well-established relationship) as well as a pattern of more night waking has also been associated with greater cancer-related fatigue at all three sampled midpoints of chemotherapy cycle in one study.[30]

■ PHARMACOLOGICAL MANAGEMENT OF SLEEP DISORDERS

Antidepressants warrant some mention here. Many of the newer-generation SSRIs are extremely beneficial to the treatment of depression in cancer patients. However, they are notoriously skilled sleep architecture modifiers,[31–34] some more so than others. More sedating ones, such as Zoloft, may be helpful for patients when insomnia is a key feature. However, highly alerting agents such as fluoxetine have been found to increase sleep onset insomnia.[32] Although the time of dosing was unknown in this study, it again suggests that the manifestation of insomnia may be complicated by other factors. Fluoxetine

may have improved fatigue, which increased daytime activity and light exposure in daytime, resetting a circadian phase delay.

Cancer patients receiving active treatment for their cancer are often on myriad medications that may influence uptake and metabolism of antidepressants. The only non-REM sleep-suppressing serotonin reuptake inhibitors on the market are nefazodone[31,35] and mirtazapine.[31] Trazodone has been used extensively in psychiatry for insomnia.[36,37] Interestingly, most sleep research suggests that it has little long-term benefit on sleep architecture, although it may increase slow-wave sleep (SWS) modestly,[38] but patient self-report has shown benefit for the long-term treatment of insomnia.[39,40] It is unlikely that the modest increase in SWS itself is responsible for this, as SWS deficiencies are typically not a key feature of insomnia. In those for whom it is a substantial contributor, lack of SWS does not explain the prevalence of sleep onset maintenance problems or that insomnia is often associated with lack of sleepiness. It is more likely that the sedating quality of trazodone as well as its antidepressant effect overall is contributing to subjective sleep quality improvement.

Many of the serotonin reuptake inhibitors are potent inhibitors of CYP3A4, an isozyme of the CYP450. They are therefore typically contraindicated in patients for whom CYP450 inhibition would impact the efficacy of the antiangiogenic treatments.[41] Paroxetine, bupropion, quinidine, and fluoxetine are strong CYP2D6 inhibitors to be avoided, particularly with patients who are undergoing aromatase inhibitor (AI) treatment (endocrine therapy) with medications such as estradiol.[42–45] Duloxetine, cimetidine, and sertraline are moderate inhibitors and if possible should also be avoided.[44,46,47] For patients using AI, many breast centers utilize venlafaxine, escitalopram, or citalopram, as they have little impact on the metabolism of AI drugs.[48] For further reading on tamoxifen and consideration of the CYP3A4 inhibitors and substrates, the reader is referred to Brauch et al.[42] Most sleep experts do not routinely recommend benzodiazepine (BZD) hypnotics or non-BZD hypnotics for chronic insomnia, as many not only may be habit forming, but in some cases may also interfere with progress with cognitive–behavioral treatment (CBT) of insomnia. A recent abstract published by Morin et al[49] suggested that a combined approach to medication and CBT was initially beneficial in alleviating symptoms, but subjects who continued maintenance CBT after initial treatment for insomnia and tapered their medication during extended therapy achieved better long-term outcomes compared with those who continued using medication intermittently.

For greater review of the BZD and non-BZD hypnotics in the treatment of insomnia, the reader is referred to Thase[32] and Perlis et al.[50] As with anxiety disorders, one of the greatest barriers to progress is the belief that one is not in control over emotions and that only outside forces (eg, medication and the behavior of others) can manage the symptoms. Lack of insight regarding how thoughts and behaviors influence insomnia (as well as general anxiety) is disabling to progress. Additionally, BZD and non-BZD hypnotics in the treatment of insomnia have not been found to be effective overall for long-term treatment of insomnia,[51] which is likely due to the fact that intense dysfunctional thoughts about sleep (which often fester during waking hours) and negative associations with sleep and the bedroom cannot be selectively pharmacologically eradicated.

The major BZDs in use at present include triazolam, temazepam, estazolam, quazepam, and flurazepam. The primary BZD receptor agonists (BZRAs) currently in use include zopiclone, eszopiclone, zolpidem, and zaleplon. In general, BZRAs are preferable to BZDs when treating insomnia as a primary symptom; BZDs often decrease SWS substantially as well as REM sleep, though less so the latter. Benefits of BZDs are that they are associated with increased total sleep time, reduced sleep onset latency, and wake time after sleep.[52] However, their longer half-life may result in greater drowsiness and fatigue. For patients who are battling daytime fatigue, this may be a highly undesirable side effect. These medications also have mild respiratory depressant properties,[53] which may be problematic in patients with sleep-related airway disease. BZRAs have less effect on sleep architecture and in general shorter half-lives. Thus, overall, BZRAs have multiple benefits to be considered prior to implementing treatment in cancer patients with insomnia: they possess shorter half-lives, have less consequent morning-after effects, and have fewer negative consequences on sleep architecture.

As cancer patients tend to have longer-term chronic difficulty with primary insomnia, most sleep specialists recommend less habit-forming sleep agents, such as ramelteon or melatonin, as first-line treatments. The lowest possible effective dose would always be the starting dose with emphasis to the patient regarding this plan and its rationale.

■ OBSTRUCTIVE SLEEP APNEA AND PSYCHIATRIC COMPLICATIONS IN CANCER

Comorbidity of airway-related sleep disturbance is extremely high in patients with head and neck cancers.[14,54,55] Airway compromise has obvious phenotypic causes in these patients. Outside the cancer population, obstructive sleep apnea (OSA; defined by Medicare guidelines as an apnea–hypopnea index of five or more respiratory events per hour) carries with it a multitude of psychiatric complaints that, although not well studied in cancer patients, is well known to be prevalent in those with OSA in general. Common complaints include depression,[56] insomnia,[57] hypersomnia,[58] fatigue,[58] and an array of neurocognitive deficits in memory and executive functioning.[59,60]

Neurohormonal factors can have a powerful impact on sleep. Patients who have been thrown into early menopause may experience serious changes in their sleep drive and circadian pattern. Additionally, testosterone is a major risk factor for OSA syndrome (one reason why OSA is more prevalent in men).[61] OSA in the non-cancer patient is associated with a high rate of depression.[62,63] Clinically, we often see anhedonia and alexithymia as well.

All head and neck and lung cancer patients should be screened for airway-related sleep disturbances. Hallmark phenotypic characteristics to look for include retrognathia, micrognathia, and midface hypoplasia. The psychiatrist and psychologist (and anyone else) concerned about an airway-related sleep disorder might keep in mind the image of our "best friend" counterparts who snore, who often sleep with us, and whose faces are easily recognizable: the pug and the Persian cat. As human caricatures, the facial morphology gives a guide with regard to what human features may be associated with an airway-related sleep disturbance: midface hypoplasia and small retrognathic chins, in addition to an often higher-than-ideal body mass index.

■ OTHER SLEEP CAUSES OF DISTURBANCE: PLMD AND RLS IN CANCER

Cancer brings with it several risk factors for sleep disturbance. One common complaint is of RLS. Comorbidity of PLMD with RLS is quite high. Although PLMD and RLS do have a strong genetic component, one common and treatable cause is iron deficiency.[64] This is not a simple relationship. Serum ferritin has been found to be abnormal in those with RLS, but substantia nigra tissue from those with RLS has revealed a complex pattern of iron-related abnormalities.[65,66] Serum ferritin levels of >50 ng/mL have been found to often be a contributor to these movement disorders. Iron deficiency is often associated with fatigue and hypersomnolence. Unfortunately, most diagnostic laboratories consider extremely low to high values to be acceptable for serum ferritin. For office staff who are not accustomed to looking at the values but rather only the ranges, this can be missed as a possible contributor. Several laboratories list values between 10 and 278 ng/mL as normal. The clinician should be conscientious of this, as it is not only sleep specialists, but also oncologists and hematologists with whom we have consulted who disagree that this range is acceptable.

PSYCHIATRIC COMORBIDITIES IN CANCER

As is outlined in various chapters of this book, psychiatric comorbidity is varied and may become pronounced in patients with cancer. Some of the greatest comorbidities include: generalized anxiety, grief, panic disorder, depression, and adjustment disorder. We will navigate through each of these to discuss how they impact sleep disturbance during and in the years following cancer treatment.

Cancer is more likely to develop in those with maladaptive lifestyles and substance abuse. Smoking has been clearly established a primary cause for lung, breast, and head and neck cancer. Alcohol use has been linked with esophageal,[67] head and neck,[68] upper gastrointestinal,[69] and breast cancer.[70] Obesity is associated with a multitude of cancers and may account for 25% to 30% of several major cancers including colon cancer,[71] endometrial cancer, kidney cancer, breast cancer,[72] and cancer of the esophagus.[73] Although poor lifestyle habits are known to be more prevalent in those with psychiatric comorbidities, trends of significant substance abuse (alcohol, nicotine, and food) do not account for the vast majority of cancer patients. However, all three of these risk factors also place patients at greater risk of sleep disturbance.

MOOD DISTURBANCE AND INSOMNIA IN CANCER PATIENTS

A wealth of research exists regarding the comorbidity of sleep disturbance with psychiatric disorders. Anxiety is possibly one of the greatest contributors to sleep disturbance in cancer. Patients face psychosocial stress of managing issues such as treatment decisions, end-of-life issues, loss of job and revenue, fertility loss, amputation (for breast cancer and osteosarcoma), disfigurement, and social role change. In a cross-sectional survey of 192 patients about to undergo chemotherapy for potentially curable cancers (breast or gastrointestinal cancers or lymphoma),[5] the Hospital Anxiety and Depression Scale was used to assess anxiety and depression and the Chemotherapy Symptom Assessment Scale was used to measure physical symptom prevalence, severity, and distress. The prevalence of anxiety was 45% and of depression was 25%. The most prevalent physical symptoms were pain (48%), feeling unusually tired (45%), and difficulty sleeping (45%). The physical symptoms rated as most severe were pain (28%), difficulty sleeping (26%), and feeling unusually tired (19%). Thus, before commencing chemotherapy, patients are already experiencing distress.

The most common psychiatric disorders that are seen in cancer patients include depression and adjustment disorder.[74] Anxiety and depression, often at their early phase, frequently co-occur with insomnia.

Although the most common insomnia diagnosis is psychophysiological insomnia, this diagnosis assumes that mood disorder is not a pervasive and significant factor influencing sleep. However, clinically, we do not experience this to be the case. General anxiety is a significant risk factor for insomnia. There is much clinical support for findings of Carney et al[75] that patients with great frequency describe a tendency to be unable to "turn off" at night.[75] Although they do not find *turning off* easier during the day typically, it is less worrisome, and in fact such hyperarousal is sometimes perceived by patients as beneficial to productivity in the workplace. As are energy and alertness, sleep is significantly impacted by psychiatric illness. If this relationship is bidirectional, which it appears to be, we should query: how does the additional stressor of a major medical illness such as cancer affect its course? Patients seem to recognize anxiety better than depression, and it appears to carry a lower stigma. Often patients indicate belief that it is only the vegetative and suicidal components of depressions that are worthy of mention.

We suggest that there may be better ways both to define the presentation of insomnia with regard to psychiatric, behavioral, and social factors and to evaluate which treatment strategies may be optimal for patients presenting with differentially weighted risk factors.

■ TREATMENT OF SLEEP DISTURBANCE IN CANCER PATIENTS

A detailed history is critical before optimal treatment of insomnia can be initiated. Despite the fact that the methods discussed below are those found to be more effective, knowing all of the contributors to the patient's sleep problem as well as what the patient has tried in the past is essential in building rapport and designing a proper program. Unlike most medical and psychiatric disorders, those with insomnia have often been faced with varying degrees of partial treatment, ineffective online self-treatment, misleading reading materials, and copious medications, creating a guarded and challenging patient by the time he or she sees us.

Patients with cancer will often use chemical means to control fatigue and associated sleepiness. Excessive caffeine to alleviate mood and to stave off sleepiness is not uncommon. As caffeine is an adenosine antagonist, the use of caffeine to control both fatigue and sleepiness makes sense. There are very few data on the use of caffeine in cancer patients to offset these conditions. However, compared with our non-cancer patients, we have seen many cancer patients, apparently self-medicating, taking excessive doses.

Cancer patients with complaint of sleep disturbance should always be queried about how they treat symptoms. Caffeine and energy drinks are common strategies. Use of a family or friend's medications are also often used, but this information is rarely offered unless the patient is specifically queried.

Strategies for modulating psychosocial effects of sleep disturbance in cancer patients are important. Cancer patients face not only the effects of their chemotherapy, cancer, radiation, and amputations, but also the biochemical changes that often accompany these interventions and the cancer itself.

■ COGNITIVE–BEHAVIORAL TREATMENT OF INSOMNIA

The first line of treatment for chronic insomnia in all cases of primary insomnia is stimulus control therapy (SCT). SCT postulates that it is the paired association with the sleep environment (bedroom) and the learned arousal that perpetuates hyperarousal and the insomnia. Detaching the association by removing oneself from the environment but not engaging in sleep outside of the bedroom is the key feature to SCT. The strategies discussed herein are identical to those that are used with otherwise healthy insomnia patients, with some minor modifications specific to cancer.

Bootzin[76] developed SCT in 1972. His theory presented the premise that reconditioning maladaptive associations with sleep and the sleep environment would dramatically alter insomnia. The NIH White Papers, in a review of insomnia treatments[77], indicate that SCT is a standard of care.[77] Additional meta-analysis and reviews suggest that there are five treatments that meet the criteria for empirically supported psychological interventions: SCT, relaxation, paradoxical intention, sleep restriction, and cognitive–behavior therapy.[78]

Although cancer patients may not have developed maladaptive associations with their bedroom or poor sleep habits until the intervening cancer, once diagnosis is made, patients face a cascade of decisions and anxieties that often results in arousal and difficulty maintaining their regular schedule. We have observed that newly diagnosed patients, who are trying to maintain routine and normalcy, will often attempt to maintain the same sleep–wake schedule. However, consequent to increased psychophysiological arousal, they will often lie in bed attempting to force sleep and will begin engaging in ruminations about their diagnosis, accommodating their lives for cancer treatments, modifying their lives, and their plans for what they anticipate their cancer may bring. Insomnia has been reported as prominent prior to diagnosis of cancer, at the time of initiating chemotherapy.[79]

Recent research has shown that the initiation of chemotherapy and subsequent treatments incrementally impair sleep–wake cycles. Savard et al[80] studied 95 women scheduled to receive neoadjuvant or adjuvant anthracycline-based chemotherapy for stage I to III breast cancer using an Actillume (Ambulatory Monitoring, Inc, Ardsley, New York) wrist actigraphy. Actigraphy uses an accelerometer device to measure minute movement in the wrist continuously over several days. These wrist movements, via their indication of activity, have been very highly correlated with overall sleep time. The American Academy of Sleep Medicine practice parameters indicate that actigraphy is a useful tool for detecting sleep in healthy individuals and for assessing specific aspects in insomnia, RLS, and circadian rhythm disorders as well as excessive sleepiness. Savard and colleagues[80] discovered transient disruption to sleep–wake cycles, with worse impairment during the first week of chemotherapy administration at each cycle and with increasing impairment with repeated administrations of chemotherapy.

Davidson et al[81] sampled 982 consecutive patients being seen in clinics for breast, gastrointestinal, genitourinary, gynecologic, lung, and non-melanoma skin cancers with a brief sleep questionnaire to assess the presence of symptoms. The most prevalent self-reported problems were excessive fatigue (44%), restless legs (41%), insomnia (31%), and excessive sleepiness (28%). SCT has been found effective in improving overall sleep in cancer patients undergoing group treatment.[81,82] Relaxation training was also found effective in improving overall sleep in each group.[81,83]

Guided imagery has not, in meta-analysis, been found to be effective in treatment of insomnia. However, we have found it effective for patients clinically in some cases. Additionally, for cancer patients, who do have benefit from guided imagery with regard to pain and nausea, these tools may be adaptable to manage insomnia as well. A likely mechanism of guided imagery is not only relaxation, but also redirecting dysfunctional and ruminative thoughts to a more productive line of focus. Patients with limited abstraction skills and poor visualization are not ideal candidates. Relaxation training through progressive muscle relaxation and guided imagery techniques has received attention both in the cancer literature and in insomnia research.[83]

These techniques have been well established as effective for cancer patients at relieving general anxiety and depression. We recommend that once guided imagery and progressive muscle relaxation is explained, patients be given the option of which they feel would be most beneficial.

CBT targeted specifically at insomnia (CBT-I) has been shown to be highly effective in modifying dysfunctional cognitions related to sleep. The cognitive–behavioral model of insomnia developed by Morin[84] identifies two mechanisms of CBT specifically for insomnia: the reduction of dysfunctional beliefs about sleep and maladaptive sleep behaviors. In cancer patients, CBT-I has been found effective in ameliorating insomnia in breast cancer patients. Tremblay et al[82] evaluated the benefits of CBT-I with breast cancer patients; they administered eight weekly group therapy sessions based on the clinical treatments developed by Morin. The approach combined SCT, sleep restriction, cognitive restructuring, sleep hygiene, and fatigue and stress management.[82] Long-term benefit was found in overall dysfunctional beliefs about sleep as well as in sleep behaviors. The reader is referred to Perlis et al[85] and to Glovinsky and Spielman[86] for more detailed descriptions of CBT-I.

■ TREATMENT OF CIRCADIAN RHYTHM DISORDERS

Patients most often present with phase-delayed sleep (falling asleep later than desired). This is most common in adolescents and in fact is a natural developmental drive found cross-culturally. Two medications are marketed specifically for clock readjustment. One is melatonin, which is available over the counter, and the other is Rozerem (*ramelteon*), which is FDA-approved for adults but not children. Caution should be used with cancer patients, given that melatonin is a neurohormone (it is produced by specialized nervous tissue, specifically the pineal gland). Many patients with phase delay problems benefit from simple sleep time modifications. For example, forcing a phase-delayed teen to rise earlier and consistently and remove stimulant substances (caffeine as well as text messaging at night) can have a profound impact. Early morning bright light and dim light at night also have a great impact on clock readjustment. The reader is cautioned that forcing wake is easier than forcing sleep when readjusting a schedule. Drive will generally intensify if the patient is woken earlier and not allowed to nap.

■ TREATMENT OF AIRWAY-RELATED SLEEP DISORDERS IN CANCER PATIENTS

Given the high incidence of OSA in head and neck and lung cancer patients, NPSG screening is extremely important in these patients. Recent data suggest that airway-related sleep disturbances are higher in many other cancers as well. Thus, in any patient presenting with classic symptoms of OSA such as snoring, obesity, waking with headache, sore throat, or observed apnea, or with other markers for OSA such as sleeping better in a recliner or feeling unrested, fatigued, and sleepy during the day, a sleep evaluation should be considered by a sleep specialist. Most cities now have sleep laboratories and centers that are credentialed by the American Academy of Sleep Medicine. We encourage practitioners to be familiar with these centers and their practitioners for referral.

■ PEDIATRIC CANCER AND SLEEP

Excessive daytime sleepiness or fatigue is frequently endorsed by both cancer patients and long-term survivors of pediatric cancer.[87] Many causes for excessive daytime sleepiness or fatigue have been identified. Both the delicate neurological balance and psychological context necessary for good sleep are at risk for disruption during and subsequent to cancer treatment.[88] The disruption may be time limited, chronic, or progressive, depending on the cause.

Research on sleep in the pediatric patient during the active phase of cancer treatment is primarily representative of children with acute lymphoblastic leukemia (ALL) and CNS tumors. In most study samples, children with cancer sleep differently. They sleep longer, have longer sleep onsets, and awaken more frequently, compared with healthy peers.[89] Gender differences in pediatric cancer patients have been reported. In one study, males awakened more frequently than females, and females slept more in the daytime.[90] The psychological context, active treatment experience, long-term treatment sequelae, and the potential impact of each on sleep will be discussed.

The Psychological Context

The diagnosis of cancer, news of relapse or progressive disease, and other health-related losses can be traumatic, sad, and anxiety-provoking. The diagnosis of cancer is life-threatening and threatening to one's physical integrity. Children experience health-related losses, such as missing school. They anticipate other losses such as dating hardships and changes in appearance. They fear the unknown, such as infertility and whether they will die from cancer. Children, adolescents, and young adults commonly experience symptoms of depression and anxiety, and the symptoms often wax and wane according to health-related events, developmental milestones, and major transitions. As with adults, depression and anxiety often manifest as sleep disruptions, including difficulty initiating sleep, difficulty sustaining sleep, or premature awakening. Hyperarousal, intrusive thoughts, muscle tension, and emotional distress are symptoms of depression and/or anxiety as well as of insomnia that perpetuate the inability to sleep. Re-experiencing events through dreams or nightmares is a further common sleep complaint for children.

Active Treatment Experience

Medical treatment, hospitalization, and cancer-related pain are elements of the active treatment experience relevant to sleep. The treatments themselves can increase risk of sleep disturbance. For example, the chemotherapy drug methotrexate requires supplemental hydration, which in turn causes frequent, nocturnal urination. Steroid medication (eg, dexamethasone), a common component of ALL treatment, is associated with increased fatigue, sleep

duration, waking minutes in bed, nighttime awakenings, and restless sleep.[89]

Hospitalized patients are frequently awakened by environmental stimuli.[91] Staff and parents traverse the patients' rooms during the sleeping hours. One sample of patients hospitalized for chemotherapy treatment of a first cancer (either acute myeloid leukemia or a solid tumor, who were not receiving steroid or sleep-related medications) had as many as 40 nocturnal awakenings per night. Number of awakenings was related to greater fatigue and longer sleep duration (likely to compensate for sleep fragmentation).[92]

Cancer-related pain increases risk of sleep disturbance. Pain can be caused by the treatment, medical procedures, or the disease process.[91] Treatments for cancer may cause acute pain (eg, mucositis, dyspepsia) and chronic pain (eg, neuropathy, avascular necrosis). Procedural pain is not always a brief experience. Bone marrow aspiration, for example, may cause lower back pain for a couple of days. The pain of the disease process may be ongoing until the antiangiogenic treatment takes effect. ALL is associated with pain in the legs, abdomen, head, neck, and back.[93] Bone pain may be localized and inhibit activity. A CNS tumor may cause headache, dizziness, and nausea. Pain may increase for those whose disease progresses; if not effectively managed, pain can disrupt sleep.

Long-term Treatment Sequelae

"Excessive daytime sleepiness has emerged as one of the most common, but often unrecognized, sleep symptoms in cancer survivors," according to Rosen et al[94] of the Pediatrics of the University of Minnesota School of Medicine. In a report from the Childhood Cancer Survivor Study (CCSS), 17% of long-term survivors have insomnia and 8% have depression,[95] which more frequently occurs in the survivor compared with the survivor's sibling. Insomnia and excessive daytime sleepiness in long-term survivors of pediatric cancer have been associated with physical conditions associated with cancer treatments, such as congestive heart failure. Some antiangiogenic medications are cardiotoxic, causing congestive heart failure. Renal insufficiencies as a result of chemotherapy can cause fragmented sleep due to nocturnal urination and/or enuresis. Sleep complaints in survivors have also been associated with cranial radiation treatment.

Long-term survivors of pediatric cancer are at risk for endocrine insufficiencies if the cancer or the cancer treatments (eg, cranial radiation, tumor resection) affected the thyroid, adrenal, pituitary, or hypothalamus.[94] Endocrine insufficiencies increase risk for sleep disturbance and obesity,[94] both of which increase risk for sleep problems. CNS involvement has been associated with differing types of sleep problems. Neuroblastoma in the context of other neurocristopathies has been associated with hypoxia and sleep apnea.[96–99] Hypothalamic damage secondary to a brain tumor has been associated with narcolepsy.[100] Brain stem damage (medulla oblongata, pons) has been associated with sleep apnea.[101]

Assessment

With regard to fatigue, one related practice guideline has been published by the Children's Oncology Group (COG). The COG *Long-term Follow-up Guidelines*[102] include a recommendation of screening for physical sources of fatigue, such as anemia, sleep disturbances, nutritional deficiencies, cardiomyopathy, pulmonary fibrosis, hypothyroidism, or other endocrinopathy. No practice guideline was found for pediatric patients during active cancer treatment.

Sleep problems may be exacerbated by cancer or triggered by cancer, and a screening assessment can begin with patient or proxy report. The clinical interview should consist of questions about sleep before and after cancer. As many sleep disorders have strong genetic components, history of family sleep disturbance is critical. Cancer has distinct challenges during the course of treatment and aftercare that may need to be parsed out during the assessment of sleep problems. Diagnosis of cancer, relapse, and progressive disease are disruptive to the psychological context. Some treatments, such as steroid medication, have an acute, time-limited impact on sleep. Chemotherapy, radiation therapy, and neurosurgery may permanently impact sleep. Chemotherapy and radiation therapy may have both a chronic and a progressive impact on sleep.

Easily disrupted by emotional distress, sleep patterns provide some transparency regarding a person's emotional state. For the cancer professional, a possible general questioning sequence may be, "How have you been sleeping? How long do you take to fall asleep? Once you are asleep, do you awaken? If so, what causes you to awaken? What is on your mind when you awaken? How are you feeling when you awaken?"

For more detailed evaluations of sleep, we recommend that specialists consider use of the Children's Sleep Habits Questionnaire (CSHQ) to evaluate sleep broadly in children.[103] This questionnaire has gained wide recognition as a screening tool for sleep disturbance. Children for whom there is suspicion of an airway-related sleep disorder should be evaluated via NPSG. Typical strategies for treating children with OSA are adenoid and tonsillectomy. Some children, particularly older ones, children with facial morphologies not conducive to surgical benefit, and children in need of supplemental nocturnal oxygen, may be better candidates for continuous positive airway pressure.

Symptom assessment scales have been designed for the pediatric cancer population, and a sleep-related question is commonly included. To complement the screening question(s), multi-item quantitative questionnaires may be helpful. The PedsQL (© 1998) Fatigue Module by Varni et al[104,105] has been extensively used in health care research, and related publications are numerous. Feasibility, reliability, and validity are well established. Both self-report and parent proxy (or accompanying caregiver) reports are available. The fatigue module consists of 18 items, and subscales include general fatigue, sleep problems, and cognitive fatigue. The fatigue module can be administered to those 5 years of age and older. Each item is scored on a Likert scale. The young child responds to a three-point Likert scale (ie, not at all, sometimes, a lot). Otherwise, the reporter responds to a five-point Likert scale (ie, never, almost never, sometimes, often, almost always). The questionnaire takes about 5 minutes to complete.

With patient or parent report of sleep problems such as insomnia or when there is clinical suspicion of sleep-related breathing abnormalities, a sleep specialist should be consulted to evaluate via clinical interview and possible testing with actigraphy or NPSG. These techniques may result in some combination of treatments. These include mechanical interventions such as continuous positive airway pressure, a snore guard, night guard (for bruxism), and positional therapy; surgical interventions such as adenotonsillectomy, rapid maxillary advancement, uvulopharyngopalatoplasty, and tongue reduction; and cognitive–behavioral interventions such as sleep hygiene, SCT, cognitive retraining, relaxation, and progressive muscle relaxation. Medications may be used for insomnia and/or to make nasal breathing easier and more productive.

Although there have been only a few articles published on the efficacy of different treatment strategies to improve sleep in children with cancer, those strategies used to treat sleep disturbance in children with other medical problems as well as in otherwise healthy children should be similarly effective. Children present with a higher incidence of some sleep disorders than do adults. They are

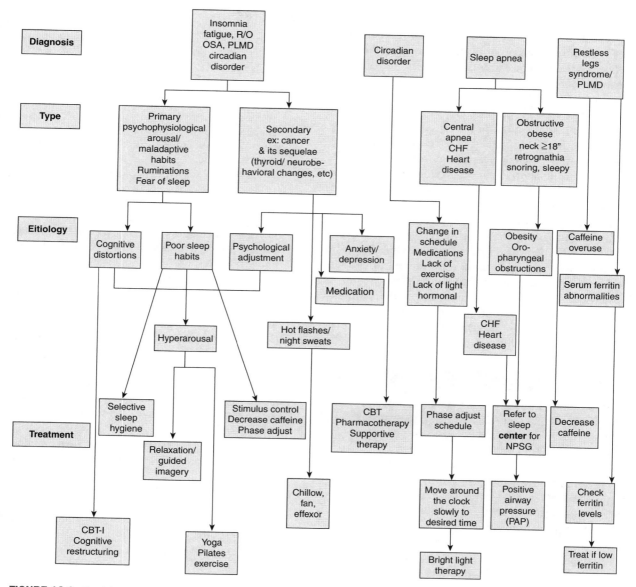

FIGURE 12-1. Decision tree: identification and treatment of sleep disorders.

more likely to have enuresis and SWS disorders such as sleep walking and night terrors. They also tend to have more frequent nightmares (generated largely during REM sleep). Behaviorally, children have more sleep refusal and teens more phase delay difficulties. For a greater review of treating children with sleep disorders, we refer the reader to Mindell and Owen's[106] *Pediatric Sleep Diagnosis and Management of Sleep Problems.*

■ SUMMARY

Cancer patients are disproportionately affected with sleep disturbance. The most common of these is insomnia, although restless legs and sleep apnea are gaining significant recognition as major sleep disturbances that negatively impact quality of life during and after cancer treatment. Facilitating change during the course of treatment is often difficult because of the patient's frustration with the sleep problem, burnout from multiple prior medical interventions for insomnia, and difficulty in divulging the range of personal issues and habits that are contributing to their distress. Through strategies used to treat insomnia, the doctor–patient relationship may also facilitate broader life changes and personal insights.

For both adult and pediatric cancer patients, the first determination to be made is the magnitude to which behavior and psychological factors are at play in the symptom complaint. Figure 12-1 outlines types of sleep disorders commonly seen in cancer patients and provides a decision tree for treatment. Modification of behavioral factors and cognitive distortions is essential when they play a significant role in the patient's sleep disturbance. Medical treatment of disorders such as OSA, RLS, and PLMD is essential and should be addressed to facilitate progress in treating general insomnia. When cognitive–behavioral interventions are indicated, the practitioner should take care to keep the patient involved in his or her treatment and to make sure the patient is on board and in agreement with any intervention.

KEY POINTS

- Sleep disturbance is a significant problem for pediatric and adult cancer patients and survivors and should be assessed during and after treatment.
- Insomnia, airway-related sleep disorders, circadian dysregulation, and movement disorders are the major sleep disturbances experienced by cancer patients.
- If sleep disturbance is reported, depression and anxiety should also be assessed.
- Cognitive–behavioral interventions are the most effective long-term treatment of insomnia, although pharmacological treatments often have benefit, particularly with comorbid mood disorder.
- Treatment of airway-related sleep disorders will likely improve not only mood, but also overall medical status.
- Cancer and its treatments may cause disturbance of hormone balance as well as iron levels, which may have a secondary and negative impact on sleep quality.

REFERENCES

1. Fiorentino L, Ancoli-Israel S. Sleep dysfunction in patients with cancer. *Curr Treat Options Neurol.* 2007;9(5):337–346.

2. Savard J, Morin CM. Insomnia in the context of cancer: a review of a neglected problem. *J Clin Oncol.* 2001;19(3):895–908.

3. Bellizzi KM, Blank TO. Predicting posttraumatic growth in breast cancer survivors. *Health Psychol.* 2006;25(1):47–56.

4. Torrente F, Gercovich D, Hirsch P, Margiolakis P, Gil Deza E, Morgenfield E, Pollola J, Rolnik B, Gercovich FG. Perspectives on psychological distress in cancer patients: comparison between expected, perceived and actual disturbances in a clinic from Argentina. *J Clin Oncol.* 2006. Annual Meeting Proceedings (Post-Meeting Edition). Vol. 24, No. 18S (June 20 suppl); 2006:18515.

5. Breen SJ, Baravelli CM, Schofield PE, Jefford M, Yates PM, Aranda SK. Is symptom burden a predictor of anxiety and depression in patients with cancer about to commence chemotherapy? *Med J Aust.* 2009;190(7 suppl):S99–S104.

6. Bellizzi KM, Blank TO. Cancer-related identity and positive affect in survivors of prostate cancer. *J Cancer Surviv.* 2007;1(1):44–48.

7. Park CL, Helgeson VS. Introduction to the special section: growth following highly stressful life events—current status and future directions. *J Consult Clin Psychol.* 2006;74(5):791–796.

8. Sateia MJ. *International Classification of Sleep Disorders.* 2nd ed. Westchester, IL: American Academy of Sleep Medicine; 2005.

9. American Academy of Sleep Medicine. *International Classification of Sleep Disorders, 2nd ed: diagnostic and Coding Manual.* 2nd ed. Westchester, Ill: American Academy of Sleep Medicine; 2005.

10. Berger AM, Wielgus K, Hertzog M, Fischer P, Farr L. Patterns of circadian activity rhythms and their relationships with fatigue and anxiety/depression in women treated with breast cancer adjuvant chemotherapy. *Support Care Cancer.* 2009;18:105–114.

11. Ohayon MM, Roth T. Place of chronic insomnia in the course of depressive and anxiety disorders. *J Psychiatr Res.* 2003;37(1):9–15.

12. Buysse DJ, Angst J, Gamma A, Ajdacic V, Eich D, Rossler W. Prevalence, course, and comorbidity of insomnia and depression in young adults. *Sleep.* 2008;31(4):473–480.

13. Tsuno N, Besset A, Ritchie K. Sleep and depression. *J Clin Psychiatry.* 2005;66(10):1254–1269.

14. Nesse W, Hoekema A, Stegenga B, van der Hoeven JH, de Bont LGM, Roodenburg JLN. Prevalence of obstructive sleep apnoea following head and neck cancer treatment: a cross-sectional study. *Oral Oncol.* 2006;42(1):108–114.

15. Davidson JR, MacLean AW, Brundage MD, Schulze K. Sleep disturbance in cancer patients. *Soc Sci Med.* 2002;54(9):1309–1321.

16. Ancoli-Israel S, Liu LQ, Marler M, et al. Fatigue, sleep, and circadian rhythms prior to chemotherapy for breast cancer. *Support Care Cancer.* 2006;14(3):201–209.

17. Berger AM, Farr LA, Kuhn BR, Fischer P, Agrawal S. Values of sleep/wake, activity/rest, circadian rhythms, and fatigue prior to adjuvant breast cancer chemotherapy. *J Pain Symptom Manage.* 2007;33(4):398–409.

18. Ohayon MM. Severe hot flashes are associated with chronic insomnia. *Arch Intern Med.* 2006;166(12):1262–1268.

19. Ahmedzai S, Brooks D. Transdermal fentanyl versus sustained-release oral morphine in cancer pain: preference, efficacy, and quality of life. The TTS-Fentanyl Comparative Trial Group. *J Pain Symptom Manage.* 1997;13(5):254–261.

20. McMillan SC. Pain and pain relief experienced by hospice patients with cancer. *Cancer Nurs.* 1996;19(4):298–307.

21. Ohayon MM. Relationship between chronic painful physical condition and insomnia. *J Psychiatr Res.* 2005;39(2):151–159.

22. Feige B, Al-Shajlawi A, Nissen C, et al. Does REM sleep contribute to subjective wake time in primary insomnia? A comparison of polysomnographic and subjective sleep in 100 patients. *J Sleep Res.* 2008;17(2):180–190.

23. Perlis ML, Smith MT, Andrews PJ, Orff H, Giles DE. Beta/gamma EEG activity in patients with primary and secondary insomnia and good sleeper controls. *Sleep.* 2001;24(1):110–117.

24. Perlis ML, Kehr EL, Smith MT, Andrews PJ, Orff H, Giles DE. Temporal and stagewise distribution of high frequency EEG activity in patients with primary and secondary insomnia and in good sleeper controls. *J Sleep Res.* 2001;10(2):93–104.

25. Bonnet MH, Arand DL. Hyperarousal and insomnia. *Sleep Med Rev.* 1997;1(2):97–108.

26. Bonnet MH, Arand DL. Insomnia, metabolic rate and sleep restoration. *J Intern Med.* 2003;254(1):23–31.

27. Bower JE, Ganz PA, Desmond KA, Rowland JH, Meyerowitz BE, Belin TR. Fatigue in breast cancer survivors: occurrence, correlates, and impact on quality of life. *J Clin Oncol.* 2000;18(4):743–753.

28. Ferentinos P, Kontaxakis V, Havaki-Kontaxaki B, et al. Sleep disturbances in relation to fatigue in major depression. *J Psychosom Res.* 2009;66(1):37–42.

29. Johns MW. A new method for measuring daytime sleepiness: the Epworth sleepiness scale. *Sleep.* 1991;14(6):540–545.

30. Berger AM, Farr L. The influence of daytime inactivity and nighttime restlessness on cancer-related fatigue. *Oncol Nurs Forum.* 1999;26(10):1663–1671.

31. Armitage R, Yonkers K, Cole D, Rush AJ. A multicenter, double-blind comparison of the effects of nefazodone and fluoxetine on sleep architecture and quality of sleep in depressed outpatients. *J Clin Psychopharmacol.* 1997;17(3):161–168.

32. Thase ME. Antidepressant treatment of the depressed patient with insomnia. *J Clin Psychiatry.* 1999;60(suppl 17):28–31.

33. Gursky JT, Krahn LE. The effects of antidepressants on sleep: a review. *Harv Rev Psychiatry.* 2000;8(6):298–306.

34. Winokur A, Gary KA, Rodner S, Rae-Red C, Fernando AT, Szuba MP. Depression, sleep physiology, and antidepressant drugs. *Depress Anxiety.* 2001;14(1):19–28.

35. Rush AJ, Armitage R, Gillin JC, et al. Comparative effects of nefazodone and fluoxetine on sleep in outpatients with major depressive disorder. *Biol Psychiatry.* 1998;44(1):3–14.

36. Becker PM. Treatment of sleep dysfunction and psychiatric disorders. *Curr Treat Options Neurol.* 2006;8(5):367–375.

37. James SP, Mendelson WB. The use of trazodone as a hypnotic: a critical review. *J Clin Psychiatry.* 2004;65(6):752–755.

38. Ware JC, Pittard JT. Increased deep sleep after trazodone use: a double-blind placebo-controlled study in healthy young adults. *J Clin Psychiatry.* 1990;51(suppl):18–22.

39. Bertschy G, Ragama-Pardos E, Muscionico M, et al. Trazodone addition for insomnia in venlafaxine-treated, depressed inpatients: a semi-naturalistic study. *Pharmacol Res.* 2005;51(1):79–84.

40. Nierenberg AA, Adler LA, Peselow E, Zornberg G, Rosenthal M. Trazodone for antidepressant-associated insomnia. *Am J Psychiatry.* 1994;151(7):1069–1072.

41. Jin Y, Desta Z, Stearns V, et al. CYP2D6 genotype, antidepressant use, and tamoxifen metabolism during adjuvant breast cancer treatment. *J Natl Cancer Inst.* 2005;97(1):30–39.

42. Brauch H, Murdter TE, Eichelbaum M, Schwab M. Pharmacogenomics of tamoxifen therapy. *Clin Chem.* 2009;55(10):1770–1782.

43. Kotlyar M, Brauer LH, Tracy TS, et al. Inhibition of CYP2D6 activity by bupropion. *J Clin Psychopharmacol.* 2005;25(3):226–229.

44. Madeira M, Levine M, Chang TK, Mirfazaelian A, Bellward GD. The effect of cimetidine on dextromethorphan O-demethylase activity of human liver microsomes and recombinant CYP2D6. *Drug Metab Dispos.* 2004;32(4):460–467.

45. Brynne N, Svanstrom C, Aberg-Wistedt A, Hallen B, Bertilsson L. Fluoxetine inhibits the metabolism of tolterodine—pharmacokinetic implications and proposed clinical relevance. *Br J Clin Pharmacol.* 1999;48(4):553–563.

46. Skinner MH, Kuan HY, Pan A, et al. Duloxetine is both an inhibitor and a substrate of cytochrome P4502D6 in healthy volunteers. *Clin Pharmacol Ther.* 2003;73(3):170–177.

47. Preskorn SH, Shah R, Neff M, Golbeck AL, Choi J. The potential for clinically significant drug–drug interactions involving the CYP 2D6 system: effects with fluoxetine and paroxetine versus sertraline. *J Psychiatr Pract.* 2007;13(1):5–12.

48. Crewe HK, Lennard MS, Tucker GT, Woods FR, Haddock RE. The effect of selective serotonin re-uptake inhibitors on cytochrome P4502D6 (CYP2D6) activity in human liver microsomes. *Br J Clin Pharmacol.* 1992;34(3):262–265.

49. Morin CM, Guay B, Ivers H, et al. Long term outcomes following cognitive behavioral therapy used singly and in combination with medication for persistent insomnia. *Sleep Res Abstr.* 2010;0587:A198.

50. Perlis M, Gehrman P, Riemann D. Intermittent and long-term use of sedative hypnotics. *Curr Pharm Des.* 2008;14(32):3456–3465.

51. Riemann D, Perlis ML. The treatments of chronic insomnia: a review of benzodiazepine receptor agonists and psychological and behavioral therapies. *Sleep Med Rev.* 2009;13(3):205–214.

52. Mendelson WB, Martin JV, Perlis M, Wagner R. Sleep and benzodiazepine receptor sub-types. *J Neural Transm.* 1987;70(3–4):329–336.

53. Mendelson WB. Drugs which alter sleep and sleep-related respiration. In: Kuna S, ed. *Sleep and Respiration in Aging Adults.* New York, NY: Elsevier; 1991:49–54.

54. Payne RJ, Hier MP, Kost KM, et al. High prevalence of obstructive sleep apnea among patients with head and neck cancer. *J Otolaryngol.* 2005;34(5):304–311.

55. Friedman M, Landsberg R, Pryor S, Syed Z, Ibrahim H, Caldarelli DD. The occurrence of sleep-disordered breathing among patients with head and neck cancer. *Laryngoscope.* 2001;111(11):1917–1919.

56. Hattori M, Kitajima T, Mekata T, et al. Risk factors for obstructive sleep apnea syndrome screening in mood disorder patients. *Psychiatry Clin Neurosci.* 2009;63(3):385–391.

57. Lavie P. Insomnia and sleep-disordered breathing. *Sleep Med.* 2007;8(suppl 4):S21–S25.

58. Chotinaiwattarakul W, O'Brien LM, Fan L, Chervin RD. Fatigue, tiredness, and lack of energy improve with treatment for OSA. *J Clin Sleep Med.* 2009;5(3):222–227.

59. Owens J, Spirito A, Marcotte A, McGuinn M, Berkelhammer L. Neuropsychological and behavioral correlates of obstructive sleep apnea syndrome in children: a preliminary study. *Sleep Breath.* 2000;4(2):67–78.

60. Bardwell WA, Ancoli-Israel S, Berry CC, Dimsdale JE. Neuropsychological effects of one-week continuous positive airway pressure treatment in patients with obstructive sleep apnea: a placebo-controlled study. *Psychosom Med.* 2001;63(4):579–584.

61. Behan M, Wenninger JM. Sex steroidal hormones and respiratory control. *Respir Physiol Neurobiol.* 2008;164(1–2):213–221.

62. Schroder CM, O'Hara R. Depression and obstructive sleep apnea (OSA). *Ann Gen Psychiatry.* 2005;4:13.

63. Ohayon MM. The effects of breathing-related sleep disorders on mood disturbances in the general population. *J Clin Psychiatry.* 2003;64(10):1195–1200.

64. Konofal E. Restless legs syndrome in children and adolescents. *Presse Med.* 2010;39(5):592–597.

65. Connor JR, Boyer PJ, Menzies SL, et al. Neuropathological examination suggests impaired brain iron acquisition in restless legs syndrome. *Neurology.* 2003;61(3):304–309.

66. Allen RP, Barker PB, Wehrl F, Song HK, Earley CJ. MRI measurement of brain iron in patients with restless legs syndrome. *Neurology.* 2001;56(2):263–265.

67. Rehm J, Patra J, Popova S. Alcohol drinking cessation and its effect on esophageal and head and neck cancers: a pooled analysis. *Int J Cancer.* 2007;121(5):1132–1137.

68. Boffetta P, Hashibe M, La VC, Zatonski W, Rehm J. The burden of cancer attributable to alcohol drinking. *Int J Cancer.* 2006;119(4):884–887.

69. Salaspuro MP. Alcohol consumption and cancer of the gastrointestinal tract. *Best Pract Res Clin Gastroenterol.* 2003;17(4):679–694.

70. Allen NE, Beral V, Casabonne D, et al. Moderate alcohol intake and cancer incidence in women. *J Natl Cancer Inst.* 2009;101(5):296–305.

71. Murphy TK, Calle EE, Rodriguez C, Kahn HS, Thun MJ. Body mass index and colon cancer mortality in a large prospective study. *Am J Epidemiol.* 2000;152(9):847–854.

72. Petrelli JM, Calle EE, Rodriguez C, Thun MJ. Body mass index, height, and postmenopausal breast cancer mortality in a prospective cohort of US women. *Cancer Causes Control.* 2002;13(4):325–332.

73. Murray L, Romero Y. Role of obesity in Barrett's esophagus and cancer. *Surg Oncol Clin N Am.* 2009;18(3):439–452.

74. Bringmann H, Singer S, Hockel M, Stolzenburg JU, Krauss O, Schwarz R. Longitudinal analysis of psychiatric morbidity in cancer patients. *Onkologie.* 2008;31(6): 343–344.

75. Carney CE, Edinger JD, Meyer B, Lindman L, Istre T. Symptom-focused rumination and sleep disturbance. *Behav Sleep Med.* 2006;4(4):228–241.

76. Bootzin RR. *A Stimulus Control for Insomnia.: American Psychological Association Proceedings.* Washington, DC: American Psychological Association; 1972:395–396.

77. Insomnia: assessment and management in primary care. National Heart, Lung, and Blood Institute Working Group on Insomnia. *Am Fam Physician.* 1999;59(11): 3029–3038.

78. Morin CM, Bootzin RR, Buysse DJ, Edinger JD, Espie CA, Lichstein KL. Psychological and behavioral treatment of insomnia: update of the recent evidence (1998–2004). *Sleep.* 2006;29(11):1398–1414.

79. Boehmke MM. Measurement of symptom distress in women with early-stage breast cancer. *Cancer Nurs.* 2004;27(2):144–152.

80. Savard J, Lianqi L, Loki N, et al. Breast cancer patients have progressively impaired sleep–wake activity rhythms during chemotherapy. *Sleep.* 2009;32(9):1155–1160.

81. Davidson JR, Waisberg JL, Brundage MD, MacLean AW. Nonpharmacologic group treatment of insomnia: a preliminary study with cancer survivors. *Psychooncology.* 2001;10(5):389–397.

82. Tremblay V, Savard J, Ivers H. Predictors of the effect of cognitive behavioral therapy for chronic insomnia comorbid with breast cancer. *J Consult Clin Psychol.* 2009;77(4):742–750.

83. Leon-Pizarro C, Gich I, Barthe E, et al. A randomized trial of the effect of training in relaxation and guided imagery techniques in improving psychological and quality-of-life indices for gynecologic and breast brachytherapy patients. *Psychooncology.* 2007;16(11):971–979.

84. Morin CM. *Insomnia: Psychological Assessment and Management.* New York, NY: Guilford Press.; 1993.

85. Perlis M, Jungquist C, Smith MT, Posner D. *Cognitive Behavioral Treatment of Insomnia: A Session-by-Session Guide.* New York, NY: Springer; 2005.

86. Glovinsky P, Spielman A. *The Insomnia Answer: A Personalized Program for Identifying and Overcoming the Three Types of Insomnia.* London: Penguin Books Ltd; 2006.

87. White AM. Clinical applications of research on fatigue in children with cancer. *J Pediatr Oncol Nurs.* 2001;18 (2 suppl 1):17–20.

88. Rosen GM, Bendel AE, Neglia JP, Moertel CL, Mahowald M. Sleep in children with neoplasms of the central nervous system: case review of 14 children. *Pediatrics.* 2003;112(1 pt 1):e46–e54.

89. Hinds PS, Hockenberry MJ, Gattuso JS, et al. Dexamethasone alters sleep and fatigue in pediatric patients with acute lymphoblastic leukemia. *Cancer.* 2007;110(10):2321–2330.

90. Sanford SD, Okuma JO, Pan J, et al. Gender differences in sleep, fatigue, and daytime activity in a pediatric oncology sample receiving dexamethasone. *J Pediatr Psychol.* 2008;33(3):298–306.

91. Jacob E, Hesselgrave J, Sambuco G, Hockenberry M. Variations in pain, sleep, and activity during hospitalization in children with cancer. *J Pediatr Oncol Nurs.* 2007;24(4):208–219.

92. Hinds PS, Hockenberry M, Rai SN, et al. Nocturnal awakenings, sleep environment interruptions, and fatigue in hospitalized children with cancer. *Oncol Nurs Forum.* 2007;34(2):393–402.

93. Van CL, Bossert E, Beecroft P, Adlard K, Alvarez O, Savedra MC. The pain experience of children with leukemia during the first year after diagnosis. *Nurs Res.* 2004;53(1):1–10.

94. Rosen GM, Shor AC, Geller TJ. Sleep in children with cancer. *Curr Opin Pediatr.* 2008;20(6):676–681.

95. Mulrooney DA, Ness KK, Neglia JP, et al. Fatigue and sleep disturbance in adult survivors of childhood cancer: a report from the childhood cancer survivor study (CCSS). *Sleep.* 2008;31(2):271–281.

96. Diez GR, Carrillo A, Bartolome M, Casanova A, Prieto M. Central hypoventilation syndrome associated with ganglioneuroblastoma. *Eur J Pediatr Surg.* 1995;5(5):292–294.

97. Masumoto K, Arima T, Izaki T, et al. Ondine's curse associated with Hirschsprung disease and ganglioneuroblastoma. *J Pediatr Gastroenterol Nutr.* 2002;34(1):83–86.

98. Rohrer T, Trachsel D, Engelcke G, Hammer J. Congenital central hypoventilation syndrome associated

with Hirschsprung's disease and neuroblastoma: case of multiple neurocristopathies. *Pediatr Pulmonol.* 2002;33(1):71–76.

99. Stovroff M, Dykes F, Teague WG. The complete spectrum of neurocristopathy in an infant with congenital hypoventilation, Hirschsprung's disease, and neuroblastoma. *J Pediatr Surg.* 1995;30(8):1218–1221.

100. Marcus CL, Trescher WH, Halbower AC, Lutz J. Secondary narcolepsy in children with brain tumors. *Sleep.* 2002;25(4):435–439.

101. Akechi T, Okuyama T, Akizuki N, et al. Associated and predictive factors of sleep disturbance in advanced cancer patients. *Psychooncology.* 2007;16(10):888–894.

102. Children's Oncology Group. *Long-term Follow-up Guidelines for Survivors of Childhood, Adolescent, and Young Adult Cancers, Version 3.0.* Arcadia, Calif: Children's Oncology Group; March 9, 2009.

103. Owens JA, Spirito A, McGuinn M. The Children's Sleep Habits Questionnaire (CSHQ): psychometric properties of a survey instrument for school-aged children. *Sleep.* 2000;23(8):1043–1051.

104. Varni JW, Burwinkle TM, Szer IS. The PedsQL Multidimensional Fatigue Scale in pediatric rheumatology: reliability and validity. *J Rheumatol.* 2004;31(12):2494–2500.

105. Varni JW, Burwinkle TM, Katz ER, Meeske K, Dickinson P. The PedsQL in pediatric cancer: reliability and validity of the Pediatric Quality of Life Inventory Generic Core Scales, Multidimensional Fatigue Scale, and Cancer Module. *Cancer.* 2002;94(7):2090–2106.

106. Mindell JA, Owens JA. *A Clinical Guide to Pediatric Sleep Diagnosis and Management of Sleep Problems.* Philadelphia, Pa: Lippincott Williams and Wilkins; 2010.

Psychosocial Approaches to Pain

• *Diane Novy and Laura M. van Veldhoven*

■ INTRODUCTION

Cancer-related pain may be experienced by 50% to 90% of patients with cancer.[1] Cancer pain shares the same neuropathophysiological pathways as non-cancer pain; however, it rarely presents as a pure neuropathic, visceral, or somatic pain syndrome. Rather, it may involve inflammatory, neuropathy, ischemic, and compression mechanisms in multiple sites. Cancer pain may be attributed to tumor progression and invasion, cancer-related surgeries and therapeutic procedures, antineoplastic chemotherapy, hormone therapy, or radiotherapy, cancer-related infections, and musculoskeletal complaints related to inactivity and generalized fatigue.[2] Cancer survivors may have persistent pain as a result of the disease or its treatment.[3] Not only affecting quality of life, but also being an important predictor of survival, cancer pain is considered to be a pathogen that can further the progression of metastatic disease.[4,5]

Cancer pain is strongly associated with psychological distress.[4,6] This association is evident across the disease spectrum, from relatively healthy outpatients to those at the end of life.[2] Pain from cancer and its treatments can result in anxiety, depression, fear, anger, helplessness, and hopelessness. Uncertainty not only about the disease, but also about the duration of pain can increase emotional distress. High levels of depression and anxiety related to a cancer diagnosis, cancer pain, or treatment side effects can influence the pain experience and can increase the level of suffering. Anxiety and tension can heighten sympathetic nervous system activity, which can lead to

muscle spasm, vasoconstriction, and other physiological changes. These changes have the potential to decrease pain tolerance, worsen the pain experience, and increase total suffering.[7] Higher levels of pain are associated with decreased social activities, lower levels of social support, reduced social functioning, and lower resiliency of the social network.[4] Patients with unrelieved cancer pain are at a high risk to consider and commit suicide.

■ PSYCHOSOCIAL ASSESSMENT FOR CANCER PAIN

Effective management of cancer pain begins with an assessment that determines the relationship between the pain and the disease, the types of mechanisms that might be sustaining the pain, and the extent to which the pain is accompanied by other symptoms or problems that might be addressed by an interdisciplinary pain team that complements expert pain management.[8] The core elements of an initial assessment include a detailed history to determine the presence of persistent pain, breakthrough pain (ie, transitory flare-up of moderate to severe pain in patients with otherwise stable persistent pain), the impact of pain on functioning, a physical examination, a diagnostic evaluation for signs and symptoms associated with common cancer pain syndromes, and a psychosocial assessment.[9]

Only in the last decade has it become standard of care in large cancer centers to have mental health clinicians available to help patients manage the psychological symptoms that can increase and maintain their pain. A

■ **TABLE 13-1. Key Assessment Dimensions**

Dimensions	Examples
Sensory/physical	Pain intensity, description of pain
Affect	Anger, anxiety, depression, frustration
Behavior	Limitations in activities
Cognition	Maladaptive patterns of thinking and self-talk

mental health clinician's background may be psychiatry, psychology, clinical social work, or psychiatric nursing. The mental health clinician often functions as part of an interdisciplinary pain team that includes pain medicine physicians and nurses.

Clinical Interview

The first role of the mental health clinician is to gather psychosocial information from a face-to-face interview with a patient and possibly from one or more of the patient's family members and/or significant others. Prior to the clinical interview, it is recommended that the mental health clinician review pertinent biomedical information. The oncologist's report provides extent of disease, medical treatment of disease and pain/symptom control, prognosis, and phase in the disease timeline. The pain medicine physician's report informs other team members about initial assessment and subsequent updated biomedical information about the patient's pain syndrome. The psychosocial clinical interview focuses on gathering information across sensory/physical, affective, behavioral, and cognitive dimensions (Table 13-1), as well as demographic and clinical information about a patient's background and current situation, including available emotional and social support. It is important to keep in mind that each of the dimensions interacts with the others. When asking a patient about one dimension, information received will be impacted by the more global construct of suffering that underlines each dimension.

There are various ways that a mental health clinician can gather information about a patient's sensory/physical experience of pain. One way is by using a numeric rating scale (0 = no pain to 10 = pain as bad as you can imagine) of present, average, highest, and lowest pain intensity during the last 24 hours. Another useful line of questioning is to probe about descriptors of the quality of the pain (eg, stabbing, aching, dull) and about the impact of pain on one's life and functioning. Probing about factors that diminish and exacerbate pain helps the mental health clinician understand the roles of various behavioral, cognitive, emotional, environmental, and physiological stimuli. Clarifying a patient's understanding of his or her condition, pain, and pain treatment helps the mental health clinician identify possible inaccuracies and barriers to various treatment modalities. It is also important to ask about the meaning of pain to a patient and his or her family and about the impact of pain on relationships within the family.

Anger, anxiety, depression, and frustration are the primary focus of the affective dimension of the psychosocial assessment. The similarity of presentation of some symptoms of depression and disease-related somatic complaints, such as decreased activity, fatigue, loss of concentration, sleep disruption, and weight loss, makes depression difficult to recognize in a patient with cancer. Because of this overlap, the mental health clinician will have to listen carefully and also take in information from behavioral observations and reports of significant others.

Although many patients with cancer adjust to the stresses of the disease and its symptoms without a diagnosable mood disorder, patients with pain report significantly more anxiety and depression than those without pain.[10] Among those who report negative emotions, most often these emotions represent acute reactions to cancer, pain, or treatment. Cancer treatment provides many opportunities for anticipatory anxiety. For example, a patient may worry about the next procedure, the next checkup, the cause of new or different pain, and the possibility of relapse. In another regard, a patient can have a long-standing mood disturbance that is exacerbated by illness or challenged by the treatment setting.

Relatively few patients with cancer commit suicide. The majority of suicides reported are among patients who had severe, inadequately controlled, or poorly tolerated pain and depression.[11] Therefore, standard assessment of affect also should include evaluation of suicide ideation.

In addition to a mental health clinician's own assessment and observation of the behavioral dimension, it is useful to ask other team members and a patient's family/significant others for their assessments of pain behavior. Of particular importance are the immediate consequences of a patient's pain behavior. This needs to be assessed to determine whether medical staff or family/significant others are reinforcing behaviors that are inappropriate or excessive. Although this is not usually the case among patients with cancer pain, pain behaviors that foster excessive dependency may be targets for psychological intervention. It also is important to assess the range of behaviors a patient is physically capable of engaging in but restricts because of pain. Frequently when a patient is asked about how he or she paces activity level, it becomes apparent that there is the tendency to overdo activities during periods of diminished pain and then suffer consequences of increased pain afterward. The mental health clinician will want to ask about which behavioral strategies (eg, distraction, relaxation, meditation, and prayer) are currently being used and their effectiveness for cancer pain management. For a patient who already uses some techniques, subsequent treatment would build on the techniques that are effective and new techniques would be introduced as well. For a patient who does not use any techniques, greater preparation will be necessary.

In the context of cancer pain, the assessment of cognition has to do with gathering information about a patient's thoughts and beliefs about his or her disease/condition and his or her ability to handle the associated problems, including pain. A range of cognitive psychological factors have been identified as modulators of pain perceptions. Included among them are expectancy, perceived controllability, appraisal processes, perceived self-efficacy, and contingencies of reinforcement.[12]

Of particular focus are maladaptive patterns of thinking that are unrealistic or distorted. Such errors in thinking have the potential to impact the maintenance and exacerbation of pain and interfere with treatment (eg, belief that there is nothing that can be done to reduce pain and belief that pain is inevitable and should be tolerated). It also is important to ask about a self-talk. This pertains to internal dialogs that reflect thoughts about the patient's condition or pain. Both the cognitive errors and self-talk can be assessed in the clinical interview and/or by asking the patient to self-monitor his or her pain and record any thoughts or feelings that accompany the pain.[13] It also is useful to query about the use and effectiveness of any cognitive coping strategies (eg, thought stopping, problem solving, and positive self-statements).

Other considerations for assessment include alterations in cognitive functioning. The term "chemobrain" has been created by the lay community to describe perceived declines in cognitive abilities assumed to be related to chemotherapy.[14] Incidence rates of cognitive declines

following cancer-related treatments remain obscure due to methodological and statistical differences utilized by researchers in this area.[15] Reduction in attention span, short-term memory loss, and inefficient information processing speed are among the most common reported changes in cognition following and undergoing chemotherapy.[16] For some, declines in cognition might be transient and resolve once treatment has ended, but for others, declines in cognition can persist following the completion of treatments.[16] Incidence rates of cognitive declines following cancer-related treatments remain ambiguous due to methodological and statistical approaches utilized by researchers in this area.[16]

In addition to "chemobrain," a cancer patient with pain might experience changes in cognition in the days immediately after starting an opioid medication or during the first few hours after taking a dose.[17,18] The effects of opioid medications on cognition often vary greatly from patient to patient as a result of multiple factors; thus, careful assessment is needed when considering opioids as a source of alterations in cognition. "Chemobrain" and potential cognitive side effects associated with opioid medications are just two examples of possible sources of changes in cognition that a cancer patient may face. Because cognitive deficits can be very troubling to a patient and these deficits can have implications on the types of psychosocial interventions chosen (eg, cognitive–behavioral techniques vs. mind–body techniques vs. supportive psychotherapy), it could be worthwhile to consult a neuropsychologist for assessment of cognitive strengths and weaknesses and for recommendations on strategies to address cognitive weaknesses. For example, if neuropsychological evaluation reveals deficits in short-term memory, it might be necessary to provide a written, step-by-step guide on how to use various pain management techniques, which the patient could frequently reference when practicing these techniques outside of the mental health provider's office. Consultation with a neuro-oncologist might also be explored, as there might be medications, such as stimulants, that could be appropriate and useful in facilitating cognitive functioning.

As previously stated, cancer pain can adversely impact sleep patterns, and, as such, assessment of a patient's sleep is also a consideration for inclusion in the psychosocial assessment. Frequently cancer patients with pain have a difficult time finding a comfortable sleeping position and can experience multiple awakenings throughout the night. It is not unusual for a patient to report that he or she is most able to sleep when seated in a recliner. Additionally, lack of activity during the day can complicate a patient's ability to maintain a typical sleep schedule. Intervention on the part of the mental health clinician might include provision of strategies to promote good sleep habits. When a patient feels well rested, he or she is better able to manage pain.

An additional psychosocial factor to assess is the economic impact of cancer and pain. Many patients find it too difficult to continue working with cancer pain. This can result in a major change in financial status of the family. It can also impact a patient's ability to maintain insurance benefits. Should these matters present problems for a patient, it may be helpful to consult social services for guidance on disability or external government support.

Lastly, the clinical interview may be supplemented with self-report questionnaires. The Biobehavioral Pain Profile is an example of a self-report tool of biobehavioral factors presumed to influence verbal report of pain, activity, and medication use.[19] It also assesses environmental situations and personal attributes related to the pain experience. Information from this tool is used for matching patient characteristics to cognitive–behavioral therapy interventions.[20] However, at times, a patient's physical condition may make it necessary to streamline the ideal assessment, which would include self-report measures, leaving the clinician with information from only the clinical interview.

◼ PSYCHOSOCIAL INTERVENTIONS FOR CANCER PAIN

The most frequently used psychosocial interventions for patients with cancer pain have been adapted from the well-researched psychosocial interventions for patients with non-cancer chronic pain syndromes.[13] Although standardized psychosocial treatment protocols have been used for research and clinical care, there is the tendency to use individually tailored treatments to fit a patient's characteristics and needs.[21] The treatments fit within four broad categories: (a) cancer pain education, (b) mind/body strategies, (c) cognitive coping skills training, and (d) supportive psychotherapy.

Cancer Pain Education

For Patients
The overall goal of education for patients with cancer and cancer-related pain is to reduce the sense of helplessness, inadequacy, uncertainty, and unpredictability stemming from a lack of knowledge, as these feelings appear to contribute to distress and suffering. Some formats for the delivery of the information are educational materials (eg, audiotapes, books, videos, and various Web sites), talking to other patients with cancer pain, and question and answer group sessions. Depending on the topic under discussion, different members of the treatment team or auxiliary staff may participate as the group leader. Educational interventions can be individually tailored to a specific patient or tailored to groups of patients with similar needs.

A number of patient, family, and health system barriers interfere with medical management of cancer pain and these barriers are often the topic of education. Patient barriers include fear of addiction, concerns about tolerance, concerns about side effects, concern that pain means disease progression, fear of distracting one's physician from treating the disease, fear of injections, fatalism, and the belief that "good" patients do not complain about pain. Research has found that the number of barriers is higher among cancer patients who are older and less educated, and have lower incomes. Patients who have more barriers have higher pain and tend to be undermedicated. Recent studies corroborate the thinking that patients' beliefs about barriers to pain management may indirectly shape their pain experience by inhibiting their willingness to report pain to clinicians or by their being less adherent with an analgesic regimen.[22,23]

Awareness of these barriers has led to important education interventions. There are now a number of educational programs to teach cancer patients about the need to report pain and take pain medications, clarify misconceptions about addiction and side effects, and encourage open communication about pain between patients and health professionals.[24,25] Evidence from three recent randomized controlled trials supports the benefit of patient-directed educational interventions and provides suggestions for treatment.[26–28]

In a study by Oliver and colleagues,[26] individualized patient education and coaching improved pain control among outpatients with cancer. In this study, 34 patients were randomly assigned to a 20-minute individualized education and coaching session to increase knowledge of pain self-management, address personal misconceptions about pain treatment, and rehearse an individually scripted patient–physician dialog about pain control. The potential misconceptions that were addressed included concerns about addiction, beliefs that pain medications simply cannot control pain, fears of being viewed as a bad patient, concerns that treating pain could distract the physician from treating the cancer, incorrect knowledge of how to take analgesics, and the assumption that analgesic side effects cannot be controlled and are worse than the pain. At 2-week follow-up, those who received the intervention had a significant decrease in their average pain as compared with 33 patients who received standardized instruction on controlling pain.

There were significant reductions in pain intensity scores, improvement in the number of appropriate analgesic prescriptions (ie, more prescriptions around the clock with needed opioids), and increases in patients' knowledge regarding pain management in a randomized clinical trial that investigated the PRO-SELF Pain Control Program versus standard care for oncology outpatients with pain from bone metastasis.[27] The PRO-SELF group received an individually tailored psychoeducation intervention that addressed the specific area of knowledge deficit. Patients who received this intervention also were taught about pain and side-effect management, how to use a weekly pillbox, and how to use a script to assist them in communicating with their physician or nurse about unrelieved pain and the need for a prescription change. This intervention lasted 6 weeks and involved home and phone visits from a study nurse. Average time spent on the intervention was 4.5 hours. Results of this study were replicated in a more recent investigation of the PRO-SELF intervention, where it was also determined that patients who experienced a 30% or more reduction in their pain (from the beginning to the end of the study) also had improvements in their mood and quality of life.[28]

The mechanism through which educational interventions affect pain management is not known. It is plausible that an increased sense of control over the process of medical care reduces anxiety and enables patients to plan, prepare, and adopt a sensible course of action for pain management. In addition, perceived self-efficacy to reduce pain may itself have an analgesic effect mediated by both opioid and nonopioid mechanisms.[29]

For Caregivers

Ward and colleagues[30] identified several barriers to medical pain management that were experienced by primary family caregivers of cancer patients who were at the end of life.[30] Caregivers were found to be concerned about side effects of medications, addiction, fear of injections, and that increasing pain corresponded to disease progression. Older caregivers noted that they were concerned that patients' reports of pain might distract the physician from treating or curing the cancer, even though curative treatment was not an option for this group of patients. When an educational intervention addressed barriers among caregivers of elderly cancer pain patients, caregivers improved in psychological functioning and social well-being, and there was an improvement in patients' reported pain intensity.[31]

For Health Care Providers

The health system has its own set of barriers to medical management of cancer pain. Like patients and their caregivers, doctors have a fear of tolerance and fear of addiction for their patients. Other doctor-related barriers are inadequate knowledge and assessment. Inadequate knowledge has to do with the roles of pharmacologic and nonpharmacologic therapy and the impact of pain on quality of life.[32] Additional health system barriers include inadequate reimbursement, rising costs of medications, restrictive regulation, and an overall health system that focuses on cure rather than on quality of life.[6]

The work of the Joint Commission on Accreditation of Healthcare Organizations'[33,34] Pain Standards has been the impetus for many health professionals and health care organizations to start actively attending to these barriers by implementing educational programs, insisting on adequate pain assessments, and expanding access to pain interventions. Other educational programs for health care professionals who treat cancer patients have addressed increased prescription of opioid medication in patients having pain related to advanced cancer and appropriate screening and prescribing of opioids for patients with chronic cancer pain who have a history of substance abuse.[35,36]

Typical Practice

Most psychological pain management for patients with cancer pain includes an educational component that is designed to address the known barriers to cancer pain management and increase knowledge.[37] Although various formats of educational interventions have been studied, including didactic sessions, role modeling, videos, and tutorials, not one stands out as being preferable to the other. In most clinical settings, the educational intervention is profile-tailored to take into account the patient's learning style and specific barriers to pain management. The intervention can be performed in an individual psychotherapy session, a session involving one or more of the patient's caregivers, or a group with other patients and their caregivers. At times, reading material is used to supplement the information given in the session.

A Specific Practice Example

At The University of Texas MD Anderson Cancer Center, patient education about cancer pain is provided by health care providers in an outpatient pain clinic and at the bedside (for hospitalized patients having acute postoperative pain or chronic pain). Extensive resources are used to complement provider–patient discussions, including written materials (eg, about pain medication side effects, sleep hygiene) and videos (eg, about procedures and implantable pain devices). Additionally, monthly pain management lectures are available for patients and their families. Patients with pain are often directed to an educational resource, "the pain pathfinder" developed by the MD Anderson Cancer Center Learning Center.[38] See Table 13-2 for examples and more material.

■ **TABLE 13-2. Key Pain Educational Resources Available at MD Anderson Cancer Center Learning Center**

Type of Material	Example
Pamphlets	Pain Control (NIH Publication 07-6287, printed 5/08)
Reference books	*Guideline for Management of Cancer Pain in Adults and Children* (American Pain Society, 2005)
Books	*Cancer Pain Management* (Fisch and Burton, 2007).[39]
Videos	Pain Control (companion to NIH Publication 07-6287)
Audios	Meditation for Optimum Health: How to Use Mindfulness Breathing to Heal (Weil and Kabat-Zinn, 2003).[40]
Internet resources	http://www.mdanderson.org/topics/paincontrol

Mind–Body Strategies for Cancer Pain

Mind–body techniques, including hypnosis, meditation, relaxation, and biofeedback, are frequently used for

■ **TABLE 13-3. Key Treatment Interventions**

Technique	Types	Purpose
Biofeedback	EEG, EMG, conductance, skin temperature	Used to teach self-regulation of physiological responses
Hypnosis	Anesthesia, direct diminution, displacement, dissociation, sensory substitution	Used to include a state of sustained attention and concentration and openness to suggestion
Relaxation	Autogenic, meditation, progressive muscle relaxation	Used to reduce skeletal muscle tension and reactivity to pain
Imagery	Guided imagery with generalization of skills to disease or pain focus	Used to help achieve a sense of control over pain
Distraction/attention diversion		Used to change the focus from pain to non-painful sensation, positive thoughts, or pleasant images
Cognitive restructuring		Used to bring awareness and a reality check into the evaluation process
Stress inoculation		Used to provide sufficient knowledge, self-understanding, and coping to facilitate better ways of handling expected stressful encounters

managing cancer pain (see Table 13-3). The research literature on the application of these interventions to address cancer pain is relatively young, and a number of different treatments have been used together. Psychological research protocols and clinical practices often combine aspects of each of these types of therapies into a "package." Depending on the specific therapeutic technique, the format may be individual, group, or family sessions. The duration of treatment ranges from brief periods, including times of crisis, to longer-term periods of time.

Hypnosis and Imagery

Hypnosis is a formal induction of a state of sustained attention and concentration, reduced peripheral awareness, and openness to suggestion.[41] The five major hypnotic techniques that have been used for the treatment of cancer pain are anesthesia, direct diminution, sensory substitution, displacement, and dissociation.[42,43] The technique of anesthesia refers to hypnotic suggestions that render a body area numb and insensitive to pain. Direct diminution and sensory substitution change the meaning of pain so that it is less important and painful (eg, turning down the volume, interpreting pain as coldness). Displacement suggestions change the location of the pain. Dissociation is used to separate pain from the patient's awareness. Posthypnotic suggestion and self-hypnosis are additional techniques that are used to extend pain relief.[42,43] Although there are shortcomings in the reported outcome studies, there are some anecdotal and controlled investigations that support the use of hypnosis to relieve cancer-related pain.[44-46]

Imagery involves having a patient develop a mental image associated with feelings of peacefulness and calmness or with a positive past experience. The patient is involved in the decision about the selection of the image. The inclusion and emphasis on various senses enhances the vividness of the image and facilitates the imagery process and relaxation.[13] Once a patient appreciates the usefulness of this technique for relaxation, he or she can generalize imagery skills to a pain-specific focus. When a patient is in a relaxed state, he or she can be instructed to focus on an image that symbolizes pain. The patient is taught to modify the image in a therapeutic manner. He or she learns that by becoming involved with the image, there is less attention available to focus on discomfort. With instruction and practice, a patient can use and terminate the imagery as needed. By so doing, he or she can experience a greater sense of control over pain.[47]

It is important to point out that the content of the image does not seem to be the important factor. Rather, the manner in which the imagery is presented, the involvement of the patient, and practice appear to be crucial. When appropriate, it may be possible to teach family members about imagery so they can help the patient use the technique when needed.

Hypnosis and imagery have the most evidence to support their use for cancer pain management. The efficacy of hypnosis and imagery in the management of acute procedural pain, anxiety, and distress was demonstrated in two separate studies involving children undergoing lumbar punctures for hematological malignancies and bone morrow biopsy.[48] Children trained in hypnosis and imagery had lower levels of self-reported pain and observer-rated behavioral distress than patients randomized to distraction or usual care. Children who were not easily hypnotizable did not achieve the same level of benefits as those who were easily hypnotizable. Further, the observed benefits of hypnosis were diminished when children were switched to self-hypnosis, thereby suggesting that other factors, such as therapist presence, may be a critical component for achieving positive effects. Several case studies have reported the successful use of hypnosis in place of general anesthesia for pediatric patients undergoing radiation therapy.[49]

A particularly important demonstration of the usefulness of hypnosis comes from a recent randomized controlled trial among 45 pediatric oncology patients from the ages 6 to 16 who required venepuncture for blood sampling.[50] The hypnosis session included an induction that was adapted to the child's age, interests, and cognitive and social development. Following several minutes of hypnotic involvement, the child was given "analgesic" suggestions, such as numbness, topical anesthesia, local anesthesia, and glove anesthesia. The session ended with a posthypnotic suggestion that the hypnotic experience would be repeated and would provide comfort during the actual medical procedure. Children in the hypnosis group were also subsequently taught self-hypnosis. The attention control group spent an identical amount of time with the same therapist. The therapist developed rapport with the child and engaged in nonmedical verbal interactions about topics such as extracurricular activities, school, and sports. While receiving the venepuncture, parents of children in both groups were instructed to stroke their child's hand not involved in the procedure. Results showed that children in the hypnosis group reported less anticipatory anxiety and less procedure-related pain and anxiety. These children were also rated as demonstrating less behavioral distress during the procedure than children in the attention control group. Children in the attention control group also experienced reduction in pain, anxiety, and distress during the actual procedure and anticipatory anxiety before the procedure, albeit to a lesser degree than those in the hypnosis group. Additionally, parents of children in the hypnosis group were less anxious than parents of children in the attention control group.

Positive results have come from other modified mind–body techniques for use with children with cancer during acute painful procedures. For example, Broome and colleagues[51] investigated the extent to which relaxation and distraction are useful for children when the techniques are learned and reinforced by a parent. They found that parents can help children practice these techniques at home and then encourage their use during painful procedures. Christensen and Fatchett (2002)[52] expanded upon this intervention by developing and implementing a parent education booklet to promote the use of relaxation and distraction during invasive procedures in the pediatric oncology setting. The booklet included developmentally age-appropriate techniques for children 3 to 18 years old. Individualized instructions to a parent of a younger child included engaging the child in medical play, singing, counting, storytelling, or pretending to blow bubbles. Suggestions for a parent of a teenager included helping the teenager use rhythmic breathing, positive affirmations, or music for relaxation and distraction. Evaluation of this intervention is ongoing, and the authors anticipate that the intervention will not only decrease the cost and risk associated with general anesthesia for lumbar punctures and bone marrow aspirations, but also add to the parent and child's repertoire of coping skills that can be used throughout the course of their treatment or during other painful procedures.

Studies with adults with acute cancer-related pain have also supported the role for hypnosis and imagery strategies for pain management. Specifically, women trained to use hypnosis for pain management prior to breast biopsy reported less postsurgical pain and distress than those receiving usual care.[53] Hypnosis also helped adult patients with acute mucositis pain associated with bone marrow transplant.[54] In a subsequent study, Syrjala and colleagues[55] reported supportive evidence for pain reduction from a relaxation and imagery intervention, with and without additional cognitive–behavioral skills training, in comparison

to standard care despite higher mucositis severity for the intervention groups. A more recent study with patients with breast cancer undergoing autologous bone marrow stem cell transplant did not confirm a reduction in pain intensity or character from a comprehensive coping skills training protocol that included guided imagery.[56]

Taking the evidence for hypnosis in alleviating pain associated with cancer as a whole, it appears beneficial to consider using hypnosis in complement with standard pharmacologic approaches for reducing treatment-related pain.[57] However, it is important to recognize that level of hypnotizability can limit the practical use and benefits of hypnosis in this context.

Relative to acute procedural pain, the role of hypnosis and imagery in chronic cancer pain has been less studied. Spiegel and Bloom[46] investigated the effectiveness of weekly group therapy with or without a hypnosis training component to reduce pain among patients with metastatic breast cancer. Their hypnosis training of 5 to 10 minutes of imaging competing sensations in the painful area was able to reduce the pain sensation and suffering from pain, but did not improve pain frequency or duration over those patients who did not use the hypnosis.

Biofeedback

Biofeedback is a collection of techniques used to teach self-regulation of physiological responses. Physiological functioning is monitored with instrumentation that can give visual and/or auditory feedback to the patient about what is happening to bodily functions that are normally unavailable to awareness. In the first phase of treatment, the patient is trained to develop an increased awareness of the specific physiological response (eg, muscular tension, hand temperature, heart rate, or blood pressure, depending on the focus of the specific biofeedback modality used). The patient is then subsequently taught to gain voluntary control of his or her physiological response(s) by means of feedback from various physiological systems. In the third phase, treatment involves employing the newly acquired voluntary controls in the natural environment.[13]

The most common types of biofeedback are electroencephalographic (EEG), electromyographic (EMG), skin conductance, and skin temperature.[58] The most typical format for biofeedback training is individual sessions. In addition to mastery of relaxation of the body, biofeedback training is thought to help a patient reduce sympathetically mediated and affective responses that induce, facilitate, or maintain pain. To date, it appears that there has been a single, randomized control study of EMG to manage cancer-related pain. Tsai and colleagues[59] randomized 24 patients with advance cancer to either receive six EMG biofeedback-assisted relaxation sessions over the course of 4 weeks or standard pain management care. Using the Brief Pain Inventory, significantly larger reductions in pain intensity from baseline were reported by those who received EMG biofeedback-assisted relaxation sessions than those who received standard care.

Relaxation Techniques

An array of relaxation techniques represents another behavioral approach to cancer pain management. Most relaxation techniques adhere to a format of individual or group sessions, several times a week, coupled with daily home practice. Patients often are given an audiotape as an adjunct to facilitate home practice. There is considerable anecdotal evidence, yet sparse collaboration by controlled randomized design research to support relaxation techniques.[60] The two most commonly used relaxation procedures are progressive muscle relaxation and autogenic relaxation.[58]

In regard to progressive relaxation, it is important to point out that this is not a single method, but a group of techniques that vary considerably in procedural detail, complexity, and length. Regretfully, although outcome studies generally support progressive relaxation, not all reviews have distinguished between the techniques.[61] The method most used for pain management consists of systematically tensing and relaxing several of the 16 major muscle groups. In contrast to progressive relaxation, autogenic training is based on passive concentration. In autogenic relaxation, the patient uses self-statements and visual images to achieve relaxation. Typical exercises begin with the image and sensation of heaviness, warmth (in some instances coolness is used), and relaxation of specific muscle groups until the whole body is involved. The heaviness is directed at muscular relaxation, whereas warmth is directed at vascular dilation. The patient concentrates on his or her body sensations without trying to directly or volitionally bring about change. In addition to helping achieve a relaxed state, autogenic training is designed to strengthen independence and to give control back to the patient.

Meditation

The practice of meditation is frequently described as achieving a deep relaxation or increased awareness as a result of maintaining focused attention on a sound, object,

the breath, or attention itself. There are many different methods of meditation and central to them is regulation of breathing and control over mental activity.[62] Transcendental meditation and mindfulness meditation are among the two most studied meditation techniques.[63] Transcendental meditation involves the repetition of a specific mantra, resulting in the quieting of mental activity and reflection upon feelings, while mindfulness meditation combines purposeful attention of feelings, perceptions, and thoughts with nonjudgmental acceptance. To date, the use of transcendental meditation to manage cancer-related pain has not yet been studied. Meditation techniques, such as Kabat-Zinn's[64] mindfulness-based stress reduction (MBSR), which involves multiple training sessions in sitting meditation, body scan, and mindful movement, have been studied in cancer populations for appropriateness in managing psychological stress, anxiety, depression, sleep disruption, and pain. Results of these studies suggest promise in managing psychological distress.[65,66] Pain was included as a quality-of-life indicator in an investigation of the effectiveness of MBSR for management of psychological distress and improvement in quality of life in breast cancer survivors. Eighty-four breast cancer survivors were randomized to either a 6-week MBSR program or standard care.[67] Improvements in physical functioning, pain, and emotional well-being were found in those who received the MBSR intervention. Further investigation of MBSR and other mindfulness techniques for the management of cancer-related pain appears warranted.

Cognitive Coping Skills

Cognitive coping skills are taught to patients with cancer pain to enhance the adequacy of their coping repertoires. Research on coping with cancer pain has shown that patients who have high self-efficacy and perceptions of control over pain experience reduced pain. In contrast, patients who focus on and exaggerate the threat value of their pain, as well as negatively evaluate their ability to deal with pain (ie, catastrophize), have a tendency to experience higher pain intensity.[68] Studies on pain coping and appraisal suggest that cognitive–behavioral techniques that focus on minimizing catastrophizing and enhancing self-efficacy lead to improved chronic cancer pain management.[2]

One of the major assumptions of cognitive approaches to pain management is that the pain experience is based partly on the appraisals and psychological significance to the individual. Negative expectation, interpretation, and anticipatory fears such as unavoidable pain, loss of control, disfigurement, and subjective perceptions of rejection are common among patients with cancer. The goal of cognitive approaches to pain management is to modify the thoughts that may be contributing to the pain problems. Specifically, cognitive techniques aim to enhance perceptions of control and resourcefulness and to reduce demoralization.[69] A related goal is to teach specific cognitive coping skills to deal with pain. Unfortunately, no study has directly tested the effectiveness of the individual cognitive techniques; however, different combinations of the techniques have demonstrated favorable results within multicomponent treatment packages. Improvements in pain and other distress symptoms persist over time when the treatment is delivered as standardized cognitive–behavioral therapy.[70,71] Short-term results seem best when the intervention is individually tailored in response to identified patient characteristics.[21] A few of the most widely used cognitive techniques are described in the following subsections. The formats used for these techniques are individual or group therapy.

Distraction and Attention Diversion

The goal of distraction and attention diversion is to change the focus from pain to nonpainful sensations, positive thoughts, pleasant images, or aspects of the environment.[13,71] To do this, the mental health clinician teaches the patient about the role that attention plays in the reduction of pain. Specifically, the clinician guides the patient to experiment with his or her awareness and helps the patient see that he or she can only be fully aware of whatever is the focus of attention at the moment. The patient learns that he or she can shift and control his or her attention focus.[13] When patients successfully use this technique, their thoughts may help to lessen their distress.

Cognitive Restructuring

Cognitive restructuring involves reconceptualization of the thoughts and feelings that have a negative effect on a patient's overall adjustment and his or her experience of pain. In stressful situations, such as dealing with cancer and cancer-related pain, deviations in the thinking process can play a major role in a patient's overall adjustment. At the same time that the nature of the situation is being evaluated, the patient is assessing (often not within awareness) his or her resources for dealing with it. This is the "risk–resources equation" that impacts a patient's response to the situation under evaluation.

Under conditions of stress and depleted resources, a patient may make an extreme, one-sided, absolutistic, and global judgment of the situation. When the appraisal tends to be extreme and one-sided, the behavioral inclination also tends to be extreme. For example, a person who is susceptible to fear reactions may interpret a body sensation deemed by the physician insignificant and unrelated to the disease in a catastrophic manner. A depression-prone person may interpret a brief physician follow-up appointment as a rejection and want to withdraw from treatment.

Reconceptualization of such deviations in thinking is accomplished by active collaboration between clinician and patient. Cognitive restructuring training seeks to bring awareness and a reality check into a patient's evaluation process. As this technique applies specifically to cancer pain, the mental health clinician will query about several things related to when pain was particularly severe. These include: what the situation was at the time of the pain; what thoughts the patient had before, during, and after the pain episode; what techniques were tried to decrease pain; and what resources are available to help deal with the pain. By examining the answers to these questions, the patient and clinician can identify negative thoughts and feelings that are not based on well-grounded evidence, and the patient can learn to develop alternative ways of responding.[13]

Stress Inoculation

Stress inoculation often is used in conjunction with cognitive restructuring and behavioral techniques. This technique is closely related to stress management and psychoeducation. As a patient identifies negative reactivity, training in stress inoculation and stress management helps him or her deal more adaptively with those situations. Since lack of preparation and surprise contribute to distressing, ineffective coping efforts, stress inoculation training bolsters a patient's preparedness and assimilatory processes. In this way, a patient can learn to pace himself or herself as he or she learns to master stressful situations gradually. The goals of this technique are to help a patient acquire sufficient knowledge, self-understanding, and coping skills to facilitate better ways of handling expected stressful encounters.[72]

Several related steps are usually followed in stress inoculation. Embedded in these steps, the clinician helps the patient appreciate the fact that his or her stress reflects a normal reaction to a difficult situation. The clinician also helps the patient reframe stressful reactions from signs of weakness to normal or adaptive reactions. In a related vein, the clinician helps the patient appreciate that there are no prescribed emotional stages that stressed individuals go through, nor is there a correct way to cope. In regard to cancer-related pain and stress, the clinician also helps a patient discover and appreciate the variable nature of certain features of the stress and pain, and how the patient unwittingly, unknowingly, and often inadvertently exacerbates and helps maintain stress reactions to certain experiences. The clinician helps the patient develop gradual mastery of stress by exposure to a more manageable reconceptualization of stress. This reconceptualization acts as the basis for coping more effectively. The patient is also taught to draw a distinction between "changeable" and "unchangeable" aspects of the stressful situations. Finally, the patient is taught to break down global stressors into specific short-term, intermediate, and long-term coping goals.

Following the reconceptualization phase of stress inoculation is a focus on individually tailored coping skills acquisition and rehearsal. The newly learned or refined coping skills are rehearsed in vivo. The final phase of stress inoculation training includes opportunities for the patient to apply the variety of coping skills on a graduated basis across other levels of stressors.

Several authors have reported the benefits of stress inoculation for patients with cancer and their families.[73,74] Jay and Elliott[75,76] developed an innovative videotape application of this technique for parents of children with pediatric leukemia who were undergoing bone marrow aspirations or lumbar punctures. Relative to parents who received a child-focused intervention, the parents who received stress inoculation training evidenced less anxiety and better coping skills.

Supportive Psychotherapy

In contrast to the didactic approaches discussed thus far, supportive psychotherapy is more "patient-centered." Supportive psychotherapy is an integration of crisis intervention and psychodynamic principles that are modified for patients with cancer pain. Feelings and fears about the pain are important topics to a patient that are often difficult to discuss with family and friends. Hence, the mental health clinician is an ideal person with whom to explore feelings that otherwise would be unexpressed. Supportive psychotherapy can be used alone and in conjunction with the other interventions discussed. Depending on the needs of the patient, the format may be individual, group, or family sessions.

Aspects of the supportive psychotherapeutic framework will vary with the exigencies of the pain. The utmost challenge lies in adapting a structure to the pain reality, even as the pain changes, without sacrificing the uniqueness of the therapeutic interaction. The uniqueness of the interaction requires flexibility in the duration, location, and scheduling of individual psychotherapy sessions according to a patient's needs. In cases involving a group format, flexibility also must be allowed. Although there has been some research on the positive impact of supportive group psychotherapy for patients with cancer, not much has focused on the pain per se.[77,78]

■ SUMMARY

Following a careful psychosocial assessment, an array of complementary psychological interventions can be individually tailored to help patients with cancer-related pain. There is a growing body of evidence to support the use of multicomponent psychological treatments. Although a greater number of research studies with increased scientific rigor are needed to fully support the treatments for cancer pain, there are an impressive number of controlled randomized studies to support the effectiveness of combinations of psychological treatments for emotional well-being.[79] Another issue for future work includes testing the efficacy of individual components of current multicomponent interventions. Research along these lines could lead to interventions that are both briefer and more economical, and could help to identify the mechanisms responsible for the therapeutic effects of the treatments.

Finally, it is important to emphasize that the psychological interventions discussed in this chapter are best thought of as part of an integrated treatment plan by an interdisciplinary team. Management of pain and other specific symptoms requires a team approach, enlisting expertise from a wide variety of clinical groups.[80] The challenge of addressing both the biomedical and psychosocial issues involved in pain is to develop rational and effective management strategies. Therapies directed primarily at psychosocial variables can also have a profound impact on nociception, and medical interventions directed at nociception can also have beneficial effects on the psychosocial aspects of pain.

> **KEY POINTS**
>
> ■ Effective management of cancer pain begins with an assessment that includes psychosocial symptoms.
>
> ■ The psychosocial clinical interview gathers information across sensory/physical, affective, behavioral, and cognitive dimensions of the pain experience.
>
> ■ Psychosocial treatments for patients with cancer pain are individually tailored to fit a patient's characteristics and needs.
>
> ■ Psychosocial treatments fit within the categories of cancer pain education, mind/body strategies, cognitive coping skills, and supportive psychotherapy.
>
> ■ There is evidence to the use of multicomponent psychological treatments.

REFERENCES

1. Miaskowski C, Clearly J, Burney R, et al. Guideline for the Management of Cancer pain in Adults and Children (Clinical Practice Guideline; No. 3). Glenview, IL: American Pain Society; 2005.

2. Keefe FJ, Abernethy AP, Campbell L. Psychological approaches to understanding and treating disease-related pain. *Annu Rev Psychol.* 2005;56:601–630.

3. Burton AW, Fanciullo GJ, Beasley RD, Fisch MJ. Chronic pain in the cancer survivor: a new frontier. *Pain Med.* 2007;8(2):189–198.

4. Zaza C, Baine N. Cancer pain and psychosocial factors: a critical review of the literature. *J Pain Symptom Manage.* 2002;24(5):526–542.

5. Page GG, Ben-Eliyahu S. The immune-suppressive nature of pain. *Semin Oncol Nurs.* 1997;13(1):10–15.

6. Portenoy RK, Thaler HT, Kornblith AB, et al. Symptom prevalence, characteristics and distress in a cancer population. *Qual Life Res.* 1994;3(3):183–189.

7. Otis-Green S, Sherman R, Perez M, Baird RP. An integrated psychosocial–spiritual model for cancer pain management. *Cancer Pract.* 2002;10(suppl 1):S58–S65.

8. Portenoy RK. Cancer pain management. *Clin Adv Hematol Oncol.* 2005;3(1):30–32.

9. Rafael J, Ahmedzai S, Hester J, et al. Cancer Pain: Part 1: Pathophysiology; Oncological, Pharmacological, and Psychological Treatments: A Perspective from the British Pain Society Endorsed by the UK Association of Palliative Medicine and the Royal College of General Practitioners.

10. Derogatis LR, Morrow GR, Fetting J, et al. The prevalence of psychiatric disorders among cancer patients. *JAMA.* 1983;249(6):751–757.

11. Massie MJ, Gagnon P, Holland JC. Depression and suicide in patients with cancer. *J Pain Symptom Manage.* 1994;9(5):325–340.

12. Turk D, Fernandez E. A cognitive-behavioral perspective. In: Watson M, Greer S, eds. *Cancer Patient Care: Psychosocial Treatment Methods.* Cambridge, UK: Cambridge University Press; 1991: PAGES.

13. Turk DC, Meichenbaum D, Genest M. *Pain and Behavioral Medicine: A Cognitive Behavioral Perspective.* New York, NY: Guilford Press; 1987.

14. Wefel JS, Lenzi R, Theriault R, Buzdar AU, Cruickshank S, Meyers CA. 'Chemobrain' in breast carcinoma?: a prologue. *Cancer.* 2004;101(3):466–475.

15. Kayl AE, Wefel JS, Meyers CA. Chemotherapy and cognition: effects, potential mechanisms, and management. *Am J Ther.* 2006;13(4):362–369.

16. Meyers CA, Abbruzzese JL. Cognitive functioning in cancer patients: effect of previous treatment. *Neurology.* 1992;42(2):434–436.

17. Chapman SL, Byas-Smith MG, Reed BA. Effects of intermediate- and long-term use of opioids on cognition in patients with chronic pain. *Clin J Pain.* 2002;18(4 suppl):S83–S90.

18. Strassels SA. Cognitive effects of opioids. *Curr Pain Headache Rep.* 2008;12(1):32–36.

19. Dalton JA, Feuerstein M, Carlson J, Roghman K. Biobehavioral pain profile: development and psychometric properties. *Pain.* 1994;57(1):95–107.

20. Dalton JA, Lambe C. Tailoring treatment approaches to the individualized needs of cancer patients with pain. *Cancer Nurs.* 1995;18(3):180–188.

21. Dalton JA, Keefe FJ, Carlson J, Youngblood R. Tailoring cognitive–behavioral treatment for cancer pain. *Pain Manag Nurs.* 2004;5(1):3–18.

22. Dawson R, Sellers DE, Spross JA, Jablonski ES, Hoyer DR, Solomon MZ. Do patients' beliefs act as barriers to effective pain management behaviors and outcomes in patients with cancer-related or noncancer-related pain? *Oncol Nurs Forum.* 2005;32(2):363–374.

23. Valeberg BT, Hanestad BR, Klepstad P, Miaskowski C, Moum T, Rustøen T. Cancer patients' barriers to pain management and psychometric properties of the Norwegian version of the Barriers Questionnaire II. *Scand J Caring Sci.* 2009;23(3):518–528.

24. Devine EC, Westlake SK. The effects of psychoeducational care provided to adults with cancer: meta-analysis of 116 studies. *Oncol Nurs Forum.* 1995;22(9):1369–1381.

25. Gordon DB, Ward SE. Correcting patient misconceptions about pain. *Am J Nurs.* 1995;95(7):43–45.

26. Oliver JW, Kravitz RL, Kaplan SH, Meyers FJ. Individualized patient education and coaching to improve pain control among cancer outpatients. *J Clin Oncol.* 2001;19(8):2206–2212.

27. Miaskowski C. Psychoeducational interventions for cancer pain serve as a model for behavioral research. *Commun Nurs Res.* 2004;37:51, 53–71.

28. Miaskowski C, Dodd M, West C, et al. The use of a responder analysis to identify differences in patient outcomes following a self-care intervention to improve cancer pain management. *Pain.* 2007;129(1–2):55–63.

29. Bandura A, O'Leary A, Taylor CB, Gauthier J, Gossard D. Perceived self-efficacy and pain control: opioid and nonopioid mechanisms. *J Pers Soc Psychol.* 1987;53(3):563–571.

30. Ward SE, Carlson-Dakes K, Hughes SH, Kwekkeboom KL, Donovan HS. The impact on quality of life of patient-related barriers to pain management. *Res Nurs Health.* 1998;21(5):405–413.

31. Ferrell BR, Grant M, Chan J, Ahn C, Ferrell BA. The impact of cancer pain education on family caregivers of elderly patients. *Oncol Nurs Forum.* 1995;22(8):1211–1218.

32. American Cancer Society. *Cancer Facts and Figures;* 2003. Available at: http://www.cancer.org/docroot/STT/stt_0_asp?sitearea=STT&level=1. May 8, 2009 approximate date that we accessed these websites on

33. Joint Commission on Accreditation of Healthcare Organizations. 1999. Available at: http://www.jcaho.org/index.htm. May 8, 2009 approximate date that we accessed these websites on

34. Caraceni A, Portenoy RK. An international survey of cancer pain characteristics and syndromes. IASP Task Force on Cancer Pain. International Association for the Study of Pain. *Pain.* 1999;82(3):263–274.

35. Passik SD, Portenoy RK, Ricketts PL. Substance abuse issues in cancer patients. Part 2: evaluation and treatment. *Oncology (Huntingt).* 1998;12(5):729–734 [discussion 736, 741–742].

36. Fishman S. *Responsible Opioid Prescribing: A Physician's Guide.* Washington, DC: Waterford Life Sciences; 2007.

37. Hanson LC, Tulsky JA, Danis M. Can clinical interventions change care at the end of life? *Ann Intern Med.* 1997;126(5):381–388.

38. "The Pain Pathfinder" developed by the MD Anderson Cancer Center Learning Center. Available at: http://www.2.mdanderson.org/app/pe/index.cfm?pageName=opendoc&docid=1592. May 8, 2009 approximate date that we accessed these websites on

39. Fisch M, Burton A. *Cancer Pain Management.* New York, NY: McGraw-Hill Medical; 2007.

40. Weil A, Kabat-Zinn J. *Meditation for Optimum Health: How to Use Mindfulness Breathing to Heal [Audio CD].* Louisville, CO: Sounds True Incorporated; 2003.

41. Barber J, Gitelson J. Cancer pain: psychological management using hypnosis. *CA Cancer J Clin.* 1980;30(3):130–136.

42. Barber J. Hypnotic analgesia. In: Holzman AD, Turk DC, eds. *Pain Management: A Handbook of Psychological Treatment Approaches.* New York, NY: Pergamon Press; 1986:151–167.

43. Margolis CG. Hypnotic interventions for pain management. *Int J Psychosom.* 1985;32(3):12–19.

44. Montgomery GH, DuHamel KN, Redd WH. A meta-analysis of hypnotically induced analgesia: how effective is hypnosis: *Int J Clin Exp Hypn.* 2000;48(2):134.

45. Spiegel D, Bloom JR, Yalom I. Group support for patients with metastatic cancer. A randomized outcome study. *Arch Gen Psychiatry.* 1981;38(5):527–533.

46. Spiegel D, Bloom JR. Group therapy and hypnosis reduce metastatic breast carcinoma pain. *Psychosom Med.* 1983;45(4):333–339.

47. Simonton OC, Matthews-Simonton S, Sparks TF. Psychological intervention in the treatment of cancer. *Psychosomatics.* 1980;21(3):226–227, 231–233.

48. Liossi C, Hatira P. Clinical hypnosis versus cognitive behavioral training for pain management with pediatric cancer patients undergoing bone marrow aspirations. *Int J Clin Exp Hypn.* 1999;47(2):104–116.

49. Bertoni F, Bonardi A, Magno L, et al. Hypnosis instead of general anaesthesia in paediatric radiotherapy: report of three cases. *Radiother Oncol.* 1999;52(2):185–190.

50. Liossi C, White P, Hatira P. A randomized clinical trial of a brief hypnosis intervention to control venepuncture-related pain of paediatric cancer patients. *Pain.* 1999;142(3):255–263.

51. Broome ME, Lillis PP, McGahee TW, Bates T. The use of distraction and imagery with children during painful procedures. *Oncol Nurs Forum.* 1992;19(3):499–502.

52. Christensen J, Fatchett D. Promoting parental use of distraction and relaxation in pediatric oncology patients during invasive procedures. *J Pediatr Oncol Nurs.* 2002;19(4):127–132.

53. Montgomery GH, Weltz CR, Seltz M, Bovbjerg DH. Brief presurgery hypnosis reduces distress and pain in

excisional breast biopsy patients. *Int J Clin Exp Hypn.* 2002;50(1):17–32.

54. Syrjala KL, Cummings C, Donaldson GW. Hypnosis or cognitive behavioral training for the reduction of pain and nausea during cancer treatment: a controlled clinical trial. *Pain.* 1992;48(2):137–146.

55. Syrjala KL, Donaldson GW, Davis MW, Kippes ME, Carr JE. Relaxation and imagery and cognitive–behavioral training reduce pain during cancer treatment: a controlled clinical trial. *Pain.* 1995;63(2):189–198.

56. Gaston-Johansson FJ, Fall-Dickson F, Nanda J, et al. The effectiveness of the comprehensive coping strategy program on clinical outcomes in breast cancer autologous bone marrow transplantation. *Cancer Nurs.* 2000;23(4):277–285.

57. Richardson J, Smith JE, McCall G, Pilkington K. Hypnosis for procedure-related pain and distress in pediatric cancer patients: a systematic review of effectiveness and methodology related to hypnosis interventions. *J Pain Symptom Manage.* 2006;31(1):70–84.

58. Jacobson P, Hann DM. Cognitive–behavioral interventions. In: Holland JC, ed. *Psycho-oncology.* New York, NY: Oxford University Press; 1998:717–729.

59. Tsai PS, Chen PL, Lai YL, Lee MB, Lin CC. Effects of electromyography biofeedback-assisted relaxation on pain in patients with advanced cancer in a palliative care unit. *Cancer Nurs.* 2007;30(5):347–353.

60. Sloman R, Brown P, Aldana E, Chee E. The use of relaxation for the promotion of comfort and pain relief in persons with advanced cancer. *Contemp Nurse.* 1994;3(1):6–12.

61. Hyman RB, Feldman HR, Harris RB, Levin RF, Malloy GB. The effects of relaxation training on clinical symptoms: a meta-analysis. *Nurs Res.* 1989;38(4):216–220.

62. Biegler KA, Chaoul MA, Cohen L. Cancer, cognitive impairment, and meditation. *Acta Oncol.* 2009;48(1):18–26.

63. Mansky PJ, Wallerstedt DB. Complementary medicine in palliative care and cancer symptom management. *Cancer J.* 2006;12(5):425–431.

64. Kabat-Zinn J. An outpatient program in behavioral medicine for chronic pain patients based on the practice of mindfulness meditation: theoretical considerations and preliminary results. *Gen Hosp Psychiatry.* 1983;4(1):33–47.

65. Carlson LE, Speca M, Patel KD, Goodey E. Mindfulness-based stress reduction in relation to quality of life, mood, symptoms of stress and levels of cortisol, dehydroepi-androsterone sulfate (DHEAS) and melatonin in breast and prostate cancer outpatients. *Psychoneuroendocrinology.* 2004;29(4):448–474.

66. Carlson LE, Speca M, Patel KD, Goodey E. Mindfulness-based stress reduction in relation to quality of life, mood, symptoms of stress, and immune parameters in breast and prostate cancer outpatients. *Psychosom Med.* 2003;65(4):571–581.

67. Lengacher CA, Johnson-Mallard V, Post-White J, et al. Randomized controlled trial of mindfulness-based stress reduction (MBSR) for survivors of breast cancer. *Psycho-Oncol.* 2009;18(12):1261–1272.

68. Bishop SR, Warr D. Coping, catastrophizing and chronic pain in breast cancer. *J Behav Med.* 2003;26(3):265–281.

69. Christensen DN. Postmastectomy couple counseling: an outcome study of a structured treatment protocol. *J Sex Marital Ther.* 1983;9(4):266–275.

70. Fawzy FI, Cousins N, Fawzy NW, Kemeny ME, Elashoff R, Morton D. A structured psychiatric intervention for cancer patients. I. Changes over time in methods of coping and affective disturbance. *Arch Gen Psychiatry.* 1990;47(8):720–725.

71. Ahles TA. Psychological approaches to the management of cancer-related pain. *Semin Oncol Nurs.* 1985;1(2):141–146.

72. Meichenbaum D. Stress inoculation training for coping with stressor. *Clin Psychol.* 1996;49:4–7.

73. Turk DC, Rennert D. Pain and the terminally ill cancer patient: a cognitive social learning perspective. In: Sobell HJ, ed. *Behavior Therapy in Terminal Care.* Cambridge, Mass: Ballinger; 1981:95–123.

74. Moore K, Altmaier EM. Stress inoculation training with cancer patients. *Cancer Nurs.* 1981;4(5):389–393.

75. Jay SM, Elliott CH. *Coping with Childhood Leukemia and Its Treatment: A Parent's Perspective* [videotape]. Urbana, Ill: Carla Medical Communication; 1986.

76. Jay SM, Elliott CH. A stress inoculation program for parents whose children are undergoing painful medical procedures. *J Consult Clin Psychol.* 1990;58(6):799–804.

77. Fawzy FI, Fawzy NW, Hyun CS, et al. Malignant melanoma. Effects of an early structured psychiatric intervention, coping, and affective state on recurrence and survival 6 years later. *Arch Gen Psychiatry.* 1993;50(9):681–689.

78. Classen C, Sephton SE, Diamond S, Spiegel D. Studies of life—extending psychosocial interventions. In: Holland JC, ed. *Psycho-oncology.* New York, NY: Oxford University Press; 1998:730–742.

79. Andersen BL. Psychological interventions for cancer patients to enhance the quality of life. *J Consult Clin Psychol.* 1992;60(4):552–568.

80. Foley KM. The treatment of cancer pain. *N Engl J Med.* 1985;313(2):84–95.

CHAPTER 14

Neurobehavioral Side Effects of Cancer and Cancer Therapy

• Mariana E. Witgert and Jeffrey S. Wefel

Advances in multimodal therapy have resulted in increased success in the management of many cancers. However, as many anticancer therapies are not highly specific, healthy tissues are also placed at risk. While traditional measures of treatment outcome have generally focused on survival time, progression-free survival, tumor response, and physiological toxicities, additional indices, including cognitive functioning and quality of life, are receiving increasing recognition as important and viable clinical endpoints. The following chapter presents evidence regarding the presence and nature of cancer- and treatment-related neurobehavioral symptoms in adult cancer patients as well as information regarding the interventions that are currently being employed against those side effects.

■ COGNITIVE IMPAIRMENT

Cancer-related Cognitive Impairment

In order to determine whether or not cancer therapies are associated with the development of cognitive impairment, it is essential to understand the presence and pattern of these symptoms prior to the initiation of treatment. Patients with brain tumors may present with a variety of cognitive complaints as tumors destroy, crowd, and infiltrate brain tissue; the nature and severity of cognitive impairments varies in association with lesion location and lesion momentum, or the rate at which tumors grow. In non-central nervous system (CNS) cancers, several studies have demonstrated cancer-related cognitive dysfunction. For example, cognitive dysfunction in at

least a subgroup of women with breast cancer has been demonstrated prior to initiation of chemotherapy, with estimates ranging from 11% 35% of patients.[1-4] The first of these studies revealed particularly frequent (18–25%) difficulties on measures assessing verbal learning and memory.[1] Pretreatment cognitive dysfunction has also been found in other patient populations, including acute myelogenous leukemia (AML) and myelodysplastic syndrome (MDS), in whom pretreatment impairments have been demonstrated in learning and memory (41–44%), cognitive processing speed (28%), aspects of executive dysfunction (29%), and upper extremity fine motor dexterity (37%).[5] Patients with small cell lung cancer have also been shown to exhibit pretreatment cognitive impairments; Meyers et al[6] demonstrated that 70% to 80% of patients with small cell lung cancer exhibited memory deficits, 38% had deficits in executive functions, and 33% showed impaired motor coordination *before* treatment was initiated.

Treatment-related Cognitive Impairment

In addition to the potential for cognitive impairment related to cancer itself, cancer therapies may have an untoward impact on cognitive functioning. This chapter will focus on the effects of chemotherapies and other agents; it is important to note that other treatment modalities, including surgery and radiation, may also result in neurobehavioral changes. In patients with brain tumors, surgery may result in damage to normal tissue that surrounds the tumor, and yield more focal cognitive impairments that may resolve over time. There is also evidence that radiation therapy may be associated with the development of neurobehavioral symptoms both during and after treatment. The acute phase develops during treatment and is characterized by transient symptoms of headache, fatigue, fever, and nausea, as well as exacerbation of preexisting neurologic deficits. Early delayed toxicity typically develops 2 to 5 months after completion of radiotherapy and has been associated with declines in information processing speed, attention, learning efficiency and memory retrieval, executive functioning, and fine motor dexterity; these symptoms may resolve spontaneously. Late-delayed toxicity can occur months to years after completion of radiation therapy and includes progressive dementia, personality changes, and leukoencephalopathy; unlike acute and early delayed effects, late-delayed toxicity tends to be irreversible.[7]

Current practice utilizes lower doses to the tumor and attempts to reduce exposure of the surrounding healthy brain tissue. It is hoped that continued advances in treatment modalities will further improve the therapeutic ratio and limit incidental brain irradiation, and that associated neurobehavioral complications will thus be minimized. However, as the most profound effects of radiation treatment may not be evident for several years posttreatment, careful monitoring of cognitive function in patients over time remains necessary.

Chemotherapy

Much of the available literature regarding chemotherapy-related side effects comes from research with patients with breast cancer; information from other cancer populations will be provided as available.

In the first prospective study to include a pretreatment neuropsychological evaluation in women with early stage breast cancer, 61% of patients evidenced decline relative to their baseline performance on one or more domains of cognitive functioning at short-term (3 weeks posttreatment) follow-up.[8] Declines were most commonly observed on measures assessing attention, learning, and processing speed. At long-term follow-up (approximately 1 year posttreatment), approximately 50% of the patients who had initially declined evidenced improvement in neurocognitive functioning, while the rest remained relatively stable. There was no statistically significant relationship between either depression or anxiety and any test of cognitive function at any time point.[8] Subsequent studies of women with breast cancer that have employed both pretreatment and posttreatment evaluations have

also reported cognitive decline, most frequently in learning and memory, attention, executive function, and processing speed, with estimates of decline ranging from 13% to 78%.[2–4,9,65] Examination of clinical and demographic characteristics has failed to consistently identify risk factors for pretreatment cognitive dysfunction or treatment-related cognitive decline.

Cognitive and emotional dysfunction associated with hematopoietic stem cell transplant (HSCT) has been reported by a number of investigators, and is thought to stem from the intense treatment regimen utilizing high-dose chemotherapy and total body irradiation during pretransplant conditioning.[10,11] While studies in this group of patients are limited by small sample size and cross-sectional design, prospective neuropsychological assessment reveals decline in executive functions[11] and memory[12] following HSCT.

Risk factors underlying neurotoxicity associated with chemotherapy Several factors that appear to increase the risk of developing neurotoxicity associated with chemotherapy have been identified. These include exposure to higher doses of chemotherapeutic agents, due to either planned use of high-dose regimens or secondary to high concentrations of the parent drug and/or its metabolite due to impaired systemic clearance and/or pharmacogenetic modulation of drug pharmacokinetics.[13] Multi-agent chemotherapy regimens may have additive effects that increase the likelihood of neurotoxicity. In addition, intrathecal administration has been associated with increased risk of neurotoxicity.[14] Medications prescribed for supportive care or symptomatic palliation during the course of cancer treatment, including adjuvant medications such as steroids, antiepileptics, and pain medications, may also cause neurobehavioral symptoms. Corticosteroids have been associated with both psychiatric and cognitive symptoms. During acute corticosteroid therapy, symptoms of mania appear to be the most common psychiatric side effect; chronic exposure to corticosteroids is more often associated with symptoms of depression. Reductions in declarative memory have been demonstrated in association with both acute and chronic use of these medications.[15] Some antiepileptic medications have known untoward effects on information processing speed, psychomotor function, attention, working memory, and executive functioning.[16] Pain medications may result in sedation, which, in turn, may be associated with reduced neurocognitive performance.

Biological Response Modifiers

Biological response modifiers (BRMs; also known as immunotherapies) are aimed at modifying the immune response of cancer patients in hopes of yielding a therapeutic effect.[17] Such agents include a wide variety of treatments, including cytokines, vaccines, monoclonal antibodies, thymic factors, and colony-stimulating factors.[18] BRMs have been demonstrated to (a) directly or indirectly augment the patient's immunologic defenses, (b) modify tumor cells such that the patient's immunologic response is increased, or (c) bolster the patient's ability to manage toxicities secondary to other cancer treatments.[19] Information regarding the association between BRMs and cognition is somewhat limited, and not all BRMs appear to have a negative effect on cognition. However, there is evidence that at least some such agents can adversely impact neurobehavioral functioning.

In normal, healthy controls, a single dose of only 1.5 million international units of the cytokine interferon-alpha (IFN-alpha) worsened reaction time at 6 and 10 hours after injection. When used as a treatment for cancers such as chronic myelogenous leukemia and melanoma, IFN-alpha is delivered at much higher doses for longer periods of time. Occasionally, the treatment results in an acute confusional state, which may be characterized by disorientation, somnolence, psychomotor retardation, expressive language difficulties, and even psychotic symptoms.[20] Posttreatment cognitive impairments have been documented on measures of verbal memory, psychomotor speed, and executive functioning, especially when used in combination with chemotherapy.[21,22] However, it should be noted that results of studies investigating the association between IFN-alpha and cognitive dysfunction have been mixed, with other studies finding no evidence of decline following treatment.[23]

Hormonal Therapies

A number of studies have described associations between hormones and cognition, with numerous reports specifically documenting the impact of estrogen and testosterone on cognitive functioning.[24,25] Hormonal treatments are commonly used in the care of breast and prostate cancer patients.

Women with estrogen receptor/progesterone receptor positive breast cancer frequently are recommended treatment with either a selective estrogen receptor modulator (SERM) such as tamoxifen (TAM) or an aromatase inhibitor such as anastrozole. However, estrogen blockade associated with these agents may adversely impact cognitive function.

It is known that TAM exerts both agonist and antagonist estrogenic effects that may partly account for the variety of side effects associated with this treatment. Although the pharmacodynamic properties of TAM, especially its CNS effects, are not well understood, there is reason to believe that TAM's hormonal and immunologic activities are related to the cognitive and emotional difficulties some women experience. As a chemopreventive agent, TAM has been found to cross the blood–brain barrier and potentially exert influence on CNS structures.[26–28] In vivo, in vitro, and animal studies suggest that in addition to its involvement with the estrogen system, TAM also affects several neurotransmitter (eg, serotonin, dopamine) and cytokine (eg, interleukin-1β, interleukin-6, interferon-γ, and tumor necrosis factor) systems that are implicated in cognitive functioning.[66–70]

Evidence that TAM has the potential to disrupt cognitive and brain function is found in both animal and human studies.[29,30] Chen et al[29] found that treatment with TAM resulted in reduced spatial memory in mice. In humans, breast cancer patients receiving hormone therapy (TAM, anastrozole, or a combination of those therapies) performed more poorly than non-cancer controls on measures of verbal memory and processing speed.[30] However, there is no consistent evidence of cognitive dysfunction associated with these agents; Schagen et al[31] found no difference between breast cancer patients who received TAM post-chemotherapy and those who did not.

In prostate cancer, LHRH agonists such as leuprolide and goserelin are the most commonly utilized hormonal therapies. Information derived from animal studies and from studies with hypogonadal men has indicated a correlation between testosterone and cognitive skills including working memory, verbal memory, and visuospatial abilities.[25] The limited number of studies that have investigated the neurocognitive impact of LHRH agonists in men with prostate cancer have yielded mixed results. The studies demonstrating adverse cognitive effects most often report alterations in visuospatial processing, including visual memory, and executive functioning, with contradictory findings with regard to verbal memory performance.[25] While group analyses utilizing a mean change often fail to demonstrate a statistically significant effect, reliable change index–based analyses have demonstrated cognitive decline in up to 50% of men treated with an LHRH agonist.[32]

Neuropsychological Profile Associated with Cancer Therapy

Research has documented that in patients with both cerebral and extracerebral malignancies, antineoplastic treatments, including chemotherapies and/or radiotherapies, are associated with a pattern of cognitive deficits suggestive of frontal–subcortical white matter dysfunction. This pattern includes impairments in executive functioning, verbal retrieval, speed of processing, and speeded motor coordination, as well as inefficiencies in learning and retrieval of stored information in the context of relatively well-preserved memory consolidation processes.[33] These impairments are manifest in patients' complaints of difficulty with short-term memory, such that they may report forgetting the details of recent conversations and events and misplacing possessions. They also frequently describe problems with sustained attention and problems with organization and multitasking. Disruption of frontal–subcortical networks has also been associated with changes in mood and personality, including depression, anxiety, and apathy.[34]

■ MOOD DISTURBANCE

In addition to presenting with cancer-related cognitive dysfunction, mood disturbance may be evident early in the disease course. Patients with brain tumors may present with neurobehavioral changes including apathy, depression, hallucinations, and disorganized thinking, especially when tumors are in the frontal or temporolimbic areas. These symptoms may occur with or without classic neurologic signs and symptoms.[35]

In addition to experiencing neurobehavioral changes that are the direct effect of cancer, patients may also experience reactive distress when diagnosed. Adjustment disorders are the most commonly encountered psychiatric problem in oncology, particularly immediately after diagnosis and early in the course of the disease and treatment, with prevalence estimates of approximately 32%. There is wide variability in estimates of the prevalence of depression, ranging from 0% to 58%.[36]

Treatment-related mood disturbance has also been documented for certain anticancer therapies, particularly in patients undergoing treatment with IFN. Psychiatric symptoms, usually increased depression, are also reported in 16% to 58% of patients receiving IFN treatment.[37] It is noted that patients with IFN-induced depression are less likely to report significant feelings of guilt as compared with nondepressed patients or depressed healthy controls. In contrast, they are more likely to report symptoms of psychomotor retardation and weight loss.[38]

Increased depression has been observed within the first month of treatment and has been linked to neurovegetative, emotional/affective, and cognitive symptoms.[37] Consistent with this, the use of IFN for the treatment of chronic myelogenous leukemia (IFN alone and in combination with chemotherapy) was shown to increase depressive symptoms independent of fatigue.[22] Both fatigue and mood alterations tend to remit following cessation of treatment, although persisting effects of each have been noted.[39–41] Several studies have demonstrated the effectiveness of antidepressant pharmacotherapies.[42–44] While antidepressants may be used prophylactically for symptom prevention/reduction in some patients, pretreatment screening in combination with close serial monitoring of a patient's mood and initiating pharmacotherapy as indicated is appropriate for many patients, allowing for avoidance of unnecessary medications and potential side effects thereof.[42,47]

In addition to symptoms of depression, the clinical picture of IFN-induced psychiatric symptoms may also vary to include "dysphoric mania," characterized by extreme irritability or agitation that is often accompanied by poor insight. In contrast to the irritability associated with depression, irritability that occurs in the context of a manic episode is unlikely to respond to treatment with antidepressants, and may even worsen in the context of such therapy. Thus, careful evaluation of psychiatric symptoms is necessary to ensure appropriate interventions are employed when necessary.[47]

The mechanisms by which IFN causes neurobehavioral effects, including possible alteration of frontal circuitry, are not fully understood.[39,45–46] Numerous studies suggest (a) changes in the endocrine system, (b) dysregulation of neurotransmitter systems, and (c) activation of secondary cytokine pathways as possible mechanisms.[45,46] The latter is supported by findings that in patients with AML and MDS, there are correlations between proinflammatory cytokine activity and cognitive dysfunction, fatigue, and ratings of quality of life.[5]

The activation of cytokine pathways in chronically ill patients has also been associated with so-called "sickness behavior," including changes in sleep and appetite, fatigue, psychomotor slowing, and cognitive changes. The presence of these symptoms as a direct consequence of illness and treatment complicates the diagnosis of depression in the context of cancer, as symptoms may overlap. However, regardless of underlying etiology, patients experiencing these symptoms are likely to benefit from intervention with antidepressants. Future effective treatments for these symptoms may target proinflammatory cytokines or inflammatory mediators directly.[47]

FATIGUE

Cancer-related fatigue (CRF) has been defined as a persistent and subjective sense of tiredness related to cancer or cancer treatment that is out of proportion to recent activity, is distressing to the patient, and interferes with usual functioning. CRF is generally less likely to be relieved by rest than the fatigue experienced by healthy individuals. It has been described by patients as the most distressing symptom associated with cancer and cancer treatment. While prevalence estimates range widely, CRF is present in approximately 50% of cancer patients at the time of diagnosis; for some patients, this is the concern that brings them to initial medical attention. CRF during cancer treatment is very common across cancer types, and has been estimated to occur in up to 60% to 96% of patients undergoing therapy.[48] It is the most frequently reported neurobehavioral symptom across trials utilizing BRMs. This side effect often persists for the duration of treatment and may result in dose reductions. In patients receiving treatment with IFN, it is estimated that between 70% and 100% of patients experience fatigue, with 10% to 40% requiring dose reduction as a result.[39]

Treatment-related fatigue tends to be most intense in the days immediately following treatment administration, with gradual improvements between courses. In some cases, however, fatigue may last well after the completion of treatment; in one study of patients with ovarian cancer, for example, approximately 33% of women who had not received any treatment for at least 6 months still reported significant fatigue.[49]

ASSESSMENT OF NEUROBEHAVIORAL SYMPTOMS

The above research highlights the findings of neurobehavioral changes associated with cancer and cancer treatments; the symptoms experienced vary across individuals, cancer types, and therapy type. Key strategies for assessment of these symptoms are summarized in Table 14-1. The utilization of baseline evaluations of neurobehavioral symptoms has allowed for the identification

■ TABLE 14-1. Key Assessment Strategies

Assessment of neurobehavioral symptoms may include
- Neuropsychological evaluation
  - Clinical interview
  - Valid and reliable tests
  - Use of alternate forms if longitudinal monitoring is anticipated
- Psychiatric assessment
  - Depends on patient/environment
  - Can range from very brief questionnaires to structured interview
- Patient self-report inventories
  - Symptom inventories
  - Functional capacity
  - Quality of life

Important considerations for neurobehavioral assessments include
- Focus on most at-risk patients
- Screening for mood disturbance/fatigue at time of
  - Initial contact
  - Identification of advanced cancers
  - Initiation and completion of chemotherapy/radiotherapy
  - Progression or recurrence
- Baseline evaluation of neurocognitive function, mood, and fatigue is ideal before initiation of known or suspected neurotoxic agents

of even subtle treatment-related neurotoxicities, as such information can prevent misclassification of patients who do experience clinically and functionally meaningful declines but continue to perform within normal limits relative to normative standards. For example, in a prospective, longitudinal study, Wefel et al[8] found that classifying patients' posttreatment cognitive performance as impaired using a conventional classification criterion (eg, 1.5 SDs below the normative mean), without consideration of their pretreatment baseline level of performance, resulted in false-negative classification errors approximately 50% of the time. Unfortunately, many studies have failed to incorporate a pretreatment evaluation; this limits their ability to distinguish cancer-related from treatment-related cognitive dysfunction and risks, yielding potentially misleading conclusions. Studies to date have often utilized small and heterogeneous samples of patients who have received different treatment regimens; appropriate control groups are frequently lacking. Additional methodological differences include variable classification criteria, assessment time points, and selection of measurements, some of which are not fully adequate to address all relevant cognitive domains with sufficient specificity and sensitivity. Appropriate neuropsychological assessment of patients with cancer includes careful selection of reliable and valid measures that are sensitive to subtle changes in functioning and are robust to practice effects.[33] The International Cognition and Cancer Task Force was established with the aim of improving research methodology in this area, and is developing guidelines to assist researchers and clinicians as well as resources for patients and caregivers seeking information about cancer and cancer therapies' impact on cognition and behavior.[50]

In addition to the above considerations, a thorough assessment of neurobehavioral symptoms includes an assessment of the direct and indirect effects of cancer on physical and emotional well-being, as well as the impact of such symptoms on cognitive functioning. Fatigue and affective distress can have an untoward impact on neurocognitive performance, particularly with regard to aspects of attention and memory. It is important to note that in cancer patients, self-report of cognitive impairment has been shown to correlate more strongly with fatigue and mood disturbance than with objective evidence of cognitive dysfunction, as assessed by standardized neuropsychological tests.[51] Thus, a thorough assessment may be needed to elucidate whether perceived difficulties are secondary to cancer- and treatment-related cognitive dysfunction and/or affective distress and fatigue.

It has been found that cancer patients often do not feel that their psychosocial needs are being met by their oncology providers and that they are frequently hesitant to initiate discussion with their oncologists regarding their mood state despite a desire to discuss their needs.[52] Patients may be more willing to initiate discussion regarding their fatigue symptoms with their providers, but studies have provided widely varied results, with 8% to 52% of patients reporting that they had never reported their fatigue to their health care provider.[52] This highlights the need for providers to initiate discussion regarding these symptoms.

It has been recommended that providers screen regularly for symptoms of fatigue; evidence suggests that screening should take place at the initial contact, for any patients with newly identified advanced cancers, and at the time of all chemotherapy visits. It has also been recommended that in patients with newly identified fatigue, assessment of depressive symptoms and insomnia also be conducted. Follow-up assessments after treatment are also suggested.[53] Understanding not only the severity of fatigue but also its course, aggravating factors, and emotional components is important in identifying potential interventions.[49]

Similarly, screening for symptoms of depression has been recommended for all newly diagnosed patients and at any time a new chemotherapy or radiotherapy is initiated, as well as when advanced disease is newly identified. In addition, studies have demonstrated a link between depressive symptoms and an expressed desire for hastened death; as a result, it is recommended that screening for depression take place at any point during the course of a patient's illness and treatment if such a desire is communicated.[53] As with any intervention, following up on the proposed treatment plan and response to therapy is important.[53] The choice of assessment tools, which range from very brief screening tools to extensive structured clinical interviews, may vary depending on the treatment setting and the patient's condition.[54]

■ INTERVENTIONS AGAINST THE NEUROBEHAVIORAL SEQUELAE OF CANCER AND CANCER THERAPY

Key intervention strategies against neurobehavioral symptoms are summarized in Table 14-2. As noted above, risk factors for treatment-related cognitive dysfunction, such as high dose and type and schedule of administration, have been identified; adjusting these factors allows for the reduction of certain neurotoxicities while maintaining adequate disease control.[14,55] Pharmacologic interventions targeted at specific underlying mechanisms of some neurotoxic side effects have been investigated; for example, treatment with the μ-opioid receptor antagonist naltrexone was effective in relieving neurotoxic side effects in seven of nine patients undergoing IFN treatment for hematological malignancies.[56] Musselman et al[57] demonstrated the benefit of pretreatment with paroxetine, a selective serotonin reuptake inhibitor, in minimizing depression in melanoma patients receiving IFN treatment. Psychostimulant medications have been shown to be effective in addressing fatigue and cognitive dysfunction in cancer patients. A commonly utilized psychostimulant is methylphenidate, which has been found to be beneficial in reducing fatigue in patients with non-CNS cancers.[58]

■ **TABLE 14-2. Key Intervention Strategies**

Behavioral interventions
- Psychoeducation/Psychotherapy
- Training in compensatory strategies
  ◦ Memory prosthesis
  ◦ Pillbox
  ◦ Alarms
  ◦ Goal management training
- Environmental alterations at work and at home
  ◦ Organizational tools
  ◦ Work accommodations
  ◦ Energy conservation
  ◦ Reduced distractions

Pharmacologic interventions
- Dose reductions of neurotoxic agents if possible
- Addressing underlying conditions that may be contributors (eg, thyroid medications, metabolic abnormalities)
- Psychostimulants
- Antidepressants
- Treatments under investigation (eg, antioxidants, donepezil)

In patients with primary brain tumors, methylphenidate was effective in combating cognitive symptoms associated with treatment-related frontal–subcortical dysfunction, such that patients demonstrated significant improvements in memory, psychomotor speed, visual-motor function, executive function, and fine motor speed.[58] Other pharmacologic interventions that have been utilized in oncology populations include modafinil to alleviate fatigue and donepezil to combat difficulties with CRF, attention, and memory.[70] The use of vitamin E has been shown to be beneficial in patients with nasopharyngeal carcinoma who had imaging evidence of unilateral or bilateral temporal lobe necrosis, such that patients who were treated with vitamin E performed better than nontreated controls on measures of verbal learning and memory, visual memory, and cognitive flexibility.[59]

Recent animal studies have identified additional potential interventions. For example, the severe memory impairment observed in rats treated with chemotherapy was fully prevented by supplementation with an antioxidant, N-acetyl cysteine.[60] Similarly, administration of the peroxisomal proliferator-activated receptor γ agonist pioglitazone prevented memory disturbance associated with whole-brain irradiation in rats.[61] Radiation-induced

memory loss was also attenuated via transplantation of human embryonic stem cells into the rat hippocampus.[62]

In addition to making adjustments to primary treatments when necessary and using psychotherapeutic and pharmacologic interventions to combat depression and fatigue, behavioral changes (such as implementing workplace accommodations and engaging in exercise) and education regarding the possible untoward effects of treatment have been identified as important intervention targets.[49,55] Goal-focused compensatory interventions and behavioral strategies may be useful in minimizing the impact of neurobehavioral symptoms on daily life in patients with cancer. Knowledge gained from traditional rehabilitation disciplines treating survivors of traumatic brain injury or stroke has yielded important information regarding evidence-based compensatory strategies that may be applicable to patients with cancer-related cognitive dysfunction. Such multidisciplinary therapeutic interventions, provided by a team of psychologists, speech/language pathologists, occupational therapists, and vocational specialists, were found to improve community independence and employment outcomes in brain tumor patients at a significantly lower cost and shorter treatment length than was typical of survivors of traumatic brain injury who took part in the same program.[63] Training in the use of compensatory strategies and attention retraining has also shown promise in addressing both cognitive complaints and mental fatigue.[64] Compensatory tools might include external memory aids such as memory notebooks, user-programmable paging systems, and medication reminder systems to assist neurologically impaired patients compensate for difficulties with forgetfulness. Psychoeducation and training in the use of energy conservation and stress management techniques have also been employed.

■ **SUMMARY**

Cancer is becoming a chronic illness, requiring ongoing symptom assessment and intervention. In association with an increased number of long-term cancer survivors, there is increased awareness of the neurobehavioral symptoms that can be associated with cancer and cancer treatment. Despite the possibility of treatment-related neurobehavioral symptoms for some patients, these agents remain a critical component in the management and eradication of many cancers. Thus, the potential side effects of these therapies must be considered in the context of the overall health benefit they provide. Continued research into the mechanisms of treatment-related cognitive dysfunction may afford opportunities for the development of neuroprotective therapies, effective adjuvant supportive pharmacotherapies, and/or modification of primary treatments. Additionally, advances in behavioral interventions will help minimize the impact of cancer and cancer therapy on neurocognitive function, mood, quality of life, and functional abilities.

KEY POINTS

- With increased success in management of many cancers, there is increased awareness of and need for information regarding neurobehavioral symptoms associated with cancer and cancer treatments.

- Cancer and cancer treatments frequently have untoward effects on cognition and neurobehavioral functioning, such as mood disturbance and fatigue.

- The cognitive profile associated with cancer- and treatment–related cognitive impairment is often suggestive of frontal–subcortical dysfunction, with deficits in aspects of learning and memory, attention, information processing speed, and executive functioning.

- Assessment of neurobehavioral symptoms allows for accurate interpretation of contributors to diminished cognitive performance and offers opportunities for early interventions.

- Pharmacologic and behavioral interventions may minimize the negative impact of cognitive dysfunction and neurobehavioral symptoms associated with cancer and cancer therapy.

REFERENCES

1. Wefel JS, Lenzi R, Theriault R, et al. "Chemobrain" in breast cancer? A prologue. *Cancer*. 2004;101:466–475.

2. Hermelink K, Untch M, Lux MP, et al. Cognitive function during neoadjuvant chemotherapy for breast cancer: results of a prospective, multicenter, longitudinal study. *Cancer*. 2007;109:1905–1913.

3. Schagen SB, Muller MJ, Boogerd W, et al. Change in cognitive function after chemotherapy: a prospective longitudinal study in breast cancer patients. *J Natl Cancer Inst*. 2006;98:1742–1745.

4. Hurria A, Rosen C, Hudis C, et al. Cognitive function of older patients receiving adjuvant chemotherapy for breast cancer: a pilot prospective longitudinal study. *J Am Geriatr Soc*. 2006;54:925–931.

5. Meyers CA, Albitar M, Estey E. Cognitive impairment, fatigue, and cytokine levels in patients with acute myelogenous leukemia or myelodysplastic syndrome. *Cancer*. 2005;104:788–793.

6. Meyers CA, Byrne KS, Komaki R. Cognitive deficits in patients with small cell lung cancer before and after chemotherapy. *Lung Cancer*. 1995;12:231–235.

7. Sheline GE, Wara WM, Smith V. Therapeutic irradiation and brain injury. *Int J Radiat Oncol Biol Phys*. 1980;6:1215–1228.

8. Wefel JS, Lenzi R, Theriault R, et al. The cognitive sequelae of standard dose adjuvant chemotherapy in women with breast cancer: results of a prospective, randomized, longitudinal trial. *Cancer*. 2004;100:2292–2299.

9. Jenkins V, Shilling V, Deutsch G, et al. A 3-year prospective study of the effects of adjuvant treatments on cognition in women with early stage breast cancer. *Br J Cancer*. 2006;94:828–834.

10. Syrjala KL, Dikmen S, Langer SL, et al. Neuropsychologic changes from before transplantation to 1 year in patients receiving myeloablative allogeneic hematopoietic cell transplant. *Blood*. 2004;104:3386–3392.

11. Ahles TA, Tope DM, Furstenberg C, et al. Psychologic and neuropsychologic impact of autologous bone marrow transplantation. *J Clin Oncol*. 1996;14:1457–1462.

12. Friedman MA, Fernandez M, Wefel JS, et al. Course of cognitive decline in hematopoietic stem cell transplantation: a within-subjects design. *Arch Clin Neuropsychol*. 2009;24:689–698.

13. Shah RR. Mechanistic basis of adverse drug reactions: the perils of inappropriate dose schedules. *Expert Opin Drug Saf*. 2005;4:103–128.

14. Keime-Guibert F, Napolitano M, Delattre JY. Neurological complications of radiotherapy and chemotherapy. *J Neurol*. 1998;245:695–708.

15. Brown ES. Effects of glucocorticoids on mood, memory, and the hippocampus. *Ann N Y Acad Sci*. 2009;1179:41–55.

16. Klein M, Engelberts NHJ, van der Ploeg HM, et al. Epilepsy in low-grade gliomas: the impact on cognitive function and quality of life. *Ann Neurol*. 2003;54:514–520.

17. National Institutes of Health. *Biological Therapy. Treatments that Use Your Immune System to Fight Cancer* [brochure]. 2003. NIH Publication No. 03-5406. NIH: https://cissecure.nci.nih.gov/ncipubs

18. Clark JW. Biological response modifiers. *Cancer Chemother Biol Response Modif*. 1996;16:239–273.

19. Mihich E. Historical overview of biologic response modifiers. *Cancer Invest*. 2000;18:456–466.

20. Raison CL, Demetrashvili M, Capuron L, et al. Neuropsychiatric adverse effects of interferon-α: recognition and management. *CNS Drugs*. 2005;19:105–123.

21. Pavol MA, Meyers CA, Rexer JL, et al. Pattern of neurobehavioral deficits associated with interferon alpha therapy for leukemia. *Neurology*. 1995;45:947–950.

22. Scheibel RS, Valentine AD, O'Brien S, et al. Cognitive dysfunction and depression during treatment with interferon alpha and chemotherapy. *J Neuropsychiatry Clin Neurosci*. 2004;16:1–7.

23. Bender CM, Yasko JM, Kirkwood JM, et al. Cognitive function and quality of life in interferon therapy for melanoma. *Clin Nurs Res*. 2000;9:352–363.

24. Maki PM, Sunderman E. Hormone therapy and cognitive function. *Hum Reprod Update*. 2009;6:667–681.

25. Nelson CJ, Lee JS, Gamboa MC, et al. Cognitive effects of hormone therapy in men with prostate cancer: a review. *Cancer*. 2008;113:1097–1106.

26. Lien EA, Wester K, Lonning PE, et al. Distribution of tamoxifen and metabolites into brain tissue and brain metastases in breast cancer patients. *Br J Cancer*. 1991;63:641–645.

27. Wilking N, Appelgren LE, Carlstrom K, et al. The distribution and metabolism of 14C-labelled tamoxifen in spayed female mice. *Acta Pharmacol Toxicol*. 1982;50:161–168.

28. McKenna SE, Simon NG, Cologer-Clifford A. An assessment of agonist/antagonist effects of tamoxifen in the female mouse brain. *Horm Behav*. 1992;26:536–544.

29. Chen D, Wu CF, Shi B, Xu YM. Tamoxifen and toremifene impair retrieval, but not acquisition, of spatial information processing in mice. *Pharmacol Biochem Behav*. 2002;72:417–421.

30. Shilling V, Jenkins V, Fallowfield L, et al. The effects of hormone therapy on cognition in breast cancer. *J Steroid Biochem Mol Biol*. 2003;86:405–412.

31. Schagen SB, van Dam FS, Muller MJ, et al. Cognitive deficits after postoperative adjuvant chemotherapy for breast carcinoma. *Cancer*. 1999;85:640–650.

32. Green HJ, Pakenham KI, Headley BC, et al. Altered cognitive function in men treated for prostate cancer with luteinizing hormone-releasing hormone analogues and cyproterone acetate: a randomized controlled trial. *Br J Urol*. 2002;90:427–432.

33. Wefel JS, Kayl AE, Meyers CA. Neuropsychological dysfunction associated with cancer and cancer therapies: a conceptual review of an emerging target. *Br J Cancer*. 2004;90:1691–1696.

34. Mega MS, Cummings JL. Frontal–subcortical circuits and neuropsychiatric disorders. *J Neuropsychiatry Clin Neurosci*. 1994;6:358–370.

35. Filly CM, Kleinschmidt-DeMasters BK. Neurobehavioral presentations of brain neoplasms. *West J Med*. 1995;163:19–25.

36. Andrykowski MA, Lykins E, Floyd A. Psychological health in cancer survivors. *Semin Oncol Nurs*. 2008;24:193–201.

37. Capuron L, Ravaud A, Miller AH, et al. Baseline mood and psychosocial characteristics of patients developing depressive symptoms during interleukin-2 and/or interferon-alpha cancer therapy. *Brain Behav Immun*. 2004;18:205–213.

38. Capuron L, Fornwalt FB, Knight BT, et al. Does cytokine-induced depression differ from idiopathic major depression in medically healthy individuals? *J Affect Disord*. 2009;119:181–185.

39. Malik UR, Makower DF, Wadler S. Interferon-mediated fatigue. *Cancer*. 2001;92(suppl):1664–1668.

40. Strite D, Valentine AD, Meyers CA. Manic episodes in two patients treated with interferon alpha. *J Neuropsychiatry*. 1997;9:273–276.

41. Meyers CA, Scheibel RS, Forman AD. Persistent neurotoxicity of systemically administered interferon-alpha. *Neurology*. 1991;41:672–676.

42. Valentine AD, Meyers CA. Neurobehavioral effects of interferon therapy. *Curr Psychiatry Rep*. 2005;7:391–395.

43. Malek-Ahmadi P, Ghandour E. Bupropion for treatment of interferon-induced depression. *Ann Pharmacother*. 2004;38:1202–1205.

44. Musselman DL, Lawson DH, Gumnick JF, et al. Paroxetine for the prevention of depression induced by high-dose interferon alpha. *New Engl J Med*. 2001;344:961–966.

45. Schaefer M, Engelbrecht MA, Gut O, et al. Interferon alpha (IFN-α) and psychiatric syndromes: a review. *Prog Neuropsychopharmacol Biol Psychiatry*. 2002;26:731–746.

46. Valentine AD, Meyers CA, Kling MA, et al. Mood and cognitive side effects of interferon-α therapy. *Semin Oncol*. 1998;25:39–47.

47. Raison CL, Miller AH. Depression in cancer: new developments regarding diagnosis and treatment. *Biol Psychiatry*. 2003;54:283–294.

48. Breitbart W, Alici Y. Pharmacologic treatment options for cancer-related fatigue: current state of clinical research. *Clin J Oncol Nurs.* 2008 12(suppl 12):27–36.

49. Stasi R, Abriani L, Beccaglia P, et al. Cancer-related fatigue: evolving concepts in evaluation and treatment. *Cancer.* 2003;98:1786–1801.

50. Vardy J, Wefel JS, Ahles T, et al. Cancer and cancer-therapy related cognitive dysfunction: an international perspective from the Venice cognitive workshop. *Ann Oncol.* 2007;19:623–629.

51. Castellon SA, Ganz PA, Bower JE, et al. Neurocognitive performance in breast cancer survivors exposed to adjuvant chemotherapy and tamoxifen. *J Clin Exp Neuropsychol.* 2004;26:955–969.

52. Fisher RE. A good life. *J Clin Oncol,* 2009;27:5298–5299.

53. Dy SM, Lorenz KA, Naeim A, et al. Evidence-based recommendations for cancer fatigue, anorexia, depression, and dyspnea. *J Clin Oncol.* 2008;26:3886–3895.

54. Vodermaier A, Linden W, Siu C. Screening for emotional distress in cancer patients: a systematic review of assessment instruments. *J Natl Cancer Inst.* 2009;101:1464–1488.

55. Valentine AD. Managing the neuropsychiatric adverse effects of interferon treatment. *BioDrugs.* 1999;11:229–237.

56. Valentine AD, Meyers CA, Talpaz M. Treatment of neurotoxic side effects of interferon-alpha with naltrexone. *Cancer Invest.* 1995;13:561–566.

57. Musselman DL, Lawson DH, Gumnick JF, et al. Paroxetine for the prevention of depression induced by high-dose interferon alpha. *New Engl J Med.* 2001;344:961–966.

58. Meyers CA, Weitzner MA, Valentine AD, et al. Methylphenidate therapy improves cognition, mood, and function of brain tumor patients. *J Clin Oncol.* 1998;16:2522–2527.

59. Chan AS, Cheung M, Law SC, et al. Phase II study of alpha-tocopherol in improving the cognitive function of patients with temporal lobe radionecrosis. *Cancer.* 2003;100:398–404.

60. Konat GW, Kraszpulski M, James I, et al. Cognitive dysfunction induced by chronic administration of common cancer chemotherapeutics in rats. *Metab Brain Dis.* 2008;23:325–333.

61. Zhao W, Payne V, Tommasi E, et al. Administration of the peroxisomal proliferator-activated receptor γ agonist pioglitazone during fractionated brain irradiation prevents radiation-induced cognitive impairment. *Int J Radiat Oncol Biol Phys.* 2007;67:6–9.

62. Acarya MM, Christie LA, Lan ML, et al. Rescue of radiation-induced cognitive impairment through cranial transplantation of human embryonic stem cells. *Proc Natl Acad Sci U S A.* 2009;106:19150–19155.

63. Scherer M, Meyers CA, Bergloff P. Efficacy of postacute brain injury rehabilitation for patients with primary malignant brain tumors. *Cancer.* 2007;80:250–257.

64. Gehring K, Sitskoorn MM, Gundy CM, et al. Cognitive rehabilitation in patients with gliomas: a randomized, controlled trial. *J Clin Oncol.* 2009;27:3712–3722.

65. Ouimet LA, Stewart A, Collins B, et al. Measuring neuropsychological change following breast cancer treatment: an analysis of statistical models. *J Clin Exp Neuropsych.* 2009;31:73–89.

66. Järvinen LS, Pyrhönen S, Kairemo KJ, et al. The effect of anti-oestrogens on cytokine production in vitro. *Scand J Immunol.* 1996;44:15–20.

67. Chaurasia CS, Chen CE, Rubin J, et al. Effects of tamoxifen on striatal dopamine and 5-hydroxytryptamine release in freely moving male rates: an in-vivo microdialysis investigation. *J Pharm Pharmacol.* 1998;50:1377–1385.

68. Sumner BE, Grant KE, Rosie R, et al. Effects of tamoxifen on serotonin transporter and 5-hydroxytryptamine (2A) receptor binding sites and mRNA levels in the brain of ovariectomized rats with or without acute estradiol replacement. *Brain Res Mol Brain Res.* 1999;73:119–128.

69. Mize AL, Young LJ, Alper RH. Uncoupling of 5-HT1A receptors in the brain by estrogens: regional variations in antagonism by ICI 182,780. *Neuropharmacology.* 2003;44:584–591.

70. Shaw EG, Rosdhal R, D'Agostino RB, et al. Phase II study of donepezil in irradiated brain tumor patients: effect on cognitive function, mood, and quality of life. *J Clin Oncol.* 2006;24:1415–1420.

Communication

Communicating with Patients and Families

• *Walter F. Baile*

■ PURPOSE AND GOALS OF PATIENT COMMUNICATION

The clinical encounter with cancer patients and their families has four specific communication aims:

(1) *Gathering information*: This is crucial not only to determining the clinical diagnosis, but also on a broader and more "patient-centered" level to determine patients' understanding of their illness, their current coping and attitude toward treatment, the role of the family and other support available to them, and factors that may present impediments to the ultimate goal of effective cancer care. Information gathering is essential not only at the initial contact with the patient and family, but also all along the cancer trajectory and especially important at milestones such as treatment failure, the development of serious complications, and transition from aggressive anticancer treatment to supportive care.

(2) *Transmitting information to the patient and family*: Patients and family members rate information as possibly the most important factor in helping them cope with their cancer.[1,2] It is also associated with positive effects on patient coping.[2–4] However, it is also probably the one need that they see as least met in their encounter with the medical team.[5] While information to the patient is important at any stage of cancer treatment, it is likely to be most sought out at the time of diagnosis, when there are complications of care, and at crucial transitions such as the initiation of new treatment.[6] Although patients may seek the maximum amount of information about their disease around the period of diagnosis when all aspects of cancer treatment may be new to them, it is likely to lessen in situations where the disease has progressed and the medical details of the "bad news" are more likely to be shunned. In these cases, a direct explanation of a treatment plan may be more valuable to patients than their seeing a CT scan with widely metastatic disease. Providing information is best conceptualized as a dialogue in which the clinician must gauge how much information a patient can process at one time, give space to the patient to ask questions, and be careful not to use jargon or "MedSpeak" in explaining information to the patient and family.

(3) *Building a trusting relationship with the patient and family*: In this case, the two key elements are the development of rapport and trust. These elements are essential in instilling patient confidence in the care provided by the clinician, achieving compliance with treatment, allowing patients to feel that the clinician has their best interest at heart and will tell them the truth about their illness, and promoting patient satisfaction with care. Paying attention to skills such as listening and attending to patient concerns is the foundation for building a relationship based on collaboration and trust.

(4) *Providing support to the patient and the family*: This is directly related to communication techniques for exploring and understanding patient concerns about treatment, demonstrating empathic understanding, providing realistic hope for the future, and reassuring patients that they will not be abandoned at the end of life.

■ **TABLE 15-1. Key Communication Concepts**

- For patients the quality of the relationship with their caregiver ranks second only to obtaining effective treatment for the disease
- Acknowledging and validating patient emotions are highly valued by patients but rarely practiced by clinicians who often try to "fix" patient emotions with reassurance or the offer of additional therapy
- The quality of this relationship determines important outcomes such as satisfaction with care, malpractice suits, and patient compliance
- Patients often complain about not getting sufficient information. This may be the fault of no one but inherent in the system. Periodically checking for patient information needs may reveal important gaps
- Among difficult communication challenges transitioning to palliative care may be the most difficult. Setting goals of care (eg, curative vs. arresting the disease) and understanding patient values (what's important to you?) early in the course of illness may facilitate the transition later on
- Difficult questions such as "Doctor, am I going to die?" often mask other concerns such as will one see one's grandson graduate from school. Exploring this further ("tell me what you are worried about") will often reveal additional statements
- Mutuality and satisfaction in the relationship with the patient (acknowledgement that to the patient the physician may represent security in the face of serious illness) can be a buffer against physician stress and burnout
- Hope is a multidimensional concept. Patients are often aware of the seriousness of their disease and hope for other social and personal milestones beyond cure and prolonged life

Table 15-1 reflects these concepts as applied in everyday communication with the patient and family.

■ WHY COMMUNICATION

It may seem alien to many practitioners to call communication a skill since at first appearance many of them seem intuitive and natural. This has led to the conceptual error that communication skills are innate and that somehow one is a "born communicator," or not. This attitude unfortunately trivializes the set of behavioral skills that form the foundation for effective communication. Moreover, just as we can objectively measure the presence or absence of pathogens in the blood, we can now accurately measure good communication. Although techniques are still being perfected, audiotaped and videotaped encounters between clinicians and families, or in some cases standardized patients, can allow us to code specific skills used, for example, in breaking bad news. For example, a recent study using audiotaped recordings of medical oncology fellows participating in a communication skills workshop demonstrated that they made significant improvements in eliciting patients' understanding of their illness and empathic response to patients.[7] Other studies using various assessments of communication skills have illuminated our understanding of communication

pitfalls occurring during the informed consent process[8] and provided insight into the aspects of conversations with patients that could predict the likelihood of a doctor being sued.[9,10]

Communication research in oncology has also contributed to a renewed understanding of the importance of the encounter with the patient and family by demonstrating the association of good communication skills with enhanced patient satisfaction, compliance with treatment, increased patient knowledge, enhanced accrual to clinical trials, better transition of patients from curative to palliative treatment, and decreased oncologist stress and burnout.[3] On the other hand, the fact that many malpractice suits are the result of ineffective communication is evidence that poor communication directly results in patient dissatisfaction and can do harm to patients by damaging hope, leaving patients feeling abandoned, or eroding the trust that patients may have in their physician.[11,12]

Despite these findings, effective communication skills training programs for practicing oncologists and fellows are still more rare than routine, and the oncology community is still largely focused on new treatments for cancer, missing opportunities to enhance the more technical skills of clinicians through promoting the interpersonal aspects of care.[13,14]

■ FUNDAMENTAL COMMUNICATION SKILLS

The Five E's: Engage, Elicit, Educate, Empathize, and Enlist

Communication skills can be thought of as *fundamental skills* that we utilize in all social encounters. *More specialized communication* skills are necessary in more complex and emotionally charged encounters such as breaking bad news or discussing errors. These essential skills are described below, and an example of how they might be incorporated in a complex communication task such as giving bad news is then described.

Engage

Engaging the patient encompasses the *physical context or setting* and the steps that are necessary to begin building rapport or a relationship with the patient. Both of these steps are important because they encourage trust on the part of the patient and family, an essential ingredient of any collaborative endeavor. They are especially important in the first encounter, during which often the most lasting impressions are formed. A few seconds spent establishing these features of the initial setup of the interview may save many minutes of frustration and misunderstanding later (for both the professional and the patient).

Space The first component is to arrange the meeting space optimally. It is easy to forget that having an important conversation with a patient and family demands thoughtfulness and sensitivity to the ambience of the environment. Try to ensure *privacy*. In a hospital setting, if a side room is not available, draw the curtains around the bed. In an office setting, shut the door. Get any physical objects out of the way—for example, move any bedside tables, trays, or other impediments out of the line between you and the patient. Ask for the television or radio to be turned off for a few minutes. If you are in an office or room, move your chair so that you are adjacent to the patient, not across the desk. There is evidence that conversations across a corner occur three times more frequently than conversations across the full width of a table.[15]

If you have the patient's chart open, make sure you look up from it and do not talk to the patient while reading the chart. If you find any of these actions awkward, state what you are doing (eg, "if you don't mind I'm going to turn off the TV so we don't have any distractions while we talk").

Giving undivided attention It is virtually impossible to assure a patient that he or she has your undivided attention and that you intend to listen seriously if you remain standing up. Only if it is absolutely impossible to sit should you try and hold a medical interview while standing. The height at which you sit can also be important; normally, your eyes should be approximately level with the patient's. If the patient is already upset or angry, a useful technique is to sit so that you are below the patient, with your eyes at a lower level. This often decreases the anger. It is best to try and look relaxed, particularly if that is not the way you feel.

Anecdotal impressions suggest that when the doctor sits down, the patient perceives the period of time spent at the bedside as longer than if the doctor remains standing. Thus, not only does the act of sitting down indicate to the patient that he or she has control and that you are there to listen, but it saves time and increases efficiency. Before starting the interview itself, take care to get the patient organized if necessary.

Seating It is important to be seated at a comfortable *distance* from the patient. This distance (sometimes called the "body buffer zone") seems to vary from culture to culture, but a distance of 2 to 3 ft between you and the patient usually serves the purpose for intimate and personal conversation.[15] This is another reason why the doctor who remains standing at the end of the bed ("six feet away and three feet up," known colloquially as "the British position") seems remote and aloof.

Make sure that whenever possible, you are *positioned* closest to the patient and that any friends or relatives are on the other side of the patient. Sometimes relatives try to dominate the interview, and it may be important for you to send a clear signal that the patient has primacy.

In almost all oncology settings, it is important to have a box of *tissues* nearby. If the patient or relative begins to cry, it is important to offer tissues, which are a way of acknowledging the appropriateness of being upset when, for example, a patient hears bad news.

Body language Try to look relaxed and unhurried. A calm demeanor is likely to be calming also to the patient. To achieve an air of relaxation, sit down comfortably with both your feet flat on the floor. Let your shoulders relax and drop. Undo your coat or jacket if you are wearing one, and rest your hands on your knees. Pay attention to your nonverbal behavior, since it may communicate that you are listening or concerned. For example, if you are listening with your hands folded in front of you, the patient may feel that you have already made your mind up about things and are not open to hearing them.

Eye contact   Maintain eye contact for most of the time while the patient is talking. Eye contact transmits interest and promotes trust.[16] If the interview becomes intense or emotionally charged—particularly if the patient is crying or is very angry—it is helpful to the patient for you to look away (to break eye contact) at that point.

Touching the patient   Touch may also be helpful during the interview if: (a) a nonthreatening area is touched, such as the hand or forearm; (b) you are comfortable with touch; and (c) the patient appreciates touch and does not withdraw.

Most of us have not been taught specific details of clinical touch at any time in our training.[17] We are, therefore, likely to be ill at ease with touching as an interview technique until we have had some practice. Nevertheless, there is considerable evidence (although the data are somewhat "soft") that touching the patient (particularly above the patient's waist to avoid misinterpretation) is of benefit during a medical interview.[18] It seems likely that touching is a significant action at times of distress and should be encouraged, with the proviso that the professional should be sensitive to the patient's reaction. If the patient is comforted by the contact, continue; if the patient is uncomfortable, stop. Touch can be misinterpreted (eg, as lasciviousness, aggression, or dominance), so be aware that touching is an interviewing skill that requires extra self-regulation.

Beginning the dialogue with the patient and family

Introductions   Ensure that the patient knows who you are and what you do. Many practitioners, including the author, make a point of shaking the patient's hand at the outset, although this is a matter of personal preference. Often the handshake tells you something about the family dynamics as well as about the patient. Frequently, the patient's spouse also extends his or her hand. It is worthwhile making sure that you shake the patient's hand before that of the spouse (even if the spouse is nearer) to demonstrate that the patient comes first, and the spouse (although an important member of the team) comes second. The "white coat syndrome" is a well-known phenomenon that describes how the medical setting induces anxiety in many patients (often even leading to blood pressure increases!), so that a friendly greeting may go a long way at putting the patient at ease. Also remember to introduce others in the room (eg, medical students, nurse) that the patient may not know. Patients may often come with several relatives. If this is a first visit and there is much work to do and explanations to be made, ask patients which one or two relatives they would like to have in the room. This will make the encounter more comfortable for you and allow patients to choose whom they want to hear the information. You can always meet with other family members later on. Some patients want to audiotape encounters. Although clinicians may be squeamish about this, it can save time by allowing other family members to be in on important aspects of patients' care such as the treatment plan. Some clinicians have found that sending a summary letter to the patient is very helpful in filling in information gaps that the patient may have.

Listening skills   As dialogue begins, the professional should show that he or she is in "listening mode."[19]

Open-ended questions   Open questions are simply questions that can be answered in any way or manner of response. In other words, the question does not direct the respondent or require him or her to make a choice from a specific range of answers. In taking the medical history, of course, most of the questions are, appropriately, closed questions ("Do you have swelling of the ankles?" and "Have you had any bleeding after your menopause?"). In therapeutic dialogue, when the clinician is trying to be part of the patient's support system, open questions are an essential way of finding out what the patient is experiencing as a way of tailoring support to the patient. Hence, open questions ("What did you think the diagnosis was?," "How did you feel when you were told that …," and "How did that make you feel?") are a mandatory part of the "nonhistory" therapeutic dialogue.

Facilitation techniques

Silence   The first and most important technique in facilitating dialogue between the patient and clinician is silence.[20] If the patient is speaking, do not talk over her. Wait for the patient to stop speaking before you start your next sentence. This, the simplest rule of all, is the one most often ignored, and it is most likely to give the patient the impression that the doctor is not listening.

Silences also have other significance: they can be—and often are—revealing about the patient's state of mind. Often, a patient falls silent when he or she has feelings that are too intense to express in words. A silence, therefore, means that the patient is thinking or feeling something important, not that he or she has stopped thinking. If the clinician can tolerate a pause or silence, the patient may well express the thought in words a moment later.

If you have to break the silence, the ideal way to do so is to say "What were you thinking about just then?," "What is it that's making you pause?," or something to that effect.

Other simple facilitation techniques Having encouraged the patient to speak, it is necessary to prove that you are hearing what is being said. The following techniques enhance your ability to demonstrate this.

In addition to silence, you can use any or all of the following simple facilitation techniques: nodding, pausing, smiling, saying "Yes," "Mmm hmm," and "Tell me more," or anything similar.

Repetition and reiteration Repetition is probably the second most important technique of all interviewing skills (after sitting down).

To show that you are really hearing what the patient is saying, use one or two key words from the patient's last sentence in your own first one ("I just feel so lousy most of the time." "Tell me what you mean by feeling lousy."). Reiteration means repeating what patients have told you, but in your words, not theirs ("Since I started those new tablets, I've been feeling sleepy." "So you're getting some drowsiness from the new tablets."). Both repetition and reiteration confirm to patients that they have been heard.

Reflection Reflection is the act of restating the patient's statement in terms of what it means to the clinician. It takes the act of listening one step further and shows that you have heard and have interpreted what the patient said ("If I understand you correctly, you're telling me that you lose control of your waking and sleeping when you're on these tablets.").

Clarifying Patients often have concerns about treatment or other issues related to their care. When not asked about them directly, they may hint or express them in nuances, protests, or questions that are not clear. Listed below are some examples of how important information may be indirectly communicated:

Statement: "I don't know how my family can take any more of this."
Patient means: "I really feel badly about being a burden."

Statement: "I just couldn't stand another round of chemo."
Patient means: "I was so upset when my hair fell out."
Statement: "Doctor, how long do you think I have to live?"
Patient means: "I wonder if I'll see my grandson graduate."
Statement: "What will the end be like?"
Patient means: "How much will I suffer?"

As the patient talks, it is very tempting for the clinician to go along with what the patient is saying, even when the exact meaning or implication is unclear. This may lead very quickly to serious obstacles in the dialogue.

It is important to be honest when we do not understand what the patient means. Many different phrases can be used ("I'm sorry—I'm not quite sure what you meant when you said …" and "When you say … do you mean that …?"). Clarification gives the patient an opportunity to expand on the previous statement or to amplify some aspect of the statement, now that the clinician has shown interest in the topic. The key to addressing questions is to use clarifying statements that get at the issue underlying the concern.

Handling time and interruptions As clinicians, we seem to have a notorious reputation for being impolite in our handling of interruptions—by phone, pager, or other people. Too often, we appear abruptly to ignore the patient we are with and go immediately to the phone or respond immediately to the pager or to our colleague. Even though we may not realize it, this appears as a snub or an insult to the patient we are with.

If you cannot hold all calls or turn off your pager (and most of us cannot), then at least indicate to the patient that you are sorry about the interruption and will return shortly ("Sorry, this is another doctor that I must speak to very briefly—I'll be back in a moment." "This is something quite urgent about another patient—I won't be more than a few minutes."). The same is true of time constraints ("I'm afraid I have to go to the O.R. now, but this is an important conversation. We need to continue this tomorrow morning on the ward round …").

Elicit

Discovering what patients understand about their illness is an important piece of information for a number of reasons. First, patients who are referred to you may have been given information about their disease that is incorrect, only partially true, or may be colored by patients' information processing or overly optimistic expectations. Asking simple questions such as "tell me what you've been told about your disease" can help you understand how much of a gap there is between the reality of the medical situation and what the patient imagines it to be. The point is that when you provide information to patients, you will need to start at the point of their understanding, so if patients have little information, you may need to start at the beginning and walk them through the medical milestones to the point where you and they are on the same page. In eliciting information key techniques are listening without interrupting, clarifying, and acknowledging what the patient says. Eliciting information is useful not only at the time of the initial visit, but also during the course of patients' treatment to ensure that you and they are "on the same page" with regard to important issues such as the goals of care. Eliciting information by allowing patients to "tell their story" may take a few more minutes, but is a powerful technique in establishing rapport and telling patients that you value their perception and opinion. Another aspect of eliciting is to understand patients' most important concerns. It is almost universal that patients will bring concerns and worries to their clinical situation that are particular to their social environment. Some patients may be worried about how to tell their children about their cancer; others may be worried about transportation or information they heard (either correctly or incorrectly!) about treatment. Studies show that patients' concerns pile up when they are unaddressed and are directly related to the risk of depression[21] with more intense and quantity of concerns being proportional to the probability of becoming depressed. Addressing them early on may prevent a psychological crisis later in treatment that interferes with patient care. Also understanding patients' viewpoint and expectations about treatment can go a long way toward preventing misunderstandings about important issues such as the goals of care, duration of treatment, and side effects of therapies.

Emotions

Emotional reactions from the patient and family are common in "high-stake" encounters such as giving a cancer diagnosis, discussing disease recurrence, and at the end of anticancer treatment when transitioning to palliative care. Strong emotions are also present when irreversible disease complications occur or at the end of life, for example, when discussing resuscitation. The axiom here is that cancer clinicians should expect emotional reactions not only from the patient and family, but also on their own part as a reaction to treatment failure, patient death, or frustrating interactions that might occur with the patient and family during the course of cancer care. The second part of this axiom is that it is beneficial to have a strategy for dealing with emotions, since they may hamper effective communication with the patient and family and may be a source of stress and burnout for the clinician. In this regard, emotions have been shown to interfere with clear thinking and ability to plan. Most clinicians have noticed that it is almost impossible to transmit information to patients while they are emotionally upset. Thus, an important goal for the clinician is to help patients "work through" an emotional reaction. This clearly has the benefit of putting patients in a better frame of mind to hear information and also allows the clinician to support patients at a time when they are feeling isolated and vulnerable. Emotions are challenging to deal with for a number of reasons: first, when they are subtle, we may not recognize them; second, when patients get upset, we may feel that we are being plunged into a situation that will take up an enormous amount of time; other barriers to addressing emotions are the fear of being responsible for the patient's problem or being blamed for failure of treatment, anxiety about the patient being plunged into a deep depression, and, as mentioned above, the clinician's own emotions.

Reminding oneself that emotions are a normal reaction to bad news or may occur as a reaction to frustration, family situations, or loss of autonomy and having a strategy to deal with them can go a long way toward allowing the physician to support patients during what for them may be a crisis in their care in which they may be feeling frightened, helpless, sad, or stunned. If you have to give bad news, assessing the situation ahead of time so that you know there is a possibility the patient will get upset will allow you to get ready to respond to an emotional reaction. Remind yourself that as bad as the patient's situation is, the patient will continue to see you as an important source of support even if occasionally you must be the messenger of bad news. This is important because feeling responsible may lead one to offer unnecessary treatment, get defensive about the care given, offer false hope or reassurance, or try and downplay the emotion by offering some fact about the cancer being less bad than the patient may imagine. So even if the bad news

■ **TABLE 15-2. Examples of Empathic Responses (The Goal is to Acknowledge the Patient's Feelings)**

Patient Says	You can Say
Defeated: "I just don't know how much I can take"	"It sound like it's been pretty rough"
Sad: "I was expecting a better result …"	"So was I, I know this comes as a shock …"
Stunned: "You mean I need more surgery?"	"I know you weren't expecting to hear this …"
Angry: "No one told me that it would take so long to recover …"	"It's been very frustrating for you"
Happy: "It's so great to have normal scan"	"I can see I've made your day"

- Give information in small chunks. Patients who are given more than three bites of information at once without an opportunity to clarify will retain less information.
- Check that the patient understands the information before going further (use phrases such as "Do you follow what I'm saying?," "Is this clear so far?, and" "Am I making sense so far?").
- Use a narrative approach to make sense of what has occurred: explain the sequence of events and how the situation seemed as events unfolded ("When you became short of breath, we didn't know whether it was just a chest infection or something more serious. So that's when we did the chest x-ray …").
- Respond to all emotions expressed by the patient as they arise. Patients may become emotional at various points during information disclosure, especially if the news is negative, so the clinician may have to shift his or her communication strategy from cognitive explanation to empathy as required.

is less bad than you think, the badness of bad news is in the eye of the beholder and dealing with the emotion first may allow you to clarify it. Simply giving the patient time to emote and respond to emotion with an empathic statement as listed in Table 15-2 can deescalate the emotion in the room and allow the patient to recover enough to begin talking about a treatment plan if one is being considered. Remember that the empathic response is about *acknowledging* the patient's emotion rather than directly feeling that emotion. Also it may take more than one empathic response to lower emotion. It is sort of a dose–response relationship: the more intense the emotion, the greater need for empathic responses. Moreover, it is really hard to overdose the patient on empathic responses.

Educate

Many patients who are diagnosed with cancer cope by seeking to master the complexities of the disease and its treatment by finding out as much as they can. In this endeavor patients and families uniformly rate their clinicians and their primary doctor as the most important source of information. Thus, medical staff can go a long way toward making sure patients comprehend information by following a few important rules:

- Begin at the level of comprehension and use the vocabulary that the patient indicated (this is called aligning).
- Use plain, intelligible English (avoid the technical jargon of the medical profession—"MedSpeak").

Enlist

Patients and families often feel a sense of helplessness about their illness. Psychologically they must travel the cognitive distance from being active members of society with responsibilities at home and work, being part of a social network that is now changed, often going from being financially independent to worrying about hospital bills and often thrust into a dependent role at home, and having entered a new world of dependency on a medical world that dictates appointments, therapies, and rules for behavior to prevent untoward events such as infection from immune suppression. All of these factors take a toll on the self-esteem of the patient, turn family relationships upside down, and challenge the patient's and family's coping. Enlisting patients in their own rehabilitation can help with transforming them from a passive participant in care to an active collaborator. Where possible, encouraging activities such as exercise, stress management, and "mainstreaming" patients wherever possible, for example, by encouraging them to continue work if they are able will aid patients' self-esteem. Families can be helped to encourage the patient in these areas also and should be told that they are an essential component of the patient's care. Two family tasks—instrumental where they might provide services to the patient such as transportation but also psychological where they provide encouragement—are crucial in helping patients adapt to a changing world. Families should however also be prepared to "give patients space" when they need it and be discouraged from pressuring patients that they need to be optimistic "all the time," since moments of sadness are almost inevitable during the journey of patients. While the role of the family is important in assisting the patient to cope, often families are dysfunctional in ways that are not helpful to the patient. A few simple questions posed to the patient such as "tell me about your family" or "whom can you rely on in your family for help" may help clarify this issue. One can also inquire of family members "how much are you prepared to help out …" that will shed light on the family's psychological and practical resources in accomplishing treatment.

Family members are also an important component of the psychological context surrounding the patient. Often they may assist the clinician in confirming the medical facts and supporting the patient as he or she responds to the information. Sometimes, however, individual family members may be at a different phase of acceptance or understanding of the medical information than the patient. This is called discordance, and it can be a serious and additional problem for the clinician. The important guideline is to seek and maintain clarity in talking to the relative. The clinician must stress that he or she is looking after the patient (not the relative), and empathic responses can be used to acknowledge and explore the emotions underlying the relative's state.

This is particularly true in a potential conflict, such as when a relative tells a clinician "My mother is not to be told the diagnosis." This is a common and awkward situation, and it requires care and effort to emphasize the primacy of the patient's right to knowledge (if that is what she wants), while at the same time underlining the relative's importance and value as part of the patient's support system.

■ APPLYING FUNDAMENTAL COMMUNICATION SKILLS

In this next section we discuss how fundamental communication skills may be applied in specific key milestones in the cancer trajectory (see Table 15-3).

Giving Bad News

Giving bad news is a frequent and significant communication challenge for oncologists, A typical oncologist in practice may give bad news as many as 20,000 times over the course of a career. Increased cancer survival now means communicating with the patient not only

■ TABLE 15-3. What's Therapeutic about the Therapeutic Relationship	
Technique	**Impact on the Patient**
Listening	Feels regarded
Clarifying concerns	Doctor is interested
Reassurance	Decreases anxiety
Encouragement	Bolsters optimism
Empathic responses	Reflects understanding
Praising the patient	Acknowledges effort

Adapted from Novack DH, *J. Gen Int Med.* 1987.[22]

information regarding the state of the disease and its response to a multitude of treatments over time, but also the adverse information related to potentially irreversible side effects, complications of the illness and the treatment, and diminished prospects for the future. This process is made difficult by several factors. First, oncologists are rarely trained in techniques for giving bad news.[23]

Second, there is an intellectual bias toward believing that communication skills including how to give bad news are somehow an innate rather than a learned skill while workshops in communication skills demonstrate that many oncologists lack fundamental competencies such as empathically responding to patient emotions.[7] Third, physicians often experience negative emotions such as anxiety and fear of being blamed when they must tell that treatment has not worked.[24]

As noted above, clinicians may react to patient emotion by offering false hope, providing premature reassurance, or omitting important information from the disclosure.[25] Fourth, many physicians fail to assess patient information prior to disclosing bad news, neglecting the point that patients may process information through a repertoire of coping strategies or styles called denial or "blunting."[26] This may include avoiding asking questions, being overly optimistic about the outcome, and distorting information to put it in a better light.

Diagnostic Disclosure and Discussions about Prognosis

At present in North America and many Western countries, there is open disclosure regarding the presence of cancer, although physicians often do not discuss the prognosis unless the patient asks. The reluctance to truthfully disclose a terminal prognosis persists in southern

Europe, including Italy and Spain.[27,28] For patients, however, not discussing the diagnosis may engender feelings of isolation, anxiety, lack of autonomy or control, psychological abandonment, mistrust, suspicion, and a sense of betrayal. On the other hand, open discussion of the diagnosis decreases uncertainty, improves participation in decisions about care, allows access to psychological support, encourages self-care, and permits the patient to begin planning for the future.[29]

Within current North American medical practice, clinicians and medical ethicists have strongly argued that for patients to make informed treatment decisions, they must have an understanding of their disease and its underlying prognosis, that is, "open awareness." With such information in hand, patients can then make informed medical decisions.[30] Reports in the literature suggest that although honest disclosure can have a negative emotional impact in the short term, most patients will adjust well over time. Gratitude and peace of mind, positive attitudes, reduced anxiety, and better adjustment are some of the benefits that patients report from having been told about their diagnosis of cancer. Because uncertainty is a major cause of emotional distress for patients, relief from uncertainty can in itself be reassuring,[31] although some theorists believe that over time patients achieve a psychosocial objective correlative of order within the context of chaos theory.[32]

Whereas most physicians in Western countries tell their patients that they have cancer, information about prognosis is less commonly presented. This often occurs despite the fact that patients often desire this information, and that it has been demonstrated that if they are actively encouraged to ask questions, prognosis is the one area in which patients ask more questions.[33] An ethical dilemma exists in that physicians and their patients with advanced cancers have a tendency to overestimate the probability of their long-term survival, which can lead to a belief that the purpose of the treatment options offered is to cure them.[30] To guide realistic treatment decisions, accurate prognostication is the key. However, statistics, which apply to groups, drive prognostics, and individuals can vary greatly in their responses to treatment. Clearly, additional research is required in the area of prognosis. It is still argued that humanistic principles should permit practitioners to temporize believing that a respect for autonomy need not imply that all information is given all of the time,[29] an approach that is at odds with the dictates of informed consent. Many specialists in palliative care have, for example, adopted a conditional approach to disclosing

terminal prognoses, indicated by use of terms such as "titrated" or through the delivery of graduated dosages of truth. Importantly, however, despite a commitment to open awareness, doctors and nurses retain control over medical information and its disclosure, which actuates ambiguity and uncertainty surrounding how open health care professionals should be.[29]

When bad news is given tactfully, honestly, and in a supportive fashion, the patient's experience of the conversation is less stressful. Friedrichsen and Strang[34] reported on patients' perception of "supporting" and "fortifying" of physician statements conveying the intention of helping patients through the course of the cancer while sentences such as "there is nothing more to do" were perceived as "abandoning" and meaning that no further support would be provided.

Not being told about the severity of their condition or not having the opportunity to express their fears and concerns may lead patients to believe that nothing can be done to help them or to understand their disease.[35] On the other hand, patients who are told bad news bluntly by a practitioner who is trying to quickly complete the difficult task of sharing bad news will likely feel extremely frightened and unsupported. Loge et al[12] surveyed 497 cancer patients regarding their experience about receiving their cancer diagnosis. Significant predictors of patient satisfaction with the conversation included perceiving the physicians as personally interested, being able to understand the information given, being informed in the proper environment (doctor's office), and having more time invested in discussing the information.[12] Although the majority of patients wish to have complete and accurate information regarding their condition, many patients feel that the news is forced upon them, unless their right to have the news given according to their preferences is acknowledged by the physician ("are you the type of person who wants to know all the details about their condition?").

In a study by Parker et al,[4] the highest rated elements of communication included the doctor being up to date on the latest research on patients' cancer, the doctor informing patients about the best treatment options and taking time to answer their questions, the doctor being honest about the severity of the condition, and the doctor using simple and clear language, giving the news directly, and giving full attention to patients. Cancer type did not predict patients' preferences. It is important for the physician to elicit patients' perspective on their condition because many incorrect beliefs can be clarified to patients' benefit.

Transition to Palliation and End-of-Life Care

For practitioners, communicating with dying patients is often complicated by countertransference issues surrounding their personal fear of dying combined with the historic tendency in Western medicine to focus on cure. Physicians who are too blunt can shatter hope for patients,[35] leaving them feeling that they have been abandoned, whereas presenting bad news in an unhurried, honest, balanced, and empathic fashion has been shown to produce greater satisfaction with communication of the news.[36] Patients also differ in how much information they want and how quickly they want to receive it.[35] American physicians fear that the revelation of a grim prognosis may psychologically damage patients' hopes and may diminish their will to survive through a form of prophecy. This is consistent with a Western cultural assumption that one needs hope to battle cancer. Physicians are also uncomfortable with putting odds on longevity, recurrence, and cure, since they do not know when or how individual patients will die.[30] In one study, hope was a constant theme of the respondents. Despite the severity of the situation, people could still feel hope, the nature of which changed with time. At the beginning of their disease, patients hoped for successful treatment, whereas later, for instance, they hoped for a little more time with their children.[38]

Patients facing death have a myriad of concerns: leaving children and other loved ones behind, decrements in socially based aspects of one's identity,[39] the end of being able to fulfill normal roles, fear of burdening loved ones,[40] loss of control, deterioration in personal appearance, needing help with intimate personal care and routine activities of daily living, worries about mental awareness,[41] pain, management of symptoms, quality of life, dignity,[42] achieving a sense of completion, having a good death, and abandonment. In fact, many patients are grateful for the opportunity to talk about questions of death, although they often have few opportunities because many patients find that the staff is afraid of or uncomfortable with talking about death and dying,[38] which exacerbates feelings of isolation and separation.

Breaking Bad News Guidelines and Strategies

Various strategies or guidelines have been proposed for having bad news consultations with patients.[24,43] Employing a specific communication strategy may more reliably result in the understanding and appropriate response to these and similar patients' doubts and fears. There have been some general guidelines and recommendations for how bad news interviews should be conducted;[4,12,24,44-46] however, these recommendations have most frequently taken the form of practical advice formulated on the basis of anecdotal experiences or opinions with little empirical foundation.[47] Two approaches[44,47] are outlined briefly in Table 15-4. As can be seen, although there are some subtle differences between these approaches, there are also many

---

■ TABLE 15-4. Strategies for Giving Bad News

By Girgis and Sanson-Fisher[47]	By Baile and Colleagues[44]
(1) Give bad news in a quiet, private place	S: Get the setting right
(2) Allow sufficient uninterrupted time for the initial consultation	P: Understand the patient's perception of the illness
(3) Assess patient's understanding and emotional status	I: Obtain an invitation to impart information
(4) Provide information simply and honestly	K: Provide knowledge and education
(5) Encourage patients to express their feelings	E: Respond to the patient's emotions with empathy, that is, responses, gestures
(6) Respond to patients' feelings with empathy	S: Provide a summary strategy, that is, respond to questions and discuss treatment options. Provide information about support services and willingness to answer questions at a future date
(7) Provide a broad time frame for the prognosis	
(8) Avoid conveying that nothing more can be done	
(9) Arrange a time to review the situation	
(10) Discuss treatment options	
(11) Offer assistance in telling others	
(12) Provide information about support services	
(13) Document the information given to the patient	

common elements. For example, each of these strategies recommends giving the news in an appropriate setting (quiet place, with uninterrupted time), assessing patients' understanding of their illness, providing the information patients want, allowing patients to express their emotions and responding appropriately, summarizing the information provided, and coming up with a plan for the next step(s). Additional research is needed to empirically support these techniques.

Importantly, research also suggests that the structure and content of the consultation influences patients' ability to remember what has been said in several ways: (1) patients usually recall facts provided at the start of a consultation more readily than those given later; (2) topics deemed most relevant and important to patients (which might not be those considered most pertinent to the doctor) are recalled most accurately; (3) the greater the number of statements made by a doctor, the smaller the mean percentage recalled by patients; and (4) items that patients do manage to recall do not decay over time as do other memories.[35]

Dealing with Hope and False Hopes

Many clinicians and patients often hedge on being completely honest when giving bad news. This may take the form of leaving out more unpalatable pieces of information, avoiding important discussions such as prognosis even when the patient desires the information, and giving chemotherapy at the end of life to avoid discussing end-of-life care.

The commonly heard excuse for this is "But you can't take away hope." Usually, the real rationale behind this is to protect the clinician from discomfort, not the patient.

Clinicians are more likely to create major problems for themselves if they promise cure when that is not possible or hold out unrealistic hopes. Supporting the patient and reinforcing realistic hopes is part of the foundation of a genuinely therapeutic relationship. Setting realistic goals for treatment early on allows you to "hope for the best while preparing for the worst."[48,49]

The important thing is not whether to tell the truth (there is a moral, ethical, and legal obligation to do so if that is what the patient wants), but how to tell the truth. Insensitive and ineffective truth-telling may be just as damaging and counterproductive as insensitive lying. In practice, the preceding protocols allow the truth to be told at a pace determined by the patient and in a way that allows recruitment and reinforcement of the patient's coping strategies.

■ COMMUNICATION AND TREATMENT DECISION MAKING

Information Needs

An area that has received significant empirical attention is identifying cancer patients' information needs. Information needs or desires mean the degree to which patients want detailed information about their cancer and the type of information they desire. Patients' information needs and preferences are mostly related to information about their disease status (eg, what is the diagnosis, what is the extent of disease) and information about treatment options or plans (eg, the best way to manage the disease).

Many patients actively seek out information and identify acquiring information as a priority. In several studies, information seeking has been found to have beneficial effects on increased compliance, increased patient satisfaction, improved quality of life, and reduced distress,[2,50–52] for example, identify six key functions of information for patients: to gain control, reduce anxiety, improve compliance, create realistic expectations, promote self-care and participation, and generate feelings of safety and security. In a study by Butow et al,[2] out of 12 specific information and support topics listed, patients expressed the greatest need for information. Of the three highest ranking topics, 97% of patients wanted more feedback on what is happening to the cancer, 88% expressed a desire for increased information on the likely future of their illness, and 91% wished for more information about their illness. Patient needs immediately after the first consultation shifted to an emphasis on support. Of the three highest ranking topics, 63% of patients wanted more assurance that they would be looked after, 59% wished for greater reassurance and hope, and 59% expressed an increased need to talk about their worries and fears.[2] Lobb et al[2,53] found that 83% of the women they interviewed wanted as much information as possible, whereas 16% wanted limited information and 91% of women wanted to know their prognosis before beginning adjuvant treatment; on the other hand, 63% wanted their oncologist to ask them whether they wanted to know their prognosis. The authors concluded that women should be given information in a staged manner that allows them the opportunity to confirm their diagnosis and prognosis and formulate questions, and that emotional support is vital when prognosis is being discussed.[54] In addition, patients' information needs may change at different points on the disease and treatment trajectory. It is often difficult for practitioners to accurately estimate or provide the amount or type of information that patients want, and patients may be dissatisfied with the amount or type of information they receive.[6,55–57] For example, in a study by Lobb et al,[6] prognostic information that was rated as most important by women with early stage breast cancer included knowing the probability of cure, disease stage, and chance of curative treatment, and receiving 10-year survival figures comparing receipt and nonreceipt of adjuvant therapy. Probability of cure and disease stage were also identified as high-priority needs in another study of women with early-stage breast cancer.[58]

Research has attempted to characterize these different information styles in a variety of ways. One of these is monitoring and blunting.[26] Monitors actively seek information, whereas blunters avoid or distract themselves from threatening information.[4,59] Thus, patients' information style may greatly affect their communication preferences and how they interact with their health care practitioners. This is an area that warrants additional study and has implications for how patients adjust to their cancer experience.

Participation Styles in Decision Making

Participation style in decision making is the degree to which patients want to be involved in the decision-making process related to their cancer. Studies of patients' desire to participate in treatment decisions have yielded conflicting results, largely depending on how participation in decision making is defined. This can range from the patient actively engaging in the decision-making process to the patient making the ultimate decision.[60] The desire to participate in treatment decisions is associated with locus of control, which describes how an individual tends to attribute control. Patients with an internal locus of control seek information to control their own destinies, whereas those with an external locus of control tend to passively accept their lot.[61]

Because research shows that a range of patients exists with respect to decision making, increasing participation for all patients may not be the most effective strategy. Various investigators have written about patient response styles.[26,62–64] Importantly, information and involvement preferences do not appear to be fixed personality characteristics, but are highly responsive to factors such as changing disease status and the behavior of the physician during consultation.[2,58] Although the categorization of

patients into various participation styles appears to offer some useful predictive power for defining communication patterns, it is clear that the issues are complex.

■ INFLUENCE OF CULTURE/ETHNICITY/ LANGUAGE ON COMMUNICATION

Developing awareness about cross-cultural practices regarding cancer disclosure issues allows the clinician to become more sensitive to the expectations of culturally and individually diverse cancer patients. When discussing diagnoses and treatment options with patients from different cultures, it is important to consider how to balance a commitment to frank discussion and a respect for the cultural values of the patient.[65] In general, patients whose dominant culture is derived from a Western philosophy subscribe to certainty, predictability, control, and obtainable outcomes.[32] This has engendered an approach that fosters self-determination and autonomy in making treatment decisions.[30] Our patient-centered society holds having fully informed patients who make accurate assessments about their health as a cultural prerogative.[65] Western cultural assumptions exist about what is good and just in medical care. One such assumption is the principle of self-determination and its importance in enabling patients to make autonomous treatment decisions.

On the other hand, patients in Italy, China, Japan,[30] Spain,[27] and Tanzania,[66] and Korean Americans and Mexican Americans believe that there is a positive value inherent in nondisclosure of diagnosis and of a terminal prognosis.[27,30] In the family-centered model of medical decision making, such as found in Mexican Americans and Korean Americans, Ethiopian refugees, and Italy, autonomy is seen as isolating.[27,30] Thus, it is essential to assess and consider patients' cultural beliefs when communicating with them about their cancer.

Communicating with the Patient's Family

Because families "can be an important resource for patients in helping them to make better decisions about their care,"[67] some believe that patient-centered approaches emphasizing patient autonomy in medical decision making should be shifted to family-centered approaches as most decision making in health care situations is carried out within the context of family care and obligation. Health care professionals are valued when they establish a structured and ongoing dialogue with family members about treatment goals, plans of care, and expectations regarding patient outcomes.[68] Caregivers report that specific and tailored direction is supportive and reduces the uncertainty they experience as they provide care.[68]

However, one must ultimately check with the patient to determine his or her desires about what level of involvement in making decisions caretakers should occupy.

Communication and Informed Consent

Traditionally, informed consent has been applied to treatment, which, unlike diagnosis, is considered to be invasive and thus liable to breach patient autonomy. Since the technological boom in medicine in recent decades, it has been realized that diagnosis too may be invasive (eg, in cardiac catheterization) and that it too requires informed consent because it may breach patient autonomy.[69] However, the physicians surveyed in one study said they were accustomed to communicating bad news verbally, in a highly individualized fashion, and find that the written nature of the form caused great difficulty for physicians who were accustomed to the flexibility and nonaccountability of verbal discussion.[70] Unfortunately, in some cases, the importance of informed consent generally drives the decision to give all information relevant to the patient regarding his or her medical condition. If patients are not given necessary information, then there may be negligence claims in the future.[29] Rudnick[69] suggests that informed consent should be sought before, not after, the diagnosis has been established, so as to avoid the patient's inference that the established diagnosis is bad news.

Communication in Palliative Care

In palliative care, communication skills are even more important than in acute care—and they may sometimes be the only therapeutic modality available to the clinician.[35] In palliative care, communication may have at least three distinct functions: (a) in taking the history, (b) in breaking bad news, and (c) as therapeutic dialogue (ie, support of the patient).

Even when the prognosis is acknowledged to be grave, there may be stages in which some hoped-for improvement or stabilization is not achieved. In these circumstances, the SPIKES protocol can be helpful, even when the clinician and the patient already have a long-standing relationship.

At other times, simply listening to the patient and acknowledging the various emotions and reactions he or she is experiencing is in itself a therapeutic intervention. This is particularly true in discussions about dying. When a patient realizes and acknowledges that he or she is dying, there is no "answer" the clinician can give. Instead, listening to the questions, issues, and emotions is a valuable service.

REFERENCES

1. Adams E, Boulton M, Watson E. The information needs of partners and family members of cancer patients: a systematic literature review. *Patient Educ Couns.* 2009;77(2):179–186.

2. Butow PN, Maclean M, Dunn SM, Tattersall MH, Boyer MJ. The dynamics of change: cancer patients' preferences for information, involvement and support. *Ann Oncol.* 1997;8(9):857–863.

3. Ong LM, Visser MR, Lammes FB, de Haes JC. Doctor–patient communication and cancer patients' quality of life and satisfaction. *Patient Educ Couns.* 2000;41(2):145–156.

4. Parker PA, Baile WF, de Moor C, Lenzi R, Kudelka AP, Cohen L. Breaking bad news about cancer: patients' preferences for communication. *J Clin Oncol.* 2001;19(7):2049–2056.

5. Harrison JD, Young JM, Price MA, Butow PN, Solomon MJ. What are the unmet supportive care needs of people with cancer? A systematic review. *Support Care Cancer.* 2009;17:1117–1128. (March).

6. Lobb EA, Butow PN, Kenny DT, Tattersall MH. Communicating prognosis in early breast cancer: do women understand the language used? *Med J Aust.* 1999;171(6):290–294.

7. Back AL, Arnold RM, Baile WF, et al. Efficacy of communication skills training for giving bad news and discussing transitions to palliative care. *Arch Intern Med.* 2007;167(5):453–460.

8. Albrecht TL, Franks MM, Ruckdeschel JC. Communication and informed consent. *Curr Opin Oncol.* 2005;17(4):336–339.

9. Spector RA. Plaintiff's attorneys share perspectives on patient communication. *J Healthc Risk Manag.* 2010;29(3):29–33.

10. Tamblyn R, Abrahamowicz M, Dauphinee D, et al. Physician scores on a national clinical skills examination as predictors of complaints to medical regulatory authorities. *JAMA.* 2007;298(9):993–1001.

11. Bedell SE, Graboys TB, Bedell E, Lown B. Words that harm, words that heal. *Arch Intern Med.* 2004;164(13):1365–1368.

12. Loge JH, Kaasa S, Hytten K. Disclosing the cancer diagnosis: the patients' experiences. *Eur J Cancer.* 1997;33(6):878–882.

13. Hebert HD, Butera JN, Castillo J, Mega AE. Are we training our fellows adequately in delivering bad news to patients? A survey of hematology/oncology program directors. *J Palliat Med.* 2009;12(12):1119–1124.

14. Hoffman M, Ferri J, Sison C, Roter D, Schapira L, Baile W. Teaching communication skills: an AACE survey of oncology training programs. *J Cancer Educ.* 2004;19(4):220–224.

15. Hall E. *The Hidden Dimension.* New York, NY: Doubleday; 1966.

16. MacDonald K. Patient–clinician eye contact: social neuroscience and art of clinical engagement. *Postgrad Med.* 2009;121(4):136–144.

17. Older J. Teaching touch at medical school. *JAMA.* 1984;252(7):931–933.

18. Buis C, de Boo T, Hull R. Touch and breaking bad news. *Fam Pract.* 1991;8(4):303–304.

19. Lipkin M Jr, Quill TE, Napodano RJ. The medical interview: a core curriculum for residencies in internal medicine. *Ann Intern Med.* 1984;100(2):277–284.

20. Frankel RM, Beckman HB. The pause that refreshes. *Hosp Pract (Off Ed).* 1988;23(9A):62, 65–67.

21. Parle M, Jones B, Maguire P. Maladaptive coping and affective disorders among cancer patients. *Psychol Med.* 1996;26(4):735–744.

22. Novack DH. Therapeutic aspects of the clinical encounter. *J Gen Intern Med.* 1987;2:346–55

23. Baile WF, Lenzi R, Parker PA, Buckman R, Cohen L. Oncologists' attitudes toward and practices in giving bad news: an exploratory study. *J Clin Oncol.* 2002;20(8):2189–2196.

24. Buckman R. Breaking bad news: why is it still so difficult? *Br Med J (Clin Res Ed).* 1984;288(6430):1597–1599.

25. Maguire P. Improving communication with cancer patients. *Eur J Cancer.* 1999;35(10):1415–1422.

26. Miller SM. Monitoring and blunting: validation of a questionnaire to assess styles of information seeking under threat. *J Pers Soc Psychol.* 1987;52(2):345–353.

27. Mitchell JL. Cross-cultural issues in the disclosure of cancer. *Cancer Pract.* 1998;6(3):153–160.

28. Surbone A. Cultural aspects of communication in cancer care. *Support Care Cancer.* 2008;16(3):235–240.

29. Arber A, Gallagher A. Breaking bad news revisited: the push for negotiated disclosure and changing practice implications. *Int J Palliat Nurs.* 2003;9(4):166–172.

30. Gordon EJ, Daugherty CK. 'Hitting you over the head': oncologists' disclosure of prognosis to advanced cancer patients. *Bioethics.* 2003;17(2):142–168.

31. Girgis A, Sanson-Fisher RW. Breaking bad news. 1: current best advice for clinicians. *Behav Med.* 1998;24(2): 53–59.

32. Mishel MH. Reconceptualization of the uncertainty in illness theory. *Image J Nurs Sch.* 1990;22(4):256–262.

33. Butow PN, Dowsett S, Hagerty R, Tattersall MH. Communicating prognosis to patients with metastatic disease: what do they really want to know? *Support Care Cancer.* 2002;10(2):161–168.

34. Friedrichsen MJ, Strang PM. Doctors' strategies when breaking bad news to terminally ill patients. *J Palliat Med.* 2003;6(4):565–574.

35. Fallowfield L, Jenkins V. Effective communication skills are the key to good cancer care. *Eur J Cancer.* 1999;35(11):1592–1597.

36. Wenrich MD, Curtis JR, Shannon SE, Carline JD, Ambrozy DM, Ramsey PG. Communicating with dying patients within the spectrum of medical care from terminal diagnosis to death. *Arch Intern Med.* 2001;161(6): 868–874.

37. Ellis PM, Tattersall MH. How should doctors communicate the diagnosis of cancer to patients? *Ann Med.* 1999;31(5):336–341.

38. Adelbratt S, Strang P. Death anxiety in brain tumour patients and their spouses. *Palliat Med.* 2000;14(6): 499–507.

39. Byock IR. The nature of suffering and the nature of opportunity at the end of life. *Clin Geriatr Med.* 1996;12(2):237–252.

40. Singer PA, Martin DK, Kelner M. Quality end-of-life care: patients' perspectives. *JAMA.* 1999;281(2):163–168.

41. Steinhauser KE, Christakis NA, Clipp EC, McNeilly M, McIntyre L, Tulsky JA. Factors considered important at the end of life by patients, family, physicians, and other care providers. *JAMA.* 2000;284(19):2476–2482.

42. Chochinov HM, Hack T, Hassard T, Kristjanson LJ, McClement S, Harlos M. Dignity in the terminally ill: a cross-sectional, cohort study. *Lancet.* 2002;360(9350): 2026–2030.

43. Baile WF, Glober GA, Lenzi R, Beale EA, Kudelka AP. Discussing disease progression and end-of-life decisions. *Oncology (Huntingt).* 1999;13(7):1021–1031 [discussion 1031–1036, 1038].

44. Baile WF, Buckman R, Lenzi R, Glober G, Beale EA, Kudelka AP. SPIKES—a six-step protocol for delivering

bad news: application to the patient with cancer. *Oncologist.* 2000;5(4):302–311.

45. Blanchard CG, Labrecque MS, Ruckdeschel JC, Blanchard EB. Information and decision-making preferences of hospitalized adult cancer patients. *Soc Sci Med.* 1988;27(11):1139–1145.

46. Fallowfield LJ, Jenkins VA, Beveridge HA. Truth may hurt but deceit hurts more: communication in palliative care. *Palliat Med.* 2002;16(4):297–303.

47. Girgis A, Sanson-Fisher RW. Breaking bad news: consensus guidelines for medical practitioners. *J Clin Oncol.* 1995;13(9):2449–2456.

48. Back AL, Arnold RM, Quill TE. Hope for the best, and prepare for the worst. *Ann Intern Med.* 2003;138(5): 439–443.

49. Von Roenn JH, von Gunten CF. Setting goals to maintain hope. *J Clin Oncol.* 2003;21(3):570–574.

50. Mills ME, Sullivan K. The importance of information giving for patients newly diagnosed with cancer: a review of the literature. *J Clin Nurs.* 1999;8(6):631–642.

51. Parker PA, Middleton MS, Kulik JA. Counterfactual thinking and quality of life among women with silicone breast implants. *J Behav Med.* 2002;25(4):317–335.

52. Siminoff LA, Ravdin P, Colabianchi N, Sturm CM. Doctor–patient communication patterns in breast cancer adjuvant therapy discussions. *Health Expect.* 2000;3(1):26–36.

53. Lobb EA, Butow PN, Meiser B, et al. Tailoring communication in consultations with women from high risk breast cancer families. *Br J Cancer.* 2002;87(5): 502–508.

54. Jenkins V, Fallowfield L, Saul J. Information needs of patients with cancer: results from a large study in UK cancer centres. *Br J Cancer.* 2001;84(1):48–51.

55. Schofield PE, Butow PN, Thompson JF, Tattersall MH, Beeney LJ, Dunn SM. Psychological responses of patients receiving a diagnosis of cancer. *Ann Oncol.* 2003;14(1):48–56.

56. Silliman RA, Dukes KA, Sullivan LM, Kaplan SH. Breast cancer care in older women: sources of information, social support, and emotional health outcomes. *Cancer.* 1998;83(4):706–711.

57. Wright EB, Holcombe C, Salmon P. Doctors' communication of trust, care, and respect in breast cancer: qualitative study. *BMJ.* 2004;328(7444):864.

58. Degner LF, Kristjanson LJ, Bowman D, et al. Information needs and decisional preferences in women with breast cancer. *JAMA.* 1997;277(18):1485–1492.

59. Ong LM, Visser MR, van Zuuren FJ, Rietbroek RC, Lammes FB, de Haes JC. Cancer patients' coping styles and doctor–patient communication. *Psychooncology.* 1999;8(2):155–166.

60. Guadagnoli E, Ward P. Patient participation in decision-making. *Soc Sci Med.* 1998;47(3):329–339.

61. Webber GC. Patient education. A review of the issues. *Med Care.* 1990;28(11):1089–1103.

62. Keating NL, Guadagnoli E, Landrum MB, Borbas C, Weeks JC. Treatment decision making in early-stage breast cancer: should surgeons match patients' desired level of involvement? *J Clin Oncol.* 2002;20(6):1473–1479.

63. Pierce PF. Deciding on breast cancer treatment: a description of decision behavior. *Nurs Res.* 1993;42(1):22–28.

64. Roberts CS, Cox CE, Reintgen DS, Baile WF, Gibertini M. Influence of physician communication on newly diagnosed breast patients' psychologic adjustment and decision-making. *Cancer.* 1994;74(1 suppl):336–341.

65. Hern HE Jr, Koenig BA, Moore LJ, Marshall PA. The difference that culture can make in end-of-life decision-making. *Camb Q Healthc Ethics.* 1998;7(1):27–40.

66. Harris SR, Templeton E. Who's listening? Experiences of women with breast cancer in communicating with physicians. *Breast J.* 2001;7(6):444–449.

67. Ballard-Reisch DS, Letner JA. Centering families in cancer communication research: acknowledging the impact of support, culture and process on client/provider communication in cancer management. *Patient Educ Couns.* 2003;50(1):61–66.

68. Given BA, Given CW, Kozachik S. Family support in advanced cancer. *CA Cancer J Clin.* 2001;51(4):213–231.

69. Rudnick A. Informed consent to breaking bad news. *Nurs Ethics.* 2002;9(1):61–66.

70. Taylor KM, Kelner M. Informed consent: the physicians' perspective. *Soc Sci Med.* 1987;24(2):135–143.

SECTION IV

Family and Cultural Issues

A Model: Supporting the Caregiver through the Crisis of Cancer

CHAPTER 16

• *Phyddy Tacchi*

■ BACKGROUND AND INTRODUCTION

Cancer caregivers are a ubiquitous, stressed, and burdened population with little social or professional support. Estimated new cancer cases in the United States in 2009 as projected by the American Cancer Society[1] will affect 1,479,350 people. Of those newly diagnosed >1 million patients, 65% will likely survive at least 5 years, a notable improvement over previous survival rates of 50% of those diagnosed from 1974 to 1976 and 54% from 1983 to 1985.[2] Not too long ago, having cancer was considered an acute disease carrying a high mortality rate. At present, many of those same cancers are treated with various therapies that may extend a patient's life beyond previous medical expectations, enabling him or her to live with a chronic disease with a fluctuating level of quality of life. Given that patients are now living longer and, in some cases, sicker, the role of and need for caregiving is extended. There are now over 22.4 million families caring for their chronically medically ill loved ones as a result of earlier hospital discharges in an attempt to control costs.[3] Because of these attempts to control medical costs by shortening hospital stays as well as lengthened survival rates, the home has become an outpatient medical care setting. The caregiver, although in most cases not formally medically trained, is providing the bulk of daily medical care from the initial diagnosis to the end of life for many patients. Caregivers are now performing complex medical tasks that not too long ago were performed solely by highly trained and experienced inpatient nurses.

A caregiver is "a person who is responsible for attending to the needs of a child or dependent adult."[4] This is a simple explanation fraught with diversified minefields, such as "a person," which likely translates into one unpaid immediate family member shouldering most of the physical, emotional, financial, and medical caregiving burden. The reference to "responsible for attending to the needs of a … dependent adult" conceals the scope of adaptations to this role change and assumption of tasks in the daily life of a caregiver. It is little wonder that the literature points to a high level of distress among cancer caregivers, who often feel overwhelmed with physical and emotional fatigue as a result of the unrelenting and cumulative burden of providing ongoing comprehensive care for their loved one. This includes assuming an array of responsibilities for provision of direct and indirect care, symptom and comfort management, synthesis of medical information, and maintenance of hope in the face of patient discouragement.[5] The assumption of these responsibilities almost always begins immediately on learning of their loved one's new cancer diagnosis. With just a few words, "your loved one has cancer," caregivers rapidly learn that life as they knew it is changed forever. Future tomorrows, mornings, afternoons, holidays, nightfalls, and summers will be colored differently from that moment on.

Caregiver distress is manifested in a variety of psychological symptoms as they vacillate between the tender fervency of hope and the tyranny of uncertainty. For example, Carter and Chang[6] found in their study of 51 caregivers that 95% expressed severe sleep problems and fatigue and over half were experiencing symptoms characteristic of clinical depression. Cameron et al[7] found among 54 caregivers that most experienced a diminished sense of emotional well-being, particularly when met with forced limitation in their ability to participate in their own valued activities and interests. Flaskerud et al[8] found, in a study involving female caregivers of people with AIDS, age-related dementias (ARD), and cancer, that the caregivers, in general, experienced distress that may affect their own mental and physical health.

A 6-year-long study by Kiecolt-Glaser et al[9] found, in 117 long-term older caregivers of dementia and Alzheimer's patients, that the caregivers had a much greater risk of developing their own serious health problems with important implications for their own morbidity and mortality than noncaregivers. They concluded that the chronic stress of caregiving places caregivers at a greater risk of disease and possibly premature aging. They found key evidence that a prolonged increased rate of IL-6 weakens the human immune system of caregivers. IL-6, a cytokine involved in a critical chemical pathway through which the immune system fights infection, is four times more likely to increase among chronic caregivers, even 3 years after their patient had died and their caregiver duties had stopped. This heightened IL-6 level, maintained over time, may predispose the caregiver to later cardiovascular disease, arthritis, osteoporosis, type 2 diabetes, and certain cancers.[9]

Caregivers report many unmet psychological needs.[10] Houts et al[11] found, in a study with 627 patients and 397 family members within 1 year of diagnosis, that psychological needs were cited as the most frequently unmet needs. Soothill et al,[12] in a 3-year study of the psychosocial needs of patients and 195 caregivers, found that caregivers report more unmet needs than patients. Caregivers report primary unmet needs for help with feelings of guilt that they may have contributed in some way to their loved one's cancer diagnosis and/or their inability to impact medical outcome, often feeling helpless while watching their loved one suffer. They also cite chronic fear and apprehension of the unknown course that their loved one's cancer might take as an unmet need for supportive help. Many caregivers state that fear of the uncertainty of their loved one's medical outcome pervades their thinking, in terms of both survivorship issues including a diminished quality of life should their loved one survive and what life will be like after their loved one dies—emotionally, physically, and financially.[12]

■ THE DYNAMICS OF CAREGIVING

Caregiver Responsibilities

The primary caregiver of a person with cancer is typically a medically untrained family member, frequently unacquainted with the rigors involved in meeting complex, often experimental, treatment demands.[13] Understandably, medical care is inherently focused on the needs, primarily physical, of the patient. Family cancer caregivers perform a myriad of concrete tasks, including tending to the emotional, physical, medical, and communication needs of the patient. Caregivers provide an endless array of services, such as provide transportation, accompany patients to appointments, manage complicated medication schedules and side effects, interact with the medical team, negotiate with insurance companies, and serve as the liaison between the patient and other family members, often while geographically displaced from the familiarities and comfort of home in order to receive treatment in a distant medical setting. Just as importantly, caregivers also provide a critical source of psychological assistance through encouragement, patience, and support. This emotional support is important in reducing anxiety and depression in the patient.[13]

Sources of Caregiver Stress

Caregiver stress varies during different stages of the disease process, that is, at the initiation of treatment versus chronicity of treatment.[14] Particularly during the chronicity of treatment, a caregiver's stress level is often proportional to the ups and downs of the patient's illness.[15] This may result in caregiver demoralization, exhaustion, inability to concentrate, and clinical depression. Moreover, the caregiver often internalizes his or her distressing feelings for fear of upsetting the patient. Caregivers complain of an overwhelming sense of loneliness as they try to hide "forbidden" emotions and thoughts from their loved one. This is done in an attempt to protect patients from the harsh realities of the loss of their former daily life once known for its predictable rhythm, now replaced with a "new normal" marked with the terror of uncertainty, pending loss, and protective hypervigilance. Caregivers often come to this role inadequately equipped with psychological tools to buffer what is experienced as an emotional "roller coaster," emotions that change from day to day or moment to moment, depending on the medical acuity of the patient.

Initiation of Treatment

On diagnosis, suddenly both the patient and caregiver are thrust into the heretofore-foreign world of oncology. This may likely include a crash course in learning the medical and technical aspects of the disease and treatment carrying the uncertainty of outcome. Along with navigation of the hospital environment, patients and caregivers find themselves interacting with multiple oncology specialists using unfamiliar terminology in discussing a patient's precarious situation precarious situation and future vulnerability. Days filled with MRIs, blood tests, appointments, treatments including surgery, chemotherapies, and radiation, ER visits, hospitalizations, medications, indwelling catheter care, interacting with insurance companies, fatigue, nausea, and pain soon become a shocking way of life for both the patient and caregiver. The caregiver often must immediately absorb these new responsibilities in addition to carrying out concurrent daily obligations, often without additional resources or a sense of practical and medical preparedness.

Chronicity of Treatment

Over time, caregiver stress increases in response to the patient's lengthy and complex medical treatment, disease recurrence, fluctuation of patient's response to treatment, and, in some instances, treatment failure. In addition to financial constraints, compounding family stressors associated with maintaining a temporary geographically remote residence to access quality care at MD Anderson Cancer Center and tending to their own medical needs, caregivers are at high risk for both emotional and physical fatigue. This may be expressed through depression, demoralization, anxiety, insomnia, social isolation, boredom, and loneliness.

Phases of Caregiver Crisis

In working with caregivers, I have found that they may enter phases of caregiver crisis, particularly as the patient's medical treatment becomes lengthier than initially expected and interlaced with periods of successful and failed responses to treatment.

Dynamic Hopefulness

In the beginning, a new caregiver typically and enthusiastically embraces the assumption that "If I just work hard enough, I can keep this person alive. If I get up early enough and stay up late enough, I can control the outcome." After the shock of the diagnosis and learning of treatment options, the caregiver mobilizes initial effort in arranging both his or her life and the patient's life around the optimistic concept of "we can, and will, beat this!" Specific organizational methods for disease research, transportation, housing, equipment, menus, medications, appointments, etc, are employed in an energetic rush to take control of the disease course and outcome. Confident predictions are made that "we will do chemo for six weeks, then return home for three weeks and back for another four weeks, etc." As long as the patient responds well to treatment, this phase can be maintained. It is only after the patient fails to respond to treatment easily that glimpses of potential failure begin to color the medical canvas. A soft alarm rings in the caregiver mind, and an early vibration of doubt begins to emerge. In its earliest stages, caregiver doubt serves as an impetus for mounting a defense with a greater sense of caregiver determination, calling, and purpose.

Determination

As the patient encounters a roller coaster response to treatment with a fluctuating constellation of physical and emotional symptoms, the caregiver often begins to focus on assuming greater responsibility for control of the disease outcome. Despite the caregiver having devoted a significant amount of effort and diligence in providing medical assistance and oversight for the patient to ensure a positive medical outcome, the patient may not respond to treatment as hoped. This may increase the caregiver's determined intent to remain vigilant and responsible in creating a better outcome, as if the patient's unsteady responsiveness to treatment is somehow attributable to faulty caregiving. This escalating cycle of caregiver effort to effect a positive medical outcome may be repeated many times during the chronicity of the patient's disease and reach a stage of caregiving crisis, including profound emotional and physical fatigue.

Doubt and Guilt

Revolving periods of hope, anger, disappointment, guilt, depression, anxiety, fatigue, fear, and persistent striving for perfection may evolve into a state of caregiver emotional fatigue, including despair and a pervasive sense of incompetence. To compensate, caregivers may resort to using emotionally charged responses in an attempt to control the "cancer chaos." This may culminate in a growing sense of caregiver guilt and ineffectiveness as the patient either continues with untoward side effects of treatment or fails to respond to treatment as planned. Vague doubts emerge, as one caregiver states, "I don't tell her, but I worry all the time that she will die. Sometimes, I feel that I don't know what to do to help. I really had it out with the doctor this morning. My wife can't eat and he doesn't seem to care."

Fear of the consequences that may result from what the caregiver perceives as patient noncompliance is expressed by irritability, with dictates to the patient to just "eat more, drink more, walk more, take your medication, etc." It is not uncommon at this time for conflict to ensue between caregiver and patient as the caregiver may perceive the patient as being obstinate and uncooperative, resulting in a power struggle of sorts. As one caregiver said, "I never know if he's not doing what he's supposed to do because he *won't* do it or he *can't* do it."

Caregiver guilt, as defined by Spillers et al,[16] "exists at the intersection of what one believes and what one does." It is when caregivers perceive that their actual care for the patient is less than what it "should" be that guilt increases. In examining their performance, caregivers often apply the following standard: if the caregiver did (or did not) do for their patient what a "good" caregiver "*should*" (or should not) do, then caregiver guilt is low. Conversely, if the caregiver did not do what a "good" caregiver should do, then caregiver guilt may be higher (Fig. 16-1).

Diminishing Reserves

As the patient continues to fail to respond to treatment or when side effects of treatment significantly interfere with patient functioning, the evolution of caregivers' emotional and physical exhaustion grows. In this stage, a caregiver's emotional reactivity heightens in response to ever-changing medical demands. The caregiver begins to overfunction for the patient. This state of hyperresponsiveness to the patient's needs further depletes the caregiver of physical and emotional energy and may cause the caregiver to question

both the patient's and his or her personal competency. This sense of hypervigilance against danger produces depletion of caregiver reserves and may have, over time, a cascading negative impact on the welfare of the patient.

Devaluing Personal Competency

Over time, as the patient physically and emotionally vacillates in response to treatment, the caregiver may begin to realize a sense of losing control over the medical outcome. In order to reestablish control and a renewed sense of safety, a caregiver may then accelerate his or her efforts in order to keep the loved one alive, as several caregivers noted: "I stay with my loved one 24/7 in the hospital, otherwise I'm afraid he'll die. As long as I'm there to keep watch, I think on some level I can prevent that from happening." "I don't sleep well and I eat my meals off his tray. Some days, I don't even have time to take a shower." "Last night I sat on the floor all night next to her bed just to make sure she didn't try to climb out and fall." "I watch every medication the nurses give her. I have caught some mistakes." "We've been here 9 months and I don't dare go back home. I don't know what he would do if I wasn't here. He doesn't remember when to take his medications, to eat or drink. I have to do it all."

In time, this extraordinary assumption of vigilant duty becomes emotionally and physically exhausting for the caregiver. As the patient continues to experience peaks and valleys of response to treatment rather than maintaining a smooth course of planned recovery, caregivers may begin to doubt the integrity and capability of their best efforts. They may begin to question their personal competency, which initiates now a new wave of emotional and physical exhaustion as they "try harder" in the face of perceived caregiver failure.

Caregiver distress may fluctuate depending on the patient's disease trajectory. As adapted from Corbin and Strauss'[17] understanding of the phases of the chronic disease process, the relationship between the chronicity of patient symptom response/lack of response and caregiver interpretation of control and effectiveness may be illustrated as shown in Table 16-1.

It may well be that caregivers' stress level peaks at phase 5 when the patient's disease symptoms fail to respond to caregiver and medical attentiveness, but then subsides as the patient cycles back to phase 1 as symptoms once again stabilize and become manageable. It is the prolonged recycling of a patient's symptomatic changes that creates a sense of caregiver emotional chaos, distress, and weariness, that is, the questioning of personal competency.

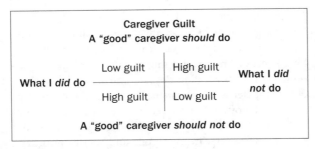

FIGURE 16-1. Caregiver Guilt.

■ TABLE 16-1. Relationship between Patient Symptoms and Caregiver Response Cycles

No.	Patient's Cycle of Symptoms	Symptom State	Caregiver Cycle of Response
1	Onset	Initial symptoms begin to present	Dynamic hopefulness
2	Crisis	Symptom dyscontrol—a potentially life-threatening situation occurs	Determination, controlled diligence
3	Acute	Symptom control sought—symptoms require control with a changed prescribed regimen	Increased effort, overfunctioning
4	Stable	Symptom control—symptoms are temporarily managed	Hypervigilance, diminishing reserves
5	Unstable	Symptom dyscontrol—symptoms become uncontrollable by the previous regimen	Helplessness, fear, self-doubt, emotional and physical fatigue

■ INTERVENTIONS FOR CAREGIVERS

Because caregivers are not the primary patient, their distress, confusion, and sense of helplessness may not be addressed by the medical staff, and they may, as a result, begin to feel a sense of loneliness and isolation with their growing concerns. They are often left to fend for themselves in a "learn as you go" process, without a compass so to speak as they navigate through the emotional chaos of caregiving.

The literature suggests that various interventions, including caregiver education in symptom management of the patient, may be effective in reducing caregiver distress. Houts et al[11] report a problem-solving educational approach teaching basic problem-solving principles using a cognitive–behavioral framework to both patients and caregivers. Their focus is primarily on symptom management and community resource support and was found to be effective in building caregiver confidence.[18]

Ideally, caregiver interventions should begin early, at the time of admission. Once a caregiver begins to question his or her own competency, a pattern of emotional reactivity may have already taken hold in an effort to avoid what the caregiver perceives as the ultimate signal of failure, that is, the patient's lack of medical responsiveness with resultant medical decline. As noted above, as the caregiver effort increases without corresponding patient symptom stability, so does caregiver emotional and physical fatigue and recurring sense of hypervigilance and fear of failure. I have found that using a model of psychoeducational interventions at this stage

of caregiving can be helpful in teaching caregivers about the concepts of emotional and physical energy conservation, and the importance of establishing a community of support and examining perceptions of control over patient responses and medical outcome. Education relative to symptoms of caregiver depression, anxiety, and insomnia is critical.[19]

Psychoeducational Intervention: The Caregiver Support Group

A primary assumption of this model is that caregivers can develop skills of emotional self-regulation as an aid for emotional health and physical energy conservation. A caregiver learns, during the group experience, that the primary source of control lies not in controlling the patient's medical outcome, but rather in self-regulation and modulation of emotional reactivity to an unpredictable medical event, instead of controlling the event itself. This can be taught by assisting the caregiver in building a sense of self-awareness and self-knowledge in a community of fellow caregivers. It is based on the premise of "The more I know about myself, the better I can regulate myself. If I can better regulate myself, I can become more effective, confident and competent ... despite the medical outcome, which I ultimately have little to no control over anyway."

This caregiver model is based, theoretically, on 5 of the 11 curative factors Yalom[20] found in his extensive work with psychotherapy groups that contribute to increased self-knowledge gained through the group experience. During our weekly caregiver psychoeducational group, designed to be an open group for caregivers who are able to attend once or more often, participants note experiences of:

- **Universality:** "I realize that I'm not alone. There are other caregivers who feel like I do."
- **Imparting of information regarding caregiver education:** "I didn't know that these thoughts and feelings are normal. I thought I was going crazy."
- **Altruism:** "Things are ok for us right now, so I'm really here to help other caregivers."
- **Catharsis (releasing pent-up negative emotion that caregivers avoid addressing with patients to protect their sense of hope):** "I can't talk with my patient about this stuff. He only wants to hear positive things. Sometimes I find myself wishing he would just go ahead and die as his suffering is unbearable to watch."
- **Existential factors in reorganization of values and priorities:** "I am sorting out my beliefs about life, death and the meaning of this cancer experience for me and for my loved one as we go through this. I realize that all those things we used to think were so important just don't really matter anymore."[20]

The six components of this model include using the above-mentioned curative factors to assist the caregiver in working, within a group setting, through a directed process of developing a new body of self-knowledge regarding emotional regulation skills (Table 16-2).

Addressing these and other related topics, for one's self-interest rather than for one's patient (a difficult task for some caregivers), may present a challenge and yet can bring a sense of deepening personal acceptance and calm. This ongoing process of sifting through and sorting out beliefs and values about the caregiver role, the medical necessity of self-care, life, and death carries the potential of redefining a realistic appraisal of caregiving function and the grander purpose of physical, emotional, and spiritual effort in providing care for another person, rather than maintaining a desperate grip over its final conclusion.

■ PSYCHOEDUCATION: SPEAKING DIRECTLY TO CAREGIVERS

Facing the Challenge Together

Are you caring for a loved one with cancer? Feeling overwhelmed? You are not alone.

The following reflects the observations of other caregivers who have been part of a similar journey. This information is intended to serve as a practical guide and an emotional survival kit to help you take care of yourself while taking care of someone else.

A caregiver has special needs, which often are quite different than those of a patient. As you probably know, caregiving brings a sudden set of new responsibilities that demand an enormous amount of time and energy. While the caregiving experience may provide opportunities for growth with positive experiences, it also can take an emotional and physical toll, at times leaving you feeling frightened, lonely, burdened, and drained.

Many people travel from near and far to receive the world-class treatment that the University of Texas MD Anderson Cancer Center offers. While this carries distinct medical advantages, the adjustments that are needed can bring unique challenges. There are many new things to learn, including navigating a large and unfamiliar setting; gaining understanding of medical terminology; building trust with a new staff; managing medications, side effects, and schedules; keeping the home fires burning from a distance, etc.

This section is designed to share with you how others have faced these challenges and the methods they used to help them get through this stressful time. We hope the guidance provided here will strengthen, soothe, and energize you—the caregiver—a pivotal member of the treatment team.

A Day in the Life of a Caregiver

I feel responsible for absolutely everything. I always think I should be leading the patient to do the right thing. I feel I'm becoming such a nag.

Life can change with just one phone call. When the words "your loved one has cancer" are heard, life changes forever for the caregiver. That moment of first hearing the news will likely live on in your memory. Suddenly, life as you knew it is gone. A whole new expansive set of responsibilities appears seemingly overnight and invades every facet of daily life, as you can see in Figure 16-2. What new responsibilities do you now have?

The Tough Times: Caregiver Doubts

I work all the time, but still feel like I'm behind.

Because of the all-encompassing duties that caregivers must absorb, fatigue and self-doubt may set in. The more

■ TABLE 16-2. Model: Building Caregiver Competency

No.	Six Building Blocks of Self-understanding	Caregiver Responses	Impact
1	Developing a personal theory of causation of cancer	"Why did my loved one get cancer?" Some believe that cancer is a punishment, a result of living unwisely, genetics, or random bad luck, etc	Acknowledges the uncertainty of the illness
2	Exploring the meaning of suffering	"Why does my loved one have to suffer?" Some believe that good people should not suffer and bad people should not be spared	Deepening understanding of "fairness"
3	Discovering spiritual sustenance	"Where is God in all of this?" Some believe that God is with them, suffering alongside the sufferer; others question why God does not cure their loved one or that God does not exist or does not care	Expanding self-soothing practices
4	Handling forbidden feelings	"Am I going crazy?" Many experience anger, guilt, fatigue, depression, hopelessness, yearning for return to a normal life, resentment, irritability, fear, or longing for one's loved one to die so as to be relieved of caregiving responsibilities	Acknowledging emotional reactivity
5	Relinquishing the illusion of control over external events	"How can I keep my loved one alive?" Many express that they are learning painful lessons in that they cannot keep this person alive, no matter how hard they work. The length of his or her life is not their decision or within their control	Monitoring one's responses to feeling helpless in interpreting one's limitations in solving difficult problems, rather than expending energy on working to change the unchangeable
6	Recognizing the capacity for internal emotional control	"How can I learn to live, really live, one day at a time?" in the midst of chronic ambivalence and uncertainty?	Establishing an internal system to confine fear to the facts at hand, appreciating the brevity of life, and regaining a sense of wonder of life's smallest joys and gifts of today

tired caregivers begin to feel, the more they may question their ability and self-confidence. Which of the following thoughts of self-doubt can you most identify with?

- "Why can't I keep up?"
- "Why can't I do everything that needs to be done?"
- "Why can't I get him/her to eat? To drink? To walk?"
- "Is there something wrong with me because I can't get him/her better?"
- "Why doesn't he/she talk with me?"
- "Why can't I control things?"
- "I'm working as hard as I can and he/she still feels bad."
- "I don't have time for anything."
- "I feel defeated and burned out."
- "My loved one is so irritable with me, I just don't know how to handle it."
- "My loved one doesn't want anyone else to care for him/her other than me. I'm just worn out."
- "My loved one won't follow my advice."
- "I let picky things get to me."

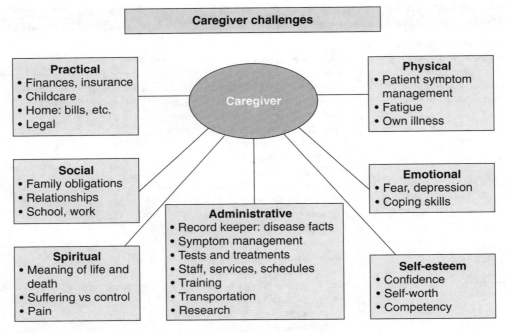

FIGURE 16-2. Adapted individual living with cancer.[21]

The Emotions of Caregiving

My loved one is so irritable with me and I'm working as hard as I can to help. All I want to do is go home.

I don't have time to take care of myself. Even if I did, I don't know where to go or what to do.

I just want things to return to normal, to the way things used to be.

Sometimes, I just have to get away.

Sound familiar? Sometimes caregivers feel as if their mood changes in relationship to managing the fluctuating nature of day-to-day medical circumstances:

Help! I'm on an emotional roller coaster and I can't get off.

Sometimes at night, I just lay there waiting for the next earthquake.

If I don't sleep at night, I end up crying the next day.

Caregivers often work overtime to provide care to their loved ones. This has its pitfalls and blessings. It is often a job requiring 24/7 attention with many physical and emotional

demands, filled with highs and lows. The most common complaints of caregivers are emotional and physical fatigue, exhaustion, and sleep deprivation. The time and effort it takes to care for your loved one each day can, over time, become very stressful with a gradual wearing down of energy.

There is a high correlation between fatigue and depression in caregivers. When you are under such tremendous chronic stress, you can experience many emotional ups and downs on any given day. One minute you feel as if you have it all together, and the next minute it seems like you are falling apart. Not only is physical fatigue a factor, but emotional overload is as well.

The Volcanic Feelings of Caregivers

Emotions to the maximum

My feelings bounce around all over the place. Sometimes they are positive and sometimes they are so painful I don't think I can stand it.

Sometimes you may feel like a virtual volcano when pressure builds without relief. Today may seem too difficult and tomorrow too uncertain. Where are you today on this spectrum of feelings?

Calm	....	Scared
Happy	....	Sad
Relieved	....	Nervous
Contented	....	Angry
Confident	....	Worried

The "Forbidden" Feelings of Caregivers

Sometimes, I can't talk to anyone about how I feel. I don't want to burden them or take away the hope of my loved one. No one understands what this is really like unless they've been through it.

It is not unusual for caregivers to have intense feelings that they are hesitant to talk about, especially to their patient as caregivers may wish to protect their loved one from hearing about their distress. These feelings can be strong and seemingly in conflict with what you are trying to do. Although others may tell you to "think positive or be optimistic," there are times when this just does not seem possible. Which of the following "forbidden" feelings can you identify with?

- Yearning for "normal"
- Resentment
- Guilt and feeling trapped
- Hopelessness
- Worry
- Grief
- Doubt
- Anger
- Fear
- Helplessness
- Sorrow
- Loneliness.

Six Basic Steps for Caregiver Self-care

In the midst of your expanded role carrying intense emotions and challenges, it is vital that you learn to take care of yourself. Many caregivers feel guilty taking time to do something for themselves while their loved one is ill. You may need to first give yourself permission to do so.

What can you do, starting today, that will make a difference for you? You do not ever have to be the same after today. People can do incredible things, unbelievable things, despite the most impossible or disastrous circumstances. You have lived all your life to come to this day, to this moment. There may be different ways to travel this road that will help you maintain your physical and mental health over the long run. Take a look at what other caregivers have found to be helpful.

Self-care: Feeding Your Body

My body is literally my caregiving machine. I have to take care of it.

Exercise: Pump up your body by walking at least 10 minutes a day.

Sleep: Rest your body for 6 to 8 hours a night.

Eat right: Feed your body, nutritionally and regularly, including breakfast. Eat lots of vegetables, fruit, and whole grains.

Drink plenty of water.

Self-care: Feeding Your Mind

I was scared all the time until I learned that the definition of fear is 'Future Events Appearing Real.' As long as I focus on the present, I keep from getting scared.

In part, our energy and mood are direct products of what we think about. During this time of stress, it is vital to control your thoughts to focus on today. Otherwise, thoughts may spin out of control with worry about what tomorrow might bring, creating a sense of chaos, fear, anxiety, and uncertainty. Our thoughts are like tools; they can be used for building up our confidence or tearing it down. Only you, not circumstances or other people, can control what you think about.

Are you using your thoughts well and productively, or do you feel victimized by them? You are what you think. You are the boss of what you think about. You are in charge of your mind—no one else.

Some caregivers find writing in a journal a good way to sort thoughts and feelings. It can serve as a soothing process to empty the mind of stress. Support groups also are useful as they provide a safe place to sort things out and to balance one's perception of reality. Others use reading, music, or meditation for thought control.

Self-care: Feeding Your Soul

Where is God in all of this?

Living a life with cancer at the forefront carries three dimensions: physical, emotional, and spiritual. Searching for spiritual sustenance is one of the exercises that many caregivers experience in their quest to make sense of this time in their lives. As their spiritual life begins to broaden in search for meaning and deeper understanding, many find that their priorities become rearranged. What was thought to be important before cancer—such as striving for material goods or worldly success—may now seem trivial and unimportant. What may emerge is the growing awareness and appreciation of the importance of faith and relationships with loved ones.

Pray and meditate—feed your soul. Seek spiritual sustenance. Learn from one caregiver who prays:

> Even though my loved one has this cancer, help me to learn to live, really live, this day.

Self-care: Preserving Your Energy

> My whole life has changed. I have no time for myself.

When possible, learn to unplug yourself from your patient and replug into something that will energize you and bring a greater sense of peace and pleasure. It is important to get away from cancer to recharge your battery so that you can come back refreshed and fortified to tend to your patient. Sometimes, just carving out 10 minutes for yourself can help rejuvenate and restore.

You have a very hard job. You likely are doing everything you reasonably can to take care of your loved one. Begin to learn to run on "premium caregiver fuel" by feeding your mind, your body, and your soul with thoughts and activities that build, nurture, comfort, and strengthen. This will conserve your energy over the long run.

Be good to yourself. You have the right and the responsibility to take care of yourself. This is not selfish; it is self-care. Taking short breaks now will give you the energy and strength to stay in this for the long haul.

This is exceedingly important, but difficult for caregivers to give themselves permission to do. Many caregivers may feel guilty when they leave the patient's bedside, when medically appropriate, to go do something pleasurable for themselves. However, as noted above, research is showing ... show that caregiver self-care is medically necessary for you to stay mentally and physically healthy and strong.

Self-care: Evaluating Your Priorities

> I started to become realistic. I didn't cause this cancer. I can't cure it or control it.

Becoming realistic can be a mind-altering experience. Starting from there, consider letting go of the idea that you are Superman or Superwoman.

- Practice being clear in your mind about what your job really is. Are you overfunctioning for your patient? Are you doing things that your loved one is capable of doing for himself or herself? This is not unusual, especially in the beginning. Be clear in your own mind what is really happening right now, not what "might" happen. Set reasonable limits with your loved one. Determine what self-care tasks he or she can do. A gentle reminder may be: do not do for your patient what he or she is capable of doing for himself or herself.

- Take stock of the things that are really important that "must" be done, not what "should" be done. As one caregiver said: "I made a list of the things that I absolutely had to do, like organize medications, schedule appointments, etc. I made another list of things that I was doing that just didn't really matter in the big picture. I just let those things slide off my back."

- If possible, delegate some responsibilities. Recruit others to help you.

- Learn some practical problem-solving techniques, such as how to manage medication side effects, organize a medication sheet, and develop strategies for symptom control of pain, nausea, or fatigue.

Self-care: Finding Your Strengths

> I've been able to do things that I never in a million years thought I could do.

- Identify your strengths. Some caregivers have a hard time doing this. Your personality is unique, and you bring talents and gifts to this demanding role of caregiving. What is it that you bring to the table that strengthens this situation that no one else can, or is willing, to do? What have you learned through this experience?

- Other caregivers have identified their strengths and you can, too. Focus on what you are good at doing.

Ten Practical Tips from Highly Effective Caregivers

1. Take time for yourself. Schedule some quiet time away from cancer, cancer, cancer. Practice blocking out worry, even for 10 minutes. Sit or walk in a

special location, imagining a sign that says, "No worry allowed." This is your "worry-free" appointment with yourself.

2. Create some distractions, such as working with puzzles, crosswords, computer games, knitting, cards, music, or yoga. Activities that have a rhythmic mechanical repetition are helpful and soothing.

3. Create a support system. Find someone who will serve as your cheerleader and your encourager, someone who will lean over the balcony, waving his or her arms as you run the race below in the arena, shouting, "You can do this. Keep pressing forward. Easy does it. First things first. You are stronger than you think."

4. Cry and laugh. These are all natural stress-buster activities. Find something to laugh about every day. It reduces stress, increases the heart rate and muscle activity, and releases feel-good chemicals into the brain. Even a smile can produce a moment of pleasure. Sometimes a good cry can discharge stress and bring relief.

5. Open up your horizon a bit. Caregiving can create a narrow, lonely, and shrinking world. Talk to someone at least once a day about anything other than cancer. Step outside and just look at the sky, even for a minute. Pray.

6. Learn to walk in beauty. Take notice of our natural world and the miracles of sunlight, fluttering leaves, bright flowers, floating clouds, a squirrel skirting across the grass, rain, thunder, a gentle breeze, morning dew, fountain sprays, and the rhythm and rotation of daylight and darkness with the promise of a new sunrise every morning.

7. As you walk, imagine energy and light traveling from your feet up into your mind, with each step visualizing its slow and healing course of travel through your legs, abdomen, torso, shoulders, and arms. Breathe in peace deeply and breathe out distress, counting to five each time. Imagine opening your heart and releasing musical notes, filling the air around you as you exhale. Practice.

8. Keep a journal of "Tiny Gratitudes." Gratitude is the number one positive emotion. Remember that life's greatest gifts sometimes arrive in small packages. Miracles really are everywhere when we look for them. Become a detective and look for and find the little things—the tiniest moment of beauty, the tiniest blessing, and the tiniest thing for which to be

grateful. Count your pulse or that of your loved one and be grateful.

9. Use positive self-talk. "I can cope. I am being held up by God. I can do this. Others have done it before me and I can do it, too. I've been through tough times before."

10. Join a support group. You do not have to go through this alone. Check out "Caregivers: I've Got Feelings, Too!" at MD Anderson's Place … of wellness. This group is designed to help broaden your perspective and horizon. Assuming the role of caregiver can be shocking and distressing. This group can provide a cushion of support from fellow comrades going through similar experiences in the war against cancer. It will help you organize the chaos in your head, sort through your feelings, and direct your goals and behaviors in ways you may not have considered.

Twelve Ways to Increase Caregiver Self-knowledge

Many caregivers find that learning more about the unique impact of caregiving on their own lives and those of their loved ones helps bring a sense of meaning to this difficult and bewildering time. How would you finish the following statements?

1. The ways this experience has been hard on me are:
2. Additional areas of stress that I'm handling are:
3. Things I've learned about myself and my family member are:
4. The skills and talents that I bring to this situation are:
5. The ways that this cancer has impacted our relationship are:
6. The thing that I'm most disappointed about in myself during this is:
7. The blessings that have come as a result of this experience are:
8. The spiritual meaning that I'm finding through all of this is:
9. What I've learned about the concept of control is:
10. The thing for which I'm most proud of myself during this is:
11. What I would recommend to someone just coming into this is:
12. The most helpful thing that my doctor or nurse said to me was:

How do you cope? What have you learned?

Preparing Yourself for Clinic Visits

1. Wear comfortable clothes and shoes. MD Anderson Cancer Center is a very large facility and you may be doing a lot of walking for appointments. Also bring a sweater, as room temperatures can be cool any time of year.
2. Bring something to do as you wait for appointments, such as a magazine or book to read, knitting, or cross-word puzzles.
3. Bring a current list of all medications that your loved one is taking, including dosages, length of time taken, prescribing doctor's name, and pharmacy telephone number.
4. Bring an organized list of questions for the doctor, as well as paper and a pen to take notes. Two people can hear two very different things and notes to refer to later will help.
6. Learn who the contact person is for your patient's doctor and collect that person's business card, in case you need to call the clinic later with questions. This may be the doctor's advanced practice nurse, physician assistant, or clinic nurse.
7. Remember that you are coming to one of the top cancer centers in the world. Take comfort in the fact that many have been through what you are dealing with now and have gone on to live productive and healthy lives. Through the experience of cancer, you may learn many good and interesting things about life, yourself, and your patient.

Caregivers Speak

Which of the following statements hits closest to home for you today?

- "I'm learning that I can get through anything."
- "I'm learning that I'm stronger than I think."
- "As long as I stay focused on the present, I can decrease my fear."
- "I have to stay connected to the outside world to keep my sanity."
- "I learned that despair is presumptuous. How do you know what's going to happen?"
- "Be good to yourself."
- "My children have seen a marriage in action during a very hard time."
- "Take power naps."
- "Through all of this, we've become closer. We're now like a tube of Super Glue."

- "Focus on today and only today. Take it one day at a time."
- "Every day, treat yourself to a good and new thing."
- "Don't watch the news. It's way too depressing."
- "Have the courage to be joyful. Laughter is like internal jogging."
- "During this time, ask 'given what is, what am I now to do? What is the lesson here?' "
- "Hug someone you love."
- "I can't fix everything, but today I can do at least one thing."
- "I'm resilient."
- "I'm the organizer. I can see the reality of things."
- "Prayer works."
- "Material things don't matter anymore."
- "Control? Ha! It doesn't exist."
- "Somehow, some way, maintain positive experiences. I try to keep a 'Positive Things Happen List' at the end of each day, no matter how small the event."
- "This whole thing has brought us closer together."
- "This is the hardest thing I've ever done in my life, but it is the most honorable."

A Caregiver's Bill of Rights

I have the right:

To take care of myself. This is not an act of selfishness. It will give me the capability of taking better care of my loved one.

To seek help from others even though my loved one may object. I recognize the limits of my own endurance and strength.

To maintain facets of my own life that do not include the person I care for, just as I would if he or she was healthy. I know that I do everything that I reasonably can for this person, and I have the right to do some things just for myself.

To get angry, be depressed and express other difficult feelings occasionally.

To reject any attempt by my loved one (either conscious or unconscious) to manipulate me through guilt, anger or depression.

To receive consideration, affection, forgiveness and acceptance for what I do from my loved one as long as I offer these qualities in return.

To take pride in what I accomplish and to applaud the courage it has sometimes taken to meet the needs of my loved one.

To protect my individuality and my right to make a life for myself that will sustain me in the time when my loved one no longer needs my full-time help.

To expect and demand that, as new strides are made in finding resources to aid physically and mentally impaired older persons in our country, similar strides will be made toward aiding and supporting caregivers.

Add your own statements of rights to the list. Read it to yourself every day.

Reprinted from "Caregiving: Helping An Aging Loved One," a book

by Jo Horne

Caregivers' ABCs

To be a good giver of care, take care of yourself every single day. Perhaps the following poetic list of reminders from a fellow caregiver will encourage and offer ways:

A	an apple each day, attend, appreciate, ask
B	breathe and remember to brush
C	cry, crosswords, crochet, climb stairs, connect
D	dream, draw, doodle, delegate
E	exhale, eye drops, exercise
F	friends and family, feelings, fresh fruit
G	giggle, gratitude, ground yourself
H	hold hands and hug, regard hope, honesty
I	intention, inhale, improvise, interact
J	jog, joke and journal writing
K	kindness, knowledge, knit
L	love, listen, laugh and live the moment
M	music, meditate, movement and muse
N	navigate, notice, nurture
O	observe objectively, remain open
P	patience, pray and read a bit of poetry aloud
Q	quiet the self, questions, quick naps
R	read, reflect, rest and relax
S	stretch, smile, sleep, shop, sushi
T	tea, time away, treasure and trust
U	unload feelings on paper
V	vitamins, vegetables and new point of view
W	walk, drink water and wash hands often
X	exercise
Y	yoga and yes to yourself
Z	zest—add flavor with enjoyment remember the zoo in Hermann Park.

Edi Klingner, caregiver, wife, poet, and artist

■ SURVIVORSHIP AND COUPLES

Many couples report greater closeness during the crisis of cancer and fear loss of this once daily life interferences and interruptions begin. There are several key issues common to many cancer survivors and caregivers. While quantity of life is most desired, so is quality of life following treatment. The impact of treatment and its aftermath affects both patient and partner in different ways.

The loss of intimacy and the fear of recurrence are two major concerns of many cancer survivors and caregivers. Both the patient and caregiver have needs, expectations, and perspectives about these issues that are unique to the individual and may be compatible with, or contrary to, their partner's. Many couples find communication about these differences to be difficult and stressful. Each is grieving in a unique way the loss of the "normal" life each had before cancer, as a couple and individually. Each may withhold thoughts and feelings about this in an attempt to protect the other's sense of hope. Adjusting to the "new normal" is not easy, and can at times result in conflict, loneliness, and misunderstandings. I often counsel patients to extend an invitation to their partner for a clear and honest discussion about the issues at hand. Many times, this effort can open the door to a meaningful dialogue. In other cases, it may require the facilitation of an objective third party to get the ball rolling.

It is my experience in working with couples that each partner desires to be given "air time" and permission to discuss one's feelings and thoughts in a safe environment, free of criticism or disapproval. A skilled marriage and family therapist who specializes in oncology can be of help in the reestablishment of closeness, support, and intimacy between the patient and loved one. For some, counseling may not be of interest initially, but perhaps it will be in future. It may be helpful to know that help is out there and one need not go through this next phase of life alone.

■ SUMMARY

With continued distress, emotional and physical fatigue may overwhelm a caregiver's initial strength and best intentions. As the patient continues to experience the chronicity of peaks and valleys of response to treatment rather than maintaining a smooth course of planned recovery, caregivers may begin to doubt the integrity and capability of their best efforts. They may begin to interpret their efforts as inadequate when the patient's progress is stalled by treatment complications. Caregivers may evolve into questioning their sense of personal competency, which initiates now a new wave of emotional and physical exhaustion as they "try harder" in the face of perceived caregiver failure.

Providing information to patients and their caregivers can assist coping and skill development.[15] The literature notes that caregivers express two primary needs—informational and psychological.[22] Northouse and Peters-Golden[22] found that caregivers report difficulty in obtaining appropriate information, particularly symptom management, from the medical team, although caregivers report that it is crucial to them. The most crucial times for information are at the time of diagnosis, during hospitalization, start of new treatments, at the time of recurrence, and during the dying phase. The quality of interaction between the caregiver, patient, and the health care team is vital. When ineffectual communication is present between the medical team and the patient and caregiver, distress and fear of uncertainty are exacerbated in both the patient and caregiver.[23] According to Given et al,[13] the caregiver's well-being must be our concern; family caregivers have a legitimate and crucial role in the cancer care team.

We believe that this psychoeducational caregiver model addresses the need for both psychological education and self-exploration in order to manage the inherent, insidious, and all too often unrecognized stress associated with prolonged caregiving. As noted above, prolonged exposure to the stressors relative to providing care for another human being may predispose caregivers to later medical consequences of their own. It is hoped that providing supportive training for emotional self-regulation may favorably impact both the present and future functioning and physical well-being of caregivers.

KEY POINTS

- A caregiver is "a person who is responsible for attending to the needs of a child or dependent adult."[4] This is a simple explanation fraught with diversified minefields, such as "a person," which likely translates into one unpaid and untrained immediate family member shouldering most of the physical, emotional, financial, and medical caregiving burden.

- Cancer caregivers are a ubiquitous, stressed, and burdened population with little social or professional support. Given that patients are now living longer, and in some cases, sicker, the role of and need for caregiving is extended. Because of the need to control medical costs and because of lengthened survival rates, the home has become an outpatient medical care setting.

- Caregivers are now performing complex medical tasks that not too long ago were performed solely by highly trained and experienced inpatient nurses. This burden, over time, produces a heightened level of chronic stress.

- With continued distress, emotional and physical fatigue may overwhelm a caregiver's initial strength and best intentions. As the patient continues to experience the chronicity of peaks and valleys of response to treatment rather than maintaining a smooth course of planned recovery, caregivers may begin to doubt the integrity and capability of their best efforts.

- Providing information to caregivers can assist coping and skill development. Our psychoeducational intervention model of building caregiver competence allows the caregiver an ongoing process of sifting through and sorting out beliefs and values about the caregiver role, the medical necessity of self-care, and other life and death issues. It carries the potential of redefining a realistic appraisal of the caregiving function, what it is and, even more importantly, what it is not.

- A primary assumption of this model is that caregivers can develop skills of emotional self-regulation as an aid for emotional health and physical energy conservation. A caregiver learns, during the group experience, that the primary source of control lies not in controlling the patient's medical outcome, but rather in self-regulation and modulation of emotional reactivity to an unpredictable medical event, instead of controlling the event itself.

REFERENCES

1. American Cancer Society Inc. *Surveillance and Health Policy Research.* 2009. John Wiley & Sons New Jersey

2. Jemal A, Tiwari RC, Murray T, et al, American Cancer Society. Cancer statistics. *CA Cancer J Clin.* 2004;54(1):10–27.

3. Holland JC, Lewis S. *The Human Side of Cancer: Living with Hope, Coping with Uncertainty*. New York, NY: HarperCollins; 2000:281.

4. *The American Heritage® Stedman's Medical Dictionary*. Retrieved June 1, 2009, from Dictionary.com.

5. Given BA, Given CW, Kozachik S. Family support in advanced cancer. *CA Cancer J Clin*. 2001;51:213–230.

6. Carter P, Chang B. Sleep and depression in caregivers. *Cancer Nurs*. 2000;23(6):410–415.

7. Cameron JI, Fanche RL, Cheung AM, Stewart DE. Lifestyle interference and emotional distress in family caregivers of advanced cancer patients. *Cancer*. 2002;94(2):521–527.

8. Flaskerud JH, Carter PA, Lee P. Distressing emotions in female caregiver of people with AIDS, age-related dementias, and advanced-stage cancers. *Perspect Psychiatr Care*. 2000;36(4):121–130.

9. Kiecolt-Glaser JK, Preacher KJ, MacCallum RC, Atkinson C, Malarkey WB, Glaser R. Chronic stress and age-related increases in the proinflammatory cytokine IL-6. *Proc Natl Acad Sci U S A*. 2003;100(15):9090–9095.

10. Hileman JW, Lackey NR, Hassanein RS. Identifying the needs of home caregiving patients with cancer. *Oncol Nurs Forum*. 1992;19:771–777.

11. Houts PS, Yasko JM, Kahn SB, Schelzel GW. Unmet psychological, social, and economic needs of persons with cancer in Philadelphia. *Cancer*. 1986;58:8–14.

12. Soothill K, Morris SM, Harman JC, Francis B, Thomas C, McIllmurray MB. Informal carers of cancer patients: what are their unmet psychosocial needs? *Health Soc Care Community*. 2001;9(6):464–475.

13. Given BA, Given CW, Kozachik S. Family support in advanced cancer. *CA Cancer J Clin*. 2001;51(4):213–231.

14. Slevin ML, Nichols SE, Downer SM, et al. Emotional support for cancer patients: what do patients really want? *Br J Cancer*. 1996;74(8):1275–1279.

15. Pasacreta JV, Barg F, Nuamah I, McCorkle R. Participant characteristics before and 4 months after attendance at a family caregiver cancer education program. *Cancer Nurs*. 2000;23(4):295–303.

16. Spillers RL, Wellisch DK, Kim Y, Matthews BA, Baker F. Family caregivers and guilt in the context of cancer care. *Psychosomatics*. 2008;49:6.

17. Corbin JN, Strauss A. A nursing model for chronic illness management based upon the Trajectory Framework. *Sch Inq Nurs Pract*. 1991;5:155–174.

18. Buchner J, Loscalzo M, Zabora J, Houts PS, Hooker C, BrintzenhofeSzoc K. Problem-solving cancer care education for patients and caregivers. *Cancer Pract*. 2001;9(2):66–70.

19. Toseland R, Blanchard C, McCallion P. A problem solving intervention for caregivers of cancer patients. *Soc Sci Med*. 1995;40:517–528.

20. Yalom I. *The Theory and Practice of Group Psychotherapy*. 4th ed. Basic Books; New York. 1995.

21. Fitch M. Psychosocial issues with a cancer diagnosis. *Hotspot Newsletter*. 1999;1(4). page 2

22. Northouse LL, Peters-Golden H. Cancer and the family: strategies to assist spouses. *Semin Oncol Nurs*. 1993;9:74–82.

23. Baile W, Buckman R, Lenzi R, Glober G, Beale EA, Kudelka AP. SPIKES—a six-step protocol for delivering bad news: application to the patient with cancer. *Oncologist*. 2000;5:302–311.

CHAPTER 17

Spirituality and Religion Perspectives on Illness and Suffering

• *David R. Jenkins*

In recent years, there has been an accumulation of empirical evidence demonstrating the positive role of religious practice and spirituality on mental health and quality of life (QOL) pertaining to coping with chronic disease. In this case, QOL generally refers to "... those aspects of life and human function considered essential for living fully."[1] Attention to holistic patient care, or "whole patient care," is now accepted as the best practice within medical care. In addition, the interdisciplinary approach to health care has a strong advocate in the Joint Commission on Accreditation of Healthcare (JCAHO), which acknowledged in 2003 that "...patients' psychosocial, spiritual, and cultural values affect how they respond to their care."[2] Nevertheless, recipients of health care in the USA report dissatisfaction with the lack of spiritually sensitive care.[3] This chapter delineates the influences that family and culture play in the patient's religious development and spiritual coping with illness and suffering. For the purpose of this discussion, "family" is defined as "... any group of people who are related biologically, legally, or emotionally."[4] Like Seaburn, I assume that all families exist within a cultural web or context that must be taken into consideration when trying to understand the decision-making process in which they are engaged. To continue Seaburn's thought: "Each family may be influenced by its own history with illness, its health beliefs, its religious tradition(s), its racial background, its nation of origin, and other vital factors that contribute to how families define themselves and make meaning of their experiences." The term "culture" is defined as "... the sum of the integrated patterns of knowledge, beliefs, and behaviors of a given community."[5] Furthermore, it can be asserted that culture "... mediates the rapport between the individual and the outer world, and it contributes to a person's identity."[6] It can also be argued that "family" is one form or context that fits the definition for culture. The family nexus functions as the most intimate relational form of culture, and thus plays a primary role in the development of personhood. Thus, the starting point for understanding how to alleviate suffering in the context of illness, taking into account the impact of family and culture on the life of the patient, is to have a basic grasp of personhood and the nature of suffering.

"Religion," for the purposes of this discussion, can be understood as the ways in which communities of faith organize and live their lives in relation to each other and the transcendent. On the other hand, spirituality is defined as: "... that human dimension that seeks meaning through intra-, inter-, and transpersonal connectedness." It should be understood that religion and spirituality are complicated constructs, often defying description in terms of how they function to bring about healing and wholeness in the context of illness and suffering. Nevertheless, religion and spirituality offer human beings the possibility of transcending life's vicissitudes, such as illness, and have the potential for transforming lives that are broken by disease and suffering. To understand how this can be so, it is necessary to first develop a basic working model of personhood.

■ THE NATURE OF PERSONHOOD

Religions, philosophy, and the sciences have all provided unique perspectives about the nature of personhood.

Cassell[7] has made the most substantive contribution to our understanding of the nature of personhood in the context of understanding illness and suffering. Dr Cassell identified approximately 13 aspects of personhood that need to be taken into consideration if illness and suffering are to be fully understood and effectively responded to by those who seek to alleviate suffering. For the purpose of this discussion, those aspects of personhood that relate directly to the person's embeddedness within family and culture are worth mentioning here. First, a person has a cultural background. "Just as a person is part of a culture and a society, these elements are part of the person."[7] Furthermore, cultural norms and definitions have an enormous impact on the sick and can be an untold source of either strength or suffering. In this respect, the intensity of ties to the family and larger culture cannot be overemphasized. To complicate matters, in the modern-day United States, many cultures and subcultures coexist, and offer individuals a myriad of possible reference groups with which to attach. This suggests that it is more difficult in our complex, dynamic, interwoven modern world to characterize any one individual in terms of the cultural matrix that informs one's worldview and experience of life. Thus, any patient–family assessment models or methodologies must resist the mistake of stereotyping or labeling, and must seek to truly understand the patient and family by letting them share how their worldviews function in the context of their illness and suffering. This requires patience and respect on the part of the caregiver, as well as a willingness to temporarily suspend all prejudgments they may have about a patient's particular culture or cultural practices that might inhibit their ability to provide compassionate care.

Second, all theories of human development, as well as religious traditions, will readily agree that, as Dr Cassell states: "No person exists without others; there is no consciousness without a consciousness of others ...." Furthermore, it is in relationships with others that the full range of human emotions and behavior finds expression. It follows then, as Dr Cassell asserts, that the extent and nature of a sick person's relationships influence the degree of suffering from a disease. The human dynamics existent within the family system, including cultural influences, have a determinative effect on the personhood of the patient. This makes the family the primary locus for human development. Not only does the family matrix impact the development of personality and personal attributes and behaviors, but also family and culture greatly influence the religious identity and spiritual development of the person-as-patient. This is particularly true because every family and every larger culture has something to impart about their respective understandings about illness and suffering, and the meaning of life. Thus, every patient comes to the place of disease and illness with a worldview about illness and suffering that is likely to be largely informed and supported by family and culture.

The patient's religious beliefs and practices, as well as views about the world, are in a very real sense "handed down" or inherited from the family and cultural matrices in which the patient is embedded. Obviously, families and cultures change over time, and thus have a dynamic impact on the patient's religious beliefs and practices. In a complex modern society, such as that of the United States, inhabitants are likely to be informed both by the "handed-down" beliefs and practices of family and by particular cultural traditions, and at the same time are free to varying degrees to assimilate religious views and practices from any number of religious and nonreligious perspectives, often arriving at the hospital or clinic with a syncretistic spiritual worldview. This is all the more reason for those charged with providing spiritual care in the context of health care to embark upon a thorough patient–family screening process that allows for the nuances of a particular patient and family to be expressed as part of the process of creating a patient history. The fact that the patient is embedded in a dynamic, ever-changing family and cultural web both complicates and enriches the possibilities for religious and spiritual development. When disease strikes and chronic illness ensues, the health crisis often includes a crisis of faith and belief. In the case of cancer, it can be said that cancer is essentially a family disease. In addition, illness, whether acute or chronic, usually creates challenges for the family, including the likelihood of disruption and discord with family and larger social circles. For example, it may be the case that the desires of the patient, for religious reasons, may or may not align with those of the family, resulting in conflict and distress. It is not unusual to see this dynamic at play when a decision about health care requires ethical considerations by the patient, family, and health care team.

Members of the health care team may become frustrated by the seemingly unending variations of religious practices and spiritual worldviews with which they come in contact through their interactions with patients and families. What is required, as a starting point, is a well-documented patient history that takes into account the religious views and practices of the patient, including any possible sources of support as well as discord within the family and cultural systems that might impact the treatment plan. In addition, the health care team needs to include, or at least be aware of, the services of chaplains, specifically trained to tease out the nuances implied in the patient's religious perspective about illness and suffering, while providing empathic support to the patient and family. Listed below are some important topics for discussion with the patient, which may help create a supportive alliance between the health care team, the patient, and the family.

It is important for the health care team to recognize that illness and suffering can be the vehicles through which spiritual growth ensues, although one should never conclude, therefore, that suffering in itself is good. The point here is that for many patients, there are inherent sources of strength within family circles and cultural/religious practices that should not be overlooked by the health care team. The roles of relational support and ritual practice carry significant power for healing and wholeness for many patients. If cancer has the potential to be a disintegrating force, certainly it can be argued and demonstrated in clinical practice that the spiritual resources that reside in family and culture have the power to reintegrate personhood, while maintaining a sense of human dignity in the context of illness.

Third, the aspect of personhood that may be of greatest importance relates to the human ability to make meaning out of life experiences, and the corresponding human capacity to experience transcendence. Dr Cassell[7] asserts: "Meaning and transcendence offer two additional ways by which the suffering associated with destruction of a part of personhood is ameliorated. Assigning a meaning to the injurious condition often reduces or even resolves the suffering associated with it." The process of meaning-making requires time and reflection. Reflection requires openness to looking at one's life circumstances, including illness, in new ways. This, in turn, may require a listening support that is attentive to the ways in which the sufferer is struggling with illness. Such a presence often comes to the patient as a result of referral to one with specific training,

such as counseling or pastoral care. However, often, family and friends can be the "listening presence" needed if one is willing to let the patient share openly without being judgmental or impatient, seeking a "quick fix" to alleviate the suffering.

"Transcendence is probably the most powerful way in which one is restored to wholeness after an injury to personhood. When experienced, transcendence locates the person in a far larger landscape." Cassell[7] continues: "Such an experience need not involve religion in any formal sense; however, in its transpersonal dimension, it is deeply spiritual." In recent years, a growing number of cancer patients have openly communicated meaning and hope through the sharing of their personal journeys as cancer survivors, often sharing transcendent life-changing moments. This in no way suggests that illness and suffering are inherently capable of producing "good" in the life of the sufferer or the community. In the deepest sense, the human capacity to experience a greater "good" out of illness and suffering is the gift of experiencing the transcendent in life.

■ THE NATURE OF SUFFERING

Over the centuries, much has been written and expressed through the arts about the nature of suffering. Human suffering, in a sense, defies any neat and easy descriptions because it comes in so many forms and reaches such depths within the human experience. This discussion will focus on suffering in the context of disease. First, it is important to distinguish between the terms "disease" and "illness." If the disease is cancer, the illness is the subjective experience of that cancer. The particular disease is a pathophysiologic process that can be described with the use of objective medical, biological, and chemical terminology. Illness, as the subjective lived experience of the disease, is difficult to describe and impossible to objectify. Much patience and empathy is required to truly grasp the extent of suffering. Suffering, in fact, may include physical pain, but is not limited to it. As Dr Cassell asserts: "Suffering occurs when an impending destruction of the person is perceived; it continues until the threat of disintegration has passed or until the integrity of the person can be restored in some other manner." An important aspect of suffering for this discussion is the fact that suffering, like hope, is often a shared experience. This is particularly true for the family of the cancer patient. It has been suggested that cancer is a family illness and recognized for the impact it has on the entire family. In fact, the findings of some empirical studies have discovered that the extent of shared suffering by family members, or entire cultures, can eclipse that of the one who suffers.[8] This is because humans can identify with the sufferer, while feeling helpless, to provide any form of alleviation.

On the other hand, human suffering often has a way of creating barriers to help that lead to the isolation of the sufferer(s). Not all human beings can respond to suffering with compassion. In fact, sometimes the professional caregivers tend to minimize the effects of disease on the integrity of the sufferer. For example, until recently, effective pain management was underreported by caregivers, that is, patient reports of pain were not taken seriously. Generally, at the conscious level, human beings are prone to avoid the suffering, and thereby cause its effects to increase. Suffering, as a human experience, is likely much more prevalent than anyone might imagine. Cassell[7] summarizes: "People suffer from what they have lost of themselves in relation to the world of objects, events, and relationships." A person has roles. People are their roles. To the extent that disease and sickness cause a diminishment of key roles, or force an unexpected change of roles, the patient suffers. This, of course, also applies to family members, who often face unwanted and/or unplanned role reversals, for example.

With respect to cancer as a disease, its complexity and chronic nature tend to increase the likelihood that suffering will be extended in time as well as among an ever-larger web of relationships, including the family and health care team. In addition, the extent of suffering is not limited to the effects of the disease and its impact on roles and relationships. In today's health care world, the financial impact of cancer as an added burden to patient and family cannot be understated. The cost of health care is not only an additional source of distress for the patient and family web, but also a source of national distress. Society is faced with ethical, political, and financial choices that may either help alleviate human suffering or actually increase the extent of suffering, even when decisions have been made with the intention to relieve suffering. There are, in fact, no signs yet that cancer as a disease is going to be eliminated as a social dilemma. On the contrary, with an aging population, the extent to which cancer is a social burden will only increase over time. Because human suffering is a shared experience, there is a very real danger that the burden of care will outstrip available resources. This is one reason why a truly interdisciplinary model of care must include family and community, as well as health care professionals.[9]

■ THE GOALS OF MEDICINE

It is in this social context that medicine's goal—to relieve suffering—must be examined. In the past, the relief of suffering was often narrowly understood as the removal of pathology, or at least the reduction of suffering if the disease could not be effectively treated. Today, the art of medicine, as it relates to the alleviation of suffering, must take into account the fullness and complexity of the human being as a unity of mind, body, and spirit. As Cassell[7] asserts: "Attempting to understand what suffering is and how physicians might truly be devoted to its relief will require that medicine and its critics overcome the dichotomy between mind and body and the associated dichotomies between subjective and objective and between person and object." In order to address its primary goal, medicine must be truly interdisciplinary. There must, for example, be ample opportunity for all disciplines that relate to human development to be involved in the alleviation of suffering. In addition, an interdisciplinary approach must include the patient and the family as members of the team. This, in fact, may be one of the most effective interventions for alleviating suffering. Dr Cassell[7] continues: "Recovery from suffering often involves help, as though people who have lost parts of themselves can be sustained by the personhood of others until their own recovers. This is one of the latent functions of physicians: to lend strength. A group, too, may lend strength. Consider the success of groups of the similarly afflicted in easing the burden of illness (e.g., women with mastectomies, people with ostomies, and even parents or family members of the diseased)." By creating a holistic health care model that views the patient as a member of a living web comprised of family and cultural influences, including religious beliefs, practices, and spiritual needs, the caregiver team positively influences the likelihood that wellness will be experienced by the patient. The ability of the health care team to take into account family and cultural religious influences can also have an empowering impact on the health care team. To that end, some key points and strategies are offered below, including a relational, interpretive patient–family assessment model.

■ GUIDING PRINCIPLES FOR A HOLISTIC PATIENT–FAMILY INTERVENTION MODEL

1. *View and treat the patient as a unity of body, mind, and spirit*. This means that all disciplines that have anything to say about these three primary aspects of personhood need to be involved at the interdisciplinary level in the treatment of the patient.

2. *Utilize a model of patient autonomy that is informed by relationships, referred to as "autonomy-in-relation."*[4] This patient care model takes into account the fact that all individuals are relational by nature. It also asserts that input from significant others is inevitable and may strengthen the patient's and family's capacities to cope with illness and suffering.

3. *Utilize spiritual assessment models that take into account the spiritual needs of both patient and family and that use a relational methodology*. Recent empirical studies illustrate that there is no significant differences between the perceived spiritual needs of patients and their caregivers.[10] It is therefore important to assess the spiritual needs of both the patient and their caregivers. The spiritual assessment model in Table 17-1 can be provided to both patients and their families.

This patient–family spiritual assessment model takes into account the primary aspects of personhood delineated above by Cassell.[7] In addition, it recognizes that not all patients are conversant or fluent in religious language, and thus can be used with patients and family members from either religious or nonreligious backgrounds. Perhaps most importantly, this model is relational, and requires a careful listening presence by the person who administers the assessment. This, in turn, has the potential to engender trust between clinic staff, patient, and family members. Obviously, it requires that clinical staff be able to listen carefully to responses in order to help the patient and family determine what is indeed important to them, in terms of religious/spiritual needs. In this respect, the categories offer concrete direction for the patient, family member(s), and staff. With this information, interventions and mutual goals can be established that will help empower the entire health care team, including the patient and family members.

Of course, there are other ways to assess religious and spiritual needs other than the semistructured interpretive approach described above. For example, another relational approach would be to organize small support groups that could focus on supporting family members where the patients have similar types of cancer. This approach often creates a sense of hope and solidarity among family members. Such groups can actually be co-led, for example, with the first half of the meeting led by a clinical staff to help families with questions and concerns related to the treatment plan. The second half could be led by a social worker or chaplain to help family members address the kinds of questions listed above in the assessment model. The emphasis is on building relationship between the patient, family members, and health care team for the sake of creating an optimum setting for trust, hope, and healing.

Another approach to this particular spiritual assessment model allows for the possibility that the assessment form simply be placed in a convenient location for patients and family members, with the understanding that it is primarily used first as a private reflection tool. Request for support would then come from the patient and/or family members as a result of perception of need, to the assigned clinical staff.

In fact, any combination of the three spiritual assessment methods mentioned above could be established by the clinical staff, increasing the likelihood for timely assessment of spiritual needs in the context of an ever-changing medical situation.

■ KEY PATIENT ASSESSMENT STRATEGIES

When possible, it is recommended to include primary family members when discussing religious needs and concerns to determine to what extent there is unanimity among the family.

When taking a patient history, determine from the patient and family specific religious practices and spiritual needs that the health care team should be aware of that may help support a positive outcome in the treatment of the disease. What, specifically, do the patient and family members need during this time of crisis?

Determine any points of potential conflict about the treatment plan that may exist within the patient–family relationships.

Keep in mind that social workers and chaplains are specifically trained and adept at helping to create a full patient assessment that takes into consideration the kinds of issues addressed here.

Determine any specific cultural needs/issues that may complicate treatment, such as dietary needs and religious ritual needs.

■ **TABLE 17-1. Themes and Categories of Spiritual Needs**

Categories	Themes/Spiritual Needs
Needs associated with relating to an ultimate other	Need to – Know God's will – Resign yourself to God being in control of your/your loved one's illness – Get right with God – Believe that God has or will heal – Remember how God has guided or helped you/your loved one – Feel that there is something out there looking after you/your loved one – Know that your/your loved one's situation is in God's hand
Need for positivity, gratitude, and hope	Need to – Have hope that you/your loved one will be well – Keep a positive outlook – Count your blessings – Tell others about the good things in your life – Just enjoy life – Have confidence/faith within yourself – Not take life for granted
Need to give and receive love from other persons	Need to – Make the world a better place – Return others' kindnesses – Protect your family from seeing you suffer – Try to help others – Get right with others (eg, forgiving or being forgiven) – Become more gracious about receiving care from other people – Know that others are praying (or thinking positive thoughts) for you – Be appreciated by others – Be with others you consider to be family – Not be a burden to others
Need to review beliefs	Need to – Review what you believe – Wonder if your beliefs about God are correct – Think about what it means to live spiritually (eg, to have faith, to forgive) – Ask "why" questions (eg, Why me/us? Or why not me? Or what did I/we do to deserve this?) – Think about the unfairness of what has been happening to you
Creating meaning, finding purpose	Need to – Get over or get past asking "why me?" – Find helpful explanations for why this illness has happened – Become aware of positive things that have come with this illness – Realize that there are other people who are worse off – Sense that there is a reason for being alive now – Try to make life count – Lessen the frustration of not being able to do meaningful things – Reevaluate your life
Religious needs	Need to – Receive prayer or a religious ritual (eg, a sacrament) from a religious leader – Participate in a religious or spiritual meeting (eg, worship at a chapel) – Listen to religious programs or music on TV or radio

Continued

Categories	Themes/Spiritual Needs
■ **TABLE 17-1. Themes and Categories of Spiritual Needs** (continued)	
Preparing for death	– Pray privately – Read scriptures or spirit-nurturing material – Have quiet time or space to reflect or meditate Need to – Make sure personal business is in order, just in case of death – Balance thoughts about dying with hoping for health – Know that there will be a purpose for your/your loved one's death, whenever it happens

Reproduced with permission from Taylor, EJ.[10]

From the perspective of the family, determine how each family member's role within the family can contribute toward a supportive atmosphere for all. Include them as members of the health care team.

■ KEY TREATMENT STRATEGIES

The treatment plan is most likely to succeed when it is developed through an interdisciplinary process that includes patient and family. With respect to addressing religious and spiritual needs, it is recommended to include a chaplain on the care team.

Allow the patient and family members opportunity to express and share their feelings and provide them with empathic support. This approach conveys respect and values their deeper hopes and fears, building trust between patient, family, and health care workers.

Whenever the health care team meets to review treatment strategies, be sure to specifically address the impact of the family and culture and pay attention to religious and spiritual sources of hope and comfort, as well as make note of any signs of discord.

KEY POINTS

■ Religious practice and spirituality have an important impact on mental health and QOL pertaining to coping with cancer.

■ When taking a patient history, pay attention to the patient's religious views and practices, including family and cultural influences that may impact the treatment plan.

■ When meeting with the patient for an initial assessment and history, always consider him or her as a member of a larger cultural web, most notably the family.

■ Take into consideration the extent to which the religious and cultural views and practices of the patient and family support a trajectory toward healing and wholeness, especially when the effects of the disease cannot be abated.

REFERENCES

1. Mor V. Cancer patients' quality of life over the disease course: lessons from the real world. *J Chronic Dis.* 1987;40(6):535–544.

2. Clark PA, Drain M, Malone MP. Addressing patients' emotional and spiritual needs. *Jt Comm J Qual Saf.* 2003;20(12):659–670.

3. Post SG, Puchalski CM, Larson DB. Physicians and patient spirituality; professional boundaries, competency, and ethics. *Ann Intern Med.* 2000;132:578–583.

4. Seaburn DB, McDaniel SH, Kim S, Bassen D. The role of the family in resolving bioethical dilemmas: clinical insights from a family systems perspective. *J Clin Ethics.* 2004;15(2):123–133.

5. Olweny C. The ethics and conduct of cross-cultural research in developing countries. *Psychooncology.* 1994;3:11–20.

6. Surbone A. The quandary of cultural diversity. *J Palliat Care.* 2003;19(1):7–8.

7. Cassell EJ. The relief of suffering. *Arch Intern Med.* 1983;143(3):522–523.

8. Humphrey LJ. New insights on the emotional response of cancer patients and their spouses: where do they find help? *J Pastoral Care*. 1995;49(2):149–156.

9. Ferrell BR. The family. In: Doyle D, Hanks GWC, MacDonald N, eds. *Oxford Textbook of Palliative Medicine*. 2nd ed. Oxford University Press. 1999: 909–917.

10. Taylor, EJ. Spiritual needs of patients with cancer and family caregivers. *Cancer Nurs*. 2003;26(4):260–266.

SECTION V

Special Populations

Children and Cancer

• *Rhonda Robert and Martha Askins*

◼ THE IMPACT OF A CANCER DIAGNOSIS AND TREATMENT

"I lost my manners after cancer."

—9 year old, posttreatment, juvenile pilocytic astrocytoma

A diagnosis of cancer is universally distressing, and most people have impaired daily functions during the first weeks after diagnosis. Most persons adjust independently of professional mental health services and report mastery over the challenges associated with diagnosis and treatment, although some (1–13%) develop a mental illness, mostly depression and anxiety disorders, and about one fourth of those diagnosed with cancer (20–25%) need a targeted intervention to foster adjustment.[1]

Children and adolescents treated with cell therapy transplantation oftentimes have had long-term illness (congenital, relapsed cancer), a guarded prognosis, stressful treatment regimen, and significant late effects. Phipps et al[2] found that even before transplantation, patients had compromised health-related quality of life. Although health-related quality of life may improve with the health gains after transplantation,[3] samples of long-term survivors have either compromised health-related quality of life[4] or developmental differences such as less autonomy, more dependence on parents, and less risk-taking behavior, for example, substance abuse and gambling.[5]

Children with bone marrow failure syndromes (BMFS) are oftentimes treated in the same centers as children with cancer. They frequent outpatient clinics and

have daily behavioral and medical prescriptions. Many are chronically ill, have medical restrictions, and are disabled. Calaminus et al[6] reported that children with BMFS have more emotional concerns than healthy controls and young adult cancer patients (>18 years of age) and an overall impaired quality of life.

Identifying those who need professional mental health services is one goal for those providing services to the pediatric cancer patient and the family. Methods for identifying patients in need of mental health services include questionnaire and interview. Structured, paper–pencil screening questionnaires, such as the PAT-2,[7] and quality of life measures (eg, Varni's PedsQL Cancer Specific and Fatigue modules[8–10]) may be utilized for this purpose. Each consists of multiple items and domains of assessment. The PedsQL modules have parallel forms for both patient and parent report. Interviewing the patient and parent may be equally as helpful. The questions can be symptom based, such as the following from the Memorial Symptom Assessment Scale[11]:

- Did you feel *sad* yesterday or today?
- Did you feel *worried* yesterday or today?
- Did you have trouble going to *sleep* the last two nights?

Interview questions may explore normal aspects of daily living, for example, How is school? ... social life?[12] Adjustment-to-illness questions have been proposed by Mack and Wolfe[13]:

- What concerns you most about your/your child's illness?

- What is your understanding of what is ahead for you/ your child?
- As you think about your/your child's illness, what are your hopes?
- As you think about your/your child's illness, what are your worries?
- As you think about your/your child's illness, what is the most important to you right now?

Many, if not most, clinical mental health services will be aimed toward adjustment, and adjustment is usually fostered by acquisition of new self-help strategies and skills. For example, Maurice-Stam and colleagues[14] have developed a group intervention to empower children and teenagers treated for cancer. The program has been well received, and participants benefit significantly. Behavioral–emotional adjustment, social competence, information-seeking skills, relaxation skills, and positive thinking were fostered. The program consists of six sessions (subprograms for 8–12 and 13–18 years of age), and interventions include communication with health care providers (giving and seeking information), cancer treatment and late effects education, relaxation, and social skill building specific to feeling or being different as a result of cancer, and positive self-talk strategies.

■ ADJUSTMENT TO CANCER

Communication

"Yeah, could I say something? After all, this conversation is about me—no? Here's an idea, if you want to know something about me—ask me. Yep, yep, that's right. Who exactly am I supposed to talk to about medical problems? And what are these people supposed to do anyways? A little information, if you please."

—31 year old, long-term survivor, suprasellar germinoma

Learning of one's cancer diagnosis is stressful and anxiety provoking. The method of communication can facilitate adjustment to the news of diagnosis. Direct and open communication about the illness is associated with healthy adjustment and may be more predictive of adjustment than the severity of the illness.[15,16] Guidelines for communicating the cancer diagnosis have been established, and the best practice standards suggest that treatment teams follow a standard communication protocol.[17] A fine example of a communication protocol for oncology professionals has been developed by Baile[18] at the University of Texas MD Anderson Cancer Center. Al-

though developed with adults in mind, the model can be adapted for children and their parents.

Some aspects of communicating a cancer diagnosis to a child versus an adult are unique. An aspect of communication unique to the pediatric patient is the negotiation with parents and child as to the possible formats for medical conversations. The format may be patient only; patient and parent simultaneously; parent first, followed by parent and patient simultaneously; or parent only. Negotiating and reevaluating the fit of the format for each family is encouraged.

Another issue specific to communicating a cancer diagnosis to a child is parents' natural desire to protect a child. However, the child needs information to understand the sensory experience of illness and treatment, as well as the new health care–related experiences. In the absence of sound information from caregivers, a child's imagination may conjure ideas far worse than the reality. Simple, accurate information will ground the child and help modulate anxiety. Open communication fosters "togetherness." Not being alone brings great comfort to persons of all ages, especially a child. Children's books can help parents initiate cancer-specific conversations:

- *"Why Charlie Brown Why:" A Story about what happens when a Friend is Very Ill*, by Charles M. Schulz (1990; New York: Ballantine Books) (available in video as well);
- *An Alphabet about Kids with Cancer*, by Rita Berglund (1994; Denver, Colo: The Children's Legacy).

Maintenance of Normal Daily Routine

"*Dear Doctor,*

… You gave me such good advice that helped me **to improve in my health side and my life side** … from your special patient …"

—18 year old, active treatment, acute lymphoblastic leukemia

The normal daily routine is referred to by the patient quoted above as "my life side." This patient being quoted became depressed during active cancer treatment if school progression was thwarted, with the depression exhibited through passive nonadherence with oral medications. The patient's parents did not want the child to feel pressured by school responsibilities and discouraged academic activities, while the patient only thrived when achieving academic milestones.

Normal daily activity may be academic achievement, peer relationships, social activities, household responsibilities, and/or participation in milestone events and ceremonies. Education should continue throughout cancer treatment with fitting accommodations that need to be negotiated between medical treatment team members, patient and family, and local school personnel. School accommodations may also be needed after cancer treatment due to delayed achievement or changes in a child's learning ability, appearance, or physical function. Neuropsychological testing facilitates the identification of changes in learning ability, from which modified achievement goals and methods for assessing academic achievement can be formulated.

Social accommodations are oftentimes needed. Repeated or protracted school absences, visible distinctions, and medical restrictions often set the child with cancer apart from peers. Interventions for both classmates and the child with cancer will foster their negotiating new social situations. The classmates learn what to expect and how to best support the classmate who is ill. These services are referred to as "school reentry programs." Some programs are developed by the mental health team at the hospital, while others are commercially available, structured programs, for example, The Kids on the Block, Inc (www.kotb.com). A philanthropically supported program titled "There's A Monkey in My Chair" (www.theresamonkeyinmychair.org) is used to explain a classmate's extended or recurring absence. Rosenbaum and colleagues[19] have demonstrated benefit of an intervention titled "The Buddy Program" in which social interaction skills are taught to classmates prior to the patient returning to school.

The child returning to school should have input regarding the personal information disclosed to classmates, the format in which the information is disclosed, persons to whom the information is disclosed, and who will disclose the information. To complement the school reentry program, the child returning to school after a health-related absence will need preparation for managing new social situations. An initial step in this skill-building process is to understand the child's interpersonal preferences. Some children prefer that classmates ask health-related questions directly, whereas other children do not want to field questions from classmates. Some children are very private and want minimal health-related information disclosed, while other children feel better understood when their classmates

have detailed information. Social skills should be taught according to the child's preferences. Commonly taught social skills include:

1. Developing a "stock" answer regarding health status:
   - vague, minimal disclosure—"I was sick";
   - specific, yet concise— "I had cancer";
   - narrative—the child's cancer story.
2. Reassuring the classmate—"I'm better now."
3. Limit setting—"I don't feel like talking about it."
4. Redirecting the conversation away from health status, toward normal, current events—"What do you want to play at recess?"
5. Identifying an ambassador, a peer who can speak on the child's behalf when the child does not want to talk, but wants peers to understand.

Some children need environmental accommodation. For example, a child who is immune-compromised may need to receive school instruction at home. Environmental accommodations are determined by the medical team but may be communicated to school personnel by the mental health professional because of the accompanying social and academic accommodations. Additional guidelines for helping pediatric cancer patients return to school have been provided by the Psychosocial Committee of the International Society of Pediatric Oncology.[20]

Maintaining normal routine as much as possible extends to social activities beyond the school day, household responsibilities, and/or participation in milestone events and ceremonies. As the child is physically able, roles in the family and community should be reestablished.

Procedural Support

"I AM IN TEARS. ... Tomorrow I see an ENT. I know this ENT will do anything and everything in order to convince me to put in another trach, or take out my vocal chords. I have thoughts of suicide. It will be the hardest to survive the night. Thoughts of anxiety surround me."

—28 year old, long-term survivor, medulloblastoma

Procedural distress is a significant concern for patients with cancer. Children learn and habituate skills quickly when presented with preparatory information and when they are engaged in covert and overt rehearsal.[21] For example, Schwarzinger and colleagues[22] developed an intervention sequence for 4- to 7-year-old children that allows for magnetic resonance imaging without anesthesia.

Three sessions, scheduled across a 1-month period, consist of (1) a parent meeting to explain intervention and treatment goal, and request the parent's collaboration, (2) a parent–child session in which a procedural picture book and a toy model of the medical equipment are presented, followed with role play, and, lastly, (3) a parent–child session in which the child is taught to employ imagination to calm and preoccupy oneself during the procedure, followed with a simulated procedure (rehearsal in the actual physical environment where the procedure will be conducted) and homework to repeat the same.

Provision of procedural information is an essential component of preparation. Procedure-specific preparation materials are readily available:

1. Procedural teaching and picture books:
   - *My Central Line Book* (undated), by Wendy Landier and Tamara Scott, available online at www.bardaccess.com, sponsored by Bard Access Systems, Salt Lake City, Utah;
   - *Cooper gets an X-ray*, by Karen Olson (2001; Atlanta, Ga: Pritchett and Hull Associates);
   - *Adam goes to the Operating Room*, by Barbara Ehreneich (1998; New York, NY: Memorial Sloan Kettering Cancer Center and Bishop Books, Inc).

2. Video:
   - www.starbrightworld.org, *Coping with Chemo*;
   - www.starbright.org provides the Starbright Explorer Series on CD-ROM, including—*Blood Tests: Exploring Our Incredible Blood* (ages 10–15), *Spotlight on IVs* (ages 6–10), *The Sickle Cell Slime-O-Rama Game* (ages 8–12), *Medical Imaging: Welcome to the Radiology Center* (ages 6–10), *Uncovering the Mysteries of Bone Marrow: Aspiration and Biopsy* (ages 10–15), and *Spinal Tap: Discovering the Secrets of Spinal Fluid* (ages 10–15).

3. Interactive games:
   - www.re-mission.net.

Scripts for building anxiety management skills, for example, visual imagery, suggestion, and relaxation techniques, are available:

- *The Moon Balloon: A Journey of Hope and Discovery for Children and Families*, by Joan Drescher (1996; Bethesda, Md: Association for the Care of Children's Health).
- *Earthlight, Starbright, Moonbeam, Sunshine, the Inner Garden, InnerSpace, and the Power of the Inner Self* is a book series by Maureen Garth (1997; New York, NY: Harper Collins Publishers).
- *Harry the Hypno-potamus: Metaphorical Tales for the Treatment of Children*, by Linda Thomson (2005; Norwalk, Conn: Crown House Publishing, Ltd).
- Progressive muscle relaxation, passive muscle relaxation, guided imagery, and scripted imagery, in *Helping Schoolchildren with Chronic Health Conditions: A Practical Guide*, by Daniel Clay (2004; New York, NY: The Guilford Press, pp. 132–135).

Parent–child interactions during procedures affect a child's emotional state. Dahlquist[23] encourages parents to:

- Focus the child's attention and behavior away from the procedure.
- Encourage positive self-talk, such as "I can do this .... I am strong .... This will soon be finished."
- Praise and recognize the child and the child's accomplishment.

Traumatic Stress: Acute Changes in Health Status and Intensive/Intrusive Treatments

"I had a breakdown. It was in the ICU. During our walk to the infirmary, I thought nothing about it. IT WAS SORT OF LIKE SOMEBODY THREW ME BACK AGAINST THE HALL WALL. But while I was in the ICU foyer, fear and a cold sweat rushed upon me. A black-and-white picture of 36 different medical machines were activating. Along with beeps, groaning sounds, hard beats on the floor and the fresh smell of burning rubber came to my mind, ears, eyes, nose, and tongue. It was all horrible. My sight, sound, smell, taste and feelings were unbearable. You would have noticed my hands were cold and clammy."

—27 year old, long-term survivor, medulloblastoma

Acute, precipitous health decline and intrusive treatments can be traumatic. Intensive care hospitalization or hospitalization for intensive interventions is more often than not traumatic for children, negatively affecting mood and triggering avoidant behavior.[24,25] Traumatic stress responses should be assessed and treated as close to the traumatic event as possible. Traumatized persons need help[26,27]:

- increasing mastery, sense of control, and absence of culpability by processing the experience through re-telling (to peers and/or caregivers);
- improving one's ability to reassess personal safety and calm oneself when in a safe environment;
- increasing family support through improved commu-nication and understanding.

Separation from parents can be more traumatic for a young child than the primary health-related event. Collaborative, family-centered care will minimize sec-ondary traumas during the critical medical interven-tions.[28,29]

Treatment Effects of Visible Distinction and Functional Loss

"I don't want to join the cancer club."

—16 year old, active treatment, alveolar rhabdosarcoma

Treatment effects may be severe and distressing. Che-motherapy causes time-limited hair loss, nausea (with a secondary effect of weight loss), and fatigue. Glucocor-ticoids cause cushingoid features and mood disturbance, earning the nickname "roid rage." Some treatment side effects are permanent and/or progressive and increase the risk of emotional maladjustment.[30] Cosmetic sequelae include multiple scars, atrophy of limbs or torso, short stature, facial or limb differences (including amputa-tion), hypogonadism, scoliosis, alopecia, and obesity. Functional sequelae include hearing impairment, sleep disorder, reduction in use of limbs, change in gait, recur-rent seizures, headaches, fatigue, small bladder capac-ity, urinary incontinence, shortness of breath, problems with concentration, poor memory, mental retardation, learning disability, loss of teeth, back tightness, chronic diarrhea, visual defect, nerve palsies, ovarian failure, and irregular menses.[31]

Psychotherapy may help the child develop compensa-tory skills and coping strategies for the functional losses, visible distinctions, and sensory experiences. Cognitive strategies, stress management techniques, self-help skills, and social boldness are a few examples of strategies to build self-confidence, decrease distress, and improve quality of life.

Children with visible distinctions will need to de-velop social skills to manage the reactions of others and build self-confidence.[32] Counseling interventions might include:

- Information on the positive functions of staring, for example, assessing safety of oneself and others, and the human drive to learn and understand anything new or different.
- Possible reactions to normal staring, for example, verbalize the observation that the person is staring; explain illness or condition; reassure others regard-ing comfort level, current status, and/or expected out-come; initiate an unrelated conversation to illustrate both safety and personal competencies; use humor; ignore.
- Information on how to distinguish aggression/bul-lying from normal staring and how to get help if bullied.

Nonadherence

"I don't like riding the little yellow bus."

—16 year old, active treatment, sickle cell disease

Nonadherence is oftentimes associated with psycho-logical processes. It may be a manifestation of avoid-ance. And, avoidance of medication or treatment may be an indicator of posttraumatic stress. In one sample of pediatric liver transplant patients, treatment adher-ence improved after a cognitive therapy intervention that focused on trauma,[33] although the intervention did not directly address the nonadherence. For members of the interdisciplinary team who wish to assess for trauma, a quick screen for traumatic stress symptoms in ill or in-jured children is available online through the National Child Traumatic Stress Network (www.NCTSNet.org). If the avoidance is driven by a traumatic stress response, then a psychological intervention would be needed for the traumatic stress.

Unresolved grief may drive nonadherence. Loss of health is to be grieved. Nonadherence may be a mani-festation of denial of loss of health—behaving as nor-mal, as opposed to grieving one's invincibility. And with the ability to forget comes the prospect of maintaining normal.

An individual's beliefs and perceptions about the pre-scribed medication regimen may drive nonadherence, including the following:

- perceived physical barriers, such as swallowing prob-lems or having a "pill phobia";
- anticipated medication side effects, which are "escaped" by not taking the medication;

- perceived environmental barriers, such as the child not wanting to be seen in the school nurse's office where the medication is administered;
- failure to plan—adolescents live in the moment, plan their activities within hours of the activity beginning, and may not have anticipated the need for medication access.

Simons and Blount[34] have developed an Adolescent Medication Barriers Scale (AMBS) and Parent Medication Barriers Scale (PMBS) to assess both the emotional barrier of "longing to be normal" and beliefs and perceptions that foster nonadherence. To complement the scale, Simons et al[35] have recommended corresponding interventions, which are largely behavioral and cognitive strategies, for example, application of salient environmental cues, communication skills, reinforcement, and positive cognitive associations.

The primary intervention may be with the parent, rather than with the patient. In a child's world, the parent oftentimes has the greatest influence. Using new parenting strategies when a child is ill may be emotionally trying for a parent. Parents are prone to feelings of guilt or fear of rejection when a child is ill. The parent's emotional well-being and parenting response to the child's nonadherence should be assessed, and parents should have access to recommended services.

Spirituality

"I am scared I am going to purgatory."

—23 year old, active treatment, advanced acute myelogenous leukemia

Over half of hospitalized pediatric patients identify having spiritual needs.[36] The effect of spiritual practices and beliefs on adult cancer patients has been well described by Kristeller with Indiana State University. Dr Kristeller et al[37] have demonstrated that spirituality (inner experience of personal meaning, inner peace, transcendence, and connectedness with a higher being with or without involvement in religious institutions or rituals) is associated with high quality of life and minimal levels of emotional distress. Parents of children in active cancer treatment who rely on religious-focused coping are more emotionally adaptive and less anxious.[38] The applicability of spiritual/religious-focused coping to children with cancer is less understood, yet a potential intervention for decreasing emotional distress.

A Special Population: Adolescents and Young Adults (AYA) with Cancer

"I don't want to live life as a loser. I'm having more and more trouble learning. If I can't go to college, I will have to live with my parents forever."

—16 year old, active treatment, adrenal cortical carcinoma

AYA patients are in transition.[39-43] Peer support and social well-being account for a significant amount of the survivor's emotional well-being.[15,30,44] AYA patients are defining themselves, individuating, moving away from dependence on parents, extending themselves beyond familial relationships, and venturing into the world of work. AYA populations need access to career and vocational counseling, fertility counseling, peer-based group support, and developmentally fitting activities and equipment available to patients during hospitalization.

Fertility is one of the top concerns for survivors. Schover,[45-47] an expert on fertility issues and cancer survivors, has found that a large majority of patients who have no children at the time of diagnosis wish to be a parent. The American Society of Clinical Oncology has recommended that age-appropriate patients (postpubertal or >14 years of age) be informed of their potential reproductive risks and fertility preservation options in a timely, thorough manner. Fertility risk and preservation options should be discussed at the earliest possible opportunity during treatment planning. Sperm and embryo cryopreservation are considered standard practice and are widely available. Guidance, financial assistance, and informational resources are available:

- *Banking on Fatherhood* is an educational, interactive CD-ROM developed by Schover. It has information for both professionals and patients. Topics include emotional concerns associated with fertility, the effect of cancer treatments on fertility, pros and cons of banking sperm, religious attitudes on reproductive assistance, facilitating semen collection, advance directives for stored semen, alternative options for parenthood, a national directory of sperm banks, and a resource list.
- *Fertilehope.org* is an online sperm banking information resource.
- *Liveonkit.com* is a resource for banking from home rather than at a sperm bank/clinic.
- *Heroes for Children* is a philanthropic organization that provides financial assistance for sperm banking.

A minority of cancer patients bank. Feelings of embarrassment and anxiety are barriers to banking.[48] AYA patients should be encouraged to address emotional issues associated with fertility and banking.

■ AFTER CANCER

Emotional and Developmental Adjustment

"I am in a deep hole I have dug out of anxiety."

—28 year old, long-term survivor,
medulloblastoma

"I don't fit in at school. Everybody else grew their wings except for me."

—29 year old, long-term survivor,
suprasellar germinoma

Many survivors report significant late effects. About two thirds of long-term survivors have at least one serious late effect.[49,50] Late effects include physical, cognitive, developmental, and emotional problems. Childhood cancer is a formative developmental experience.[51] Childhood memories, personality, interpersonal style, lifestyle, personal philosophy, and religious beliefs are some of the areas believed to be affected. The cancer experience may have a disequilibrating effect on identity formation, leaving survivors feeling different and vulnerable—weak, yet prematurely aged and mature. Some evidence suggests that survivors are family-focused rather than peer-focused later into their adult years compared with their peers, delaying separation from parents and development of extrafamilial relationships.[52,53]

Persistent emotional problems include unresolved grief, identity problems, limited peer and love relationships, interpersonal insecurity, ambivalent parent–child attachment, low self-esteem, and negative mood states.[54] Pediatric cancer survivors are more likely to have symptoms of anxiety and depression compared with their siblings[1,55] and are more anxious than their peers.[56,57] Prevalence estimates of emotional problems in survivors vary. One of the first reports came from Koocher and O'Malley,[58] and the participants were on average 12 years posttreatment. Forty-seven percent of those sampled reported symptoms of mental disorders. Eleven percent presented with six to nine symptoms and reported impaired daily function, while 36% reported two to five symptoms, which did not interfere with daily function.

Cancer is surprising, random, unpredictable, and life-threatening. These characteristics of the diagnosis and treatment are traumatic.[59] Long-term losses are associated with the primary trauma, such as infertility, growth problems, cardiac dysfunction, and cognitive changes, which may be traumatic as well.[60] Lifetime posttraumatic stress disorder prevalence rates of pediatric cancer survivors range from 5% to 35%, with intrusive thoughts and avoidant behavior commonly reported.[59,60] Traumatic responses and maladjustment to cancer are associated with[61,62]:

- higher subjective appraisal of life threat;
- experience of treatment as "hard" or "scary";
- coping style;
- overall high anxiety level;
- history of stressful experiences;
- higher perceived stress;
- recent completion of treatment;
- female gender;
- lack of family and social support;
- chaotic family environment;
- parental maladjustment;
- unresolved family conflict or parent–child relationship problems;
- low socioeconomic status;
- multiple late effects.

Those who appear to be more insulated from long-term effects or buffered from insults are optimistic and report positive social support and self-esteem.[63] For some survivors, family interactions are more closely associated with trauma symptoms than the cancer diagnosis and treatment.[64] Trauma is less likely to occur within the context of adaptable and flexible family environments in which autonomy is fostered.[65,66] During adolescence and early adulthood, families reorganize boundaries to accommodate teenagers' flexible movement into and out of the family system, which is even more exaggerated when the adolescent has special health care needs. Families who support the teenager by fostering independence with a flexible "safety net" facilitate greater adjustment in the maturing young adult.

Survivors need information about possible late effects, rehabilitation services, medical follow-up, possible effect on social life, and psychosocial support and services. Practice guidelines, health links, and educational sheets on survivorship are available through the Children's Oncology Group. Emotional, educational, and chronic pain issues are addressed. The information is updated regularly and based on available research findings. These resources are thoughtfully written, free, and easily accessed at www.survivorshipguidelines.org. They can be especially helpful for non-M.D. mental health professionals because physical conditions associated with survivorship may be mistaken for a mental disorder, for example, urinary incontinence secondary to an alkylating chemotherapy agent versus enuresis.

Neurocognitive Abilities

"I have a meeting with my son's teachers tomorrow morning. They are considering keeping his 504 Plan active, as he is having some trouble completing tests on time. He has some problems with processing, but if given enough time, he does extremely well with his school work. The school counselor has requested that his doctor write a brief note stating that there is sometimes mental confusion or processing difficulties resulting from chemotherapy. I don't like the term, 'chemobrain' but I know that's the phrase often used to describe the symptoms."

—Mother of a 12-year-old patient, active treatment, acute lymphoblastic leukemia

Such a request is common, and the request may be the first and only information a mental health professional has regarding a patient. The urgency of the parent meeting with school professionals, "the next day," is not fitting with the best process for determining educational recommendations. Providing a parent and school personnel with general information, temporary recommendations, and a plan to conduct neuropsychological testing to thoroughly answer the question may be the start of an important service.

Cancer and some of the cancer treatments have a negative effect on learning. The effect can be pervasive, negatively affecting overall intelligence (IQ), or specific aspects of cognition.[67–69] Attention, memory, processing speed, and perceptual and motor skills are commonly affected by cancer treatments. The changes may be subtle and gradual. By having thorough baseline and follow-up neuropsychological evaluations, tailored recommendations can be made based on the testing results, to the school personnel, patient, and others who help the patient learn. Factors that increase the risk of neurocognitive impairment include[70]:

- Patient factors:
  - young age at time of treatment (birth to 7 years of age);
  - female sex.
- Disease factors:
  - metastatic or primary CNS disease.
- Treatment factors:
  - intrathecal chemotherapy;
  - cranial or total body irradiation;
  - neurological compromises.

Cancer survivors are more likely to be unemployed or work less than half-time, compared with their siblings.[55,71] Early identification of learning differences extrapolated from the neuropsychological testing may maximize the individual's opportunity for academic and vocational achievement. Neurocognitive deficits may be exhibited in poor social behavior. For children with social problems, social skills training may be needed.[72]

■ THE DYING CHILD

"I am scared of what will happen to my mother after I die."

—14 year old, active treatment, advanced acute myelogenous leukemia

Relapse increases illness burden and is associated with lower quality of life, compared with survivors without relapse.[73] Similarly, children with advanced cancer are at increased risk for maladjustment, including anxiety and depression.[74] Good communication between patient, family, and treatment team providers; collaborative, treatment decision making; and social support help patients with advanced cancer and their parents.

Talking about death and end-of-life decisions can be helpful to both the dying child[75] and parents.[76] Parents who acknowledged the incurability of the disease, actively participated in treatment decision making at end-of-life, and planned the location of their child's death felt better than parents who did not.[77–79] In contrast, parents who did not talk to their child about death experienced regret.[80]

Social support facilitates the grieving process.[76] Parents were more likely to have worked through their grief if they had shared their problems with others during the child's illness and had access to psychological services during the last month of their child's life.

Initiating an end-of-life talk with a child is a major milestone. When a loving adult provides information, a child develops trust, knows what to expect, and shares the experience with loved ones. Children learn that loved ones have each other and the beloved are never alone, not even in death. With modeling of how persons are helped regardless of circumstance, death need not be feared. In preparation for an end-of-life discussion, parents may need information and the opportunity to rehearse their disclosure, which might be facilitated by a member of the treatment team.

Most children adjust best when provided with a safe environment in which they are encouraged to ask questions, voice concerns, and participate in care. Parents should be encouraged to look and listen for cues that a child is ready to participate in discussions about end-of-life issues. Cues may be:

- Vague reference to death, for example, a past experience and reference to a movie with a death theme.
- Expressed afterlife wish: "When I die, I want …."
- Anticipated grief: "What if this medicine doesn't work? … I am scared of dying …. Does it hurt when you die?"
- Voiced suspicion or supposition: "I have a death sentence."
- New types of questions about cancer, treatment, God, and afterlife, for example, "What is heaven like? … Will I see grandma in heaven?"
- New assertions: "I don't want any more chemo."
- Expression with double meanings: "I want to go home" and "I'm tired of all this."
- Sleeplessness and/or fear of dying while sleeping.
- Nightmares about separation from loved ones, threat to oneself, or death.
- Observation of health decline, for example, "I'm losing weight. Look at my arm."
- Catastrophically expressed truth: "I am dying!"

A child may use a cue to initiate a conversation, hoping to protect parents' feelings. Once cued, parents should assume they need to initiate the conversation. How the conversation is initiated will depend on the developmental age of the child.

Preschool-age children understand physical discomfort and look to parents for soothing. They have a limited ability to project into the future—hours and days, rather than weeks and months. They do not have "issues to resolve" or "need closure" before death. An end-of-life discussion may consist of a reference to the illness, followed by parents' reassurance of their loving presence.

Young school-age children are growing into understanding death. The concept that all living things will die and that one day death will happen to the child is a helpful foundation to establish before having an end-of-life discussion. Children's books can help parents lay this foundation, such as:

- *Gentle Willow*, by Joyce C. Mills;
- *The Fall of Freddy the Leaf*, by Leo Buscaglia;
- *Water Bugs & Dragonflies: Explaining Death to Young Children*, by Doris Stickney;
- *When Dinosaurs Die: A Guide to Understanding Death*, by Laurie Krasny Brown;
- *Sad isn't Bad: A Good-grief Guidebook for Kids dealing with Loss*, by Michaelene Mundy.

End-of-life information should be simple, concrete, and proximal to death. Young school-age children may look to themselves (their misbehavior) as the cause of death. Magical thinking, the misattribution of cause and effect, will need to be dispelled by the provision of correct information regarding cause of death. A young school-age child may ask very concrete questions, such as questions about bodily functions after death. Death may be believed to be temporary and reversible. Parents can be encouraged to provide simple, corrective information, for example, when a person dies, the body stops working; the person neither eats, nor hurts, nor comes back.

Older school-age children and adolescents have a broad range of concerns and need for information. They need explicit permission to voice concerns. Some may need to hear examples of commonly experienced concerns, as most are apprehensive to disclose private thoughts about death. They may need a neutral party with whom to disclose concerns, wanting to protect loved ones from sadness. Common concerns include:

1. what dying feels like and if dying is painful;
2. what happens after death, with special concern regarding separation from loved ones
3. how others will fare

Many parents fear that their crying will be a barrier to these important conversations. Parents should be encouraged to talk through their tears and explain, "I am crying because I am sad." Thereafter, the parent can return to the primary conversation.

Young patients are capable of participating in treatment decision making[81] and have important opinions and beliefs. Some youth place importance on having an advance directive.[82] Parents should be encouraged to ask older school-age children and adolescents about their wishes in the event that parents need to act on the child's behalf. Older children and adolescents should be invited to talk about their wishes, followed with open-ended question, such as, "If you get too sick and cannot speak for yourself, what do I need to know?" A guide for documenting an advance directive, *My Wishes*, is available through Aging with Dignity (www.agingwithdignity.com). Wiener and colleagues[83] are studying the effect of using a written tool for advanced care planning with chronically ill AYA. To date, most study participants believed advanced care planning to be important and were especially interested in asserting how they wanted to be treated and remembered.

Siblings will need timely information regarding major changes in the ill child's health status and prognosis. The guidelines described above for talking with the ill child can be applied to siblings. Siblings should be given permission to visit the ill child, although not coerced. Prior to the visit, siblings should be apprised of changes in hospital room, such as new medical equipment, and changes in the ill sibling's appearance and function. Siblings may not tolerate a lengthy visit. Parents should be guided to monitor siblings for signs to end the visit, for example, fidgeting, withdrawal, and comfort-seeking behaviors.

Once a child dies, siblings will need information regarding funereal or memorial events. Siblings should be invited to participate in the events, for example, selecting pictures or music and giving something special to the child who died. An adult caregiver is recommended for each sibling, to monitor and accommodate the sibling's needs, which may change quickly during the course of the event. A child may exhibit intense signs of grief, followed by a request to play.

Survivors should be informed of community-based grief support groups. National organizations available to facilitate identification of local bereavement resources include:

- *Compassionate Friends* (www.compassionatefriends. org) is a national organization for bereaved parents. Local chapters provide parent support groups.
- *Dougy Center* (www.dougy.org) is a bereavement organization that provides an international listing of services for bereaved siblings.

■ CANCER AND THE FAMILY

Parents

"We are walking through the Valley of the Shadow of Death."

—Quotation from the 23rd Psalm. Mother of 6-year-old patient, active treatment, acute lymphoblastic leukemia

Parents are deeply affected emotionally by their child's cancer and are at risk to experience episodic anxiety, depression, and insomnia. In one sample of families, 99% of families had one family member reporting posttraumatic stress symptoms.[84] Neamtu and colleagues[85] measured depressive symptoms in parents with children in active treatment for brain or bone tumor, and 72% of parents reported symptoms of depression (38% mild, 21% moderate, and 13% severe depression). Parents of children undergoing cell therapy transplantation (both autologous and allogeneic) have persistent depressive symptoms, which appear to abate 2 years after transplantation.[86] Insomnia is also common. In one sample of parents whose children were outpatients and 6 months into active cancer treatment (all types of cancer), 48% had sleep problems, compared with 15% in a normal control group.[87] Parents felt unrested on awakening, awakened during the night because of emotional distress, and had nightmares.

Parents may need help in the adjustment process before they are able to foster their child's adjustment. For example, parents who rely on coping strategies that are not focused on emotion are less anxious.[38] Parents trained in stress reduction techniques prior to their child's admission for bone marrow transplantation had positive outcomes.[88] In addition to onsite mental health services for teaching parents coping and stress reduction strategies, referrals in the family's home community may be complementary. Mental health professionals can be found through online registries and licensee rosters, such as The National Registry of Health Service Providers at www. findapsychologist.org. Also on the Internet, state licensing boards provide licensee rosters by city or zip code. The key search words are "State Board of Examiners of …. (Psychologists, Psychiatrists, Licensed Professional Counselors, or Social Workers)."

Parents should be encouraged to identify sources of social support. Parents of children in active cancer treatment who search for social support are less anxious,[38]

and their children are better adjusted.[89] Incumbent with social support is decision making regarding disclosure of the child's health-related information. What the parent discloses will have an effect on all family members. For example, the patient may want more privacy than a parent, or a sibling may want to avoid having classmates know about the ill sibling. Parents should be encouraged to talk with immediate family members regarding their privacy preferences before disclosing significant health information. Parents may need to review conversational skills in which they lead the discussion away from medical information. For example, supportive others want to help. Although they may pose the question, "How is your child?," the primary message is, "I am interested and available to help." Parents should be encouraged to interpret questions as an invitation for help rather than an expectation for parents to disclose medical details. Asking for help may initially be difficult, but the support from help received will benefit all family members. Parents may benefit emotionally by feeling more loved and less lonely, while also being relieved of a responsibility. Having an assignment can relieve supportive others of their feelings of helplessness. *Lots a Helping Hands* is a private, web-based caregiving coordination service that allows family, friends, neighbors, and colleagues to create a community to assist a family caregiver with the daily tasks that become a challenge during times of need (www.lotsahelpinghands.com).

Parents might also be encouraged to appoint a family spokesperson and/or consider electronic means of communication to:

- provide written updates via the Internet, for example, www.caringbridge;
- record an update on the telephone voicemail greeting.

In some instances, supportive others may not agree with the immediate family's treatment decision making. Parents may be encouraged to consider feedback during the decision-making process. However, once a decision has been made, feedback may be experienced as criticism and assertiveness skills may need to be reinforced.

Siblings

"I (my cancer) caused my brother's drug problem."

—18 year old, active treatment, acute lymphoblastic leukemia

Siblings are affected acutely, and some siblings are affected long term. They are at risk for less emotional support during the patient's active treatment phase.[90] About one third of siblings internalize their problems, engage in pessimistic thinking, and withdraw from sources of social support.[91]

Given the sibling's unique needs, a best practices paper has been published through the International Society of Pediatric Oncology **Psycho-Oncology Committee**,[90] which provides thoughtful recommendations for parents who are faced with the dilemma of caring for both a well and a sick child. Siblings need consistent, trustworthy information regarding the ill sibling, while maintaining familiar routines. They need contact with their parents and ill sibling throughout the course of medical care, including end-of-life. School and peer-based activities need to continue. When parents are unable to sustain these routines, surrogate caregivers should be identified to help. Suggestions for parenting a healthy child when another child in the family is ill are provided by the parent support organization Candlelighters (www.candlelighters.org) and the sibling support organization Supersibs (www.supersibs.org).

Cell Therapy Transplantation
Minor Related Donors

"If it doesn't work is it my fault?"

—13-year-old minor sibling donor, pre-stem cell

Minor donors are asked to participate in medical procedures for the sole purpose of benefiting a family member. The psychological outcome literature that exists suggests negative changes in pediatric cell therapy donor emotions, learning, and behavior.[92–95] Minor donors are at risk to feel overwhelmed with responsibility when asked to donate, which can lead to psychological distress. Although having an ill sibling affects all siblings, some distinctions have been made between the minor sibling donor and minor sibling nondonor experience of emotional distress. Minor sibling donors have higher anxiety, lower self-esteem, and variable school performance compared with siblings who do not donate. They more commonly express somatic complaints, feelings of guilt, sleep difficulties, and behavior problems and avoid topics related to the sibling's illness and donation process. Some overachieve in school, while others misbehave in school. No literature is available on children donating for their ill parent. The information available about the minor sibling donor is based on retrospective surveys with a limited sample, roughly 7 years after transplantation. Psychosocial adjustment during the donation-related events is not known. Much of what is described in the literature is based on one sample of 21 donors. Wendy Packman, a clinical psychologist in Palo Alto, California, thoroughly assessed patients from the University of California Medical Center in San Francisco, which accounts for a significant portion of the available literature.

Given what is known about the minor sibling donor experience, early intervention has been recommended to prevent or minimize potential donor distress. Psychosocial services may foster minor donor adjustment, including:

- Preparatory information, modeling, and/or medical role play, for example, the illness, why and how transplantation works, precollection tests, and preparation for the collection process. A pictorial teaching booklet may ensure consistent presentation of information, for example, Neupogen shot instruction, physical examination, operating and recovery rooms, venipuncture (number of sticks, numbing tools), anesthesia, amount of marrow taken, hospital admission, postoperative pain management, talking with the physician, G-CSF injections and side effects of bone pain and flulike symptoms, peripheral IV or central line access, femoral Quinton catheter, bilateral cannulae, apheresis, and cell separation. For younger children, a patient puppet and medical equipment may be complementary.
- Allegorical children's story, that is, *The Gift: For Children who are Bone Marrow Donors*, by S. Heiney and S. Lamphier (1996; Columbia, SC: Richland Memorial Hospital).
- Coaching tour of persons and the involved facility (ie, apheresis area).
- Sharing information with the donor's supervising adults, for example, teacher and scout leader.
- Facilitation of a discussion regarding the donor's feelings about being a donor and dispel common myths and questions.
- Teaching anxiety management coping strategies, for example, deep breathing, progressive muscle relaxation, imagery, and positive self-talk.

Children of Adult Patients

"I was afraid to ask. I knew something bad was going on."

—13-year-old child of adult patient with advanced cancer

Mental health providers who work within a hospital that serves both children and adult cancer patients will likely be called upon to help children of adult patients. Children of adult patients are at risk for mental health problems, primarily symptoms of anxiety and depression.[96] The parent's emotional adjustment is more closely associated with the child's adjustment to the parent's cancer diagnosis than the parent's illness parameters, for example, duration of illness, prognosis, chemotherapy status, physical impairment, and family.[97] A depressed parent is less communicative, supervises the child less, disciplines inconsistently, and is more hostile, irritable, and coercive when interacting with family members. Children of depressed mothers with cancer report emotional distress and low self-esteem.[98] In contrast, children of well-adjusted parents with cancer report less avoidance, open communication, positive parent–child relationship, and high self-esteem.[99] Health-specific information is associated with the positive adjustment of children and adolescents of adult cancer patients, whereas lack of information is associated with emotional distress for both children[100,101] and adolescents.[102]

Interventions may initially be focused on the parent's emotional adjustment and thereafter directed toward the child. Suggested interventions for the child of an adult cancer patient include: (1) provision of health-specific information, (2) normalizing feelings, (3) teaching distress management skills, and (4) finding support. A self-help guide for adolescents has been published by the National Cancer Institute, *When Your Parent has Cancer*, and may be requested online at www.cancer.gov or by telephone at 1-800-4-CANCER (1-800-422-6237). A parent guide, *When a Parent has Cancer: How to Talk to Your Kids*, has been developed by the Cancer Council of New South Wales and the Pam McLean Communication Centre, Woolloomooloo, Australia, and is available online at www.nswcc.org.au. Support group curriculums for children and adolescents of adult cancer patients have been developed and appear to be helpful.[103–105]

KEY POINTS

- Patients needing professional mental health services postcancer diagnosis will need to be identified, as not all patients will need the services.

- Adjustment to health-related stressors can be fostered by communicating directly and clearly with the patient about the illness and treatment.

- Although health and safety are the priorities, normal daily activities should be maintained as much as possible throughout active cancer treatment.

- Patients frequently need mental health services specific to:
  - new or intrusive medical procedures;
  - precipitous health decline or intensive medical care;
  - visible distinction and functional loss, including acute and long-term effects of cancer and treatment.

- Patients oftentimes need to talk about death, and explicit permission should be provided for patients with advanced cancer.

- Professional mental health services may be needed by other family members and should be included in the treatment plan.

REFERENCES

1. Derogatis LR, Morrow GR, Fetting J, et al. The prevalence of psychiatric disorders among cancer patients. *JAMA*. 1983:249(6):751–757.

2. Phipps S, Dunavant M, Garvie PA, et al. Acute health-related quality of life in children undergoing stem cell transplant: I. Descriptive outcomes. *Bone Marrow Transplant*. 2002:29(5):425–434.

3. Barrera M, Atenafu E, Pinto J. Behavioral, social, and educational outcomes after pediatric stem cell transplantation and related factors. *Cancer*. 2009:115(4):880–889.

4. Lof CM, Forinder U, Winiarski J. Risk factors for lower health-related QoL after allogeneic stem cell transplantation in children. *Pediatr Transplant*. 2007:11(2):145–151.

5. Vrijmoet-Wiersma CM, Kolk AM, Grootenhuis MA, et al. Child and parental adaptation to pediatric stem cell transplantation. *Support Care Cancer*. 2009:17(6):707–714.

6. Calaminus G, Heimpel H, Niemeyer C, et al. Quality of survival in patients with bone marrow failure syndromes (BMFS): a flashlight of the results of the first evaluation within the BMFS network. *Pediatr Blood Cancer*. 1990:53(5):722.

7. Kazak AE, Cant MC, Jensen MM, et al. Identifying psychosocial risk indicative of subsequent resource use in families of newly diagnosed pediatric oncology patients. *J Clin Oncol*. 2003:21(17):3220–3225.

8. Varni JW, Limbers CA, Bryant WP, et al. The PedsQL Multidimensional Fatigue Scale in type 1 diabetes: feasibility, reliability, and validity. *Pediatr Diabetes*. 2009:10(5):321–328.

9. Varni JW, Burwinkle TM, Katz ER, et al. The PedsQL in pediatric cancer: reliability and validity of the Pediatric Quality of Life Inventory Generic Core Scales, Multidimensional Fatigue Scale, and Cancer Module. *Cancer*. 2002:94(7):2090–2106.

10. Varni JW, Burwinkle TM, Seid M. The PedsQL as a pediatric patient-reported outcome: reliability and validity of the PedsQL Measurement Model in 25,000 children. *Expert Rev Pharmacoecon Outcomes Res*. 2005:5(6):705–719.

11. Portenoy RK, Thaler HT, Kornblith AB, et al. The Memorial Symptom Assessment Scale: an instrument for the evaluation of symptom prevalence, characteristics and distress. *Eur J Cancer*. 1994:30A(9):1326–1336.

12. Baile WF, Glober GA, Lenzi R, et al. Discussing disease progression and end-of-life decisions. *Oncology (Huntingt)*. 1999:13(7):1021–1031 [discussion 1031–1036, 1038].

13. Mack JW, Wolfe J. Early integration of pediatric palliative care: for some children, palliative care starts at diagnosis. *Curr Opin Pediatr*. 2006:18(1):10–14.

14. Maurice-Stam H, Silberbusch LM, Last BF, et al. Evaluation of a psycho-educational group intervention for children treated for cancer: a descriptive pilot study. *Psychooncology*. 2009:18(7):762–766.

15. Fritz GK, Williams JR, Amylon M. After treatment ends: psychosocial sequelae in pediatric cancer survivors. *Am J Orthopsychiatry*. 1988:58(4):552–561.

16. Mack JW, Hilden JM, Watterson J, et al. Parent and physician perspectives on quality of care at the end of life in children with cancer. *J Clin Oncol*. 2005:23(36):9155–9161.

17. Masera G, Chesler MA, Jankovic M, et al. SIOP Working Committee on Psychosocial Issues in Pediatric Oncology: guidelines for communication of the diagnosis. *Med Pediatr Oncol*. 1997:28(5):382–385.

18. Baile WF, Aaron J. Patient–physician communication in oncology: past, present, and future. *Curr Opin Oncol.* 2005:17(4):331–335.

19. Rosenbaum PL, Armstrong RW, King SM. Improving attitudes toward the disabled: a randomized controlled trial of direct contact versus Kids-on-the-Block. *J Dev Behav Pediatr.* 1986:7(5):302–307.

20. Masera G, Jankovic M, Deasy-Spinetta P, et al. SIOP Working Committee on Psychosocial Issues in Pediatric Oncology: guidelines for school/education. *Med Pediatr Oncol.* 1995:25(6):429–430.

21. Pressdee D, May L, Eastman E, et al. The use of play therapy in the preparation of children undergoing MR imaging. *Clin Radiol.* 1997:52(12):945–947.

22. Schwarzinger S, Leiss U, Leitner D. Development of a psychological training to prepare children aged from 4 to 7 for magnetic-resonance-imaging without anesthesia. *Pediatr Blood Cancer.* 2009:53(5):875.

23. Dahlquist LM. Commentary on "Treatments that work in pediatric psychology: procedure-related pain". *J Pediatr Psychol.* 1999:24(2):153–154.

24. Rees G, Gledhill J, Garralda ME, et al. Psychiatric outcome following paediatric intensive care unit (PICU) admission: a cohort study. *Intensive Care Med.* 2004:30(8):1607–1614.

25. Mintzer LL, Stuber ML, Seacord D, et al. Traumatic stress symptoms in adolescent organ transplant recipients. *Pediatrics.* 2005:115(6):1640–1644.

26. Foa EB. Psychosocial therapy for posttraumatic stress disorder. *J Clin Psychiatry.* 2006:67(suppl 2):40–45.

27. Kazak AE, Rourke MT, Alderfer MA, et al. Evidence-based assessment, intervention and psychosocial care in pediatric oncology: a blueprint for comprehensive services across treatment. *J Pediatr Psychol.* 2007:32(9):1099–1110.

28. Wolfram RW, Turner ED, Philput C. Effects of parental presence during young children's venipuncture. *Pediatr Emerg Care.* 1997:13(5):325–328.

29. Wolfram RW, Turner ED. Effects of parental presence during children's venipuncture. *Acad Emerg Med.* 1996:3(1):58–64.

30. Joubert D, Sadeghi MR, Elliott M, et al. Physical sequelae and self-perceived attachment in adult survivors of childhood cancer. *Psychooncology.* 2001:10(4):284–292.

31. Lackner H, Benesch M, Schagerl S, et al. Prospective evaluation of late effects after childhood cancer therapy with a follow-up over 9 years. *Eur J Pediatr.* 2000:159(10):750–758.

32. Rumsey N, Harcourt D. Body image and disfigurement: issues and interventions. *Body Image.* 2004:1(1):83–97.

33. Shemesh E, Lurie S, Stuber ML, et al. A pilot study of posttraumatic stress and nonadherence in pediatric liver transplant recipients. *Pediatrics.* 2000:105(2):E29.

34. Simons LE, Blount RL. Identifying barriers to medication adherence in adolescent transplant recipients. *J Pediatr Psychol.* 2007:32(7):831–844.

35. Simons LE, McCormick ML, Mee LL, et al. Parent and patient perspectives on barriers to medication adherence in adolescent transplant recipients. *Pediatr Transplant.* 2009:13(3):338–347.

36. Feudtner C, Haney J, Dimmers MA. Spiritual care needs of hospitalized children and their families: a national survey of pastoral care providers' perceptions. *Pediatrics.* 2003:111(1):e67–e72.

37. Kristeller JL, Rhodes M, Cripe LD, et al. Oncologist Assisted Spiritual Intervention Study (OASIS): patient acceptability and initial evidence of effects. *Int J Psychiatry Med.* 2005:35(4):329–347.

38. Kohlsdorf M, Junior ALC, Coutinho S. Analysis of coping strategies adopted by parents of children and adolescents undergoing leukemia treatment. *Pediatr Blood Cancer.* 2009:53(5):873.

39. Albritton K, Bleyer WA. The management of cancer in the older adolescent. *Eur J Cancer.* 2003:39(18):2584–2599.

40. Corey AL, Haase JE, Azzouz F, et al. Social support and symptom distress in adolescents/young adults with cancer. *J Pediatr Oncol Nurs.* 2008:25(5):275–284.

41. Kuwabara SA, Van Voorhees BW, Gollan JK, et al. A qualitative exploration of depression in emerging adulthood: disorder, development, and social context. *Gen Hosp Psychiatry.* 2007:29(4):317–324.

42. Soliman H, Agresta SV. Current issues in adolescent and young adult cancer survivorship. *Cancer Control.* 2008:15(1):55–62.

43. Zebrack B. Information and service needs for young adult cancer survivors. *Support Care Cancer.* 2009:17(4):349–357.

44. Felder-Puig R, Formann AK, Mildner A, et al. Quality of life and psychosocial adjustment of young patients after treatment of bone cancer. *Cancer.* 1998:83(1):69–75.

45. Schover LR. Patient attitudes toward fertility preservation. *Pediatr Blood Cancer.* 2009:53(2):281–284.

46. Schover LR, Brey K, Lichtin A, et al. Knowledge and experience regarding cancer, infertility, and sperm banking in younger male survivors. *J Clin Oncol.* 2002:20(7):1880–1889.

47. Schover LR, Rybicki LA, Martin BA, et al. Having children after cancer. A pilot survey of survivors' attitudes and experiences. *Cancer.* 1999:86(4):697–709.

48. Edge B, Holmes D, Makin G. Sperm banking in adolescent cancer patients. *Arch Dis Child*. 2006:91(2):149–152.

49. Geenen MM, Cardous-Ubbink MC, Kremer LC, et al. Medical assessment of adverse health outcomes in long-term survivors of childhood cancer. *JAMA*. 2007:297(24):2705–2715.

50. Oeffinger KC, Mertens AC, Sklar CA, et al. Chronic health conditions in adult survivors of childhood cancer. *N Engl J Med*. 2006:355(15):1572–1582.

51. Gray RE, Doan BD, Shermer P, et al. Psychologic adaptation of survivors of childhood cancer. *Cancer*. 1992:70(11):2713–2721.

52. Stam H, Grootenhuis MA, Last BF. The course of life of survivors of childhood cancer. *Psychooncology*. 2005:14(3):227–238.

53. Kepak T, Radvanska J, Bajciova V, et al. Long term survivors of childhood cancer: cure and care. The ERICE statement. *Klin Onkol*. 2009:22(2):77–79.

54. Hudson MM, Mertens AC, Yasui Y, et al. Health status of adult long-term survivors of childhood cancer: a report from the Childhood Cancer Survivor Study. *JAMA*. 2003:290(12):1583–1592.

55. Zeltzer LK, Chen E, Weiss R, et al. Comparison of psychologic outcome in adult survivors of childhood acute lymphoblastic leukemia versus sibling controls: a cooperative Children's Cancer Group and National Institutes of Health study. *J Clin Oncol*. 1997:15(2):547–556.

56. Bauld C, Anderson V, Arnold J. Psychosocial aspects of adolescent cancer survival. *J Paediatr Child Health*. 1998:34(2):120–126.

57. Arvidson J, Larsson B, Lonnerholm G. A long-term follow-up study of psychosocial functioning after autologous bone marrow transplantation in childhood. *Psychooncology*. 1999:8(2):123–134.

58. Koocher G, O'Malley J. *Facing the Sword of Damocles*. Boston, Mass: Dana-Farber Cancer Institute; 1981.

59. Pelcovitz D, Libov BG, Mandel F, et al. Posttraumatic stress disorder and family functioning in adolescent cancer. *J Trauma Stress*. 1998:11(2):205–221.

60. Hobbie WL, Stuber M, Meeske K, et al. Symptoms of posttraumatic stress in young adult survivors of childhood cancer. *J Clin Oncol*. 2000:18(24):4060–4066.

61. Stuber ML, Kazak AE, Meeske K, et al. Predictors of posttraumatic stress symptoms in childhood cancer survivors. *Pediatrics*. 1997:100(6):958–964.

62. Phipps S, Larson S, Long A, et al. Adaptive style and symptoms of posttraumatic stress in children with cancer and their parents. *J Pediatr Psychol*. 2006:31(3):298–309.

63. Kamibeppu K, Sato I, Honda M, et al. Posttraumatic growth among survivors of childhood cancer. *Pediatr Blood Cancer*. 2009:53(5):754.

64. Kazak AE, Boyer BA, Brophy P, et al. Parental perceptions of procedure-related distress and family adaptation in childhood leukemia. *Child Health Care*. 1995:24(3):143–158.

65. Hauser S, Jacobson A, Milley J, et al. Ego development paths and adjustment to diabetes: longitudinal studies of preadolescents and adolescents with insulin dependent diabetes mellitus. In: Susman E, Feagans L, Ray W, eds. *Emotion, Cognition, Health, and Development in Children and Adolescents*. Hillsdale, NJ: Erlbaum; 1992:133–152.

66. Levin Newby W, Brown RT, Pawletko TM, et al. Social skills and psychological adjustment of child and adolescent cancer survivors. *Psychooncology*. 2000:9(2):113–126.

67. Ronning C, Sundet K, Due-Tonnessen B, et al. Persistent cognitive dysfunction secondary to cerebellar injury in patients treated for posterior fossa tumors in childhood. *Pediatr Neurosurg*. 2005:41(1):15–21.

68. Grill J, Viguier D, Kieffer V, et al. Critical risk factors for intellectual impairment in children with posterior fossa tumors: the role of cerebellar damage. *J Neurosurg*. 2004:101(2 suppl):152–158.

69. Grill J, Kieffer V, Kalifa C. Measuring the neuro-cognitive side-effects of irradiation in children with brain tumors. *Pediatr Blood Cancer*. 2004:42(5):452–456.

70. Moore BD 3rd. Neurocognitive outcomes in survivors of childhood cancer. *J Pediatr Psychol*. 2005:30(1):51–63.

71. Kupst MJ, Natta MB, Richardson CC, et al. Family coping with pediatric leukemia: ten years after treatment. *J Pediatr Psychol*. 1995:20(5):601–617.

72. Barrera M, Schulte F. A group social skills intervention program for survivors of childhood brain tumors. *J Pediatr Psychol*. 2009:34(10):1108–1118.

73. Essig S, Rebholz C, Strippoli M-PF, et al. Long-term survivors of childhood ALL: is health-related quality of life reduced in those who had suffered a relapse? *Pediatr Blood Cancer*. 2009:53(5):856.

74. Wolfe J, Friebert S, Hilden J. Caring for children with advanced cancer integrating palliative care. *Pediatr Clin North Am*. 2002:49(5):1043–1062.

75. Hinds PS, Drew D, Oakes LL, et al. End-of-life care preferences of pediatric patients with cancer. *J Clin Oncol*. 2005:23(36):9146–9154.

76. Kreicbergs UC, Lannen P, Onelov E, et al. Parental grief after losing a child to cancer: impact of professional and social support on long-term outcomes. *J Clin Oncol*. 2007:25(22):3307–3312.

77. Wolfe J, Klar N, Grier HE, et al. Understanding of prognosis among parents of children who died of cancer: impact on treatment goals and integration of palliative care. *JAMA*. 2000:284(19):2469–2475.

78. Mack JW, Nilsson M, Balboni T, et al. Peace, Equanimity, and Acceptance in the Cancer Experience (PEACE): validation of a scale to assess acceptance and struggle with terminal illness. *Cancer*. 2008:112(11):2509–2517.

79. Dussel V, Kreicbergs U, Hilden JM, et al. Looking beyond where children die: determinants and effects of planning a child's location of death. *J Pain Symptom Manage*. 2009:37(1):33–43.

80. Kreicbergs U, Valdimarsdottir U, Onelov E, et al. Care-related distress: a nationwide study of parents who lost their child to cancer. *J Clin Oncol*. 2005:23(36):9162–9171.

81. Hinds PS, Oakes L, Furman W, et al. End-of-life decision making by adolescents, parents, and healthcare providers in pediatric oncology: research to evidence-based practice guidelines. *Cancer Nurs*. 2001:24(2):122–134 [quiz 135–136].

82. McAliley LG, Hudson-Barr DC, Gunning RS, et al. The use of advance directives with adolescents. *Pediatr Nurs*. 2000:26(5):471–480.

83. Wiener L, Ballard E, Brennan T, et al. How I wish to be remembered: the use of an advance care planning document in adolescent and young adult populations. *J Palliat Med*. 2008:11(10):1309–1313.

84. Kazak AE, Barakat LP, Meeske K, et al. Posttraumatic stress, family functioning, and social support in survivors of childhood leukemia and their mothers and fathers. *J Consult Clin Psychol*. 1997:65(1):120–129.

85. Neamtu M, Neamtu S, Somlea C. Psychiatric morbidity among parents of children suffering from central nervous system and bone tumors. *Pediatr Blood Cancer*. 2009:53(5):873.

86. Barrera M, Atenafu E, Hancock K. Longitudinal health-related quality of life outcomes and related factors after pediatric SCT. *Bone Marrow Transplant*. 2009:44(4):249–256.

87. Sachdeva A, Yadav SP, Kalra M, et al. Study of sleep disorders in parents of childhood cancer patients. *Pediatr Blood Cancer*. 2009:53(5):737.

88. Streisand R, Rodrigue JR, Houck C, et al. Brief report: parents of children undergoing bone marrow transplantation: documenting stress and piloting a psychological intervention program. *J Pediatr Psychol*. 2000:25(5):331–337.

89. Sloper P. Predictors of distress in parents of children with cancer: a prospective study. *J Pediatr Psychol*. 2000:25(2):79–91.

90. Spinetta JJ, Jankovic M, Eden T, et al. Guidelines for assistance to siblings of children with cancer: report of the SIOP Working Committee on Psychosocial Issues in Pediatric Oncology. *Med Pediatr Oncol*. 1999:33(4):395–398.

91. Massie K, Barrera M. Internalizing behavior problems in siblings of children with cancer: influence of social support and cognitive appraisal. *Pediatr Blood Cancer*. 2009:53(5):722.

92. Packman W. Psychosocial impact of pediatric BMT on siblings. *Bone Marrow Transplant*. 1999:24(7):701–706.

93. Packman WL, Crittenden MR, Schaeffer E, et al. Psychosocial consequences of bone marrow transplantation in donor and nondonor siblings. *J Dev Behav Pediatr*. 1997:18(4):244–253.

94. Wiley FM, Lindamood MM, Pfefferbaum-Levine B. Donor–patient relationship in pediatric bone marrow transplantation. *J Assoc Pediatr Oncol Nurses*. 1984:1(3):8–14.

95. Weisz V, Robbennolt JK. Risks and benefits of pediatric bone marrow donation: a critical need for research. *Behav Sci Law*. 1996:14(4):375–391.

96. Visser A, Huizinga GA, Hoekstra HJ, et al. Emotional and behavioural functioning of children of a parent diagnosed with cancer: a cross-informant perspective. *Psychooncology*. 2005:14(9):746–758.

97. Cummings EM, Davies PT. Maternal depression and child development. *J Child Psychol Psychiatry*. 1994:35(1):73–112.

98. Armsden GC, Lewis FM. Behavioral adjustment and self-esteem of school-age children of women with breast cancer. *Oncol Nurs Forum*. 1994:21(1):39–45.

99. Lewis FM, Zahlis EH, Shands ME, et al. The functioning of single women with breast cancer and their school-aged children. *Cancer Pract*. 1996:4(1):15–24.

100. Issel LM, Ersek M, Lewis FM. How children cope with mother's breast cancer. *Oncol Nurs Forum*. 1990:17(3 suppl):5–12 [discussion 12–13].

101. Zahlis EH. The child's worries about the mother's breast cancer: sources of distress in school-age children. *Oncol Nurs Forum*. 2001:28(6):1019–1025.

102. Huizinga GA, van der Graaf WT, Visser A, et al. Psychosocial consequences for children of a parent with cancer: a pilot study. *Cancer Nurs*. 2003:26(3):195–202.

103. Heiney SP, Lesesne CA. Quest. An intervention program for children whose parent or grandparent has cancer. *Cancer Pract*. 1996:4(6):324–329.

104. Hoke LA. A short-term psychoeducational intervention for families with parental cancer. *Harv Rev Psychiatry*. 1997:5(2):99–103.

105. Lewis FM, Casey SM, Brandt PA, et al. The enhancing connections program: pilot study of a cognitive–behavioral intervention for mothers and children affected by breast cancer. *Psychooncology*. 2006:15(6):486–497.

CHAPTER 19

Cancer and the Older Person

• *Sriram Yennurajalingam*

■ INTRODUCTION

In the United States, as the life expectancy increases there would be an increase in older individuals in terms of both absolute numbers and proportions of the total population.[1-4] By 2050 it is expected that there would be approximately 70 million individuals over 65 years of age.[1] This older population has a high risk for cancer and also a higher cancer mortality rate.[3] This increase in incidence and mortality would mean better understanding of the disease and the consequences of the disease in the older population so as to provide optimal care. An older person's ability to tolerate treatment to prolong life or cure cancer or have quality of life depends on a complex assessment of interaction of individual person's physiological aging process, comorbidities, psychosocial, environmental factors, cancer, and cancer treatment itself.[5] In this chapter the author plans to review the challenges confronting older patients who are coping with cancer and to discuss various strategies to manage these challenges effectively.

■ AGING AND CANCER

Older population has a high risk for cancer and also a higher cancer mortality rate. An age-adjusted cancer mortality rate is 1068/100,000 for those over 65 years of age as compared with 67/100,000 for those under 65.[3] Various reasons have been proposed to explain the increased individual risk, including genetic factors and environmental factors[6-8] such as DNA damage by reactive oxygen species,

toxic agents, and UV rays, epigenetic alteration, differential gene expression, telomere shortening, stem cell loss of function, and death. The following factors may also increase susceptibility of aging tissues to carcinogens: (1) cumulative exposure to environmental toxins and free radicals (carcinogens) and (2) immunological (diminished tumor surveillance).[6-8]

Key physiological changes due to aging that impact cancer and treatment include the following:

(a) There is a decrease in total body water and lean body mass. This is coupled by increase in body fat (eg, benzodiazepines, gabapentin).[9] There may be also a decreased protein binding (phenytoin) and a decreased rate of oxidation/reduction (phase I) reactions (eg, benzodiazepines, tricyclics, SSRIs). Overall hepatic metabolism of many drugs through the cytochrome P-450 enzyme system decreases with aging.[9-13]

(b) There is a decrease in GFR due to decreased renal mass and renal blood flow.[9]

(c) Vision problems increase with age, including the risk for glaucoma, cataract, and age-related macular degeneration.

(d) Hearing issues increase, including otosclerosis, presbycusis, and tinnitus.

(e) Cardiovascular system: aberrant heart rhythms and extra heart beats become more common. The baroreceptors that monitor blood pressure become less sensitive. Quick changes in position may cause dizziness from orthostatic hypotension.[10]

(f) Respiratory: the total lung capacity remains constant but vital capacity decreases and residual volume increases.

(g) Gastrointestinal: the liver is less efficient in metabolizing drugs and repairing damaged liver cells. Reduced peristalsis of the colon can increase risk for constipation.

(h) Urinary system: kidney mass decreases by 25% to 30% and the number of glomeruli decrease by 30% to 40%. These changes reduce the ability to filter and concentrate urine and to clear drugs. With aging, there is a reduced hormonal response (vasopressin) and an impaired ability to conserve salt, which may increase risk for dehydration. Bladder capacity decreases and there is an increase in residual urine and frequency. These changes increase the chances of urinary infections, incontinence, and urinary obstruction.[9]

(i) Endocrine system: insulin resistance may result in glucose intolerance.

(j) Nervous system: the incidence of cognitive impairment increases with age so that by age 85, up to one third of older persons have some degree of cognitive impairment. The cognitive abilities of older adults vary tremendously both within individuals and across age groups and are determined by comorbidities such as those that increase the risk for dementia.

To summarize, the impact of these physiological changes on cancer and treatments options in older patients includes the following: (a) effect on function is observed due to changes in vision, hearing, memory, and bladder (eg, nocturia, frequency) and (b) effects on cardiovascular, respiratory, gastrointestinal, and immune system may increase the risk for cancer, infections, and their treatments.

■ KEY ISSUES IN CANCER CARE DUE TO OLDER AGE

In older patients, physiological aging is determined by genetic factors, comorbidities, presence of geriatric syndromes, impaired physical function, malnutrition, and a higher amount of psychosocial distress rather than chronological age alone.

Physiological aging can increase the cancer risk, impact the tolerance to treatment, and effect physical and psychological consequences of cancer and treatment. Hence, it is important to determine a more accurate physiological age and identify factors contributing to reduced physiological age (diminished physiological reserve). This can be determined by use of appropriate assessment methods such as comprehensive geriatric assessment and symptom assessment tools such as Edmonton symptom assessment scale (ESAS). Psychosocial distress is contributed by the following factors: (i) poor physical and psychological symptom control, (ii) independence and function, (iii) dementia, (iv) urinary incontinence, (v) abuse and neglect, (vi) psychosocial, spiritual, and emotional concerns, (vii) social isolation, (viii) economic and logistical concerns including transportation, (ix) environmental assessment, (x) comorbidities, (xi) caregiver and communication issues, (xii) psychosocial issues in elderly with cancer, and (xiii) polypharmacy.

Pain and Other Symptoms

Assessment and Management of Pain and Other Symptoms in Older Patients with Cancer

Pain and other symptoms are typically underreported and undertreated in individuals living with cancer.[14] Patients over 70 years were among those at greatest risk for receiving inadequate analgesia. Barriers to the assessment and provision of adequate pain and symptom management may be patient- or physician-related, with culture and generational beliefs often playing a prominent role in older individuals.[15] Ineffective treatment of pain may be associated with depression, social isolation, immobility, sleep disturbances, increased health care costs, and severe caregiver strain.[16] More globally, inadequate pain and symptom control may negatively impact health and quality of life, which affects adherence to oncological treatment.[17,18]

Optimal symptom control is contingent upon expert assessment of the multiple domains impacting the patient's symptom experience, thereby integrating the symptom report into a more comprehensive understanding of the individual's experience. In addition to general medical, oncological, psychosocial, and spiritual histories and physical examination, key components of the symptom history include a systematic symptom survey and a symptom-specific history. For pain, the latter includes intensity, severity, associated distress, location and sites of radiation, relieving and exacerbating features, as well as prior treatment modalities and their outcome. Similar parameters may be assessed for nonpain symptoms. The information derived from the symptom experience is then used to synthesize a working diagnosis related to the underlying etiology and pathophysiology. The treatment plan targets primary therapy at the underlying causes, nonspecific symptom-directed therapy, and interventions directed at other needed areas of care.

Validated measures should be used whenever possible to enhance reporting consistency and communication effectiveness with other clinicians and researchers. Symptom assessment tools may be unidimensional or multidimensional and may assess multiple or single symptoms. Numerous symptom batteries exist, including the ESAS,[19–21] the MD Anderson Symptom Inventory, the Memorial Symptom Assessment Scale, which has pediatric-specific versions, and the Rotterdam Symptom Checklist,[21] among others. The ESAS is an example of a unidimensional symptom battery measuring symptom intensity, while the Memorial Symptom Assessment Scale and the MD Anderson Symptom Inventory are multidimensional tools measuring several components of the symptom experience. The Memorial Symptom Assessment Scale and its derivatives look at frequency, intensity, and associated distress of individual symptoms, while the MD Anderson Symptom Inventory can be performed over the telephone by incorporating interactive voice response technology. Among the scales measuring specific symptoms, pain is the best developed. Unidimensional tools for measurement of pain intensity include a variety of numeric and verbal ratings, as well as visual analog and face scales. The Brief Pain Inventory,[21] validated in numerous languages, includes a measure of pain impact on a variety of functions. An analogous scale, the Brief Fatigue Inventory, has been developed for fatigue, and is commonly used in clinical and research settings.[21]

Because of the multidimensional nature of the symptom experience, health care workers assessing a patient's symptom level of pain should keep in mind the "production–perception–expression" model of symptoms.[22] This model builds on that proposed by the renowned Dame Cicely Saunders, who first described the construct of "total pain."[22] The cascade model addresses the different levels of symptom development that result in an individual rating of the patient's suffering. It focuses on the patient's expression of the suffering, rather than on production or perception of a symptom. This model emphasizes that affective dimensions, such as agitation, catastrophizing, somatization, depression, and anxiety, can have a considerable impact on this expression and may thereby worsen the pain. If affective dimensions are suspected, they should be further investigated by using highly specific assessment tools and then treated along with pain, as necessary. This model can also be extrapolated to nonpain symptoms.

Symptom Assessment of Patients with Cognitive Impairment

Cognitive impairment is commonly found in patients with advanced cancer, occurring in up to 85% in the period before death.[23] Cognitive impairment may be a consequence of delirium, dementia, or both.

Since symptom expression requires cognition, patient self-report should not be relied upon if cognitive impairment is suspected. The example of pain will be used, as this is the more frequently studied symptom. Patients with dementia are less likely to recall, interpret, and articulate their experiences with pain than those without, even those who are communicative. Consequentially, they are less likely to report pain than patients without delirium.[15,16]

Elderly patients with dementia have difficulty with commonly used tools such as a visual analog scale (VAS), likely due to decreased memory, poor orientation, as well as visual and spatial skills.[15,16] These deficits strongly impact pain ratings in cognitively impaired patients. For older adults with mild to moderate cognitive impairment, the Faces Pain Scale and a verbal descriptor scale rating are among the scales of choice, as compared with a vertical VAS, a 21-point Numeric Rating Scale, and an 11-point Verbal Numeric Rating Scale. VAS are 100-mm lines with anchors at either end describing the characteristic to be measured, for example, "no pain" and "the worst pain imaginable." The individual makes a mark perpendicular to the line, which, when measured from the anchor, provides a quantitative estimate of symptom intensity. Additional validated assessment tools are needed for pain and nonpain symptoms, as well as for patients with dementia who cannot communicate. The latter rely predominantly on behavioral measures and require third-party or proxy raters, complicated by the need for interpretation of another individual's experience.

Pain management Good pain control regimens are typically multimodal. Salient features of optimal therapy involve identifying the specific syndrome to target pharmacological and other interventions at specific etiologies whenever possible, minimizing drug interactions, and incorporating nonpharmacological approaches to enhance symptom control, function, and sense of autonomy. Older individuals are less likely to tolerate aggressive pharmacotherapeutic interventions than younger individuals due to physiological changes altering drug pharmacokinetics and pharmacodynamics, resulting in a narrowed therapeutic index, with an increased risk of toxicity and drug–drug interactions. Low plasma protein levels, decreased volume of distribution, dehydration, and concomitant clinical problems make advanced geriatric cancer patients particularly vulnerable to drug interactions. The best-known drug interactions occur as a result of induction or inhibition of the cytochrome P450 (CYP) isoenzymes, seen with many drugs commonly used in the cancer population, with the potential for toxic or subtherapeutic drug levels. Fentanyl and methadone are metabolized primarily by CYP 3A4, and to a lesser extent by other isoenzymes such as CYP1A2, CYP2D6, CYP2C9, and CYP2C19.[11,12] For a highly potent drug such as methadone, with a long half-life, awareness of the potential for drug interactions is especially important. While not a contraindication to drug combinations, the narrowed therapeutic index and increased risk of drug interactions in older individuals requires cautious prescribing. Therefore, use of non-pharmacological approaches such as physical therapy, rehabilitative approaches, and cognitive behavioral therapy, in conjunction with pharmacotherapy, assumes even greater relevance in the older population than in younger individuals with similar symptoms. For the small minority in whom pain control remains inadequate, a variety of neurolytic procedures, neurosurgical techniques, and improved catheter and pump systems for spinal delivery of opioids, nonopioid analgesics, and local anesthetics may facilitate pain control when used as part of a multimodal treatment plan.

The selection of opioid depends on patient and drug factors, with intensity of pain influencing selection of the initial opioid prescribed. Moderate pain is usually treated with a weak opioid (codeine), and severe pain with a strong opioid (morphine), according to steps 2 and 3 of the World Health Organization ladder for management of pain. Antiemetic and laxative regimens should be commenced with the initiation of the opioids. A prokinetic agent, such as metoclopramide, is usually effective for nausea when given regularly around the clock with breakthrough doses as needed for the first 3 days and as needed thereafter. A combination of sennoside (senna) and docusate is commonly used for prevention of constipation. Opioid side effects should be identified proactively and treated appropriately. When dose-limiting toxicity to opioid analgesia precludes adequate pain control or when escalation to very high doses makes administration difficult, rotation to an alternative opioid may be an effective treatment strategy. Extreme care must be taken when rotating to methadone, as its equianalgesic ratio to other opioids varies highly with the individual's preexisting degree of opioid tolerance. For clinicians without significant experience using methadone, the assistance of an experienced clinician should be sought.

Delirium

Delirium in older cancer patients is due to treatments of cancer or comorbidities. The etiology is a multifactorial process.[24] Significant causes include dehydration, medications, infections, hypoxia, central nervous system involvement by the cancer, renal failure, and hepatic failure.[24] Risk factors identified for delirium are advanced age, prior cognitive impairment, illness severity, and burden of comorbidities.[24]

Delirium, associated with an increased mortality rate, is underrecognized, misdiagnosed, and undertreated. Characterized by degrees of behavioral activity, the hyperactive and mixed subtypes come to medical attention more frequently than the hypoactive subtype, due to disruptions caused by the patient's agitation. Frequently, delirium is misdiagnosed as either depression or dementia, especially when hypoactive.[24] Failure to recognize agitated delirium as such is of particular concern owing to the distress it causes the patient, family members, and medical staff.

Physicians may fail to recognize delirium as a potential medical emergency, although delirium in elderly patients may be the sole manifestation of a life-threatening illness, such as sepsis. Management involves identifying and correcting reversible risk factors and treating the symptoms of delirium. Psychotropic medications such as haloperidol, olanzapine, and risperidone are the mainstay of treatment. The intensity of the search for causative factors for delirium and of the treatment strategies used in the end-of-life setting must be individualized, according to the clinical situation and goals of care. When possible, correction of possible opioid toxicity, dehydration, infection, medication interactions or side effects, and metabolic disturbances may help to reverse delirium. Environmental manipulation strategies such as reorientation, limiting staff changes, and reducing noise stimulation can also be tried.

Fatigue

Fatigue is one of the most prevalent and distressing symptoms with cancer and its treatment.[25] It is characterized by unusual and profound tiredness after minimal effort, accompanied by unpleasant sensation of generalized weakness. A well-validated tool such as Brief Fatigue Inventory can be used to measure fatigue. Major etiological categories include direct tumor effects (ie, brain metastasis), tumor-induced products (ie, cytokines), and tumor-accompanying factors (ie, paraneoplastic phenomena, treatment-related side effects). In a different model, factors associated with the disease or its treatment, intercurrent systemic disorders, sleep disorders, immobility, lack of exercise, chronic pain, centrally acting drugs, anxiety disorders, and depression have all been invoked as potential causes.[25]

Because of the paucity of the data, interventions are empirically directed at the potential reversible mechanisms, as determined by individual patient assessment in conjunction with symptomatic therapy. Pharmacological approaches include the use of psychostimulants, such as methylphenidate, corticosteroids, and antidepressants. Nonpharmacological approaches involve patient education, exercise, modification of activity and rest patterns, cognitive therapies, and attention to nutrition factors.

Anorexia–Cachexia Syndrome (ACS)

ACS causes severe distress for patients and their families, along with its attendant social implications. It is caused by direct tumor effects on lipolysis and protein catabolism, resulting in anorexia and metabolic abnormalities. A recent review describes the role of cytokines, such as tumor necrosis factor, IL-1, and IL-6, in the causation of anorexia.[25] Profound anorexia adds a nutritional deprivation component to the metabolic abnormalities induced by the cancer itself. Anorexia is worsened by nausea caused by tumor byproducts, decreased gastric emptying, bowel obstruction, constipation, and pain medications.

Management involves a combination of nutritional and pharmacological approaches, as well as education about realistic treatment expectations. A main challenge in management is defining the outcome for nutritional and pharmacological approaches, as these interventions are ultimately unlikely to reduce weight loss in most patients. Potential pharmacological interventions include the prokinetic metoclopramide doses prior to meals (up to 60 mg per day), melatonin, and short-term use of corticosteroids and megestrol acetate.

Dyspnea

Dyspnea is defined as uncomfortable awareness of breathing. It is a subjective sensation, which cannot be measured by any physical abnormality, such as respiratory rate or accessory muscle use. There are multiple causes of dyspnea in the elderly with colorectal cancer, including lung metastasis, pleural effusions, infections, anemia, pulmonary embolism, deconditioning, psychological distress, abdominal distension due to ascites or bowel obstruction, and general medical conditions such as heart failure and chronic obstruction pulmonary disease.

Many of the causes of dyspnea improve with treatment of the underlying condition, such as antibiotics for pneumonia, anticoagulation for pulmonary embolism, or transfusions for anemia. Corticosteroids are effective in the management of dyspnea associated with carcinomatous lymphangitis. The symptoms of dyspnea are treated with oxygen, opioids, and behavioral strategies.[26]

Independence and Function

Physical function can predict survival, dependency, and ability to tolerate cancer treatment.

Functional Impairment

Functional impairment involves the inability of an older person to perform daily life activities normally. A recent survey indicated that 10% to 13% of older persons between the ages of 65 and 69 have difficulty getting out of bed, and 6% to 10% need help with routine care. As older people age, this need increases, with 24% to 29% of those over age 80 requiring help to get out of bed, and 29% to 42% requiring help with routine care.[67]

Functional impairment can also affect cancer care. For example, having to depend on someone for transportation may contribute to difficulty in keeping appointments. In older patients with functional impairments, one must also consider the impact of the patient's disease and treatment on caregiver burden. Appropriate referral to social workers or community-based services may help reduce stress on the caregiver and enable continued care over a longer period of time.

Functional Assessment

Identification of functional disability using comprehensive geriatric assessment using tools such as activities of daily living (ADLs), instrumental activities of daily living (IADLs), gait speed, get-up-and-go, etc, is helpful in maintaining or restoring independence and useful in cancer treatment planning and provision of appropriate psychosocial support. Functional assessment instruments, such as the Karnofsky Performance Scale or Index and Eastern Cooperative Oncology Group (ECOG) Performance Status (PS) Scale, are widely used to help predict prognosis in cancer patients.[27,28] Studies have demonstrated that these two scales are highly correlated and have predictive validity.[35,36] Functional status is also used as an outcome measure to gauge response to cancer treatment. For example, ECOG values are followed frequently over the duration of therapy.

The Karnofsky Performance Scale has been evaluated in a geriatric outpatient population and compared with the traditional functional assessment measures, ADLs and IADLs. ADLs are a measure of six basic functions: bathing, dressing, toileting, continence, transferring, and feeding.[30] IADLs are a measure of eight higher-level functions: using the telephone, traveling, shopping, preparing meals, laundry, doing housework, taking medicine, and managing money.[31] A study in 134 patients showed that the above three measures were highly correlated with one another.[32]

Correlation of Geriatric and Oncological Scales

Assessment of function is an interesting topic in older cancer patients. The ECOG PS or Karnofsky Index is widely used by oncologists. However, there is a "natural" adaptation of this score with age. We do not expect the patient who is 80 years old to meet the same criteria for an ECOG score of 1 as the patient who is 20 years old. Trying to mitigate this problem, geriatricians have developed task-based tools such as the various versions of the ADL and IADL scales. Although the basic ADL is relatively gender-indifferent, IADL scales may present significant gender biases. Such is the case for Lawton's 8-item IADL scale; Lawton himself designed a 9-item version of his scale to address this problem.[33]

It is also important to ask whether the patient can do a task, rather than whether he or she actually does it.[33] Geriatric scales have an interesting potential in oncology. Whereas only 20% of elderly patients achieve an ECOG score of 2 or more, more than half display some dependence in their IADL.[35] This suggests that, in well-functioning patients such as those receiving chemotherapy, the IADL may be more sensitive to change than the ECOG PS.

The Karnofsky score and ECOG PS are closely correlated (Spearman $r = 0.87$).[5] However, despite being more detailed, the Karnofsky Index does not appear to have a higher predictive power.[36]

More targeted measurements such as geriatric scales (ADL, IADL) may fare better. Two studies have assessed the correlation between oncological and geriatric scales.[34,35,32] One is mentioned by Naeim and Reuben, and evaluates the Karnofsky Index;[35,37] the other, a study of ECOG performance status, was conducted by Externman's group.[32] Naeim and Reuben suggest a screening tool for use in primary care setting. The tool they highlight, developed by Moore and Siu,[37] or similar one developed by Lachs et al,[38] would be convienient aid to a busy oncologist. Patients screening positively on these tools could benefit from further assessment, ideally by a multidisciplinary geriatric or oncogeriatric team. It is pleasing to note that as a fruitful dialogue continues between geriatrics and oncology, user-friendly tools are being developed, and both specialties will benefit from a common understanding of their patients—who, after all, are the ultimate beneficiaries of the process.

In patients where the diminished physical function cannot be alleviated, measures that turn the focus from physical functioning to other enjoyable nonphysical activities may be considered. Patients may benefit from physical therapy evaluation and orthotics, wheelchairs, walkers, and physical therapy to improve function, which can enhance quality of life.[39,40]

Important factors that are associated with independence and function in older patients are the Geriatric syndromes, most important among which are dementia, delirium, urinary incontinence, pressure ulcers, and falls. These have to be identified early as a part of assessment methods such as comprehensive geriatric assessment and managed accordingly.

Dementia

Dementia is defined as memory loss and one or more of the following cognitive difficulties: disorientation (aphasia, apraxia [difficulty performing coordinated movements], and agnosia [difficulty recognizing familiar objects] and disturbance of executive functions.

Various types of dementia have been described. These include Alzheimer's disease characterized by amyloid plaques and neurofibrillary tangles, vascular dementia with history of cortical or subcortical infarctions, leukoaraiosis (white matter changes), Lewy body distinguished by alpha-synuclein protein, and frontotemporal (Pick's disease) characterized by tau protein.

Assessment of dementia can be performed by instruments such as Folstein's Mini Mental State Exam (MMSE), Clox 2 by Royall, Cordes, and Polk (1998), Mini-Cog by Scanlon et al (2000), or Word list generation, Letter WLG—"FAS," and Category WLG—"animals."[41,42,43]

Management of Older Cancer Patients with Dementia

Cancer treatment should be individualized based on a comprehensive geriatric assessment. Patients and their health care proxies should be involved in the decision making with a clear emphasis to explain them the prognosis and clinical course of their cancer in context to the dementia. This would reduce distressing symptoms to patients and avoid burdensome interventions.[44] Patients and families would benefit from an access to a palliative care team.

Urinary Incontinence

Incontinence may have a significant impact on a patient's quality of life. The prevalence of incontinence in the elderly varies considerably. In the community, the incidence of incontinence ranges from 15% to 30%, but in the nursing home setting, as many as 50% to 60% of patients are incontinent.[45]

Metastatic disease to the brain or spinal cord can interfere with nerve pathways needed for normal micturition and cause incontinence.[46,47] Furthermore, incontinence is sometimes an early indication of an underlying urinary tract infection, which may lead to sepsis in older cancer patients. The treatment of cancer may also precipitate or worsen incontinence. Fluids and diuretics are often administered in conjunction with chemotherapy and can exacerbate the symptoms of incontinence, making mild symptoms moderate or severe, and, thereby, adversely affecting quality of life.[48]

The history and physical examination are essential in distinguishing transient from chronic causes of incontinence. Transient causes of incontinence include delirium, urinary tract infections, atrophic vaginitis, use of certain medications (eg, benzodiazepines, alcohol, diuretics, anticholinergic agents), psychological disorders, endocrine disorders, restricted mobility, and stool impaction.[49] The postvoidal residual (PVR) test measures residual urine after the patient voids via catheterization or ultrasound. Typically a PVR >200 mL suggests detrusor weakness or bladder outlet obstruction; even a PVR >50 mL can be sufficient to exacerbate stress or urge incontinence.

Abuse and Neglect

Elderly abuse and neglect is another syndrome that has a significant prevalence (1.3–7.4%, but probably underreported) and goes largely unrecognized, due to both patient underreporting and the reluctance of physicians to engage in questioning that could lead to time-consuming and disagreeable consequences. However, most of the time, both patient and caregivers go to great lengths to ensure the patient's relative independence in a personal home environment. A correct assessment of the patient's social situation, including the caregiver's major health problems or limitations, will help to identify risky situations and prevent potentially dramatic complications of treatment.

Psychosocial, Spiritual, and Emotional Concerns

Older patients with cancer commonly experience spiritual and existential concerns. They may ponder the meaning of their illness, their suffering, their relationship to God, and their possible death. Socially, patients are stressed by the arduous treatment procedures used to achieve control of the disease or cure. The long period of treatment and rehabilitation and continuing surveillance can also exhaust insurance and require significant out-of-pocket expenses. It may cause the loss of employment for patient and caregiver and interruptions in academic preparation.

Older adults commonly turn to spirituality and religion when they encounter difficult life-changing events and experience personal losses. Several studies of spirituality and health have been conducted. One study found that religiosity is positively associated with health-enhancing attitudes and behaviors, and inversely associated with health-compromising behaviors and adverse health-related outcomes.[50] Oncologists need to be aware that religion may assume more importance as a person ages, and that formal instruments to assess its importance are being developed.

Social Isolation

Social isolation is the lack of contact and interaction with other people. Subjectively, it is the feeling of loneliness or lack of companionship or close and genuine communication with others. Loneliness is the perception of being alone and can be experienced even when one is in contact with others.[51] Although older persons can live alone without being socially isolated or feeling lonely, living alone is a leading indicator of the potential for social isolation.

There are a number of potential causes of social isolation, the most important of which include role loss, living alone, widowhood, health problems, poverty, and the aging baby boomer. Interventions that help to reduce social isolation, including group interventions such as discussion, self-help, exercise, and skills training, have shown to be effective in non-cancer settings.[52]

Economic and Logistical Concerns Including Transportation

Economic and logistical concerns including transportation can be distressful to patients and caregivers. This would have significant impact on compliance to treatment and management of disease and treatment-related symptoms.

Environmental Assessment

Environmental Hazards

The physical environment can play a major role in the day-to-day functioning and health of older patients. Mismatches between a patient's capabilities and environmental demands can result in disability. There is a high prevalence of environmental hazards in the homes of older persons. One population-based study showed that there were loose throw rugs and obstructed pathways, respectively, in nearly 80% and 50% of the homes of older persons with physical disabilities.[53] Some studies suggest that between 35% and 45% of falls are attributed to home hazards, such as poor lighting, inadequate bathroom grab rails and stairway banisters, exposed electrical cords, clutter on the floors, and throw rugs.[54]

Home Assessment

It can be helpful to have a visiting physician, nurse, or social worker perform a home assessment using a home safety checklist provided by the National Safety Council such as a knowledge of (a) the patient and caregivers on how to report an emergency and (b) the correct use of the equipment as applicable such as the wheelchair, oxygen supplies, and Bipap (noninvasive ventilator).[55] Home assessment can also provide other valuable information on nutritional adequacy, sanitary conditions, medication use and misuse, social interactions, and elder abuse and neglect.[54]

Comorbidities including Under/Untreated Psychosocial Issues such as Alcoholism, Smoking, Personality, and Psychiatric/Maladaptive Disorders

Older cancer patients are also more likely than younger patients to present with concurrent comorbid conditions (ie, presence of multiple, concurrent health conditions) and/or functional disabilities.[56,57] Comorbidity can become a major confounder in oncological practice and studies in the elderly. Comprehensive assessment of comorbidity can be performed using various scales such as Charlson Index, Kaplan–Feinstein Index, and NIA/NCI cancer and comorbidity measure. Comorbidity can be factored into various oncological practices such as screening,[58] treatment decisions,[59] clinical trial participation,[60] and cancer care.

Older cancer patients may have developed more effective skills to manage stress, tend to be less depressed than younger patients, and show a reduced vulnerability concerning mental health and psychological functioning.[59,61] It was also demonstrated that the elderly respond positively to conservative organ-sparing treatments,[62] and it has also been demonstrated that there is no difference in quality of life as a function of age.

Caregiver and Communication Issues

Decision making (eg, transition of treatment plan from disease-specific treatment to palliative care only) and symptom distress such as delirium-related symptoms can cause severe distress in both patients and family members. Good communication is a solid foundation for creating an atmosphere of sensitivity and compassion for optimal therapeutic outcome. It promotes honesty and openness between families and health care providers. Better communication and better interpersonal care translate into improved patient satisfaction, compliance with medical recommendations, and health outcomes. Ong et al[63] found that doctor–patient communication during oncological consultation is related to patients' quality of life and satisfaction. The affective quality of the consultation seems to be the most important factor in determining these outcomes.[64]

Communication allows empowerment of the family and the patient by involving them in decision-making with regard to treatment. These issues should be addressed directly with them. Treatment should be explained in adequate detail so that they can give informed consent or refusal, and facilitate a continuing sense of their being in control.

Improving Communication Strategies

Elderly patients usually require a longer visit time. It would allow the patients to express their emotions and give the clinician time to listen, recognize, and respond to the emotion accordingly. A split meeting with patient and caregiver may facilitate a more open discussion of concerns and distressing issues.

Caregiver Distress

Prior studies found that the caregiver distress is more severe with the number and severity of symptoms such as pain and fatigue and advanced nature of the disease in the patients.[65] Adult children caregivers experience distress and anxiety related to role change (from taking care to giving care) and task overload with multiple role demands from their work and family life. Older spouses, on the other hand, suffer from role changes in the relationship, the loss of support, and anticipation of future loss and change. Age-related impairments in the healthy partner could also add considerable stress and limit their caregiving capacity. Caregiver tasks with older cancer patients may involve one or more of the following activities: (a) medication dispensing and monitoring, (b) symptom management, (c) monitoring of side effects and adverse events, (d) meal preparation and nutritional balance, (e) care decisions and problem solving, (f) skin care and infection control, (g) management of highly technical equipment, (h) management of medical procedures such as catheters and wound care, (i) bill paying, (j) transportation and errands, and (k) advocacy with health professionals and within the health care system.[66]

Factors found to be helpful in alleviating the distress include interdisciplinary interventions such as supportive counseling for patients and caregivers, information and education about illness, treatments, costs, and services available, and providing access to supportive cancer care that includes active and longitudinal management of patients' symptoms related to cancer and treatment including anxiety, depression, and provision of modalities to improve nutritional status and physical performance by provision of physical and occupational therapy.

Psychosocial Issues in Elderly with Cancer

Older adults diagnosed with cancer face a multitude of psychosocial issues. In addition to coping with common grief and loss responses related to their mortality, finances, role changes within their families, and changes in their cognitive and physical abilities, older cancer patients are often faced with common challenges brought about by advanced aging such as chronic comorbid conditions. Key issues in older cancer patients include those given in the following subsections.

Coping and Psychiatric Treatment

Overall, older patients appear to cope with cancer better than younger patients. However, it is more difficult to assess psychiatric distress in the elderly (Patricia Ganz). On initial diagnoses, an initial shock and disbelief is followed by a period of turmoil, anxiety, depression, irritability, and neurovegetative symptoms.

These symptoms are usually self-limited and resolve over days to weeks with support of family, friends, and doctors. Hypnotics or anxiolytics can be helpful in extreme situations but need to be given based on individuals' risk benefit profile of drug interactions.

However, when depressive or anxious symptoms do not improve after a few weeks and are maladaptive, such as impaired social and/or occupational functioning, emergence of suicidal ideations, or request for physician-assisted suicide, special interdisciplinary psychiatric should be considered. Few points should be considered in the management of psychiatric complications. These include the following: (a) many elderly patients, especially men who have never had psychiatric treatment, are less willing to accept psychiatric treatment in the cancer setting, when needed; (b) psychotherapy and psychiatric medications can be very helpful, but may need to be modified to accommodate the elderly and end-of-life; (c) however, family and social resources must be taken into account to achieve successful psychiatric treatment in the elderly.

Depression

The frequency estimates in the elderly with depression range from 36% to 50%.

Risk factors include (a) loss of spouse, (b) functional disability, (c) inadequate emotional support, (d) other life stresses or losses, (e) uncontrolled pain and advanced illness, (f) poor physical conditioning, (g) previous history of depression, (h) family history of depression or suicide, and (i) medications (eg, steroids) and metabolic abnormalities (eg, hypercalcemia).

Risk of depression plateaus from the ages of 65 to 75 but then increases again with advancing age. Mood disorder with depressive features due to cancer, and delirium need to be ruled out as they are other common symptoms in older cancer patients.

Screening and Diagnoses

One method of assessment using a single-item interview for assessing mood, "Have you been depressed most time for the past two weeks?," can be very useful. Other instruments include a two-item interview assessing depressed mood and loss of interest in activities, VAS for depressed mood (ESAS), and Beck depression inventory-13 item. Key symptoms diagnostic may include (a) hopelessness, (b) excessive guilt, (c) worthlessness, (d) feeling one is being punished, and (e) suicidal ideation.

Polypharmacy

Polypharmacy is defined as the concurrent use of several different medications, including more than one medication from the same drug classification.[12] In a study based on Ohio Cancer Incidence Surveillance System (OCISS), there were 282 patients with incident breast cancer, 111 patients with prostate cancer, and 259 patients with colorectal cancer having a median age of 73, 74, and 75 years, respectively[13]; nearly 45% were prescribed at least one type of medication in the month preceding cancer diagnosis. Of those with any prescription in that time period, nearly 49% were prescribed five or more types of medications. Polypharmacy (five or more types of medication) was present in more than 22% of patients in this study population.

Older patients with cancer are especially vulnerable to the risks associated with polypharmacy. Their heightened use of drugs to treat cancers and increasing chronic illnesses, the availability of nonprescription medications, the tendency to self-treat, and the prohibitive costs of some anticancer medications are among the various reasons that can promote polypharmacy. The consequences of polypharmacy involve adverse drug reactions, drug interactions, higher medication costs, and noncompliance. Polypharmacy is often recognized after it has occurred.

The key to the prevention of polypharmacy is to incorporate prevention methods prior to its occurrence: (1) education of the medical community as well as the elderly population is an effective prevention method; (2) communication among medication prescribers reduces the number of medications used; (3) the use of the "essential medication only" premise to medication treatment in the elderly population will also aid in the prevention of polypharmacy; (4) cost factors, therapeutic endpoints, nondrug therapy through health promotion, and communication among the older patient and all prescribers involved in medical care are vital components

to the main goal of decreased medication use in the senior population with cancer.

■ SUMMARY

Physiological aging can increase the cancer risk, impact the tolerance to treatment, and effect physical and psychological consequences of cancer and treatment. Hence, it is important to determine a more accurate physiological age and identify factors contributing to reduced physiological age. This can be determined by use of appropriate assessment methods such as comprehensive geriatric assessment and symptom assessment tools. Appropriate management of these factors would assist in effective prevention of complications of cancer, cure, prolonged survival, and improvement of quality of life with preservation of functional independence.

KEY POINTS

- Physiological aging can increase the cancer risk, impact the tolerance to treatment, and effect physical and psychological consequences of cancer and treatment.
- Elderly cancer patients usually require a longer visit time. It would allow the patients to express their emotions and give the clinician time to listen, recognize, and respond to the emotion accordingly.
- Factors found to be helpful in alleviating the caregiver distress include interdisciplinary interventions such as supportive counseling for patients and caregivers.
- Older patients appear to cope with cancer better than younger patients.

REFERENCES

1. National Center for Health Statistics. *Health, United States 2007*. Washington, DC: US Department of Health and Human Services; 2007. DHHS publication 2007-1232.

2. Muss HB. Cancer in the elderly: a societal perspective from the United States. *Clin Oncol (R Coll Radiol)*. 2009;21(2):92–98 [Epub December 6, 2008].

3. Berger NA, Savvides P, Koroukian SM, et al. Cancer in the elderly. *Trans Am Clin Climatol Assoc*. 2006;117:147–155 [discussion 155–156].

4. Ershler WB. Cancer: a disease of the elderly. *J Support Oncol.* 2003;1(4 suppl 2):5–10.

5. Albert SM, Im A, Raveis VH. Public health and the second 50 years of life. *Am J Public Health.* 2002;92:1214–1216; Satariano WA, Silliman RA. Comorbidity: implications for research and practice in geriatric oncology. *Crit Rev Oncol Hematol.* 2003;48:239–248.

6. Calvanese V, Lara E, Kahn A, Fraga MF. The role of epigenetics in aging and age-related diseases. *Ageing Res Rev.* 2009;8(4):268–276.

7. Marques FZ, Markus MA, Morris BJ. The molecular basis of longevity, and clinical implications. *Maturitas.* 2009;65(2):87–91.

8. Fraga MF. Genetic and epigenetic regulation of aging. *Curr Opin Immunol.* 2009;21(4):446–453.

9. Beck LH. The aging kidney. Defending a delicate balance of fluid and electrolytes. *Geriatrics.* 2000;55:26–32.

10. Pugh KG, Wei JY. Clinical implications of physiological changes in the aging heart. *Drugs Aging.* 2001;18:263–276.

11. Corcoran M. Polypharmacy in the older patient with cancer. *Cancer Control.* 1997;4:419–428.

12. Tam-McDevitt J. Polypharmacy, aging, and cancer. *Oncology (Huntingt).* 2008;22(9):1052–1055 [discussion 1055, 1058, 1060].

13. Koroukian SM, Owusu C, Madigan E, et al. Polypharmacy in elders with cancer: an analysis of the Ohio Medicaid population. 2007 ASCO Annual Meeting Proceedings. *J Clin Oncol.* 2007;25(18S):19550.

14. Deandrea S, Montanari M, Moja L, Apolone G. Prevalence of undertreatment in cancer pain. A review of published literature. *Ann Oncol.* 2008;19(12):1985–1991.

15. Farrell MJ, Katz B, Helme RD. The impact of dementia on the pain experience. *Pain.* 1996;67:7–15.

16. Porter FL, Malhotra KM, Wolf CM, et al. Dementia and response to pain in the elderly. *Pain.* 1996;68:413–421.

17. Turner NJ, Muers MF, Haward RA, Mulley GP. Psychological distress and concerns of elderly patients treated with palliative radiotherapy for lung cancer. *Psychooncology.* 2007;16(8):707–713.

18. Hill KM, Amir Z, Muers MF, Connolly CK, Round CE. Do newly diagnosed lung cancer patients feel their concerns are being met? *Eur J Cancer Care (Engl).* 2003;12(1):35–45.

19. Bruera E. Research into symptoms other than pain. In: Doyle D, Hanks GW, MacDonald N, eds. *Oxford Textbook of Palliative Medicine.* 2nd ed. New York, NY: Oxford University Press; 1998:179–185.

20. Chang VT, Hwang SS, Feuerman M. Validation of the Edmonton Symptom Assessment Scale. *Cancer.* 2000;88:2164–2171.

21. Kirkova J, Davis MP, Walsh D, et al. Cancer symptom assessment instruments: a systematic review. *J Clin Oncol.* 2006;24(9):1459–1473.

22. Bruera E, Kim HN. Cancer pain. *JAMA.* 2003;290(18):2476–2479.

23. Pereira J, Hanson J, Bruera E. The frequency and clinical course of cognitive impairment in patients with terminal cancer. *Cancer.* 1997;79:835–842.

24. Lawlor PG, Bruera ED. Delirium in patients with advanced cancer. *Hematol Oncol Clin N Am.* 2002;16:701–714.

25. Yennurajalingam S, Bruera E. Palliative management of fatigue at the close of life: "it feels like my body is just worn out". *JAMA.* 2007;297(3):295–304.

26. Reddy SK, Parsons HA, Elsayem A, Palmer JL, Bruera E. Characteristics and correlates of dyspnea in patients with advanced cancer. *J Palliat Med.* 2009;12(1):29–36.

27. Ostchega Y, Harris TB, Hirsch R, et al. The prevalence of functional limitations and disability in older persons in the US: data from the National Health and Nutrition Examination Survey III. *J Am Geriatr Soc.* 2000;48:1132–1135.

28. Oken MM, Creech RH, Tormey DC, et al. Toxicity and response criteria of the Eastern Cooperative Oncology Group. *Am J Clin Oncol.* 1982;5:649–655.

29. Karnofsky DA. Determining the extent of the cancer and clinical planning for cure. *Cancer.* 1968;22:730–734.

30. Katz S, Downs TD, Cash HR, et al. Progress in development of the index of ADL. *Gerontologist.* 1970;10:20–30.

31. Avlund K, Schultz-Larsen K, Kreiner S. The measurement of instrumental ADL: content validity and construct validity. *Aging (Milano).* 1993;5:371–383.

32. Crooks V, Waller S, Smith T, et al. The use of the Karnofsky Performance Scale in determining outcomes and risk in geriatric outpatients. *J Gerontol.* 1991;46:M139–M144.

33. Lawton MP. Scales to measure competence in everyday activities. *Psychopharm Bull.* 1988;24(4):609–614, 789–791.

34. Naeim A, Reuben D. Geriatric syndromes and assessment in older cancer patients. *Oncology* (Williston Park). 2001;15(12):1567–77.

35. Extermann M, Overcash J, Lyman GH, et al. Comorbidity and functional status are independent in older cancer patients. *J Clin Oncol.* 1998;16:1582–1587.

36. Buccheri G, Ferrigno D, Tamburini M. Karnofsky and ECOG performance status scoring in lung cancer: a

prospective, longitudinal study of 536 patients from a single institution. *Eur J Cancer.* 1996;32A:1135–1141.

37. Moore AA, Siu AL. Screening for common problems in ambulatory elderly: clinical confirmation of a screen instrument. *Am J Med.* 1996;100:438–443.

38. Lachs MS, Feinstein AR, Cooney LM Jr, et al. A simple procedure for general screening for functional disability in elderly patients. *Ann Intern Med.* 1990;112(9): 699–706.

39. Oldervoll LM, Loge JH, Paltiel H, et al. The effect of a physical exercise program in palliative care. *J Pain Symptom Manage.* 2006;31:421–430.

40. Neuenschwander H, Bruera E, Cavalli F. Matching the clinical function and symptom status with the expectations of patients with advanced cancer, their families, and health care workers. *Support Care Cancer.* 1997;5:252–256.

41. Royall DR, Cordes JA, Polk M. CLOX: an executive clock drawing task. *J Neurol Neurosurg Psychiatry.* 1998;64(5):588–594.

42. Borson S, Scanlan J, Brush M, Vitaliano P, Dokmak A. The Mini-Cog: a cognitive "vital signs" measure for dementia screening in multi-lingual elderly. *Int J Geriatr Psychiatry* 2000.

43. Giovannetti-Carew TG, Lamar M, Cloud BS, et al. Impairment in category fluency in ischaemic vascular dementia. *Neuropsychology* 1997;11:400–412.

44. Mitchell SL, Teno JM, Kiely DK, et al. The clinical course of advanced dementia. *N Engl J Med.* 2009;361(16): 1529–1538.

45. Diokno AC. Epidemiology and psychosocial aspects of incontinence. *Urol Clin North Am.* 1995;22:481–485.

46. Voigt JC, Kenefick JS. Sacrococcygeal chordoma presenting with stress incontinence of urine. *S Afr Med J.* 1971;45:557.

47. Ehrlich RM, Walsh GO. Urinary incontinence secondary to brain neoplasm. *Urology.* 1973;1:249–250.

48. Diokno AC, Brown MB, Herzog AR. Relationship between use of diuretics and continence status in the elderly. *Urology.* 191;38:39–42.

49. Johnson TM, Busby-Whitehead J. Diagnostic assessment of geriatric urinary incontinence. *Am J Med Sci.* 1997;314:250–256.

50. Oleckno WA, Blacconiere MJ. Relationship of religiosity to wellness and other health-related behaviors and outcomes. *Psychol Rep.* 1991;68:819–826.

51. Wegner GC, Davies R, Shahtahmasebi S, Scott A. Social-isolation and loneliness in old-age: review and model refinement. *Aging Soc.* 1996;16:333–358.

52. Cattan M, White M, Bond J, Learmouth A. Preventing social isolation and loneliness among older people: a systematic review of health promotion interventions. *Aging Soc.* 2005;25:41–67.

53. Rubenstein LZ, Josephson KR, Robbins AS. Falls in the nursing home. *Ann Intern Med.* 1994;121:442–451.

54. Rubenstein LZ. Preventing falls in the nursing home. *JAMA.* 1997;278(7):595–596.

55. Gillespie LD, Gillespie WJ, Robertson MC, Lamb SE, Cumming RJ, Rowe BH. Interventions for preventing falls in elderly people. *Cochrane Database Syst Rev.* 2003;(4):CD000340.

56. Kennedy BJ. Aging and cancer. *Oncology.* 2000;14: 1731–1733.

57. Yancik R, Havlik RJ, Wesley MN, et al. Cancer and co-morbidity in older patients: a descriptive profile. *Ann Epidemiol.* 1996;6:399–412.

58. Parnes BL, Smith PC, Conroy CM, Domke H. When should we stop mammography screening for breast cancer in elderly women? *J Fam Pract.* 2001;50:110–111.

59. Fleming C, Wasson JH, Altertson PC, Barry MJ, Wennberg JE. A decision analysis of alternative treatment strategies for clinically localized prostate cancer. *JAMA.* 1993;269:2650–2658.

60. Kemeny MM, Peterson BL, Kornblith AB, et al. Barriers to clinical trial participation by older women with breast cancer. *J Clin Oncol.* 2003;21:2268–2275.

61. Extermann M. Measurement and impact of comorbidity in older cancer patients. *Crit Rev Oncol/Hematol.* 2000;35(3):181–200.

62. Ngeowa J, Leonga SS, Gaob F, et al. Impact of comorbidities on clinical outcomes in non-small cell lung cancer patients who are elderly and/or have poor performance status. *Crit Rev Oncol/Hematol.* 2009;(December). 2010;76(1):53–60. In press.

63. Ong LM, Visser MR, Lammes FB, de Haes JC. Doctor–patient communication and cancer patients' quality of life and satisfaction. *Patient Educ Couns.* 2000;41(2):145–156.

64. World Health Organization. *National Cancer Programs: Policies and Managerial Guidelines.* 2nd ed. Geneva: World Health Organization; 2002:83–91.

65. Greenberg J, Seltzer M, Brewer E. Caregivers to Older Adults. 2006;17:339–355.

66. Wolff. J. *Health-related Responsibilities Assumed by Informal Caregivers.* In Institute of Medicine. (2008). *Retooling for an aging America: Building the health care workforce.* Washington, DC: National Academies Press, 2007. Accessed as of Feb 2010, from: http://www.iom.edu/)

Survivorship

• *Karin Hahn*

▦ CANCER SURVIVORSHIP IN THE UNITED STATES

According to the National Cancer Institute (NCI), a cancer survivor is "one who remains alive and continues to function during and after overcoming a serious hardship or life-threatening disease. A person who has been diagnosed with cancer is considered to be a survivor from diagnosis until the end of life."[1] The *President's Cancer Panel 2003–2004 Annual Report*[2] entitled "Living beyond Cancer: Finding a New Balance" defined the term "survivor" as any person who has ever been diagnosed with cancer. There are those, however, who believe that a cancer survivor is someone who is "cancer-free" 5 years after his or her diagnosis of cancer, and others who reject the "label" of being a "cancer survivor" altogether.[3] At the University of Texas MD Anderson Cancer Center (MDACC), we follow the NCI definition of a cancer survivor and consider a cancer survivor to be a person who has ever been diagnosed with cancer.

Advances in cancer diagnosis and treatment have increased the number of cancer survivors who live for long periods of time.[1] In 2005, there were about 11 million cancer survivors living in the United States. Approximately 23% of these survivors had been diagnosed with breast cancer, 19% with prostate cancer, and 11% with colorectal cancer. Approximately 5% of these 11 million cancer survivors were longer-term survivors that had been diagnosed at least 29 years earlier. According to the 2007 NCI's Cancer Trends Progress Report, the total economic burden of cancer in the United States in 2004 was estimated at $190 billion. Direct medical expenditures, which included cancer screening and treatment, accounted for about $90 billion of the estimated $190 billion total economic burden of cancer. The $100 billion difference included indirect costs such as losses in time and economic productivity resulting from cancer-related illness and death.

The magnitude of the qualitative burden of cancer survivorship, however, has been much more difficult to elucidate.[4] Surveys of survivors that explore the psychosocial impact of cancer diagnosis and treatment, such as the Internet survey reported by the Lance Armstrong Foundation (LAF) in 2004, have been limited by selection bias and the underrepresentation of minority and/or underserved populations.[5,6] The City of Hope Beckman Research Institute quality of life (QOL) model applied to cancer survivors has four domains: physical well-being and symptoms, psychological well-being, social well-being, and spiritual well-being.[7] The items in psychological well-being domain of this model include control, anxiety, depression, enjoyment/leisure, pain, distress, happiness, fear of recurrence, cognition/attention, overall perception of QOL, and distress of diagnosis and treatment. The social well-being domain includes the following items: family distress, roles and relationships, affections/sexual function, appearance, isolation, employment, and finances. Given the depth and breadth of the items in these domains, it is not surprising that addressing the psychosocial needs of cancer survivors involves a multidisciplinary approach and a diversity of services to meet these needs.[8]

■ THE PSYCHOSOCIAL NEEDS OF CANCER SURVIVORS

In 2008 the Institute of Medicine[8] (IOM) published a report on cancer care that focused on meeting the psychosocial health needs of cancer survivors. Psychosocial problems can result from or be exacerbated by cancer diagnosis and treatment. Failing to address these issues could result in needless patient and family suffering, obstruction of the provision of quality health care, and a potential effect on the course of disease.[8] Stress, untreated mental health problems, social isolation, and other social factors can add to cancer survivors' emotional distress as well as their ability to adhere to recommended treatment plans and engage in behaviors that promote their health and well-being.

Breast Cancer Survivors

Given the large percentage of breast cancer survivors, it is not surprising that the vast majority of research on the psychosocial needs of cancer survivors has been focused on breast cancer survivors. In fact, the IOM[9] published an entire report on meeting the psychosocial needs of women with breast cancer. Research on the QOL of breast cancer survivors has been obtained from focus groups, individual interviews, as well as mail and telephone surveys. This research has sought to determine not only the psychosocial impact of breast cancer diagnosis and treatment, but also whether there are risk factors such as age at diagnosis and type of breast cancer treatment that affect the magnitude of that impact.

Research on the psychosocial aspects of breast cancer suggests that most women adjust well to the diagnosis and treatment of breast cancer.[10,11] This research has been conducted using a number of methodologies including focus groups, structured and semistructured interviews, and surveys conducted in person, by telephone or mail.[12–20] For example, Ganz et al[15] conducted a study that examined health-related QOL and sexual functioning among breast cancer survivors from Los Angeles, California, and Washington, DC, who were disease-free; this study was conducted on average 3 years after the diagnosis of breast cancer. When the mailed survey results of the 864 breast cancer survivors were compared with those of healthy, age-matched women, breast cancer survivors had: highly favorable levels of general health perceptions and physical, emotional, and social functioning; low to average levels of depression; and good quality of marital/

partner relationships. Despite these reassuring results, among the breast cancer survivors Ganz et al[15] surveyed, about 23% had scores on the Center for Epidemiologic Studies-Depression Scale (CES-D) compatible with a potentially significant level of depression. In another study, Kornblith et al[20] reported on the long-term adjustment of breast cancer survivors after adjuvant chemotherapy. Of the 153 breast cancer survivors interviewed using standardized measures, 5% of survivors had scores suggestive of clinical levels of distress and 15% reported two or more posttraumatic stress disorder (PTSD) symptoms. However, in this study it is difficult to determine whether these survivors' overall psychological state is significantly different from that of individuals without a cancer history because only breast cancer survivors were interviewed.

Although the majority of breast cancer survivors appear to cope with their psychosocial distress, a number of risk factors have been identified that may make a breast cancer survivor more vulnerable to this distress. Some of these factors include younger age at diagnosis, preexisting mental illness or psychological distress, limited social support, and comorbid conditions.[11] For example, Cimprich et al[21] found that long-term breast cancer survivors who had been diagnosed at 65 years of age or older showed significantly worse QOL outcomes in the physical domain of the Quality of Life-Cancer Survivors (QOL-CS) instrument. Those diagnosed with breast cancer between ages 27 and 44 years had worse QOL scores in the social domain than the other age groups examined in this study. When Maunsell et al[17] evaluated potential risk factors for the development of psychological distress after initial treatment for breast cancer, those survivors with a history of depression were significantly more likely to have high levels of psychological distress than those who had no such history, 63.1% and 14.3%, respectively. They also found that a high level of psychological distress in survivors was associated with an increasing number of stressful life events in the 5 years preceding breast cancer diagnosis. In another study of breast cancer survivors, their amount of social support, perception of family cohesiveness, and amount of social contact had direct effects on coping.[22] More recently, Yang and Schuler[23] reported that breast cancer survivors in stable, distressed relationships appeared to have worse psychological outcomes, poorer health, and a steeper decline in physical activity compared with breast cancer survivors in stable, nondistressed relationships.

Although there has been a fair amount of research on the psychosocial impact of breast cancer diagnosis and treatment, the ability to generalize these findings to minority or underserved populations is limited. The majority of these studies have been conducted among Caucasian women who have access to health care. In a systematic review of QOL research on African American breast and prostate cancer survivors published in 2007, Powe et al[24] identified only four breast cancer studies and two prostate cancer studies that met their inclusion criteria. However, these authors concluded that they could not adequately describe the QOL of African American cancer survivors given the limited and conflicting research as well as inconsistent measurements and methodologies used in this research.

Subsequently, Paskett et al[25] analyzed the data from the Women's Health Initiative Observational Study to compare the health-related quality of life (HRQOL) of African American and white breast cancer survivors. In multivariate regression analysis comparing the HRQOL of African American ($N = 465$) and white ($N = 4446$) breast cancer survivors, African American breast cancer survivors reported poorer physical functioning and general health and greater role limitations due to emotional health. They did not, however, find any significant differences in vitality, social functioning, emotional well-being, or depression. In the Health, Eating, Activity, and Lifestyle (HEAL) Study, African American breast cancer survivors ($N = 198$) had statistically significantly lower physical functioning scores when compared with non-Hispanic white ($N = 463$) and Hispanic ($N = 86$) breast cancer survivors.[26] Although African American breast cancer survivors in this study had higher mental health scores than non-Hispanic white breast cancer survivors, this difference did not reach statistical significance in their fully adjusted model ($P = .06$). Additional research into the impacts of race or ethnicity, including Hispanic breast cancer survivors, and being medically underserved on the psychosocial aspects of breast cancer survivorship is needed.

Other Cancer Survivors

Research on the psychosocial needs of cancer survivors who have not been diagnosed with breast cancer is much more limited. Among the 4636 survivors of adult-onset cancer of 5 or more years who responded to the National Health Interview Survey (NHIS) from 2002 to 2006, breast cancer survivors and survivors of cancer of the cervix/uterus/other female genital organs represented almost 50% of respondents, 22.9% and 25.2%, respectively.[27] Survivors of cancer of the male genital organs (prostate and testicular cancer) and colorectal cancer accounted

for 13.9% and 9.6% of survey respondents, respectively. In this analysis, the prevalence of serious psychological distress was significantly higher among cancer survivors than among the 122,220 NHIS respondents who were never diagnosed with cancer (5.6% vs. 3%; $P < .001$). Unfortunately, these results were not further analyzed by type of cancer.

However, in a study of 180 long-term cancer survivors 60 years of age or older who had been diagnosed with breast (41.4%), colorectal (32.2%), or prostate cancer (26.7%), no significant differences were found in the six dimensions of psychological distress analyzed or the PTSD total score.[28] Although most of the survivors in this analysis did not demonstrate clinical levels of PTSD, 25% appeared to have clinical levels of depression. They found that current cancer-related symptoms were the strongest predictors of depression and the PTSD subdimension of hyperarousal. A subsequent study of coping among 321 long-term breast, colorectal, and prostate cancer survivors over 60 years of age found no significant differences in the coping strategies used based on cancer type.[29]

We will now examine in more depth the research on the psychosocial needs of survivors of four tumor types with a high prevalence in the United States: prostate, colorectal, and cervical cancer as well as non-Hodgkin's lymphoma (NHL).[30] On January 1, 2006, in the United States, there were approximately 2.2 million prostate cancer survivors, 1.1 million colorectal cancer survivors, 250,000 cervical cancer survivors, and 500,000 NHL survivors.

Prostate Cancer Survivors

Bloom et al[31] performed a systematic review of studies published in English between 1998 and October 1, 2006 that examined QOL among adult-onset cancer survivors 5 or more years from diagnosis where QOL was the primary outcome. They only included studies that had sample sizes of 30 or more participants and those using QOL measurement instruments commonly used and recognized as reliable. Among the 10 studies of prostate cancer survivors' psychological QOL that met their criteria, some reported no differences in long-term mental health measures between survivors and controls or between those who had a radical prostatectomy and those who had an external beam radiation therapy.[32–34] Two of the studies in this systematic review reported higher levels of distress in prostate cancer survivors with higher levels of urinary dysfunction.[34,35] A subsequent study by Sanda et al[36] compared QOL and satisfaction with outcome among prostate cancer survivors treated with prostatectomy, brachytherapy, or external beam radiation, some of whom also had androgen suppression therapy. In this study, the results for the QOL domain "vitality or hormone function," which included hot flashes, breast problems, depression, lack of energy, and weight gain, were worse after radiation therapy or brachytherapy among those who received androgen suppression therapy.

Bloom et al[31] also identified two studies that explored the role of race or ethnicity on QOL among prostate cancer survivors. These studies found that African American prostate cancer survivors were more bothered by their level of sexual functioning than Euro-American men.[37,38] One of these two studies also reported that African American men scored lower on both the physical component and the mental component of the SF-36, a multipurpose, short-form health survey with only 36 questions.[37]

Colorectal Cancer Survivors

Only three articles, from two different studies, met the criteria of Bloom et al[31] for their systematic review of studies examining QOL in colorectal cancer survivors. In the first study, female long-term survivors of colorectal cancer appeared to report HRQOL comparable to that of similarly aged women in the general population.[39] For these survivors, the mental component of the SF-36 was negatively influenced if they had a greater number of comorbidities or less formal education. The survivors in this study had better scores on the mental component if they had larger social networks, saw more social ties at least once a month, and had more overall social connectedness.[40] The second study identified by Bloom et al[31] found male and female colorectal cancer survivors to have a relatively high and uniform QOL, but that both non-cancer-related comorbidities and low income status had a negative impact on HRQOL.[41] A later study by Krouse et al[42] recently reported that when male and female long-term rectal cancer survivors who had permanent ostomies were compared with those without ostomies, it was the female survivors with ostomies who had significantly worse overall HRQOL and psychological well-being.

Cervical Cancer Survivors

Among the research on long-term survivors of cervical cancer, Bloom et al[31] found only two studies that met their criteria for inclusion in their systematic review. The first study by Wenzel et al[43] compared the QOL of 51 long-term cervical cancer survivors who had been diagnosed during their child-bearing years to 59 age-matched controls. In this case–control study, cervical cancer survivors reported QOL comparable to normative data as the control subjects. In this study, cervical cancer survivors reported better mental component scores on the SF-36 if they had less cancer-specific distress, better social support, better spiritual well-being, better sexual functioning, or fewer reproductive concerns. In the other study identified by Bloom et al, Bradley et al[44] also found no significant differences in QOL between cervical, endometrial, and healthy "controls" (not age-matched) as measured by the SF-36. Although no significant differences were found in depressive symptoms between the three groups, they found that cervical cancer survivors reported significantly more anxiety, depressive symptoms, anger, and confusion than endometrial cancer survivors. Cervical cancer survivors also had more anger and confusion when compared with healthy subjects. No differences were noted between groups with regard to vigor, fatigue, or total mood disturbance.

A subsequent study at MD Anderson compared the QOL of cervical cancer survivors treated with a radical hysterectomy, to those treated with radiation as well as to age- and race-matched controls.[45] In multivariate analysis, there were no significant differences between these three groups on the mental health component of the SF-12 or on emotional distress as measured by the Brief Symptom Index-18. Of note, in all three of these studies,[43–45] the majority of cervical cancer patients were of non-Hispanic white race/ethnicity (90.2%, 95%, and 69%, respectively).

Non-Hodgkin's Lymphoma Survivors

Although there were more NHL survivors than Hodgkin's lymphoma survivors in the United States in 2006, Bloom et al[30,31] did not include NHL survivors in their review of QOL among long-term adult cancer survivors, although they did include survivors of Hodgkin's lymphoma. However, Smith et al[46] examined the health status and QOL among those with active NHL, disease-free short-term survivors (2–4 years postdiagnosis), and long-term survivors (≥5 years postdiagnosis). Not surprisingly, those with active disease had worse physical and mental functioning, worse QOL, and less positive and more negative impacts of cancer compared with disease-free survivors. In this study, no significant differences were observed between short- and long-term survivors. When the mental health component scores of the SF-36 from disease-free

NHL survivors were compared to their age-stratified normative scores, the survivors' scores were close to the general population norms, although some differences existed among some age groups, particularly the 25- to 34-year age group.

Another study by Smith et al[47] examined posttraumatic stress outcomes in those with active NHL as well as in those who were disease-free. In this study, the adjusted prevalence for full PTSD was 7.9%, and for partial PTSD it was 9.1%. In multiple linear regression analysis, partial or full PTSD was associated with having less education, being closer to time of diagnosis, more comorbidities, less social support, insurance/employment issues related to cancer, and a higher appraisal of life threat and treatment intensity score. In both of these studies almost 86% to 87% of all survivors were Caucasian.[46,47]

■ ADDRESSING THE PSYCHOSOCIAL NEEDS OF BREAST CANCER SURVIVORS

The Institute of Medicine Report 2008

In 2008, the IOM[8] published a report entitled *Cancer Care for the Whole Patient: Meeting Psychosocial Health Needs.* In this report, they provided a list of the psychosocial needs of cancer survivors and which health services could address those needs. In addition to the formal health services that they outlined in their report, they acknowledged that informal sources of support including family members and friends are key providers of psychosocial health services for cancer survivors.

Some of the psychosocial needs identified by the IOM[8] included obtaining information and coping with emotions about illness and treatment, help with managing illness, as well as managing disruptions in patients' personal and professional lives, assistance with changing health behaviors, material and logistical needs such as transportation, and financial advice and/or assistance. They also provided examples of possible formal health services to help cancer patients cope with these needs. For example, they suggested that health services to help deal with the emotions accompanying cancer diagnosis and its treatment could include peer support programs, individual or group counseling/psychotherapy, and/or pharmacologic management of depression and/or anxiety. Clearly a diversity of services is needed to help patients cope with the psychosocial impact of being a cancer survivor. We will now discuss the ways in which MDACC strives to meet the psychosocial needs of cancer survivors.

The University of Texas MD Anderson Cancer Center Survivorship Patient Care and Support Programs

Patient Care Programs

In an effort to meet the medical and psychosocial needs of cancer survivors, MDACC has developed seven cancer type–specific survivorship clinics. There are clinics for survivors of cancer of the breast, genitourinary tract, head and neck, thyroid, gynecologic tract, as well as survivors of childhood cancer and stem cell transplantation.[48] In addition to monitoring for cancer recurrence and recommending appropriate screening for other malignancies, each clinic strives to identify and address the needs of long-term cancer survivors. Addressing these needs often involves a multidisciplinary or multimodality approach.

Our Psychiatry Department provides expertise on the psychiatric aspects of cancer and cancer treatment for our cancer center and its patients through integrated, high-quality programs in patient care, research, and education.[48] Our psychiatrists and advanced practice nurses provide counseling and, when appropriate, pharmacologic treatment for those with psychological distress from or exacerbated by cancer diagnosis and/or its treatment including long-term cancer survivors.

Supportive Programs

The Anderson Network This is a cancer support group of more than 1500 current and former MDACC patients.[48] The Anderson Network takes a personalized approach to supporting both cancer patients and caregivers, and one such program they offer tries to match a cancer patient with a Network member who has had the same diagnosis and treatment. Their resources include a patient and caregiver telephone support line, weekly educational forums featuring MD Anderson and community experts, a quarterly newsletter with information of interest to cancer patients as well as inspirational stories, and a yearly conference targeting the needs of cancer survivors.

Place ... of wellness The Place ... of wellness provides programs that focus on the mind, body, and spirit and could complement medical care.[48] Their mission is to provide authoritative, accurate, and current information for cancer patients, caregivers, and health care professionals; to offer complementary therapies such as yoga and meditation that may be used in addition to usual medical care to manage symptoms, relieve stress, and enhance QOL;

and to conduct research using intervention programs that could improve QOL and clinical outcomes.

Department of Social Work The licensed clinical social workers at MD Anderson are available to help our patients, as well as their families and friends, cope with their cancer, and to assist them in dealing with psychological or social barriers to their cancer treatment.[48] Our social work counselors conduct numerous support groups for MDACC patients, their family members, friends, and/or caregivers that focus on a variety of topics including emotional support and specific diseases or treatments. Our clinical social workers also provide individual short-term counseling on subjects that include: adjustment to diagnosis and treatment, coping with life changes, family counseling, and sexuality and intimacy counseling for couples and individuals.

National Efforts

The Office of Cancer Survivorship[49] at the NCI conducts and supports research that studies and addresses the long- and short-term effects of cancer for both pediatric and adult cancer survivors and their families. In addition to its research mission, the Office of Cancer Survivorship promotes the dissemination of information regarding the needs of cancer survivors and their families to professionals who treat cancer patients as well as the general public.

A number of national advocacy groups seek to identify and address the needs of cancer survivors. The oldest survivor-led cancer advocacy organization in the United States, the National Coalition for Cancer Survivorship,[50] advocates for quality cancer care and the empowerment of cancer survivors through legislative advocacy and patient education. In addition to the educational information provided through its main Web site, the American Cancer Society offers cancer survivors support through its American Cancer Survivors Network®.[51] This Network enables cancer survivors a private, secure way to find and communicate with other cancer survivors who share their interests and experiences. The LAF strives to improve the QOL of cancer survivors through education and research as well as advocacy.[5]

A number of cancer site–specific foundations and organizations are focused on providing education and support for cancer survivors. Some of the organizations that also fund research that could improve the QOL of cancer survivors include the Susan G. Komen for the Cure,[52] National Colorectal Cancer Research Alliance,[53] Prostate Cancer Foundation,[54] Leukemia and Lymphoma Society,[55] and the Gynecologic Cancer Foundation.[56] These cancer site–specific organizations are also engaged in educating the public about the needs of cancer survivors and their families.

KEY POINTS

- According to the NCI, a cancer survivor is "one who remains alive and continues to function during and after overcoming a serious hardship or life-threatening disease. A person who has been diagnosed with cancer is considered to be a survivor from diagnosis until the end of life."

- In 2005, there were about 11 million cancer survivors living in the United States.

- Surveys of survivors that have explored the psychosocial impact of cancer diagnosis and treatment have been limited by selection bias and the underrepresentation of minority and/or underserved populations.

- According to the 2008 IOM report *Cancer Care for the Whole Patient: Meeting Psychosocial Health Needs*:

  1. Psychosocial problems can result from or be exacerbated by cancer diagnosis and treatment.

  2. Failing to address these issues could result in needless patient and family suffering, obstruct the provision of quality health care, and potentially affect the course of disease.

  3. Stress, untreated mental health problems, social isolation, and other social factors can add to cancer survivors' emotional distress as well as their ability to adhere to recommended treatment plans and engage in behaviors that promote their health and well-being.

  4. In addition to formal health services, informal sources of support including family members and friends are key providers of psychosocial health services for cancer survivors.

  5. Psychosocial needs include obtaining information and coping with emotions about illness and treatment, help with managing illness, as well as managing disruptions in patients' personal and professional lives, assistance with changing health behaviors, material and logistical needs such as transportation, and financial advice and/or assistance.

REFERENCES

1. www.cancer.gov.

2. The President's Cancer Panel: Leffall LD Jr, Armstrong L, Kripke ML. *President's Cancer Panel 2003–2004 Annual Report*. Bethesda, Md: National Institutes of Health; May 2004.

3. Committee on Cancer Survivorship: Improving Care and Quality of Life, National Cancer Policy Board, Hewitt M, Greenfield, Stovall E, eds. *From Cancer Patient to Cancer Survivor: Lost in Transition*. Washington, DC: The National Academies Press; 2006.

4. Wolff SN. The burden of cancer survivorship: a pandemic of treatment success. In: Feuerstein M, ed. *Handbook of Cancer Survivorship*. New York, NY: Springer Science+Business Media; 2007:7–18:chap 2.

5. www.livestrong.org.

6. Hewitt M, Breen N, Devesa S. Cancer prevalence and survivorship issues: analyses of the 1992 National Health Interview Survey. *J Natl Cancer Inst.* 1999;91:1480–1486.

7. Ferrell BR, Hassey Dow K, Grant M. Measurement of the quality of life in cancer survivors. *Qual Life Res.* 1995;4:523–531.

8. Institute of Medicine (IOM). In: Adler NE, Page AEK, eds. *Cancer Care for the Whole Patient: Meeting Psychosocial Health Needs*. Washington, DC: The National Academies Press; 2008.

9. Institute of Medicine (IOM). In: Hewitt M, Herdman R, Holland J, eds. *Meeting Psychosocial Needs of Women with Breast Cancer*. Washington, DC: The National Academies Press; 2004.

10. Kornblith AB, Ligibel J. Psychosocial and sexual functioning of survivors of breast cancer. *Semin Oncol.* 2003;30:799–813.

11. Ganz PA. Psychosocial and social aspects of breast cancer. *Oncology.* 2008;22:642–652.

12. Ferrell BR, Grant M, Funk B, et al. Quality of life in breast cancer: part I: physical and social well-being. *Cancer Nurs.* 1997;20:398–408.

13. Ferrell B, Grant M, Funk B, et al. Quality of life in breast cancer: part II: psychological and spiritual well-being. *Cancer Nurs.* 1998;21:1–9.

14. Ganz PA, Coscarelli A, Fred C, et al. Breast cancer survivors: psychosocial concerns and quality of life. *Breast Cancer Res Treat.* 1996;38:183–199.

15. Ganz PA, Rowland JH, Desmond K, et al. Life after breast cancer: understanding women's health-related quality of life and sexual functioning. *J Clin Oncol.* 1998;16: 501–514.

16. Hanson Frost M, Suman VJ, Rummans TA, et al. Physical, psychological and social well-being of women with breast cancer: the influence of disease phase. *Psychooncology.* 2000;9:221–231.

17. Maunsell E, Brisson J, Deschênes L. Psychological distress after initial treatment of breast cancer. *Cancer.* 1992;70:120–125.

18. Dorval M, Maunsell E, Deschênes L, et al. Long-term quality of life after breast cancer: comparison of 8-year survivors with population controls. *J Clin Oncol.* 1998;16:487–494.

19. Coscarelli Schlag CA, Ganz PA, Polinsky ML, et al. Characteristics of women at risk for psychosocial distress in the year after breast cancer. *J Clin Oncol.* 1993;11:783–793.

20. Kornblith AB, Herndon JE II, Weiss RB, et al. Long-term adjustment of survivors of early-stage breast carcinoma, 20 years after adjuvant chemotherapy. *Cancer.* 2003;98:679–689.

21. Cimprich B, Ronis DL, Martinez-Ramos G. Age at diagnosis and quality of life in breast cancer survivors. *Cancer Pract.* 2002;10:85–93.

22. Bloom JR. Social support, accommodation to stress and adjustment to breast cancer. *Soc Sci Med.* 1982;16:1329–1338.

23. Yang H-C, Schuler TA. Marital quality and survivorship. *Cancer.* 2009;115:217–228.

24. Powe BD, Hamilton J, Hancock N, et al. Quality of life of African American cancer survivors. *Cancer.* 2007;109 (2 suppl):435–445.

25. Paskett ED, Alfano CM, Davidson MA, et al. Breast cancer survivors' health-related quality of life. *Cancer.* 2008;113:3222–3230.

26. Bowen DJ, Alfano CM, McGregor BA, et al. Possible socioeconomic and ethnic disparities in quality of life in a cohort of breast cancer survivors. *Breast Cancer Res Treat.* 2007;106:85–95.

27. Hoffman KE, McCarthy EP, Recklitis CJ, et al. Psychological distress in long-term survivors of adult-onset cancer. *Arch Intern Med.* 2009;169:1274–1281.

28. Deimling GT, Kahana B, Bowman KF, et al. Cancer survivorship and psychological distress later in life. *Psychooncology.* 2002;11:479–494.

29. Deimling GT, Wagner LJ, Bowman KF, et al. Coping among older-adult, long-term cancer survivors. *Psychooncology.* 2006;15:143–159.

30. http://seer.cancer.gov.

31. Bloom JR, Petersen DM, Kang SH. Multi-dimensional quality of life among long-term (5+ years) adult cancer survivors. *Psychooncology.* 2007;16:691–706.

32. Hoffman RM, Gilliland FD, Penson DF, et al. Cross-sectional and longitudinal comparisons of health-related quality of life between patients with prostate carcinoma and matched controls. *Cancer.* 2004;101:2011–2019.

33. Korfage IJ, Essink-Bot M-L, Borsboom GJJM, et al. Five-year follow-up of health-related quality of life after primary treatment of localized breast cancer. *Int J Cancer.* 2005;116:291–296.

34. Potosky AL, Davis WW, Hoffman RM, et al. Five-year outcomes after prostatectomy or radiotherapy for prostate cancer: the prostate cancer outcomes study. *J Natl Cancer Inst.* 2004;96:1358–1367.

35. Dalkin BL, Wessells H, Cui H. A national survey of urinary and health-related quality of life outcomes in men with an artificial urinary sphincter for post-radical prostatectomy incontinence. *Am Urol Assoc.* 2003;169:237–239.

36. Sanda MG, Dunn RL, Michalski J, et al. Quality of life and satisfaction with outcome among prostate-cancer survivors. *N Engl J Med.* 2008;358:1250–1261.

37. Jenkins R, Schover LR, Fouladi RT, et al. Sexuality and health-related quality of life after prostate cancer in African-American and white men treated for localized disease. *J Sex Marital Ther.* 2004;30:79–93.

38. Johnson TK, Gilliland FD, Hoffman RM, et al. Racial/ethnic differences in functional outcomes in the 5 years after diagnosis of localized prostate cancer. *J Clin Oncol.* 2004;22:4193–4201.

39. Trentham-Dietz A, Remington PL, Moinpour CM, et al. Health-related quality of life in female long-term colorectal cancer survivors. *Oncologist.* 2003;8:342–349.

40. Sapp AL, Trentham-Dietz A, Newcomb PA, et al. Social networks and quality of life among female long-term colorectal cancer survivors. *Cancer.* 2003;98:49–58.

41. Ramsey SD, Berry K, Moinpour C, et al. Quality of life in long term survivors of colorectal cancer. *Am J Gastroenterol.* 2002;97:1228–1234.

42. Krouse RS, Herrinton LJ, Grant M, et al. Health-related quality of life among long-term rectal cancer survivors with an ostomy: manifestations by sex. *J Clin Oncol.* 2009;27:4664–4670.

43. Wenzel L, DeAlba I, Habbal R, et al. Quality of life in long-term cervical cancer survivors. *Gynecol Oncol.* 2005;97:310–317.

44. Bradley S, Rose S, Lutgendorf S, et al. Quality of life and mental health in cervical and endometrial cancer survivors. *Gynecol Oncol.* 2006;199:479–486.

45. Frumovitz M, Sun CC, Schrover LR, et al. Quality of life and sexual functioning in cervical cancer survivors. *J Clin Oncol.* 2005;23:7428–7436.

46. Smith SK, Zimmerman S, Williams CS, et al. Health status and quality of life among non-Hodgkin lymphoma survivors. *Cancer.* 2009;115:3312–3323.

47. Smith SK, Zimmerman S, Williams CS, et al. Post-traumatic stress outcomes in non-Hodgkin's lymphoma survivors. *J Clin Oncol.* 2008;26:934–941.

48. www.mdanderson.org.

49. http://cancercontrol.cancer.gov/ocs/about.html.

50. http://www.canceradvocacy.org/about/.

51. http://csn.cancer.org/.

52. www.komen.org.

53. http://www.eifoundation.org/programs/eifs-national-colorectal-cancer-research-alliance.

54. www.prostatecancerfoundation.org.

55. www.lls.org.

56. www.thegcf.org.

CHAPTER 21

Body Image and Disfigurement

• *Michelle Cororve Fingeret*

Body image is a critical psychosocial issue for individuals with cancer as the disease and its treatment can result in significant changes in physical appearance and bodily functioning. Although adjustment to bodily changes can vary significantly depending on the patient, it is important to recognize that all patients with cancer regardless of tumor site, stage, or treatment modality undergo a process of body image adaptation. Similar to other medical patients, individuals with cancer can experience many possible cosmetic and functional changes, some of which are temporary, while others are more permanent. The degree to which these changes are accompanied by significant distress and difficulties with emotional, social, and occupational functioning is influenced by a host of personality, medical, and treatment-related factors. This chapter focuses on how to better identify, evaluate, and treat psychosocial difficulties stemming from body image concerns in the oncology setting. In order to fully appreciate the complex process of adjusting to bodily changes, considerable attention is being given to defining the construct of body image and discussing its theoretical underpinnings. Unique body image issues that arise in the oncology setting are also an important focus here. This chapter concludes with practical suggestions and advice for health care professionals on how to work more effectively with patients exhibiting body image concerns, and ways to alleviate and/or prevent more serious behavioral and psychosocial problems through early recognition and intervention.

■ DEFINITION OF BODY IMAGE

It has been argued that the lack of clear and consistent definition of body image in psychosocial oncology research is a significant barrier to conducting conceptually driven research and theoretically informed psychological assessments and treatment.[1] Body image is a complex and multidimensional construct that encompasses a range of experiences, yet much existing research in the oncology setting relies on loosely constructed or simplistic definitions. Body image cannot be adequately captured with a single-item measure or by merely asking about patient satisfaction with cosmetic outcome.

Body image is a multifaceted concept involving perceptions, thoughts, and feelings about the entire body and its functioning.[2] When one conceptualizes body image in this comprehensive manner, it is clear that the range of bodily changes cancer patients may undergo prior to, during the process of, or following treatment are encompassed here. This includes but is not limited to scarring, swelling, skin discoloration, hair loss, tooth loss, sensory changes (eg, numbness, tingling, burning), functional alterations (eg, changes in speech, swallowing, articulation, hearing, eyesight, bowel/bladder incontinence), sexuality/fertility effects, weight gain, weight loss, loss of mobility, and use of prosthetic devices. While changes to physical appearance are an important component of body image, it is critical to emphasize that body image experiences extend well beyond perception of appearance.[3]

A fundamental element of body image experiences is that they are subjective and, as such, do not reflect the objective reality of the body.[3] This point is underscored by a wealth of research showing that response to disfigurement cannot be adequately explained by disease characteristics or severity of disfigurement alone.[2,4,5] The fact that patients with even small and unnoticeable appearance changes can experience significant distress, and those with more extensive defects can adjust poorly or well to bodily changes suggests that it is vital to attend to patients' perception of body image rather than what is more readily observed by others.

A broader understanding of the complex process of body image development can be obtained by reviewing theoretical models developed by Cash[6] and White,[1] who draw heavily from cognitive and behavioral paradigms in psychology. According to Cash,[6] body image experiences are initially shaped by historical/developmental influences but clearly are further influenced by proximal events and processes. Historical factors refer to past events, attributes, and circumstances that predispose or influence how people think, act, or feel about their body. The most salient historical/developmental factors identified by Cash include cultural socialization concerning values and standards of appearance, experiences tied to social interactions, and one's actual physical characteristics. Proximal processes entail current events that trigger and maintain body image experiences. Cancer diagnosis and its treatment are proximal events that active processing of information about and self-evaluations of one's own physical appearance and bodily functioning. This can be especially problematic for individuals who place a high degree of importance on physical attributes (ie, those with a high degree of appearance investment). White[1] argues that patients with high levels of appearance investment are more likely to direct attention, encode, and interpret stimuli related to bodily experiences in a negative fashion. White's heuristic model of body image dimensions was specifically developed to conceptualize further research, clinical assessment, formulation, and treatment of body image problems among cancer patients. According to this model, cancer patients with perceived or actual appearance changes, which threaten their own personal body image ideals, will experience negative appearance-related assumptions, thoughts, emotions, and behaviors if the discrepancy between their perceived and body image ideals relates to a physical attribute in which they have significant personal investment. In other words, patients who value the way they look will have trouble adjusting to alterations (whether perceived or actual) that deviate from the way they ideally want to look. This also applies to the value or personal meaning attached to functional aspects of the body, such that alterations in or loss of function will be most distressing to those who place a great deal of importance and value on specific aspects of bodily integrity. Taken together, the body image models delineated by Cash and White identify a number of important concepts that should be taken into account when assessing and treating body image problems in the oncology setting. This includes obtaining an understanding of overall satisfaction/dissatisfaction with various aspects of the body (appearance, sensory, functional), importance/value placed on appearance and bodily functions compromised by cancer, and associated emotions, thoughts, and behaviors.

■ UNIQUE BODY IMAGE ISSUES IN THE ONCOLOGY SETTING

Unlike patients with psychiatric disorders who can experience inaccurate distortions of body image or become excessively preoccupied with imagined defects in appearance, it is important to recognize that patients with cancer undergo objective and oftentimes extensive changes to their physical appearance and bodily functioning. An important distinction to be made with patients in any medical context, but especially within the oncology setting, is that body image disturbance should not necessarily be considered pathological in nature. Because the majority of cancer patients are expected to experience body image discomfort related to their disease and treatment, it can be useful to consider body image concerns as existing on a continuum (see Fig. 21-1). This model is consistent with previous work describing a broad array of medical patients[3] and has also been specifically applied to patients with cancer.[7] In the center of the continuum are patients experiencing what is considered to be an average or normative amount of body image concerns. These patients have realistic expectations for cosmetic and functional outcomes but acknowledge some difficulties in adjusting to body image changes as a result of their illness and/or treatment. They may experience some intrusive thoughts about body image discomfort and feel self-conscious in social situations, but do not significantly limit or curtail their daily activities due to body image concerns. At the far right of the continuum are patients with extreme or

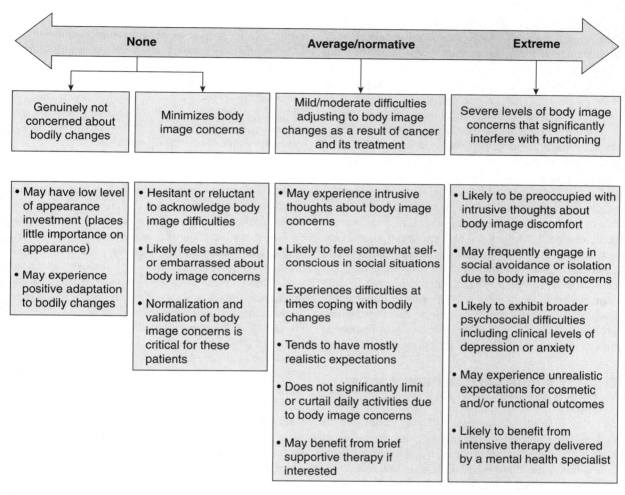

None		Average/normative	Extreme
Genuinely not concerned about bodily changes	Minimizes body image concerns	Mild/moderate difficulties adjusting to body image changes as a result of cancer and its treatment	Severe levels of body image concerns that significantly interfere with functioning
• May have low level of appearance investment (places little importance on appearance) • May experience positive adaptation to bodily changes	• Hesitant or reluctant to acknowledge body image difficulties • Likely feels ashamed or embarrassed about body image concerns • Normalization and validation of body image concerns is critical for these patients	• May experience intrusive thoughts about body image concerns • Likely to feel somewhat self-conscious in social situations • Experiences difficulties at times coping with bodily changes • Tends to have mostly realistic expectations • Does not significantly limit or curtail daily activities due to body image concerns • May benefit from brief supportive therapy if interested	• Likely to be preoccupied with intrusive thoughts about body image discomfort • May frequently engage in social avoidance or isolation due to body image concerns • Likely to exhibit broader psychosocial difficulties including clinical levels of depression or anxiety • May experience unrealistic expectations for cosmetic and/or functional outcomes • Likely to benefit from intensive therapy delivered by a mental health specialist

FIGURE 21-1. Continuum of body image concerns.

severe levels of body image concerns that significantly disrupt and interfere with daily functioning. These patients are likely to be preoccupied with intrusive thoughts about body image discomfort and frequently engage in social avoidance or isolation. They are also very likely to exhibit broader psychosocial difficulties and clinical levels of depression and/or anxiety that may require immediate psychiatric treatment. Unrealistic expectations for cosmetic and functional outcome can further contribute to body image disturbance. Finally, it is important to further understand the select group of cancer patients on the far left of the continuum who deny the existence of any body image concerns. This group includes patients with a range of observable bodily changes, and it is believed that appearance investment plays an important role in

determining the degree to which these changes induce distress or contribute to psychosocial impairment. Patients who are generally not concerned about or invested in their appearance may very well experience no salient body image concerns even when confronted with significant disfigurement. It is also possible that some patients experience positive adaptation to bodily changes such that they consider cancer to be a "blessing in disguise" or view their scars as a "badge of honor." However, it is critical to recognize that some patients may be minimizing their concerns and feel uncomfortable discussing body image issues with their health care provider. It is not uncommon for patients with cancer to worry about being seen as "vain" and experiencing shame and embarrassment about their body image concerns. Moreover, health care providers must be vigilant about the manner in which they can unknowingly or unintentionally invalidate body image concerns for patients with cancer. A well-meaning physician or nurse who repeatedly tells patients how "good" or "wonderful" they look can make patients feel as if their body image concerns are insignificant or trivial.

Body image issues in the oncology setting are further complicated by the nature of cancer treatment that can involve a combination of various modalities such as surgery, radiation, and/or chemotherapy. Each type of treatment is associated with its own set of bodily changes, which can be acute (as in the case of surgery), gradual (e.g., with radiation and/or chemotherapy), and in some cases may involve late effects that emerge or worsen at the completion of treatment. It is also important to note here that surgical treatment is not necessarily a single event. Individuals may require multiple surgical procedures over time depending on the extent and severity of their tumor, whether the tumor is recurrent, and/or whether additional cancers develop over time. It is the ongoing process of adjusting to bodily changes that can present unique challenges in the oncology setting.

■ BODY IMAGE AND SPECIFIC CANCER POPULATIONS

Although a comprehensive review of body image research that has been conducted with specific cancer populations is beyond the scope of this chapter, it is important to provide an overview of published findings in this area. Readers are asked to keep in mind that a host of methodological issues have been recognized with respect to the manner in which body image has been evaluated and conceptualized in past research. This includes not only the use of loosely constructed or simplistic definitions of body image, but also the use of poorly validated measures and failure to distinguish body image from related constructs such as sexuality, self-esteem, stigma, and self-consciousness.[8] Careful attention to methodology is therefore required when interpreting results from individual studies.

Women with breast cancer have clearly received the most amount of attention with respect to evaluation of body image outcomes in the oncology setting. Adverse body image outcomes have been consistently documented among women who undergo a mastectomy, especially when compared with those who undergo a lumpectomy.[9,10] Considerable attention has been given to ascertaining whether patients are satisfied with reconstructive outcomes. Medical factors that appear to be of particular importance for enhancing patient satisfaction in women undergoing breast reconstruction are type and timing of procedures. Although findings are mixed, research generally favors more positive body image outcomes for patients receiving immediate versus delayed reconstruction.[11–13] Additional research has demonstrated greater general and aesthetic satisfaction with autologous-based procedures compared with implant-based procedures.[14,15]

Body image issues for patients with cancer in the head and neck region have received a modest amount of attention. Patients with head and neck cancer encounter unique body image challenges due to the visible nature of the facial region and its inclusion of functionally critical structures including the eye, ear, nose, nasal cavity, mouth, and oral cavity. The social significance of the face must be recognized here, as it is intimately associated with identity, communication abilities, and interpersonal functioning. Research with a broad array of head and neck patients identifies a number of psychosocial difficulties associated with appearance-related changes, including worsened relationships with partners, impaired sexuality, high levels of anxiety and depression, and increased social isolation.[16,17] For surgical patients in particular, preoperative expectations and anticipatory anxiety have been found to significantly influence subsequent adjustment to body image changes. Both the anticipation of disfigurative surgery and inaccurate expectations for postoperative appearance have been significantly related to overall distress and low levels of coping effectiveness following surgery.[18–20] The degree to which disease and treatment characteristics as well as individual factors (e.g., demographics, personality variables) influence adjustment to bodily changes associated with head and neck cancer is still not well understood.[21]

Additional research on body image issues in the oncology setting is spread across various other patient groups, while other work focuses on body image issues stemming from specific procedures or treatment modalities. Although it is clear that bodily changes can have devastating psychosocial effects for any cancer patient, a final group of patients being given specific attention is children and adolescents with cancer. It is critical to recognize that children and adolescents must deal with the effects of cancer and its treatment during a particularly vulnerable period in their body image development. Heightened awareness of physical changes and social relationships begin to emerge during this time, which can result in much greater attention being placed on appearance and physical attractiveness. Some research has pointed to the devastating impact that visible and functional differences such as amputation, hair loss, stunted growth, dramatic weight change, and scarring can have on self-image, particularly for adolescents.[22] Fan and Eiser[23] conducted a systematic literature review of studies examining body image issues in children and adolescents. Not surprisingly, they noted a host of methodological issues among the studies conducted in terms of heterogeneity of body image measures, sample characteristics, and research methods. Overall, they found consistent effects of gender and age such that females seemed to have more difficulty coping with appearance changes than males, and adolescents expressed more body image concerns than younger children. Significant correlations were observed between body image and psychosocial adjustment. Body image difficulties in this population were associated not only with higher levels of anxiety and depression, but with increased behavioral problems as well. Additional research supports the beneficial role social support can have in mitigating the adverse effects of body image on self-esteem and adjustment.[23]

■ ASSESSMENT TOOLS/STRATEGIES

There are a number of current obstacles to identifying appropriate tools and strategies for evaluating body image concerns in the oncology setting. It is important to recognize that the field of body image is historically rooted in identifying and treating patients at risk for or experiencing eating disorders. As a result, most instruments in this field have been developed for women and focus on evaluating weight/shape concerns. It is only recently that attention has been given to developing tools for assessing the body image experiences of patients with other medical conditions, including cancer. These tools play a critical role in helping to identify and address the body image suffering of medical patients because these issues too often go unrecognized by physicians or other health care providers. Pruzinsky[3] believes that the "benign neglect" of body image issues in most medical treatment contexts is the result of physicians being uncomfortable with and/or unskilled at addressing such issues. In order for body image tools to be clinically useful, it is argued here that they must be brief and feasible to administer to patients in a medical setting, have established reliability and validity for the specific population of interest, have empirically determined cut points to accurately identify

patients in need of treatment, and be sensitive to changes in body image that result from disease progression and effects of treatment.

Prior to reviewing available body image tools, it is first important to discuss general ways to promote increased communication with patients about body image and other psychosocial concerns. Relying on patients to volunteer information about their body image concerns or any other psychosocial difficulties is woefully insufficient. Health care providers are urged to directly inquire about whether patients are experiencing body image difficulties, regardless of whether they conduct formalized screening with established assessment tools. It has been stressed previously in this chapter that all patients with cancer are at risk for experiencing body image disturbance due to appearance and functional changes that result from their illness and its treatment. Therefore, routine questioning about body image concerns is warranted in the oncology setting. This type of inquiry can be accomplished in three easy steps, referred to here as the 3 C's (see Fig. 21-2). In the first step, patients are reminded that it is very *common* to experience body image difficulties as a result of cancer and its treatment. Normalizing body image concerns is a critical component of this model because it reduces shame, embarrassment, and stigma about these issues. Next, patients are asked about what types of *concerns* or difficulties they are experiencing as a result of changes to appearance and bodily functioning. This is asked in an open-ended fashion to facilitate useful information to better understand patients' needs. If necessary, prompts can be offered to determine whether difficulties involve physical, social, or emotional functioning. Finally, patients are asked about the *consequences* of body image difficulties, or the manner in which these issues are interfering with their daily functioning. Again, it is recommended that this first be asked in an open-ended fashion, with prompting as necessary to ascertain whether there are specific aspects of functioning affected (eg, occupational, social activities). Examples of specific questions that can be asked are provided in Figure 21-2.

It is recognized that clinicians may argue that this approach requires too much time, and they are fearful of what to do when patients have a strong emotional reaction to discussing these issues (ie, they start crying). A few practical tips are offered with respect to these concerns. Clinicians must be accepting and understanding of negative emotions as they are often a routine part of the cancer experience. It is acceptable for patients to cry

---

Common

- Make certain to mention to patients that it is common for individuals with cancer to experience some difficulties adjusting to bodily changes

Example (at a pretreatment visit): Mr. Doe, it may be important for you to know that many of our patients experience concerns about the types of body changes they are about to undergo as a result of surgical treatment. Most do not completely know what to expect and are anxious about how they will look, especially when they have a cancer that affects their face.

Example (at a follow-up visit): Mrs. Smith, it is not uncommon that even after the completion of radiation and chemotherapy that patients continue to experience difficulties adjusting to the changes their body has undergone as a result of treatment. Because you just completed these treatments within the last month, you should expect to see continued improvement but you may have particular worries or concerns that you'd like to discuss today.

Concerns

- Ascertain the types of concerns patients have with respect to their body image, try to keep your inquiry open-ended if possible to allow the patient to elaborate.

Example (open-ended): What, if any, body image concerns are you experiencing today?

- If warranted, follow-up on the response given by the patient to get more information.

Example: Tell me more about aspects of your physical appearance you are dissatisfied with or concerned about.

Example: Tell me more about your specific concerns about the functional changes to your ___ (e.g., eye, speech, swallowing)

Consequences

- Obtain specific information on how the body image concerns are interfering with functioning and quality of life.

Example (open-ended): In what way are these concerns affecting your day to day life?

- If warranted, prompt to obtain an understanding of how these concerns are impacting social, occupational, and emotional functioning

Example: Are you having emotional difficulties or problems coping with these body image concerns? In what way?

Example: Are you restricting your social activities specifically because of your body image concerns. How so?

FIGURE 21-2. Key assessment strategies for oncologic health care professionals.

and experience negative emotions—just by listening to the patient you are providing a supportive and helpful treatment experience. This will promote more effective patient–provider communication and can contribute to compliance with treatment recommendations and satisfaction with overall care. Some limitations can be placed on this discussion as the clinician is recognized to have to go through a complete view of systems during a typical examination. Most patients understand that this is only one aspect of their care, and there are other issues that need to be addressed and discussed. In the next section, attention will be given to providing appropriate referrals and resources in the event that body image difficulties are recognized as being problematic for the patient. Having these resources handy will also facilitate the discussion.

An alternative approach to evaluating body image issues within the clinic setting is to have patients complete a brief self-report questionnaire while waiting to be seen and to follow up with them during the clinic visit on any items that have been endorsed. This approach is similar to what has been presented in the 2007 Institute of Medicine Report[24] focusing on optimal strategies for meeting the psychosocial health needs of cancer patients. Utilizing a body image screening instrument has been noted to have a number of specific advantages. Pruzinsky[3] explains that this type of assessment, when given as part of routine preconsultation paperwork, can help normalize the body image evaluation process if patients understand that they are not being singled out to discuss these potentially sensitive issues. He further notes that being able to report concerns in writing may facilitate the evaluation process in the event that patients are reticent to verbally express these concerns in the exam room. An additional advantage to utilizing a more formalized screening tool at each patient visit is that valuable data can be obtained and used to track body image difficulties over time.

Returning to the challenges inherent in identifying appropriate body image tools for the oncology setting, it is noted here that while there are a number of potential instruments available for use, each is associated with its own drawbacks. A brief overview of selected tools will be provided to familiarize readers with these instruments. The only tool developed for routine use in clinical practice that will be mentioned here is the Distress Thermometer. The Distress Thermometer (discussed in greater detail in Chapter 4) is a well-known validated screening instrument that includes a single item to capture general distress as well as 35-item Problem List, which encourages patients to identify specific difficulties they are having across a number of psychosocial domains. Included in the Problem List is an item about body image, and if endorsed can prompt a discussion using the 3 C's. The use of this measure is supported through guidelines established by the National Comprehensive Cancer Network.[25] The advantages of using this measure include its brevity, established psychometric properties, and empirically derived cut points. Because it was developed to capture a broad range of psychosocial difficulties, it does not recognize the multifaceted nature of body image difficulties and merely asks about the presence or absence of body image problems in a simplified fashion. This measure does not specify or evaluate dimensions of body image that may be central to the patient's specific medical condition.

Other assessment tools to be discussed here were developed within a research context and not necessarily for clinical use per se. As mentioned earlier, there are a number of criteria that need to be considered to determine whether any given body image measure is clinically useful. To reiterate, these criteria include brevity and ease of administration and having established psychometric properties and empirically derived cut points. It is also important to capture the multifaceted nature of body image by evaluating perceptions, thoughts, behaviors, and emotions about the body and its functioning. Unfortunately, it is believed that at the present time none of the instruments presented below meet these minimum requirements. However, it is worthwhile to become familiar with some of the existing tools that have been developed for evaluating body image concerns to demonstrate some of the different approaches that have been taken. Table 21-1 provides a list of a variety of body image instruments that have been developed within the general population, specifically for patients with cancer, or for patients with other medical conditions. These measures were selected because they are believed to have some potential for use within the oncology setting. A brief description of each of these instruments is offered along with what is known about their respective psychometric properties. Selective instruments will be highlighted below to illustrate some of their unique or distinctive features.

The Body Image Scale (BIS) has a clear advantage for use in the oncology setting because it was specifically designed for patients with cancer and evaluates body image concerns in relation to illness and its treatment.[26] This measure is geared toward evaluating concerns after initiation of treatment. Because it can be used with a broad range of patients (regardless of site and form of treatment), it has wide-ranging applicability. The body image instruments (BII) is particularly valuable because it focuses on evaluating body image issues for a highly vulnerable cancer population, namely adolescents and children.[27] Another distinct advantage of the BII is that it focuses on appearance as well as functional concerns by incorporating items on physical strength, stamina, and coordination. With respect to disease-specific instruments, it is not surprising that considerable attention has been given to developing body image tools for breast cancer patients. Disease-specific instruments purportedly have the advantage of capturing unique body image issues related to a specific medical illness and provide a more refined approach to assessment. For example, the Body Image after Breast Cancer Questionnaire (BIBCQ) includes a subscale specific to evaluating arm concerns due to functional and sensory changes that can result from breast cancer treatment.[28] Another disease-specific instrument for breast cancer patients described in Table 21-1 is the Breast Evaluation Questionnaire.[29] It is worth noting here that there are a number of other disease-specific tools focusing on broader quality of life issues for cancer patients that incorporate questions about

■ **TABLE 21-1.** Select Tools for Evaluating Body Image Concerns

Name of Instrument	Brief Description	Psychometric Properties	Population
Body image tools designed specifically for cancer patients			
Body Image Scale (BIS)	10 items; designed to evaluate satisfaction/dissatisfaction with appearance changes resulting from cancer and its treatment	Validated only with breast patients; internal consistency (0.93); sensitive to change over time	Considered applicable for patients with any cancer site and any form of cancer therapy
Body Image after Breast Cancer Questionnaire (BIBCQ)	45-Item disease-specific scale, recognizes the multidimensional nature of body image; evaluates functional difficulties, satisfaction with body shape and appearance, body stigma	Test–retest reliability (0.77–0.88) for all six scales; convergent validity, distinguished between women with lumpectomy and those with mastectomy, between women with breast cancer and controls	Women with breast cancer
Breast Evaluation Questionnaire	55-Item disease-specific scale; designed to assess breast satisfaction, comfort with general appearance, and specific appearance of the breast	Test–retest reliability 0.89 to 0.97 across three scales; internal consistency 0.90 to 0.97	Women with breast cancer
Body Image Instrument (BII)	28-Item measure with five subscales; evaluates concerns about physical appearance, body competence (physical strength, stamina, coordination), importance of appearance, concerns about others' reaction	Concurrent validity with other QOL measures; internal consistency (0.68–0.85) for different scales	Designed for adolescents and young adults with cancer
Body image tools designed for other medical groups			
Derriford Appearance Scale	59- or 24-item measure (short form) designed to evaluate distress and difficulties experienced in living with problems of appearance; widely used in research	Short form: internal consistency (0.92), test–retest reliability (0.82), and criterion validity with the DAS59 (0.88)	Developed for medical and nonmedical populations
Satisfaction with Appearance Scale (SWAP)	15-Item measure; focuses on subjective body image distress as well as the social impact of body image dissatisfaction	Internal consistency (0.87); test–retest reliability (0.59), convergent and discriminant validity with measures of body image, depression, anxiety, PTSD, and QOL	Developed to assess body image in disfigured medical populations

Continued

■ TABLE 21-1. Select Tools for Evaluating Body Image Concerns (continued)

Name of Instrument	Brief Description	Psychometric Properties	Population
Other body image tools (designed and/or tested in the general population)			
Multidimensional Body–Self Relations Questionnaire (MBSRQ)	Widely used assessment of broad dimensions of body image in clinical research; 69 items; includes seven factor scales to evaluate attitudes and behaviors relevant to physical appearance, fitness, and health/illness. Also includes three subscales to evaluate satisfaction with body areas and weight concerns	Established convergent, discriminant, and construct validity with other body image and psychosocial measures	General population, adolescents and adults (15 years or older)
Body Image Coping Strategies Inventory	29 items, evaluates strategies that women and men employ to manage or cope with body image threats or challenges; three subscales: Appearance Fixing, Positive Rational Acceptance, Avoidance	Cronbach's alpha ranges from 0.74 to 0.91 for individual subscales; convergent validity with other body image scales	Designed for use with persons with body image difficulties
Appearance Schemas Inventory-Revised	20 items; evaluates the importance, meaning, and influence of appearance in one's life (body image investment)	Internal consistency (0.90); convergent validity with other measures of body image and psychosocial functioning	Developed in the general population; separate norms for men and women
Body Satisfaction Scale	16-Item scale evaluating satisfaction with body parts; half involving the head and the other half involving the body	Internal consistency (0.79–0.89) depending on sample; discriminates between general population and individuals with eating disorders	Developed for the general population; also used for patients with weight-related difficulties
The Situational Inventory of Body Image Dysphoria (SIBID)	20-Item short form or 48-item long form; designed to evaluate negative body image emotions in specific situational contexts; can provide helpful targets for behavioral treatment	Internal consistency (0.96); test–retest reliability (0.80); established convergent and discriminant validity, responsive to body image therapy	Developed in the general population, designed for use in persons with body image difficulties and disorders

Continued

■ **TABLE 21-1. Select Tools for Evaluating Body Image Concerns (continued)**

Name of Instrument	Brief Description	Psychometric Properties	Population
Other body image tools (designed and/or tested in the general population)			
Body Esteem Scale	35-Item scale designed as a measure of body dissatisfaction that has separate factor structures for males and females; evaluates satisfaction with upper body strength, physical conditioning, sexual attractiveness, and weight concern	Coefficient alphas range from 0.78 to 0.87 for the different factors; convergent and discriminant validity	Designed for men and women in the general population
Body Image Ideals Questionnaire (BIQ)	Evaluates body image from the perspective of Self-Discrepancy Theory—assesses the degree of discrepancy of self-perceived and idealized physical attributes while considering the importance of each of the physical ideals of the person	Internal consistency (0.75–0.79) for men and women; responsive to therapeutic body image interventions	Developed in the general population, designed for individuals with body image difficulties
Body Image Quality of Life Inventory	19-Item instrument designed to quantify the impact of body image in specific life contexts (eg, social situations, sexual encounters, work/other daily activities)	Internal consistency (0.95), test–retest reliability (0.79), convergent validity	Developed in the general population, designed for those with body image difficulties
Body Image Avoidant Questionnaire (BIAQ)[41]	19-Item measure of behaviors that often occur with body image disturbance (eg, avoiding looking in mirrors, social isolation)	Internal consistency (alpha = 0.89), test–retest reliability (r = 0.87)	Developed to measure avoidant behaviors for persons with body image difficulties or disorders
Body Image Disturbance Questionnaire (BIDQ)	7-Item measure evaluating preoccupation with appearance-related concerns, distress, and impairment in important areas of functioning, and behavioral avoidance	Convergent validity with other measures of body image	Developed for use with various clinical groups (patients with BDD, eating disorders)

body image difficulties. Examples include the Functional Assessment of Cancer Therapy (FACT)-Head and Neck,[30] Head and Neck Survey,[31] Skin Cancer Index,[32] and FACT-Breast[33] to name a few.

Additional attention is given to describing body image tools that were not initially developed for cancer patients, but may nonetheless be useful in the oncology setting. The Derriford Appearance Scale and Satisfaction with

Appearance Scale are examples of two measures designed for use with medical populations that appear to capture salient body image issues and concerns for patients with cancer. The DAS was specifically designed to capture difficulties for individuals feeling self-consciousness in relation to their appearance,[34,35] and the SWAP includes items to evaluate nonweight-related body image dissatisfaction at multiple body sites and social discomfort related to appearance.[36] There are a number of additional instruments worth mentioning that focus on important components of body image but were developed in the general population. The Appearance Schemas Inventory-Revised[37] and Appearance Orientation subscale of the Multidimensional Body Self-Relations Questionnaire[38] evaluate the core factor of appearance investment. The Body Satisfaction Scale assesses the evaluative component of satisfaction/dissatisfaction with body parts and includes items involving the head and the body.[39] The Situational Inventory of Body Image Dysphoria[40] and Body Image Avoidance Questionnaire[41] tap into the important dimensions of behavioral avoidance and can help clinicians identify problematic situations that trigger body image distress. The Body Image Coping Strategies Inventory is unique in that it identifies potentially adaptive and maladaptive strategies used by patients to deal with body image distress.[42] A final measure worth specific mention is the Body Image Disturbance Questionnaire (BIDQ) because it taps into multiple body image domains.[43] The BIDQ contains seven items and evaluates appearance-related concerns, mental preoccupation with these concerns, associated experiences of emotional distress, resultant impairment in social occupational or other importance areas of functioning, interference with social life or school, job or role functioning, and consequential behavioral avoidance. Five additional items ask for open-ended clarification of responses, which can be informative in clinical contexts or qualitative research. Other questionnaires more fully described in Table 21-1 include the Body Esteem Scale,[44] Body Image Ideals Questionnaire,[45] and Body Image Quality of Life Inventory.[46]

◼ TREATMENT STRATEGIES/APPROACHES—ONCOLOGIC HEALTH CARE TEAM

To facilitate a discussion of appropriate treatment strategies for patients having difficulty adjusting to bodily changes as a result of cancer and its treatment, we must revisit the body image continuum model presented in Figure 21-1 as well as the 3 C's assessment approach presented in Figure 21-2. Treatment strategies can be appropriately tailored depending on the nature and extent of patients' body image concerns and the degree to which these concerns are interfering with their daily functioning. Patients with mild-to-moderate levels of distress arising from body image concerns may benefit from brief supportive therapy or community resources. However, those who are preoccupied with intrusive thoughts about appearance and bodily changes, engage in a high degree of behavioral avoidance, and/or significantly limit or curtail daily activities due to body image concerns are likely in need of a more intensive therapy. Another important factor to consider when planning an intervention for body image difficulties is the patient's stage of treatment. Patients in the preoperative or pretreatment stage may be facing difficult treatment decisions that will affect their bodies, while others may simply have to deal with coming to terms with bodily changes associated with the only treatment options available to them. A critical intervention at this stage of treatment is to help patients realistically prepare for the bodily changes they are about to experience by developing appropriate expectations for cosmetic and functional outcomes. Patients who are in the midst of treatment require assistance coping with the actual bodily changes they are experiencing and the manner in which these alterations are interfering with their life. Those who have completed treatment must face long-term or permanent changes in their bodies and work toward body image acceptance.

Routine questioning about body image concerns as discussed with the 3 C's approach is the first important step in providing an appropriate intervention for body image difficulties in the oncology setting. Health care professionals without specialty mental health training can provide effective and critical support to patients experiencing problems adjusting to bodily changes as a result of cancer and its treatment. A primary way to assist patients with these difficulties is to provide empathic listening to patients and their families and encourage open discussion of body image concerns. This requires listening to what is being said and responding in a way that allows the patient to feel understood and accepted. Even if the patient's body image complaints are excessive and unrealistic, the health care provider needs to try and view the situation from the perspective of the patient and acknowledge that he or she is feeling upset or unsatisfied and that body image concerns are significantly interfering with the quality of life. A second key treatment strategy that needs to be employed by all health care professionals is to normalize or validate body image concerns within the oncology setting. Patients need to hear that it is common to experience difficulties adjusting to bodily changes, even if their body image concerns are on the extreme end of the continuum. This information may carry particular weight when coming directly from the treating oncologist. Finally, health care providers have the ability to offer vital knowledge to patients that can assist with adjustment to bodily changes. After obtaining an understanding of the types of body image concerns patients are experiencing and understanding the manner in which these concerns interfere with daily functioning, health care providers are in an optimal position to educate patients about what to expect in terms of cosmetic improvement and functional recovery. For patients who have unrealistic/unreasonable expectations and express particular dissatisfaction with what is recognized by the treatment team as an optimal or satisfactory outcome, health care providers must be sensitive to approaching this situation and educating patients in an objective manner. These treatment strategies are summarized in Table 21-2.

A critical mistake that is made by health care professionals is to immediately and instinctively comment to patients about how "good" they look or how "well" they are doing. This type of introductory statement can unknowingly serve to frustrate and upset patients who are experiencing adjustment difficulties. Moreover, this type of statement can invalidate their body image concerns and make them much more reluctant to openly discuss these problems and obtain needed support. It is strongly recommended that health care providers first ask patients about whether they are having any cosmetic or functional concerns and go from there. In this way, they can be more responsive to patients' concerns and better prepared to approach delicate situations such as when a patient is exceedingly unsatisfied with a satisfactory or optimal outcome.

Consider the following vignette: Sally is a 43-year-old woman with a history of breast cancer who underwent a double mastectomy with immediate reconstruction using tissue expanders. Following the expansion process, she underwent a procedure to replace the tissue expanders with silicone-based implants. She returns for a postoperative visit 7 days following this procedure.

■ **TABLE 21-2. Key Treatment Strategies for Managing Distress Arising from Body Image Concerns in the Oncology Setting**

Health care providers in the oncology setting
- Utilize empathic listening
- Validate body image concerns
- Educate patients about expected outcomes
- Provide patients with community resources to assist them in coping with body image difficulties (see Table 21–3)
- Refer patients to a mental health specialist when needed for brief or intensive therapy
- Follow-up with patients about body image concerns at each clinic visit

Mental health specialists
- Educate patients to promote realistic expectations
- Assist with treatment decision making and problem solving
- Promote body image acceptance
- Identify and challenge problematic appearance-related assumptions
- Behavioral activation strategies to reduce social isolation and avoidance
- Coaching on social/interpersonal skills
- Mind–body relaxation strategies

Although the nurse's instinctive reaction is to comment on how good Sally looks since there is minimal swelling and how great she is doing since they will be able to remove the drains today, she reminds herself that it is first important for her to check in with the patient. She asks Sally how she has been doing since the surgery. Sally launches into a litany of complaints about pain, scarring and swelling, breast asymmetry, and how she feels "horribly disfigured." During this clinic visit, the nurse and doctor take the time to help Sally realize that most breast cancer patients experience difficulties adjusting to bodily changes. They discuss with her the way in which her outcome compares favorably to other patients, and that she will continue to experience improvement with further recovery time. Sally is also reminded that she will have the opportunity to undergo surgical revision in several months to correct minor issues with breast asymmetry. A frank discussion ensues about her expectations for final cosmetic outcome taking time to explain again that scars may fade over time but not completely disappear, and that size and shape of her breasts will not necessarily approximate what she looked like before—but the goal is to get them to look as similar to each other as possible.

The vignette described above intended to demonstrate a way of approaching patients that normalizes and validates body image concerns. In this type of scenario, the sensitive way in which questions are asked and information is conveyed may in itself serve to alleviate distress associated with body image concerns. It is noted here that there is often a need to repeat information presented at previous clinic visits—which can be a source of frustration for some clinicians. Patients vary in the degree to which they are receptive to listening and comprehending information provided to them depending on where they are in the treatment process. In this case, Sally may have been so overwhelmed during her presurgical consultation that she did not attend to or process information related to the postoperative healing process. Having this information repeated in an objective and straightforward manner may be extremely important for this patient. As mentioned above, this type of brief clinical intervention may provide what is needed to assist the patient. Let us add a few wrinkles to this scenario and see how this would change the approach being recommended.

Sally explains rather adamantly that she expected to look "almost back to normal" after this procedure. She remains upset about her appearance changes, and notes that she is having difficulty viewing herself in the mirror and doubts she will ever be able to resume sexual activity with her husband again. At this point, Sally is provided with some information about counseling services available through the American Cancer Society (ACS) as well as a referral to a mental health specialist in the area. She is reminded that it is not uncommon for patients to experience these types of difficulties, and that she would likely benefit from talking with trained specialists about her concerns.

Having psychosocial resources available for patients experiencing body image difficulties is considered vital. A number of helpful resources will be reviewed here to familiarize clinicians with community organizations that have programs or services designed to help ameliorate distress arising from appearance changes (see also Table 21-3). Changes Faces is a national organization based in the United Kingdom that supports and represents people who have disfigurements of the face or body from any cause. This organization provides support for children, young people, adults, and families by providing advice, information (booklets, videos, self-help guides), and counseling. The Changing Faces program has developed a variety of useful educational handouts available for purchase and/or can be downloaded from their Web site (see Table 21-3) on topics such as ways to handle other people's reaction to facial disfigurement, how to talk with health care professionals about disfigurement, strategies for communicating successfully when you have a disfigurement that affects your eye, and how to manage the effects of facial paralysis. One practical suggestion is to purchase these educational materials for use in the clinic and offer them to patients if a particular issue is relevant. The ACS can help identify local resources to provide assistance with cancer patients' appearance difficulties and has several specific programs targeting these concerns. Looking Good … Feeling Better is a free, national public service program administered by ACS designed to help women offset appearance-related changes from cancer treatment. This includes educating women on beauty techniques to enhance appearance and self-image during treatment. Small group programs, one-on-one salon consultations, and self-help materials are also available. The Lance Armstrong Foundation is a nonprofit organization that provides practical information and tools people with cancer need to live their life on their own terms. Specific information on coping with physical and emotional effects of cancer and practical tips on adapting to body image changes are available. There are two specific programs designed to provide assistance to breast cancer patients that are worth highlighting here. Network of Strength, formerly known as the Y-Me Breast Cancer Organization, is a national nonprofit organization that provides a hotline to give emotional support and information about breast cancer. This organization is unique in that all newsletters, publications, and brochures are available in English and Spanish. Their Web site offers information in Chinese, Russian, Vietnamese, and Korean, and they have interpreters available to provide services in over 150 languages. Network of Strength also has a survivor and partner match program to pair

■ **TABLE 21-3. Contact Information for Community Resources**

Name of Organization	Purpose	Contact Information
American Cancer Society (ACS)	Provides a wealth of cancer-related educational resources and support groups to people around the country	www.cancer.org (1-800-227-2345)
ACS Looking Good ... Feeling Better Program	Specifically assists cancer patients having difficulty coping with appearance-related changes	www.lookinggoodfeelbetter.org (1-800-395-5665)
American Psychosocial Oncology Society (APOS)	Promotes the practice of psychosocial care for people with cancer; can help patients find counseling services in their own community	www.apos-society.org (toll-free hotline: 1-866-276-7443)
CancerCare	Provides counseling, education, financial assistance, and practical help for patients with cancer	www.cancercare.org (1-800-813-HOPE (4673))
Changing Faces	Provides support and resources to people who have disfigurements of the face or body from any cause	www.changingfaces.org.uk
Gilda's Club	Offers support and networking groups, seminars, specialized programs, and social events in a nonresidential homelike setting	www.gildasclub.org (1-888-GILDA-4-U)
Lance Armstrong Foundation (LAF)	Provides practical information and tools for people with cancer; including counseling programs	www.livestrong.org (1-866-673-7205)
National Cancer Institute, Cancer Information Service	Provides education about cancer prevention, risk factors, early detection, symptoms, diagnosis, and treatment	www.cancer.gov (1-800-4-CANCER)
National Coalition for Cancer Survivorship	Survivor-led cancer advocacy organization; has a free audio program called the Cancer Survivor Toolbox that teaches skills to help cancer survivors	www.canceradvocacy.org (1-877-622-7937)
Network of Strength (formerly known as the Y-Me Breast Cancer Organization)	Provides counseling and resources to patients with breast cancer; services available in over 150 languages, Web site offers information in English, Spanish, Russian, Vietnamese, Korean, and Chinese	www.networkofstrength.org (1-800-221-2141)
People Living with Cancer (associated with the American Society of Clinic Oncology)	A patient information Web site that provides timely oncologist-approved information to help patients and families make well-informed health care decisions	www.plwc.org (1-886-651-3038)
Shop Well with You	Web site that offers resources on body image and clothing-specific needs of cancer survivors	www.shopwellwithyou.org (1-800-799-6790)
The Wellness Community	Offers special groups and wellness classes for cancer survivors at centers around the country; also offers online support groups	www.thewellnesscommunity.org (1-888-793-WELL)

patients and family members with individuals who have experienced similar challenges. Shop Well with You is a not-for-profit organization that offers a number of resources on their Web site including articles on body image and information on clothing-specific needs of cancer survivors. The site provides general tips on fabrics, styles, and cuts that offer the most comfort for specific conditions.

There are, of course, a number of other organizations that provide a broad range of psychosocial services. These include CancerCare, National Cancer Institute, Cancer Information Service, National Coalition for Cancer Survivorship, American Psychosocial Oncology Society, The Wellness Community, People Living with Cancer, and Gilda's Club, to name a few. Relevant contact information for each of these organizations is provided in Table 21-3. Interested readers are encouraged to contact these organizations directly for more information on available services for patients with cancer.

Returning to the case vignette presented above, mental health specialists can provide critical support and assistance to patients with body image difficulties especially for those motivated and interested in treatment and for those with poor coping skills, inadequate social support, preoccupation with appearance-related issues, and high levels of anxiety and/or depression. Services provided by mental health specialists can range from brief supportive therapy to more intensive therapy. Clinical integration of psychosocial services with onsite mental health professionals is described as an ideal health care model in the 2007 IOM report. This model is believed to facilitate patient follow-through on referrals and has been found to improve treatment outcomes. Moreover, this approach can promote optimal collaborative care and management of patients, allowing treating physicians to obtain rapid feedback on psychosocial concerns and behavioral health issues of referred patients. Regardless of whether psychosocial services are integrated into the medical care setting or referred to providers offsite, following up with patients after a referral is an important element of quality care that must not be overlooked.

■ TREATMENT STRATEGIES/ APPROACHES—MENTAL HEALTH SPECIALIST

There are a variety of treatment strategies and approaches that a well-trained mental health specialist can deliver to target body image difficulties of cancer patients

(see also Table 21-2). Although there is a dearth of research involving body image treatment specifically for cancer patients, cognitive–behavioral therapy (CBT) has been established as an effective and empirically sound intervention for individuals with body image difficulties in the general population as well as for those with psychological disturbances such as eating disorders and body dysmorphic disorder. Treatment with CBT in these groups has shown positive effects on self-esteem, social functioning, and other psychological variables such as anxiety and depression.[6,47] Body image CBT programs focus largely on identifying, labeling, and challenging maladaptive appearance assumptions about the self and others. Additional attention is given to altering patterns of behaviors that are the foundation of distress and disruptive body image experiences. The varied treatment strategies that can be used include teaching adaptive coping skills, improved problem solving, relaxation techniques, and coaching on social/interpersonal skills.

Cash[48] has developed a particularly helpful resource to assist mental health professionals in working with patients experiencing body image difficulties. This empirically validated CBT-based program can be easily adapted for patients with cancer and is found in *The Body Image Workbook: An Eight Step Program for Learning to Like Your Looks.*[48] Basic elements of this program include (1) conducting a self-assessment of the various facets of body image to evaluate strengths and weaknesses, (2) exploring historical influences on body image through expressive writing exercises, (3) promoting mindful awareness of body image experiences, (4) identifying problematic appearance-related assumptions, (5) challenging maladaptive thinking through cognitive restructuring, (6) confronting body image avoidance through exposure-based exercises, (7) challenging and disruptive problematic appearance fixing rituals, and (8) promoting positive body–self relations through pleasurable activities.

> Consider the following vignette: Max is a 35-year-old man with a history of squamous cell carcinoma of the right base of tongue who has undergone chemotherapy, radiation, and then a bilateral neck dissection. This patient now suffers from neck soft tissue deformity that has greatly impacted his life and body image as he wears a bandana at all times, even when he is home alone. His plastic surgeon has referred him to a clinical psychologist to assist with his adjustment difficulties. Max explains to the psychologist the

manner in which his preoccupation with appearance and distress is adversely affecting his daily functioning. He completes self-report questionnaires that reveal scores in the problem range for behavioral avoidance, high level of negative appearance-related thoughts, and extremely poor evaluation of his appearance. It is noted that he does experience positive thoughts about some aspects of appearance. His treatment plan consists of examining the role appearance played in his life prior to being diagnosed with cancer to help him better understand factors contributing to his high level of appearance investment, identify and challenge his numerous appearance-related assumptions, and engage in gradual exposure of removing his bandana in social situations. By the end of treatment, Max was able to tolerate removing his bandana entirely at home, and for increasingly longer periods of time during the day. He also was regularly engaging in pleasurable activities to promote health and fitness and other sensate-enhancing activities such as exercising and massage therapy.

■ SUMMARY

This chapter addresses an extremely important, yet often neglected, psychosocial issue that affects a broad range of cancer patients. Body image concerns, which can range from mild to severe in intensity, can negatively impact quality of life in a variety of ways. All patients with cancer are at risk for experiencing difficulties adjusting to bodily changes as a result of disease and its treatment. It is argued here that health care providers in the oncology setting can and should be more sensitive to the body image concerns of their patients. In this chapter, particular emphasis has been given to demonstrating the multidimensional nature of body image, which encompasses perceptions, thoughts, behaviors, and emotions about the entire body and its functioning. Oncologists are reminded that body image is entirely subjective, and, as such, they must directly talk with their patients to understand their perspective, which may differ from objective reality. Practical suggestions and advice are offered here to assist with the identification, assessment, and treatment of body image difficulties in the oncology setting. It is important to stress that research on body image issues in the oncology setting is in its infancy, and therefore much additional knowledge is needed to refine our understanding of the unique body image challenges of this patient group. Current treatment recommendations are based on data from other patient groups. Ideally, future research should concentrate on developing and validating tailored interventions to address the unique body image challenges faced by patients with different types of tumors.

KEY POINTS

- Body image is a complex and multidimensional construct.
- Body image is inherently subjective and does not only refer to physical appearance.
- Body image disturbance in the oncology setting is not necessarily pathological.
- Body image concerns are best understood to exist on a continuum.
- Beware of minimizing/invalidating body image concerns.
- Body image research and treatment in medical populations is in its infancy.

REFERENCES

1. White CA. Body image dimensions and cancer: a heuristic cognitive behavioural model. *Psychooncology.* 2000;9:183–192.

2. Pruzinsky T. Social and psychological effects of facial disfigurement: quality of life, body image and surgical reconstruction. In: Weber RW, Goepfert H, Miller MJ, eds. *Basal and Squamous Cell Carcinomas Skin Cancers of the Head and Neck.* Philadelphia PA: Williams & Wilkins; 1996:357–362.

3. Pruzinsky T. Enhancing quality of life in medical populations: a vision for body image assessment and rehabilitation as standards of care. *Body Image Int J Res.* 2004;1:71–81.

4. Rumsey N, Clarke A, White P, Wyn-Williams M, Garlick W. Altered body image: appearance-related concerns of people with visible disfigurement. *J Adv Nurs.* 2004;48:443–453.

5. Newell R. *Body Image and Disfigurement Care.* New York, NY: Taylor & Francis Group; 2000.

6. Cash TF. Cognitive–behavioral perspectives on body image. In: Cash TF, Pruzinsky T, eds. *Body Image: A Handbook of Theory, Research, and Clinical Practice.* New York, NY: The Guilford Press; 2002:38–46.

7. Fingeret MC. Psychosocial impact of skin cancer treatment. In: Weber RS, Moore BA, eds. *Cutaneous Malignancy of Head & Neck: A Multidisciplinary Approach*. San Diego, CA: Plural Publishing. In press.

8. White CA. Body images in oncology. In: Cash TF, Pruzinsky T, eds. *Body Image: A Handbook of Theory, Research & Clinical Practice*. New York, NY: The Guilford Press; 2002:379–386.

9. Yurek D, Farrar W, Andersen BL. Breast cancer surgery: comparing surgical groups and determining individual differences in postoperative sexuality and body change stress. *J Consult Clin Psychol*. 2000;68:697–709.

10. Rowland JH, Desmond KA, Meyerowitz BE, Belin TR, Wyatt GE, Ganz PA. Role of breast reconstructive surgery in physical and emotional outcomes among breast cancer survivors. *J Natl Cancer Inst*. 2000;92:1422–1429.

11. Frierson GM, Andersen BL. Breast reconstruction. In: Sarwer DB, Pruzinsky T, Cash TF, Goldwyn RM, Persing JA, Whitaker LA, eds. *Psychological Aspects of Reconstructive and Cosmetic Plastic Surgery: Clinical, Empirical, and Ethical Perspectives*. Philadelphia, Pa: Lippincott Williams & Wilkins; 2006:173–188.

12. Al-Ghazal SK, Sully L, Fallowfield L, Blamey RW. The psychological impact of immediate rather than delayed breast reconstruction. *Eur J Surg Oncol*. 2000;26:17–19.

13. Wilkins EG, Cederna PS, Lowery JC, et al. Prospective analysis of psychosocial outcomes in breast reconstruction: one-year postoperative results from the Michigan Breast Reconstruction Outcome Study. *Plast Reconstr Surg*. 2000;106:1014–1025 [discussion 1026–1027].

14. Alderman AK, Wilkins EG, Lowery JC, Kim M, Davis JA. Determinants of patient satisfaction in postmastectomy breast reconstruction. *Plast Reconstr Surg*. 2000;106:769–776.

15. Alderman AK, Kuhn LE, Lowery JC, Wilkins EG. Does patient satisfaction with breast reconstruction change over time? Two-year results of the Michigan Breast Reconstruction Outcomes Study. *J Am Coll Surg*. 2007;204:7–12.

16. Gamba A, Romano M, Grosso IM, et al. Psychosocial adjustment of patients surgically treated for head and neck cancer. *Head Neck*. 1992;14:218–223.

17. Katz MR, Irish JC, Devins GM, Rodin GM, Gullane PJ. Psychosocial adjustment in head and neck cancer: the impact of disfigurement, gender and social support. *Head Neck*. 2003;25:103–112.

18. Cassileth BR, Lusk EJ, Tenaglia AN. Patients' perceptions of the cosmetic impact of melanoma resection. *Plast Reconstr Surg*. 1983;71:73–75.

19. Dropkin MJ. Postoperative body images in head and neck cancer patients. *Quality of Life-A Nursing Challenge*. 1997;5:110–113.

20. Dropkin MJ. Body image and quality of life after head and neck cancer surgery. *Cancer Pract*. 1999;7:309–313.

21. Fingeret MC, Vidrine DJ, Reece GP, Gillenwater AG, Gritz ER. A multidimensional analysis of body image concerns among newly diagnosed patients with oral cavity cancer. *Head Neck*. 2010;32:301–309.

22. Abrams AN, Hazen EP, Penson RT. Psychosocial issues in adolescents with cancer. *Cancer Treat Rev*. 2007;33:622–630.

23. Fan SY, Eiser C. Body image of children and adolescents with cancer: a systematic review. *Body Image*. 2009;6:247–256.

24. Institute of Medicine. *Cancer Care for the Whole Patient: Meeting Psychosocial Health Needs*. Washington, DC: The National Academic Press; 2008.

25. *The NCCN Clinical Practice Guidelines in Oncology™ Distress Management (Version 2.2009)*. © 2009 National Comprehensive Cancer Network Inc. Available at: NCCN.org. Accessed June 26, 2009.

26. Hopwood P, Fletcher I, Lee A, Al Ghazal S. A body image scale for use with cancer patients. *Eur J Cancer*. 2001;37:189–197.

27. Kopel SJ, Eiser C, Cool P, Grimer RJ, Carter SR. Brief report: assessment of body image in survivors of childhood cancer. *J Pediatr Psychol*. 1998;23:141–147.

28. Baxter NN, Goodwin PJ, McLeod RS, Dion R, Devins G, Bombardier C. Reliability and validity of the body image after breast cancer questionnaire. *Breast J*. 2006;12:221–232.

29. Anderson RC, Cunningham B, Tafesse E, Lenderking WR. Validation of the breast evaluation questionnaire for use with breast surgery patients. *Plast Reconstr Surg*. 2006;118:597–602.

30. List MA, D'Antonio LL, Cella DF, et al. The Performance Status Scale for Head and Neck Cancer Patients and the Functional Assessment of Cancer Therapy-Head and Neck Scale. A study of utility and validity. *Cancer*. 1996;77:2294–2301.

31. Gliklich RE, Goldsmith TA, Funk GF. Are head and neck specific quality of life measures necessary? *Head Neck*. 1997;19:474–480.

32. Rhee JS, Matthews BA, Neuburg M, Logan BR, Burzynski M, Nattinger AB. Validation of a quality of life instrument for nonmelanoma skin cancer patients. *Arch Facial Plast Surg*. 2006:314–318.

33. Brady MJ, Cella DF, Mo F, et al. Reliability and validity of the Functional Assessment of Cancer Therapy-Breast quality-of-life instrument. *J Clin Oncol.* 1997;15:974–986.

34. Carr T, Harris D, James C. The Derriford Appearance Scale (DAS-59): a new scale to measure individual responses to living with problems of appearance. *Br J Health Psychol.* 2000;5:201–215.

35. Carr T, Moss T, Harris D. The DAS24: a short form of the Derriford Appearance Scale DAS59 to measure individual responses to living with problems of appearance. *Br J Health Psychol.* 2005;10(pt 2):285–298.

36. Heinberg LJ, Kudel I, White B, et al. Assessing body image in patients with systemic sclerosis (scleroderma): validation of the adapted Satisfaction with Appearance Scale. *Body Image.* 2007;4:79–86.

37. Cash TF, Melnyk SE, Hrabosky JI. The assessment of body image investment: an extensive revision of the Appearance Schemas Inventory. *Int J Eat Disord.* 2004;35:305–316.

38. Cash TF. *Multidimensional Body–Self Relations Questionnaire Users' Manual.* Norfolk, VA: Old Dominion University; 2000.

39. Slade PD, Dewey ME, Newton T, Brodie D, Kiemle G. Development and preliminary validation of the Body Satisfaction Scale (BSS). *Psychol Health.* 1990;4:213–220.

40. Cash TF. The situational inventory of body-image dysphoria: psychometric evidence and development of a short form. *Int J Eat Disord.* 2002;32:362–366.

41. Rosen JC, Srebnik D, Saltzberg E, Wendt S. Development of a Body Image Avoidance Questionnaire. *Psychol Assess.* 1991;3:32–37.

42. Cash TF, Santos MT, Williams EF. Coping with body-image threats and challenges: validation of the Body Image Coping Strategies Inventory. *J Psychosom Res.* 2005;58:190–199.

43. Cash TF, Phillips KA, Santos MT, Hrabosky JI. Measuring "negative body image": validation of the Body Image Disturbance Questionnaire in a nonclinical population. *Body Image.* 2004;1:363–372.

44. Franzoi SL, Shields SA. The Body Esteem Scale: multidimensional structure and sex differences in a college population. *J Pers Assess.* 1984;48:173–178.

45. Cash TF, Szymanski ML. The development and validation of the Body-Image Ideals Questionnaire. *J Pers Assess.* 1995;64:466–477.

46. Cash TF, Fleming EC. The impact of body image experiences: development of the body image quality of life inventory. *Int J Eat Disord.* 2002;31:455–460.

47. Jarry JL, Berardi K. Characteristics and effectiveness of stand-along body image treatments: a review of the empirical literature. *Body Image.* 2004;1:319–333.

48. Cash TF. *The Body Image Workbook: An Eight Step Program for Learning to Like Your Looks.* 2nd ed. Oakland, CA: New Harbinger Publications Inc; 2008.

Physical Medicine and Rehabilitation

• *Benedict Konzen*

■ INTRODUCTION

Ultimately the goal of physical medicine and rehabilitation is to restore an individual to the highest level of function. By definition, functioning is usually thought of in mechanical terms—walking, running, and climbing. In the sports world, it is a question of swimming, soccer, basketball, cycling, skiing, skating, etc. We often take for granted movement or the daily activities of getting dressed, bathed, or going to the restroom—that is, until we no longer have the ability to perform these tasks independently.

In much the same way as an infant begins to roll from abdomen to back, sit, utter a first word, crawl, stand, cruise, and eventually walk, the passage of activities in the cancer patient is characterized by milestones. The determination, practice, and energy that went into these activities are often forgotten.

The same concentration and fortitude are required when attempting to meet the needs of any medical patient. Characteristically, the physician is required to interview a patient in depth and understand that patient's medical background, his or her historical family, and the interplay between different biopsychosocial elements. From a physical medicine and rehabilitation perspective, a patient's overall function requires a detailed personal interview and an understanding of who the patient is—physically, socially, intellectually, motivationally, and spiritually. Sound physical and mental functioning demand harmony between these different features.

Where there is homeostatic malalignment, function suffers, and the patient becomes ill-equipped to meet the challenges of both his or her work and social environment. Maladaptive behaviors may ensue. What previously was an acceptable means of societal interchange—the 40-hour work week, washing the car on Saturday, the family weekend picnic or barbecue, socializing with friends and family, sending cards and letters, and reading books—today, has given way to instant communication, pagers, texting, and blackberries. We are overly integrated and saturated with work, politics, and instant news. Like the cancer patient, we often demonstrate a limited ability to properly and adequately digest, process, sort, categorize, and plan appropriate responses and strategies. Rather in today's world, we need to be constantly vigilant—everything at a moment's notice.

Is it any surprise that older institutions of coping—the afternoon drive, a trip to the cinema, having a cup of coffee and an afternoon chat, and talking to one's spiritual advisor—have been left on the shelf? Gainful employment, meeting social/financial obligations, and maintenance of one's livelihood currently entail competition, potentially a difficult work week, poor sleep, poor nutrition, limited exercise, and, possibly, alcohol/tobacco/pharmacologic coping. In this environment, marriages/relationships may falter, and these unopposed stressors may inadvertently lead to poor overall functioning and diminished individual productivity.

Adding to these stressors is the issue of disease. Cancer patients are not immune from everyday life and functioning—yet, they have the added burden of fighting what is often construed as the "Big C"—a compendium of diseases felt to be laced with a more tangible mortality. Treating cancer involves a multimodal approach. In addition, the cancer patient requires a comprehensive network of friends' and familial supports. Patients seek a definitive cure. Expectations may be unrealistically optimistic. Reality may be altogether different.

The role of rehabilitation medicine has always been to facilitate and support individuals to function at their highest potential. In cancer care, functioning depends inherently on a well-working biopsychosocial interchange. The interplay of physiatry and psychiatry often becomes tantamount.

This chapter will focus on the role of physiatry in caring for the cancer patient. Initially it is important to understand the objectives of the patient being treated, his or her support network, and, most importantly, hopes/aspirations. Next, one needs to understand the interchange between the treating physician and the patient. Following this is realizing what treatment will mean physically, socially, economically, emotionally, and spiritually. Optimally, rehabilitation medicine addresses all of these issues—in an inpatient as well as outpatient setting.

■ WHO IS THE CANCER PATIENT?

From a rehabilitation perspective, any individual who enters the hospital or is tentatively planning on undergoing consultation with his or her physician would benefit from an in-depth evaluation. An initial assessment involves a comprehensive history—centering on current functioning and how this has changed over the past few weeks to months. Of particular interest is whether or not the patient lives alone or has a close base of support—spouse, children, neighbors, or friends. Has the patient been independent in the home? Is the home one or multilevel? Is there a bathroom with standard toilet and tub shower? The emphasis is on returning the patient to his or her highest premorbid level of care—with awareness of limitations and instituting a safe home structure and family supports.

In cancer patients, treatments may involve chemotherapy, surgery, radiation, or a combination of the above. Chemotherapy, especially with the taxanes or platin-based agents, may result in a neuropathy.[1] Neuropathy may physically present as altered or loss of sensation at the distal digits of the hands or feet. A person's proprioception, vibration, or temperature sense may be changed. This may functionally present as an inability to button clothing effectively, use the zipper on a garment, tie a belt or shoelaces, grasp an object, and twist or close a jar lid. Bruising, falls, fractures, and burns may be the eventual result.

In cases of surgery, a patient may find that while a tumor may have been excised, an organ system has inadvertently been disrupted. In squamous cell carcinomas of the oropharynx, portion of the mandible may need to be removed. This leads at times to limitations in nutrition, hydration, weight loss, and increased debility. In these cases concomitant treatment with chemotherapy may exacerbate nausea and impaired sensation. Radiation may lead to a mucositis of the oropharynx and esophagus and further contribute to a slower recovery. Superimposed bacterial and fungal infections of these regions can lead to an aspiration pneumonia and sepsis.

In patients with extensive disease of the spine—whether from idiopathic sources such as schwannoma, ependymoma, chordoma, or medulloblastoma or from a metastatic source such as melanoma, breast, lung, colon, or prostate cancer—there may be alterations in neurologic transmission of sensation (pain, temperature, touch), motor functioning (ambulation, balance), and bowel/bladder functioning. Patients with nonmetastasizing tumors of the brain—astrocytomas/glioblastoma and oligodendrogliomas—may likewise have problems of seizure disorder, cognition, impaired memory, limited insight, aphasias, dysphagias, and/or paresis/paralysis.[2]

During the active treatment phase, cancer patients often mirror a compilation of effects—poor nutritional intake; the effects of pain, fatigue, and poor sleep; nausea, emesis, constipation, diarrhea, and, frequently, immobility.

With involvement of each organ system, overall functioning becomes impeded. Lung disease limits respiratory functioning. This directly affects cardiovascular functioning. Hepatic and renal involvement tends to disrupt the body's ability to detoxify drugs. With liver failure there will be elevation in ammonia levels and encephalopathy. This can lead to seizure activity. Hepatic dysfunction may produce hypoalbuminemia, impaired enzymatic activity, and peripheral edema. Impaired renal functioning may lead to anemia, proteinuria, electrolyte imbalance, and eventual dialysis.

Immobility in and of itself may make a patient prone to bedsores at key pressure points—shoulder joints, sacrum/coccyx, and heels. Immobility may lead to pneumonia, deep venous thrombosis, and pulmonary embolus.[3]

WHERE DOES THE CANCER PATIENT COME FROM?

Cancer is ubiquitous. While the hope is that it may one day be cured, the reality is that it affects every segment of society—the poor and affluent; well-educated and illiterate. Wealth and insurance may enhance access to care. However, at least currently in the United States patients from all strata still acquire cancer and require access to medical care. While a patient's treatment may be superficially covered by private insurance, Medicare/Medicaid, ultimately, the economic costs may be staggering. However, social implications also are present.

As is often the case after acute treatment, patients will likely depend on a caregiver. While wealth may obviate the immediate need for physical, hands-on care, success in treatment depends on a dynamic interchange between financial arenas, creativity, and deep, loving connections with the patient.[4]

One dilemma facing many cancer patients who seek specialized cancer care is economics.[5] While there may be oncologists throughout the nation, protocol therapy and surgical expertise may require an individual to travel to a regional cancer facility. There are incumbent costs, however, to the patient and his or her family. Adult patients come with additional responsibilities—they may be married, employed, have children, and, indeed, may be on a limited budget. Staying at a metropolitan center likely will require lodging, food, parking fees, and miscellaneous costs. Unforeseen complications of chemotherapy and surgery may require additional time spent in the hospital that may further tax a patient's economic resources.

Many individuals are accompanied by family members to these treatment centers. In cases of stem cell transplantations, individuals may be in the hospital from 2 to 3 months. A family member is required to be in attendance during that time period as well as in the post-transplant phase. Apartments often need to be acquired. While individuals now are linked to home by phone, e-mail, and/or texting, there still can be a sense of isolationism from one's base of support.

EXPECTATIONS

In many cases, patients present to regional centers hoping for a cure—that many times cannot be acquired in their locale. There is the expectation that the big, metropolitan center with ongoing research, superspecialists, protocol treatment, stem cell transplantations, and innovative technologies in radio imaging, radiation therapy, surgery, and chemotherapy will be able to affect a cure.

Patients often leave home believing that they have nothing to lose in their quest for cure. There is a sense that accepting the finality of a local physician's counsel or current treatment may not be enough. Patients simply may not be willing "to give up." There is a wide host of emotions that characterize patients at this time—initially beginning with hope. Hope often continues through treatment and rehabilitation. However, as patients begin to understand their disease process and the additive effects of treatment, they may come to a deeper realization of what the physical and psychological implications of their disease are. They may have to reassess and redefine their initial goals of care and cure.

For many patients, dealing with their disease follows a progression:

1. **Defining the disease:** Patients or their support network tend to search the Web, journals, articles on their disease, treatment options, and physician specialists. Outlining the disease and a strategy for cure is a coping mechanism.

2. **Mobilizing all resources to combat the disease:** Patients often tend to enlist the aid of their physicians, employers, coworkers, and spiritual contingent and may even maintain a working rapport with their insurance case managers.

3. **Integration of care specialties:** Once in the hospital and in treatment, often hospital staff—physicians, nursing, therapists, chaplaincy, social work, and case management—become an integral part of ongoing care support.

4. **Viewing the patient holistically:** Rehabilitation with its close daily encounters with the patient, perceived investment in a patient's physical and mental functioning, well-being, and overall health and advocacy round out this process.

And as in any family situation, where there is crisis due to the uncertainty of disease, limited finances, or emotional support, the patient and his or her immediate contingent may critically focus on perceived shortcomings/limitations in treatment and care. They may reach out for additional guidance and social assistance.

Eventually, once the acute aspects of treatment are addressed, there is the need to get the patient home. The concept of home, however, may be redefined by the ongoing medical requirements of the patient. In cases of leukemia, a stem cell transplant, or where additional protocol interventions will be required, the patient may need to stay within the environs of the treating center. Each round of chemotherapy may lead to cyclic debility, recovery, and eventually additional treatment. This is where rehabilitation often becomes involved in both the hospital and outpatient setting.

◼ INTERFACING WITH CANCER PATIENTS

Rehabilitation typically requires evaluation of prior baseline functioning. Everyday activities require us to get out of bed, toilet, shower/bathe, groom, and dress. The mundane tasks of putting on jeans, tying one's shoe, buttoning, and even brushing one's teeth are often force of habit. Then it is off to the kitchen to get a cup of coffee and a piece of toast before climbing into the car and zipping off to work. While driving, we defensively have to watch out for people changing lanes, speeding through yellow lights, and swerving unexpectedly to make the exit ramp. Once at work, we busily answer the phone, text, e-mail, and interact with colleagues. We are constantly thinking about a myriad of subjects, making memories and planning new strategies. Finally, there is home and dinner at the end of the day. All of these activities require exquisite coordination of mind and body.

Any injury—secondary to fall, trauma, or lesion such as tumor—alters the homeostatic balance. Any stressor may lead to muscle tension or strain. For any human being, receiving "bad news" leads to heightened anxiety. This may induce "irrational" fears or expectations. Resulting stressors may then spill over and affect all aspects of life. Patients may experience societal withdrawal. Ultimate outcomes may include depression characterized by alterations in nutrition and coping strategies. Physically, stress may be seen in trapezial myofascitis, muscle tightness leading to shoulder dysfunction, and a concurrent greater occipital neuralgia. Cancer patients experience baseline biomechanical disruption and overuse injuries involving shoulder, wrist, hip, and knee joints. They experience occupational stressors, too. But, in addition, they have cancer- and treatment-induced issues as well.

Cancer with metastatic involvement of the spine (eg, breast, lung, prostate, gastrointestinal tumors, hematopoietic, melanoma) may lead to pain and immobility of a joint, but in addition, there may be difficulties with urinary bladder and bowel incontinence. There may be accompanying paraparesis/plegia as well.

◼ UNDERSTANDING THE DISEASE PROCESS HOLISTICALLY

It is essential that treating clinicians assist the patient and his or her family with understanding the disease process—the principal tumor type; its typical pattern of behavior (ie, local vs. metastatic spread); typical treatment options, and eventually the side effects of treatment—physiologic; psychologic; and in terms of functioning. In an effort to explain—but not overwhelm a patient and his or her family—physicians often tend to look at a particular aspect of the disease. Focusing initially on treatment may allow patients to accept their disease state while affording an initial strategy on dealing realistically with their disease. Ultimately, a physician, however, needs to look holistically at how treatment may alter function and what this will mean to the patient and his or her family/caregiver.[6]

From a physical medicine standpoint, integration of disease, treatment, and ongoing functioning is critical. As circumstances change, the ultimate goal is to anticipate change in mobility, activities of daily living, and even alterations in perception, memory, executive decision making, and overall reasoning. Pulling in family members and friends to assist in supervising or caring for an individual may be necessary. Understanding the goals of the patient, and his or her prior background, work, value, and belief system provides the patient with a support system that may be essential during the peritreatment and posttreatment phase of care.

The approach of the rehabilitation team is multidisciplinary. The team often comprises a physiatrist, nurse practitioner, the rehabilitation nurse, physical therapist, occupational therapist, speech pathologist, neuropsychologist; nutritionist, chaplain, social worker, and case manager. The team—in close collaboration with the patient and his or her family—is essential in detailing a customized course of treatment for each patient. Goals need to be clear and achievable in the short term. Short-term goals can then be expanded into long-term goals that often occur in the outpatient setting.[7]

From a cancer perspective, short-term goals often include building up nutrition, hydration, and endurance. Patients will need to be able to mobilize from their beds, transition to sitting and standing with assistive equipment such as a cane/walker. Toileting may initially require use of a bedside commode before transitioning to the toilet and eventually the shower. Promoting activity limits morbidity related to bedsores, pneumonia, contractures, deep venous thromboses, and/or pulmonary emboli.

Goals for rehabilitation, therefore, are divided into four stages:

1. the acute hospitalization or acute rehabilitation stage;
2. the immediate posthospitalization period;
3. the subacute period;
4. recovery and maintenance programs.

As noted above, the acute phase of care often involves therapists visiting patients in their rooms or bringing patients down to the rehabilitation gym. The goal is taking patients at their current level of functioning and eventually preparing them for the discharge home. Ideally, a patient will successfully be able to discharge home if certain preconditions are met:

1. Patients have achieved at least supervision or contact guard level of functioning in their mobilization and self-care.
2. There is a caregiver who can assist with overseeing patients' mobility in the home setting and supervise their activities of daily living—eating, grooming, dressing, bathing, toileting, communication, social interaction, and memory.
3. Patients have the ability to access transportation—car, bus, taxi, or airplane.
4. Patients can continue their rehabilitation by in-home therapy services, access to outpatient therapy services, or continuation of a home exercise program.
5. Patients have economic resources that can allow both them and their caregiver a security of home and sustenance.
6. There exists a balance of sound reasoning on the part of patients/caregivers, economic security, and genuine concern for patients.
7. There exists a means to defuse increased anxiety, frustration, and exhaustion that may lead potentially to caregiver burnout and possible patient neglect/abuse.

The immediate posthospitalization period likely will require ongoing supervision in the home. Caretakers who have taken family leave may no longer have payable benefits. What previously may have been a financially stable dual-income household is now subject to severe economic stress. The caretaker may have no choice but to return to work and attempt to enlist the help of neighbors, friends, or religious institutions to assist. Often patients remain unattended for periods throughout the day, and family members attempt to remain in contact through cell phones at a patient's bedside. Patient-alert systems, meals-on-wheels, visiting nurses, and adult day care programs may be other options of care. If a patient has multiple ongoing medical and care needs in the immediate postsurgical or chemoradiation period, a discharge directly to home may be contraindicated. If the patient is unable to participate at an acute inpatient rehabilitation level of care secondary to increased fatigue and pain, or decreased levels of endurance or participatory effort or ongoing medical care needs (eg, intravenous antibiotic therapy, radiation therapy needs, wound care requirements—wound VACs/dressing changes—etc), he or she may require placement in a subacute/skilled nursing level of care.

Once home, a patient often is transitioned to outpatient physical and occupational therapies. The goal is building upon what was previously learned in the hospital setting. Patients with either a well-implemented home exercise program or continued outpatient (or in-home) therapies will likely continue to increase their overall functioning, endurance, and strength. In the outpatient setting, patients often will visit with their therapists two to three times a week for an additional 1 to 2 months. During this time period, the patient's home exercise program is established and modified—based on the future achievement of goals. Eventually, the patient is transitioned to a maintenance program. During all of these phases in rehabilitation care, it is crucial that the physiatrist remains in communication with the patient's therapists and sees the patient back at regular intervals. The close overall interaction with therapies and the rehabilitation physicians is often viewed by patients as a meaningful continuation of care and concern by their health care team.

At times, patients who have limited transportation resources or live in more rural districts may require in-home therapies. While this is not necessarily optimal, patients nevertheless can continue to make progress in overall functioning. Visiting therapists allow a patient to conserve energy—avoiding excessive car travel, parking, transferring in and out of the car; or waiting periods prior to their visit with the therapists. A patient, indeed, who has limited energy secondary to recovery from surgery or chemotherapy, may find in-home therapies beneficial. The traveling therapist may actually allow a more functional recovery in the short term. Additionally, the home layout may be evaluated first-hand by a patient's therapists. Interventions with reference to entrance safety (stairs/ramps), removal of fall-inducing items (unsecured rugs or exposed electrical cords), placement of hand grip devices/rails on the walls/toilet, and evaluation of lighting may actually assist patients as they continue in their outlined treatment plans.

In caring for the patient with cancer, the issue of impairment secondary to surgical treatment or chemoradiation is often raised. Patients who previously were defined by their professions, creativity, and/or productivity may now be facing an inability to return to their prior duties. Not only does this have financial repercussions, but it may also alter/jeopardize an individual's insurance benefits. Many cancer treatments are costly and ongoing. Patients require serial reimaging involving CT scans, MRIs, and PET/CT scans. Surgery may involve not only resection, but also extensive reconstruction, prolonged healing periods, wound care, and antibiotic management. Stem cell transplantations involve immunosuppression. Patients need to be treated with immunosuppressive agents, and antibiotics, antifungal, and antiviral agents. Often patients have pancytopenia, necessitating frequent transfusion of blood products and serial blood count monitoring. Medical comorbidities often exist—drug reactions, nausea, emesis, diarrhea, graft-versus-host disease, fistulas, abscesses, malnutrition, infection, blood clots, pressure sores, and pulmonary emboli.

In order to successfully rehabilitate a patient, the patient must have a realistic understanding of his or her disease process. There must be a close interaction between the patient's physician, oncologist, additional treating specialists, and therapists. Communication—while often purported as crucial—is often missing in the equation of care.

Treating physicians frequently feel that they have taken adequate time to educate their patients. However, all too often there is a disconnect between what was presented and what the patient/family members understand. In this regard, it is helpful to have family members accompany cancer patients to their clinic appointments. Patients may be overwhelmed by the psychological implications of their disease and altered physical appearance (colostomy, urostomy, or lymphedema), or they may simply be unable to mentally process—secondary to cognitive changes, fatigue, or pain—what they have been told. Physicians may feel that they have clearly explained options of treatment along with concurrent benefits/side effects. A patient may "appear" to understand, but actually may be confused—and too embarrassed to ask questions or reticent to take any additional time when asking for clarification.[8]

In cases where there has been a brain injury secondary to primary brain tumors (astrocytoma, oligodendroglioma, ependymoma) or metastatic lesions (from lung, gastrointestinal, breast primaries), chemoradiation and surgery are often prescribed courses of treatment. Side effects may include memory deficits, alterations in cognition, and executive decision making. As a result, the patient—who once may have been quite functional in both social and working circles—now begins to demonstrate difficulties with initiation/completion of tasks. There are behavioral changes including emotional lability, outbursts, or depression. This may jeopardize working relationships and future job viability, and potentially lead to wrongful dismissal.

Safeguards currently exist to protect the privacy of a patient. No longer are employers necessarily privy to the myriad of medical and family-based concerns that their employees have. This, unfortunately, is a two-edged sword. On the one hand, one's personal/medical issues remain confidential. On the other hand, if a patient does not recognize changes in his or her behavior and personality due to illness or treatment thereof; or there is no input from a treating physician as to causation, a patient's livelihood may be seriously compromised. The goal of the cancer specialist or rehabilitationist is, therefore, simple. Serial reevaluations need to look at acute changes in behavior, memory, work performance, and social interactions with others. Where cancer specialists may feel that evaluation of social function is outside the scope of their practice, they need to consult with other physicians whose operational practice makes use of the biopsychosocial model, for example, physiatrists, psychiatrists, neuropsychologists, and palliative care physicians.

A number of functional assessment tools currently exist that may be of benefit when evaluating cancer patients including the FIM,[9] Karnofsky,[10] and Edmondton Symptom Assessment scores.[11] Within the realm of cancer care, physical and occupational therapists are often confronted with issues of pain and fatigue in their patients.[12] A multiteam approach involving therapists in close collaboration with primary, rehabilitation, and symptom control physicians becomes important. Tumor-based pain may be alleviated by surgery or palliative radiation. However, if there is persistent or metastatic disease, both acute and ongoing chronic pain management becomes necessary. Pain needs to be characterized and quantified. Treatment may require multimodal interventions—pharmacologic, surgical, or radiation.

Characteristically, pain may be visceral, somatic, or neuropathic. It may begin acutely and continue chronically with altered manifestations. Pain limits function when left untreated or undertreated. Likewise, overtreatment may lead to lethargy, somnolence, mental status changes/obtundation, and constipation. Fatigue, likewise, may be the result of a change in the physiologic state of a patient. It may have its antecedents in modified neurophysiologic pathways (ie, alterations in neurotransmission or gonadotropin release). Ultimately a patient's functioning requires close monitoring of these parameters along with concurrent and progressive—but supervised—levels of activity.[13]

■ HOW DOES CANCER REHABILITATION DIFFER FROM MAINSTREAM REHABILITATION?

The practice of physical medicine and rehabilitation by convention embodies a comprehensive approach to care. When possible, the physiatrist attempts to restore an individual to the highest level of prior functioning. Common physiatric interventions have arisen as the result of stroke, traumatic brain injury, myocardial infarction, cardiac transplant, COPD, degenerative joint disease, and/or trauma related to the shoulder joint, hips, knees, feet, and spinal cord. Ultimately, when dealing with these patients, a physiatrist interacts with medical specialists. Of great import, however, is the concomitant interaction with a team of therapists—physical, occupational, and speech therapies. Social reintegration is often accomplished with the assistance of social work, case management, psychology, or chaplaincy. Evaluations are often initiated in the outpatient setting. Acute illness may require a hospitalization followed by acute inpatient rehabilitation. Eventually, the patient either is transitioned to home independently or is followed as a patient with outpatient therapies.

Within cancer rehabilitation, the above objectives remain the same. Indeed, the overall framework of care is similar. The patient, however, often has a progressive disease process that ultimately may limit overall function. The goal of rehabilitation is also different. Many individuals will not be returning to work. Their life expectancy may be shortened and the associated morbidity of treatment heightened. The point of emphasis is simple—returning the patient home safely and as functional as possible. To do this requires an understanding of one's disease, realistic future functioning, shortcomings to treatment, modifying activity goals, and working in unison with the patient, family, and treating physicians, nurses, and therapists.

Ultimately, success is achieved in rehabilitation when there is a realistic balance between goals in treatment, function, and family supports.

KEY POINTS

■ In cancer rehabilitation the patient often has a progressive disease process that ultimately may limit overall function.

■ The goal of physical medicine and rehabilitation has always been restoring an individual to the highest premorbid level of function.

■ Integration of disease, treatment, and ongoing functioning is critical.

■ Rehabilitationists must anticipate a patient's change in mobility, activities of daily living, and even alternations in perception, memory, executive decision making, and overall reasoning.

■ The rehabilitation team is multidisciplinary. It must work closely with the patient and his or her family.

■ Patients may be overwhelmed by the psychological implications of their disease and altered physical appearance, or they may simply be unable to mentally process what they have been told—secondary to cognitive change, fatigue, or pain.

■ In order to successfully rehabilitate a patient, the patient must have a realistic understanding of his or her disease process.

■ There must be a close interaction between that patient's physician, oncologist, additional treating specialists, and therapists.

■ Communication—while often purported as crucial—is often missing in the equation of care.

REFERENCES

1. Sioka C, Kyritsis AP. Central and peripheral nervous system toxicity of common chemotherapeutic agents. *Cancer Chemother Pharmacol.* 2009;63(5):761–767.

2. Pytel P, Lukas RV. Update on diagnostic practice: tumors of the nervous system. *Arch Pathol Lab Med.* 2009;133(7);1062–1077.

3. Dib M. Pressure ulcers: prevention and management. *J Med Liban.* 2008;56(2):112–117.

4. Silveira MJ, Given CW, Given B, Rosland AM, Piette JD. Patient–caregiver concordance in symptom assessment and improvement in outcomes for patients undergoing cancer chemotherapy. *Chronic Illn.* 2010;16(1):46–56.

5. Schickedanz A. Of value: a discussion of cost, communication, and evidence to improve cancer care. *Oncologist.* 2010;15(suppl 1):73–79.

6. Haylock PJ. Living to the end: merging holistic and evidence-based strategies and meet the needs of people living with advanced cancer. *Oncology (Huntingt).* 2009;23(8 suppl):35–40, 51–52.

7. Palacio A, Calmels P, Genty M, Le-Quang B, Beuret-Blanquart F. Oncology and physical medicine and rehabilitation. *Ann Phys Rehabil Med.* 2009;52(7–8):568–578.

8. Shields CG, Coker CJ, Poulsen SS, Doyle JM, Fiscella K, Epstein RM, Griggs JJ. Patient-centered communication and prognosis discussions with cancer patients. *Patient Educ Couns.* 2009;77(3):369–378.

9. FIM instrument. In: *Uniform Data Systems for Medical Rehabilitation: Guide for the Uniform Data Set for Medical Rehabilitation.* Buffalo, NY: State University of New York at Buffalo; 1997.

10. Karnofsky DA, Abelmann WH, Craver LF, Burchenal J. *Karnofsky Scale.* 1948. Available at: www.anapsid.org/cnd/files/karnofskyscale.pdf.

11. Bruera E, Kuehn N, Miller MJ, Selmser P, Macmillan K. The Edmonton System Assessment System (ESAS): a simple method for the assessment of palliative care patients. *J Palliat Care.* 1991;7:6–9.

12. Shun SC, Lai YH, Hsiao FH. Patient-related barriers to fatigue communication in cancer patients receiving active treatment. *Oncologist.* 2009;14(9):936–943.

13. Borneman T. Reducing patient barriers to pain and fatigue management. *J Pain Symptom Manage.* 2010;39(3):486–501.

Integrative Medicine

Integrative Medicine in Cancer Care

• *Richard Tsong Lee, M. Kay Garcia, M. Alejandro Chaoul, Laura Baynham-Fletcher, Lisa M. Gower, and Lorenzo Cohen*

■ INTRODUCTION

Integrative medicine seeks to merge conventional medicine and complementary therapies in a manner that is comprehensive, personalized, evidence-based, and safe in order to achieve optimal health and healing. Although applying the concept of integrative medicine to cancer care is still in its formative years, a number of comprehensive cancer centers in the United States are trying to put this concept into practice under the term *integrative oncology*. As a result of this growing interest in integrative medicine in cancer care, the National Cancer Institute formed the Office of Cancer Complementary and Alternative Medicine (OCCAM), the American Cancer Society (ACS) dedicated a portion of its Web site to assessment of complementary therapies, the Consortium of Academic Centers for Integrative Medicine created an oncology working group, and the Society for Integrative Oncology (SIO) was formed. The SIO mission is to study and facilitate cancer treatment and recovery through the use of integrated complementary therapeutic options, including natural and botanical products, nutrition, acupuncture, massage, mind–body therapies, and other complementary modalities (www.integrativeonc.org). This chapter will review the role of integrative oncology in cancer care with an emphasis on a comprehensive approach, an overview of the evidence, educational resources to guide health care providers and patients, and guidelines for creating a comprehensive, integrative treatment plan for cancer patients.

■ DEFINITIONS

Complementary and alternative medicine (CAM) has been defined by the National Center for Complementary and Alternative Medicine (NCCAM)[1] and major US surveys as "… diverse medical and healthcare systems, practices, and products that are not presently considered to be part of conventional medicine." Although evidence may exist for some of these modalities, it may not be sufficient to bring them into the realm of *conventional* medicine, and other CAM modalities may have no scientific support for their use. Strictly speaking, *alternative* medicine by definition is when a patient makes use of a nonconventional treatment modality in place of conventional medicine whether or not there is evidence for its efficacy. *Complementary* medicine, on the other hand, is when a patient makes use of a CAM modality in combination with conventional medicine.

The terms *alternative, complementary*, and *conventional* focus on types of treatment modalities. In the last few years, the term *integrative* medicine or complementary and integrative medicine (CIM) has become more prevalent in medical settings. CIM is more about a philosophy of medical practice that merges both conventional and complementary medicine. The Consortium of Academic Health Centers for Integrative Medicine[2] has defined this term as "the practice of medicine that reaffirms the importance of the relationship between practitioner and patient, focuses on the whole person, is informed by evidence, and makes use of all appropriate therapeutic approaches, healthcare professionals and disciplines to achieve optimal health and healing." In this way, integrative medicine makes use of both conventional and complementary treatment modalities using an interdisciplinary approach to health care. Practitioners of all disciplines should be knowledgeable and aware of all treatment options and open to communication with other types of practitioners. In contrast to simply receiving two or more different treatment modalities (conventional and complementary) with fractionated medical care, an integrative medicine approach evaluates the risks and benefits of the individual therapies and, when used in combination, increases communication between health professionals, and creates a coordinated, comprehensive treatment plan to optimize outcomes. Throughout this chapter the term CIM is used in favor of CAM or other terms.

The NCCAM has created five categories of CIM: (1) whole medical systems such as traditional Chinese medicine (TCM), homeopathy, and Ayurveda; (2) mind–body approaches such as meditation, guided imagery, music, art, and other expressive arts and behavioral techniques; (3) biologically based approaches such as those centered on nutrition, herbs, plants, animals, minerals, or other products; (4) body-manipulative approaches such as massage and reflexology; and (5) energy-based therapies such as yoga, tai chi, qigong, Reiki, and healing touch. Some therapies naturally overlap into more than one category such as yoga, which also contains mind–body effects. Several different types of specialty health care providers offer CIM therapies, and these may include physicians, nurses, physical therapists, psychiatrists, psychologists, chiropractors, massage therapists, and naturopaths who are operating within the guidelines of their licenses or accrediting organizations.

■ UTILIZATION

The World Health Organization (WHO) estimates that up to 80% of people in developing countries rely on nonconventional traditional medicines for their primary health care. People in more developed countries also seek out complementary medicine and practices. A 1997 survey of US adults found CIM use (excluding self-prayer) varied from 32% to 54%.[3] A 2007 survey by the US Centers for Disease Control found that 38% of adults had used CIM therapies during the last 12 months.[4]

Among patients and families touched by cancer, the use of CIM is even higher than that in the general population. An estimated 40% to 69% of US patients with cancer use CIM therapies,[5–7] and percentages increase if spiritual practices are included and among specific populations of cancer patients, such as those involved in phase I clinical trials.[7,8] Complementary therapies are used in 70% of all oncology departments engaged in palliative care in Britain.[9,10] A survey of five clinics within a US comprehensive cancer care center found that CIM therapies were used by 68.7% of patients (excluding psychotherapy and spiritual practices).[7] Breast cancer patients have been found to have an elevated use of CIM when compared with other cancer types, and two reviews on the topics have found prevalence range of 17% to 87% with one study reporting a mean prevalence of 45%.[11–13] This range of prevalence patterns reflect differences in the patient population studied.

In most cases, people who use CIM are not disappointed or dissatisfied with conventional medicine but want to do everything possible to regain health and improve their quality of life.[14–21] Patients use CIM to reduce side effects such as organ toxicity, improve quality of life, protect and stimulate immunity, or prevent further cancers or recurrences. Whether or not patients use CIM therapies to treat cancer or its effects, they may also use them to treat other chronic conditions such as arthritis, heart disease, diabetes, chronic pain, and other conditions.

■ COMPLEMENTARY AND INTEGRATIVE THERAPIES—AN EVIDENCE-BASED APPROACH

The field of integrative oncology is a constantly evolving set of disciplines. As such, the evidence at any point in time becomes dated as quickly as new modalities for specific conditions are found to be either effective or ineffective and either incorporated into conventional medicine or dismissed. There has been a dramatic increase in research in integrative oncology within conventional scientific journals, including two journals specifically dedicated to integrative oncology: the *Journal of the Society for Integrative Oncology* and *Integrative Cancer Therapies*, both of which are peer-reviewed, Medline indexed journals dedicated to publishing original research and to education within the field of integrative oncology.

Below we list some of the key findings to date in integrative oncology in the main areas of CIM where there is sufficient evidence to recommend the therapies as part of the standard of care: mind–body treatments, massage, and acupuncture. These CIM therapies should be considered in conjunction to physical activity and nutrition, which were briefly discussed earlier in this chapter. Although there is ongoing research in many other areas such as healing touch, homeopathy, natural products, and special diets, there is insufficient evidence to recommend these within the standard of care at this point in time. Until there is evidence for the safety and efficacy of specific natural products (eg, soy), they should not be used as alternatives to mainstream care, and patients should be encouraged to seek out the whole food source and use it in moderation, and avoid extracts or purified formulations with the purported "active" ingredient. Cancer prevention studies of beta-carotene, vitamin E, and selenium have been unsuccessful and have highlighted some of the dangers of prolonged use of such supplements.[22–37] The SIO *Integrative Oncology Practice Guidelines* provides comprehensive, detailed up-to-date evidence in these other areas and is an excellent resource.[38]

Acupuncture

Acupuncture is a common treatment modality that is part of TCM and has been practiced in China for thousands of years. It is one of the most popular TCM therapies outside of China and is used in at least 78 countries.[39] The traditional theory behind the benefits of acupuncture is that the placement of needles, heat, or pressure at specific places on the body can help to regulate the flow of qi (vital energy).

The most common form of acupuncture involves the placement of solid, sterile, stainless steel needles into various points on the body that are believed to have reduced bioelectrical resistance and increased conductance.[40,41] Different techniques can be used to stimulate the needles, including manual manipulation or electrical stimulation.[40–42] For some patients, acupressure may be used, which involves applying heat or pressure to acupoints instead of puncturing the skin. Stainless steel or gold (semipermanent) needles, or "studs," are also sometimes placed at specific points on the ears and left in place for several days.

There is good scientific evidence that acupuncture is effective for managing both postoperative and chemotherapy-related nausea and vomiting.[43–47] An NIH consensus statement in 1997[43] supported this use, stating that the level of evidence was sufficient. Further research has substantiated this claim, and the American

Cancer Society (ACS)[48] now states that clinical studies have found acupuncture may help treat nausea caused by chemotherapy drugs and surgical anesthesia. In addition, specific neuroimaging research of patients while undergoing acupuncture treatments using nausea points has helped to delineate the neural mechanisms of action.[49]

There is also good evidence that certain types of acupuncture are effective for both postoperative and chronic pain in cancer patients.[126–128] The primary mechanisms involved are believed to include enhanced conduction of bioelectromagnetic signals, activation of opioid systems, and activation of the autonomic and central nervous systems, causing the release of various neurotransmitters and neurohormones.[40]

One well-controlled randomized, blinded, placebo-controlled trial[50] investigating the use of acupuncture for chronic pain among cancer patients compared active auricular acupuncture with two placebo groups: group 1 had ear studs placed at active acupuncture points; group 2 had ear studs placed at inactive acupuncture points; and group 3 had ear seeds placed at inactive points. Mean (SD) scores on a 0 to 100 visual analog scale (VAS) for the active acupuncture group, sham acupuncture group, and sham ear seed group were 37 + 19, 55 + 24, and 58 + 20, respectively. Thus, pain scores were significantly lower in the active treatment group ($P < .001$).[50]

Methodological rigor is improving, and initial research suggests acupuncture is beneficial and, in some cases, can have a lasting effect. A number of clinical trials, both controlled and uncontrolled, are growing and indicate benefit from acupuncture for radiation-induced xerostomia, hot flashes, and aromatase-induced arthralgias.[129–133] A recent study by Walker et al randomized women to acupuncture versus venlafaxine and reported similar reductions in hot flash severity and frequency at 12 weeks. A randomized, sham-controlled trial of acupuncture for aromatase inhibitor–associated arthralgias found significant reduction in the true acupuncture arm at 3 weeks.[51] These studies suggest acupuncture as a reasonable option for xerostomia, hot flashes, and aromatase-induced arthralgias, especially among women who have refractory symptoms despite medication use. Large definitive randomized clinical trials are still needed.

For the management of other treatment- or cancer-related symptoms, the evidence is not as strong as that for pain and nausea. Nevertheless, there is some preliminary and anecdotal evidence to suggest that acupuncture may be useful in the treatment of anxiety, depression, fatigue, constipation, loss of appetite, peripheral neuropathy, insomnia, dyspnea, and leucopenia.[52,53] The quality of the research for these symptoms remains weak, however, and further studies are needed.

When performed correctly, acupuncture has been shown to be a safe, minimally invasive procedure with very few side effects. The most commonly reported complications are fainting, bruising, and mild pain. Infection is also a potential risk, although very uncommon.[54,55] Acupuncture should only be performed by a health care professional with an appropriate license and preferably one who has had experience in treating patients with malignant diseases.

Although the mechanisms are not well understood, for symptoms such as chemotherapy-related and postoperative nausea, vomiting, and pain, there is good evidence to support the use of acupuncture. Data of efficacy are currently lacking for the control of other cancer- and treatment-related symptoms, but as a very low-risk and cost-effective option, acupuncture may be a helpful adjunct to conventional treatment for patients suffering from cancer and from side effects of treatment that are poorly controlled.[56] At MD Anderson Cancer Center, patients may receive acupuncture through physician referral.

Massage

Massage for relaxation and to help manage pain and discomfort has been used for thousands of years. There are various forms of massage, and they all typically apply some degree of pressure to muscle and connective tissue and, in some cases, work with specific pressure points. A clinical form of massage known as manual lymph drainage has been shown to decrease lymphedema when combined with elastic sleeves or bandaging for patients with arm edema after breast cancer surgery.[57] However, this is a detailed and lengthy process and self-massage with this technique has not been found to be as effective as either that performed by a trained therapist or simulation by a specially designed pump.

Research to date suggests that massage is helpful at relieving pain, anxiety, fatigue, distress, and increasing relaxation.[58–61] A challenge of course in conducting massage therapy research is having a placebo control group. It is therefore not clear what the exact mechanisms are for the benefits of massage in an oncology setting. Despite some of the imperfections in research design, the current findings are encouraging. Moreover, massage is generally safe when it is conducted by a licensed practitioner

who has also had some training in working with cancer patients. In general, cancer patients should not receive deep tissue massage, and patients with bleeding tendencies should only receive light touch. Obviously, areas that have recently had surgery or radiation should be avoided. Therapeutic benefit can also be derived from simply receiving a massage to the feet, hands, and head as these areas are especially sensitive to tactile stimulation and can result in providing relaxation and an increase in general well-being.[62,63]

Mind–Body Practices

Mind–body practices are defined as a variety of techniques designed to enhance the mind's capacity to affect bodily function and symptoms.[1] Mind–body techniques include relaxation, hypnosis, visual imagery, meditation, biofeedback, cognitive–behavioral therapies, group support, autogenic training, and spirituality and expressive arts therapies such as art, music, or dance. Therapies such as yoga, tai chi, and qigong often fall into the CIM category of energy medicine, as they are intended to work with bodily "energetic fields" (eg, meridians or subtle channels and *qi* [pronounced chee—China], *lung* [pronounced loong—Tibet], *prana* [India], and *ki* [pronounced kee—Japan]). However, they are also likely to exert strong effects through a mind–body connection and as such fall into the mind–body medicine category. Some of these therapies are no longer considered "alternative," and they are well integrated into conventional medicine and most medical settings (hypnosis, biofeedback, cognitive–behavioral therapy, and group support). As research continues, the treatments that are found beneficial will hopefully become integrated into conventional medical care.

Research has shown that after being diagnosed with cancer, patients try to bring about positive changes in their lifestyles, often seeking to take control of their health.[64] Techniques of stress management that have proven helpful include progressive muscle relaxation,[65,66] diaphragmatic breathing,[67,68] guided imagery,[69–71] social support,[72,73] and meditation.[74,75] Participation in stress management programs prior to treatment has enabled patients to tolerate therapy with fewer reported side effects.[76–79] Supportive expressive group therapy has also been found to be useful for patients with cancer.[80–82] Psychosocial interventions have been shown to specifically decrease depression and anxiety and to increase self-esteem and active approach coping strategies.[83–86]

A meta-analysis of 116 studies found that mind–body therapies could reduce anxiety, depression, and mood disturbance in cancer patients, and assist their coping skills.[87] Newell and colleagues[88] reviewed psychological therapies for cancer patients and concluded that interventions involving self-practice and hypnosis for managing nausea and vomiting could be recommended, but that further research was suggested to examine the benefits of relaxation training and guided imagery. Further research was also warranted to examine the benefits of relaxation and guided imagery for managing general nausea, anxiety, quality of life, and overall physical symptoms.[88] More recently, Ernst et al[89] examined the change in the state of the evidence for mind–body therapies for various medical conditions between 2000 and 2005 and found that there is now maximal evidence for the use of relaxation techniques for anxiety, hypertension, insomnia, and nausea due to chemotherapy.

Research examining yoga, tai chi, and meditation incorporated into cancer care suggests that these mind–body practices help to improve aspects of quality of life including improved mood, sleep quality, physical functioning, and overall well-being.[86,90–92] Hypnosis, and especially self-hypnosis, has been found to be beneficial to help reduce distress and discomfort during difficult medical procedures.[93] An NIH Technology Assessment Panel[77] found strong evidence for hypnosis in alleviating cancer-related pain. Hypnosis effectively treats anticipatory nausea in pediatric[95] and adult cancer patients,[96] reduces postoperative nausea and vomiting,[97] and improves adjustment to invasive medical procedures.[98–100]

■ EDUCATIONAL RESOURCES

The rapidity with which a comprehensive review can become out of date and the ease of Internet publishing have fostered the growth of comprehensive scientific review organizations that provide electronic access to their reviews. Below we list seven Web sites we believe are especially useful for health care professionals as a resource for seeking out information relevant to specific therapies cancer patients may be using or are seeking information on their benefits (see Table 23-1).

Natural Medicines Comprehensive Database (www.naturalmedicinedatabase.com)[101] provides the largest number of evidence-based reviews of complementary therapies (over 1000). The majority of its authors

■ TABLE 23-1. Recommended Web Sites for Evidence-based Resources

Organization/Web Site	Address/URL
Bandolier	http://www.medicine.ox.ac.uk/bandolier/
Cochrane Review Organization	www.cochrane.org
Memorial Sloan-Kettering Cancer Center Integrative Medicine Service	http://www.mskcc.org/aboutherbs
Natural Medicines Comprehensive Database	http://www.naturaldatabase.com/
Natural Standard	http://www.naturalstandard.com/
NCI Office of Cancer Complementary and Alternative Medicine (OCCAM)	http://www.cancer.gov/cam
University of Texas MD Anderson Cancer Center Complementary/Integrative Medicine Education Resources	www.mdanderson.org/CIMER

and editors are Doctors of Pharmacy, and their reviews include scientific names, uses, safety, effectiveness, mechanisms of action, adverse reactions, interactions, dosage, and administration. Full access requires an individual or institutional subscription. It has received top ratings in comparative evaluations for answering questions about herbal and dietary supplements.[102–104] However, these one- to two-page reviews do not provide background or in-depth assessments of the evidence on which their conclusions are based.

The oldest and most comprehensive of the scientific review organizations for conventional therapies is the Cochrane Review Organization (www.cochrane.org).[105] Founded in 1993 as an international nonprofit independent organization, it now provides over 2000 systematic reviews and has recently added the complementary therapies of massage, acupuncture, and chiropractic. Its review process includes searches of multiple bibliographic databases by professional librarians. At least two blinded independent reviewers evaluate studies according to standard sets of questions with discrepancies resolved through conferences with attempts to contact authors for resolution of remaining questions. A statistician and an editorial board join with reviewers for development and summation of final conclusions. Abstracts of Cochrane reviews are free, but completed reviews require either individual or institutional subscription.[105,106]

Modeling itself on the Cochrane organization, Natural Standard (www.naturalstandard.com)[107] formed a multidisciplinary, multi-institutional initiative dedicated to the review of complementary and alternative therapies. It follows a similar process to build in-depth evidence- and consensus-based analysis of scientific data in addition to historic and folkloric perspectives. It now provides several hundred authoritative reviews. Access requires an institutional subscription, but some subscribing institutions have also purchased summaries of reviews for public access.

The NCI OCCAM has reviewed about a dozen complementary therapies (http://www.cancer.gov/cam).[108] These "PDQ" Cancer Information Summaries provide extensive details and citations for health professionals including background, history of development, proposed mechanisms of action, and relevant laboratory, animal, and clinical studies.

Memorial-Sloan Kettering Cancer Center provides over 200 evidence-based reviews on herbs (www.mskcc.org/aboutherbs).[109] These are written by either an oncology-trained pharmacist with expertise in botanicals or a cancer nutrition specialist with secondary reviews by at least two other editors or panel advisors.

Bandolier, a monthly journal about evidence-based health care produced by scientists at Oxford University, provides a subset of complementary therapy in-depth analyses, commentaries, and meta-analyses found in searches of the Cochrane Library and PubMed (http://www.medicine.ox.ac.uk/bandolier/).[110]

The University of Texas MD Anderson Cancer Center's Web site for complementary/integrative medicine (www.mdanderson.org/cimer)[111] provides reviews that include in-depth assessments of the background and evidence by their own staff plus purchased summaries of some of the previously described reviews by Natural Standard, Natural Medicines Comprehensive Database, and the Cochrane Library and access to all reviews by the NCI OCCAM and Memorial Sloan Kettering. Their own methodology includes searches by library personnel, reviews by staff with expertise in laboratory, clinical, and population studies, and secondary reviews by appropriate faculty members or outside advisors.

Searching these seven Web sites may be efficiently accomplished by physicians or delegated to appropriate clinic personnel. Patients or caregivers can then be given specific recommendations, printed summaries, or the names of these or other prescreened Web sites. Questions generated from this information can then be brought back for discussion with the physician or other clinic professional.

Although the National Cancer Institute, the American Cancer Society (ACS), and the MD Anderson Cancer Center Web sites also provide links to other reliable Web sites, patients or caregivers may wish to investigate independently. If so, they should be encouraged to look for Web sites that subscribe to the principles of the Health on the Net Foundation[112] and carry its "HONcode" seal. This nongovernmental organization is supported by the State of Geneva in Switzerland, the Swiss Institute of Bioinformatics, and the University Hospitals of Geneva. It screens Web sites for compliance with its eight principles of authority: medically trained and qualified professionals, support of the patient/site visitor and his or her physician, confidentiality, clear references to source data, claims supported by appropriate and balanced evidence, transparency of authorship, transparency of ownership, and honesty in advertising and editorial policy.[112] The HONcode is displayed by two of the above-mentioned seven Web sites for health care professionals: the National Cancer Institute and the MD Anderson Cancer Center.

■ ESTABLISHING AN INTEGRATIVE ONCOLOGY APPROACH WITH PATIENTS

Integrative Oncology Model

The process of creating an integrative approach for cancer should address several principles: comprehensive, personalized, evidence-based, and safe. The traditional model of cancer treatment involves three different disciplines (surgery, radiation, chemotherapy), and integrative oncology aims to expand the interdisciplinary approach to include other therapies such as acupuncture, yoga, meditation, diet, exercise, and other modalities. This is in response to the concept of treating the whole patient in all domains. Engel's[113] biopsychosocial model of health care, first published in *Science* over 30 years ago, describes these domains of patient care and their importance in the treatment of all patients. We have proposed an integrative oncology model as a framework to

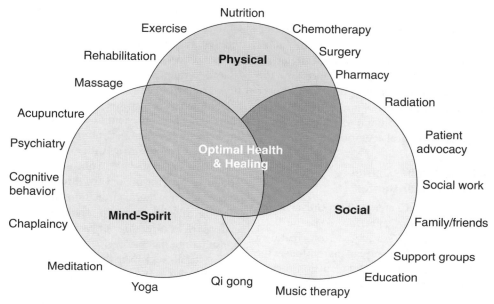

FIGURE 23-1. The Lee–Thomas integrative oncology model.

assist in creating comprehensive integrative care plans (Fig. 23-1). Without comprehensive assessment and appropriate attention given to patient needs, patients may perceive gaps in their care. Although symptoms such as severe pain or nausea are traditionally thought of as purely physical symptoms, if symptoms remain severe and chronic, they will often impact the psychosocial dimensions of health as patients may become more fatigued due to insomnia, irritable, and unable to remain socially active. By creating a comprehensive care plan, patients will have a cancer treatment plan that addresses all of their needs in a more seamless manner that has the greatest potential for improving their overall health and well-being. The concept of overall health and well-being is analogous to performance status. Assessment of performance status remains one of the most consistent prognostic factors for cancer. Similarly, quality of life has been also shown to predict survival in cancer patients.[114] A study by Quinten et al[114] included a meta-analysis of 30 randomized clinical trials from 11 different types of cancer and found performance status to be predictive of survival that provided a better model than known clinical factors alone. These basic comprehensive evaluations are an aggregate of many different components and addressing issues of nutrition, physical activity, symptom control, and other factors will undoubtedly help

improve the performance of cancer patients throughout the continuum of care.

Physical Well-being

Although this book focuses primarily on psychosocial aspects of cancer care, we will briefly discuss the growing importance of physical activity and nutrition in the health of cancer patients. These types of health behaviors have been correlated with improved clinical outcomes. The Women's Intervention Study (WINS)[115] reported that a 24% reduction in fat intake reduced recurrence rates. The Women's Healthy Eating and Living (WHEL)[116] randomized women to increase fruit and vegetable intake as well as a reduction in dietary fat, but did not find a significant reduction in breast cancer events; however, when secondary analyses were performed including physical activity, an increased survival of approximately 50% was found among women who were physically active *and* maintained a diet high in fruits and vegetables.[117] Similar associations are beginning to be reported in colon cancer.[118,119] The American Institute for Cancer Research and the World Cancer Research Fund have created a combined report for guidelines regarding nutrition and physical activity to prevent cancer, and the American Cancer Society (ACS) has published guidelines for those with cancer.[120,121] Additionally, a recent study examining obesity during neoadjuvant chemotherapy for breast cancer patients found obesity was correlated with decreased survival,[122] and a different study found obesity predicts a second primary on the contralateral breast.[123] Patients need to be encouraged to follow the ACS guidelines and/or the American Institute for Cancer Research/World Cancer Research Fund (AICS/WCRF) guidelines for cancer prevention and to adopt healthful behaviors in regards to physical activity and diet.

The Integrative Medicine Center at MD Anderson Cancer Center

The Integrative Medicine Center at The University of Texas MD Anderson Cancer Center, located in the Texas Medical Center in Houston, Texas, focuses on creating a comprehensive and integrative care plan that addresses the whole person with cancer. The Center's mission focuses on three areas: clinical delivery, education, and research. The main objectives of these areas are as follows:

1. *Clinical*: To provide the highest-quality integrative medicine therapies to patients and their families by using a patient-centered approach. The therapies are provided in concert with mainstream care to manage symptoms, relieve stress, and enhance quality of life.
2. *Education*: To offer reliable information on integrative medicine treatment options to patients, families, and medical staff of MD Anderson.
3. *Research*: To advance knowledge on the outcome and effectiveness of these therapies through peer-reviewed, mixed-methodology research.

The Integrative Medicine Center is housed within the Division of Cancer Medicine that includes all of the medical oncology departments at MD Anderson. Below we present details on the clinical and educational aspects of our Center.

The Integrative Medicine Center at MD Anderson is an important component of the mission to treat the whole person—from prevention and treatment to survivorship.[107] Ongoing research is examining intervention programs and treatments that can improve quality of life and clinical outcomes. Educational programs provide authoritative, accurate, and current information to our faculty, staff, students, trainees, and the public about complementary and alternative approaches.

Cancer patients use CIM for a variety of reasons including to reduce side effects and organ toxicity, protect and stimulate immunity, or prevent further cancers or recurrences. Patients often do not report their use of CIM therapies to their health care team, and mixing of different therapies without clear knowledge regarding the risks and benefits of such an approach has the potential to lead to unintentional harm.[3] This gap in communication results from patients' perception that their physicians are indifferent or negative toward CIM[125] or from physicians' emphasis on scientific studies and evidence-based medicine rather than patient preferences. The Integrative Medicine Center at MD Anderson offers integrative oncology consultation with an oncologist with CIM training and focuses on the use of CIM throughout the continuum of cancer care. These consultations are initiated by the primary oncologist similar to a referral to another subspecialty such as cardiology or gastroenterology. During this consultation, the oncologist will not only review the particular details regarding the cancer history and treatment plan, but also gain an understanding of each patient, covering topics such as goals of care, fears, what is most important to the patient, and reasons for CIM interest. This discussion ranges from researching reliable information sources related to CIM therapies to providing expertise in natural products, including nutritional supplements, vitamins, and herbs, to incorporating mind–body techniques such as music therapy and meditation. Other topics may focus on managing pain, stress, and anxiety, and other symptoms resulting from illness and/or treatment side effects. The goals of this visit are to help patients obtain optimal health and healing through a treatment plan that is comprehensive, integrative, personalized (both the person, type of cancer, and treatment plan), evidence-based, and safe. The consultation strives to collaborate with the primary oncology team in order to achieve these goals and communicates with them regularly. Recommendations are always placed within the context of the patient's goals of care. The recommendations provided often emphasize the three dimensions of well-being (physical, psychospiritual, and social) and better ways in which to achieve optimal health and well-being through more natural approaches such as improved dietary foods and mind–body techniques rather than through the use of unproven herbs, which often lack quality scientific data on efficacy and safety. These treatment plans commonly involve multiple health practitioners including dieticians, meditation instructors, chaplains, physical/occupational therapists, acupuncturists, massage therapists, yoga instructors, music therapists, and others. For challenging cases, these are discussed at a weekly multidisciplinary team meeting so that treatment plans can be formulated and coordinated. The team communicates with the primary oncology team regarding the recommendations.

The Integrative Medicine Center also provides educational and group therapy sessions to patients and caregivers. These programs began with a vision in 1995 that later became Place … of wellness in 1998. The mission of the Integrative Medicine Center (formally the Place … of wellness) *is an environment where all persons touched by cancer (patients, family members, and personal caregivers, and friends in their support system and regardless of where they received treatment) may enhance their quality of life through programs that complement medical care and focus on the mind, body, and spirit.* Therapies offered can enhance patients' quality of life through programs that complement medical care and focus on the mind, body, and spirit such as guided imagery, meditation, yoga, tai chi, music therapy, acupuncture, massage, and cooking and tea classes. Faculty, staff, and community practitioners credentialed in their respective areas of expertise facilitate the programs. Most programs are offered free of charge, except acupuncture and full body massage, which are provided for a fee.

The Integrative Medicine Center now offers over 100 program opportunities each month in the following categories: support groups, expressive arts, music therapy, massage, acupuncture, movement (eg, yoga, qigong, tai chi, pilates), energy, relaxation/meditation, educational forums, and spirituality. Should a therapist identify a particular issue, such as a rotator cuff or lymphedema problem, we refer the patient to Physical Medicine and Rehabilitation Services for further assessment. In addition to these services, which are conducted in our facilities, we also serve participants in the in-patient setting, the Ambulatory Treatment Centers, waiting areas, and others on request. Waiting areas can be places of high anxiety—waiting for results, waiting to start a treatment, waiting to visit a family member who is in the Critical Care Center, waiting for a family member's surgery to be completed, etc. Having a 10-minute relaxation massage in the waiting area, learning a guided imagery or relaxation technique, or making a paper flower can be of great comfort and support.

Funding

We sometimes hear business operations, and others say that they are considering opening an integrative medicine center given the demand and how much is spent each year on complementary medicine. Using this model, most are expected to fully recover their costs and be self-sustaining. What they do not realize is that unless you charge for all services, broaden the scope to serve the community for fee-for-service, or sell products, integrative medicine will most likely not be a revenue leader for the institution. Although the revenue we receive from medical consultation, full-body massage, and acupuncture does contribute to our Division, it does not cover the expenses incurred. As for downstream revenue, we do track referrals made to other services, but many of them are also to nonrevenue services (eg, nutritional counseling, chaplaincy, etc). We are fortunate that our institution has chosen to provide much of the funding for our clinical programming. We also rely on philanthropy and internal organizations through which we can apply for funding for some clinical services, start-up services, equipment, special events, or other expenditures. We have found that funding opportunities for clinical services and programming are quite limited. Most of our services and programs are for patients with any cancer diagnosis, which further limits funding, as there are foundations that fund diagnosis-specific efforts but do not fund efforts for general cancer populations. The philosophy of our institution is that integrative medicine services are provided for our patients and families because it is the right thing to do. We continue to incorporate fee for service or billing as appropriate when supported by the field.

Other Key Operational Areas

Documentation is an essential part of the delivery of integrative medicine services. Not only is it an institutional policy and a requirement of the Joint Commission on Accreditation of Healthcare Organizations, but it is also an excellent way to educate an institution's clinical personnel about the services provided and outcomes. Our CIM practitioners make notes in the medical records of patients and complete progress notes for nonpatients, which are kept in our clinic files.

Participant satisfaction and quality assurance is another key operational area. A preprogram and postprogram survey has been developed for our music therapy, massage therapy, and acupuncture services. Basic information on common cancer- and treatment-related symptoms is tracked before and after each treatment session (eg, fatigue, pain, distress, nausea, etc). In addition, we collect participant feedback for the first six sessions of every new program and then randomly twice per year for an entire month for all programs and services. The most valuable feedback results from asking the question "would you recommend this program to a friend" and asking participants to name three things they liked best about the program, what they would change, and what services they would like added.

SUMMARY

Integrative oncology is a rapidly expanding discipline that holds tremendous promise for additional treatment options and more effective symptom control. An integrative approach also provides patients with a more personalized system of care for meeting their needs. The majority of patients are either using complementary medicines or want to know about them, so it is incumbent on the conventional medical system to provide appropriate education and clinical services. The clinical model for integrative care requires a patient-centered approach with attention to patient concerns and enhanced communication skills. In addition, it is essential that conventional and nonconventional practitioners work together in developing a comprehensive, integrative care plan. In this way, cancer patients will be receiving the best medical care making use of all appropriate treatment modalities to achieve optimal clinical outcomes.

KEY POINTS

- The majority of cancer patients use some form of complementary or alternative medicine treatments during their cancer journey. Patients' utilization of these modalities is idiosyncratic, often involves therapies with uncertain efficacy and/or safety, and is not implemented as part of a well-designed, integrated treatment plan.

- Integrative medicine seeks to merge conventional medicine and complementary therapies in a manner that is comprehensive, personalized, evidence-based, and safe in order to achieve optimal health and healing.

- Clinicians should ask all of their patients about the use of CAM in a manner that is open-minded and collaborative. These discussions will often strengthen the relationship with patients and reveal unmet needs.

- There are a number of comprehensive scientific review organizations that provide electronic access to the reviews of complementary medicine treatments (www.naturalmedicinedatabase.com, www.cochrane.org, www.naturalstandard.com, www.mskcc.org/aboutherbs, www.cancer.gov/cam, www.mdanderson.org/cimer).

- There are a number of complementary medicine strategies that can help patients manage side effects and improve clinical outcomes: (1) mind–body approaches such as meditation, yoga, guided imagery, expressive arts such as music therapy or art therapy, behavioral techniques, support groups, and social support; (2) acupuncture; (3) nutrition; (4) physical activity; and (5) massage.

REFERENCES

1. NCCAM. *National Center for Complementary/Alternative Medicine of the National Institutes of Health. What is Complementary and Alternative Medicine?* June 24, 2008. Available at: http://nccam.nih.gov/health/whatiscam/. Accessed June 12, 2010.

2. CAHCIM. June 24, 2008. Available at: http://www.imconsortium.org/cahcim/about/home.html. Accessed June 12, 2010.

3. Eisenberg DM, Davies RB, Ettner SL, et al. Trends in alternative medicine use in the United States, 1990–1997: results of a follow-up national survey. *JAMA.* 1998;280(18):1569–1575.

4. Barnes PM, Bloom B, Nahin RL. Complementary and alternative medicine use among adults and children: United States, 2007. *Natl Health Stat Rep.* 2008;(12):1–23.

5. Navo MA, Phan J, Vaughan C, et al. An assessment of the utilization of complementary and alternative medication in women with gynecologic or breast malignancies. *J Clin Oncol.* 2004;22(4):671–677.

6. Mao JJ, Farrar JT, Xie SX, Bowman MA, Armstrong K. Use of complementary and alternative medicine and prayer among a national sample of cancer survivors compared to other populations without cancer. *Complement Ther Med.* 2007;15(1):21–29.

7. Richardson MA, Sanders T, Palmer JL, Greisinger A, Singletary SE. Complementary/alternative medicine use in a comprehensive cancer center and the implications for oncology. *J Clin Oncol.* 2000;18(13):2505–2514.

8. Dy GK, Bekele L, Hanson LJ, et al. Complementary and alternative medicine use by patients enrolled onto phase I clinical trials. *J Clin Oncol.* 2004;22(23):4810–4815.

9. Ernst E. Complementary therapies in palliative cancer care. *Cancer.* 2001;91(11):2181–2185.

10. White P. Complementary medicine treatment of cancer: a survey of provision. *Complement Ther Med.* 1998;6: 10–13.

11. Astin JA, Reilly C, Perkins C, Child WL; Susan G. Komen Breast Cancer Foundation. Breast cancer patients' perspectives on and use of complementary and alternative medicine: a study by the Susan G. Komen Breast Cancer Foundation. *J Soc Integr Oncol.* 2006;4(4):157–169.

12. DiGianni LM, Garber JE, Winer EP. Complementary and alternative medicine use among women with breast cancer. *J Clin Oncol.* 2002;20(18 suppl):34S–38S.

13. Morris KT, Johnson N, Homer L, Walts D. A comparison of complementary therapy use between breast cancer patients and patients with other primary tumor sites. *Am J Surg.* 2000;179(5):407–411.

14. Eisenberg DM, Kessler RC, Van Rompay MI, et al. Perceptions about complementary therapies relative to conventional therapies among adults who use both: results from a national survey. *Ann Intern Med.* 2001;135(5):344–351.

15. Richardson MA, Mâsse LC, Nanny K, Sanders C. Discrepant views of oncologists and cancer patients on complementary/alternative medicine. *Support Care Cancer.* 2004;12(11):797–804.

16. Crocetti E, Crotti N, Feltrin A, Ponton P, Geddes M, Buiatti E. The use of complementary therapies by breast cancer patients attending conventional treatment. *Eur J Cancer.* 1998;34(3):324–328.

17. Kappauf H, Leykauf-Ammon D, Bruntsch U, et al. Use of and attitudes held towards unconventional medicine by patients in a department of internal medicine/oncology and haematology. *Support Care Cancer.* 2000;8(4): 314–322.

18. Miller M, Boyer MJ, Butow PN, Gattellari M, Dunn SM, Childs A. The use of unproven methods of treatment by cancer patients. Frequency, expectations and cost. *Support Care Cancer.* 1998;6(4):337–347.

19. Morant R, Jungi WF, Koehli C, Senn HJ. Why do cancer patients use alternative medicine? *Schweiz Med Wochenschr.* 1991;121(27–28):1029–1034.

20. Oneschuk D, Fennell L, Hanson J, Bruera E. The use of complementary medications by cancer patients attending an outpatient pain and symptom clinic. *J Palliat Care.* 1998;14(4):21–26.

21. Wyatt GK, Friedman LL, Given CW, Given BA, Beckrow KC. Complementary therapy use among older cancer patients. *Cancer Pract.* 1999;7(3):136–144.

22. Bairati I, Meyer F, Gelinas M, Fortin A, Nabid A, Brochet F, et al. A randomized trial of antioxidant vitamins to prevent second primary cancers in head and neck cancer patients. *J Natl Cancer Inst.* 2005;97(7):481-488.

23. Clark LC, Combs GF, Jr., Turnbull BW, Slate EH, Chalker DK, Chow J, et al. Effects of selenium supplementation for cancer prevention in patients with carcinoma of the skin. A randomized controlled trial. Nutritional Prevention of Cancer Study Group. *JAMA.* 1996;276(24):1957–1963.

24. Clark LC, Dalkin B, Krongrad A, Combs GF, Jr., Turnbull BW, Slate EH, et al. Decreased incidence of prostate cancer with selenium supplementation: results of a double-blind cancer prevention trial. *Br J Urol.* 1998;81(5):730–734.

25. Combs GF, Jr., Clark LC, Turnbull BW. An analysis of cancer prevention by selenium. *Biofactors.* 2001;14(1-4):153–159.

26. Combs GF, Jr. Status of selenium in prostate cancer prevention. *Br J Cancer.* 2004;91(2):195–199.

27. Duffield-Lillico AJ, Dalkin BL, Reid ME, Turnbull BW, Slate EH, Jacobs ET, et al. Selenium supplementation, baseline plasma selenium status and incidence of prostate cancer: an analysis of the complete treatment period of the Nutritional Prevention of Cancer Trial. *BJU Int.* 2003;91(7):608–612.

28. Duffield-Lillico AJ, Slate EH, Reid ME, Turnbull BW, Wilkins PA, Combs GF, Jr., et al. Selenium supplementation and secondary prevention of nonmelanoma skin cancer in a randomized trial. *J Natl Cancer Inst.* 2003;95(19):1477–1481.

29. Finley JW. Reduction of cancer risk by consumption of selenium-enriched plants: enrichment of broccoli with selenium increases the anticarcinogenic properties of broccoli. *J Med Food.* 2003;6(1):19–26.

30. Huff J. Re: Selenium supplementation and secondary prevention of nonmelanoma skin cancer in a randomized trial. *J Natl Cancer Inst.* 2004;96(4):333–334.

31. Klein EA, Thompson IM, Lippman SM, Goodman PJ, Albanes D, Taylor PR, et al. SELECT: the selenium and vitamin E cancer prevention trial. *Urol Oncol.* 2003;21(1):59–65.

32. Klein EA, Lippman SM, Thompson IM, Goodman PJ, Albanes D, Taylor PR, et al. The selenium and vitamin E cancer prevention trial. *World J Urol.* 2003;21(1):21–27.

33. Klein EA. Clinical models for testing chemopreventative agents in prostate cancer and overview of SELECT: the

Selenium and Vitamin E Cancer Prevention Trial. *Recent Results Cancer Res.* 2003;163:212–225.

34. Moyad MA. Selenium and vitamin E supplements for prostate cancer: evidence or embellishment? *Urology.* 2002;59(4 suppl 1):9-19.

35. Reid ME, Duffield-Lillico AJ, Garland L, Turnbull BW, Clark LC, Marshall JR. Selenium supplementation and lung cancer incidence: an update of the nutritional prevention of cancer trial. *Cancer Epidemiol Biomarkers Prev.* 2002;11(11):1285–1291.

36. Vinceti M, Malagoli C, Bergomi M, Vivoli G. Correspondence re: Duffield-Lillico et al., Baseline characteristics and the effect of selenium supplementation on cancer incidence in a randomized clinical trial: a summary report of the Nutritional Prevention of Cancer Trial. 11: 630-639, 2002. Cancer Epidemiol Biomarkers Prev 2003 Jan;12(1):77.

37. Whanger PD. Selenium and its relationship to cancer: an update. *Br J Nutr.* 2004;91(1):11–28.

38. Deng GE, Frenkel M, Cohen L, et al. Evidence-based clinical practice guidelines for integrative oncology: complementary therapies and botanicals. *J Soc Integr Oncol.* 2009;7(3):85–120.

39. WHO. *WHO Traditional Medicine Strategy 2002–2005.* World Health Organization: Geneva; 2002.

40. Helms JM. *Acupuncture Energetics: A Clinical Approach for Physicians.* Berkeley, Calif: Medical Acupuncture Publishers; 1997.

41. Mittleman E, Gaynor JS. A brief overview of the analgesic and immunologic effects of acupuncture in domestic animals. *J Am Vet Med Assoc.* 2000;217(8):1201–1205.

42. Altman S. Techniques and instrumentation, electroacupuncture. In: Schoen AM, ed. Veterinary Acupuncture—Ancient Art to Modern Medicine. St. Louis: Mosby; 1994. Edited by Allen M. Schoen; Publisher is Goleta, CA: American Veterinary Publications. St. Louis: Mosby; 1994.

43. Acupuncture. *NIH Consens Statement.* 1997;15(5):1–34.

44. Ezzo J, Vickers A, Richardson MA, et al. Acupuncture-point stimulation for chemotherapy-induced nausea and vomiting. *J Clin Oncol.* 2005;23(28):7188–7198.

45. Lee A, Done ML. The use of nonpharmacologic techniques to prevent postoperative nausea and vomiting: a meta-analysis. *Anesth Analg.* 1999;88(6):1362–1369.

46. Lee A, Done ML. Stimulation of the wrist acupuncture point P6 for preventing postoperative nausea and vomiting. *Cochrane Database Syst Rev.* 2004;3:CD003281.

47. Vickers AJ. Can acupuncture have specific effects on health? A systematic review of acupuncture antiemesis trials. *J R Soc Med.* 1996;89(6):303–311.

48. *American Cancer Society: Acupuncture.* June 15, 2008. Available at: http://www.cancer.org/docroot/ETO/content/ETO_5_3X_Acupuncture.asp?sitearea=ETO. Accessed June 12, 2010.

49. Wu MT, Hsieh JC, Xiong J, et al. Central nervous system pathway for acupuncture stimulation: localization of processing with functional MR imaging of the brain—preliminary experience. *Radiology.* 1999;212:133–141.

50. Alimi D, Rubino C, Pichard-Léandri E, Fermand-Brulé S, Dubreuil-Lemaire ML, Hill C. Analgesic effect of auricular acupuncture for cancer pain: a randomized, blinded, controlled trial. *J Clin Oncol.* 2003;21(22):4120–4126.

51. Crew KD, Capodice JL, Greenlee H, Brafman L, Fuentes D, Awad D, et al. Randomized, blinded, sham-controlled trial of acupuncture for the management of aromatase inhibitor-associated joint symptoms in women with early-stage breast cancer. *J Clin Oncol.* 2010;28(7):1154–1160.

52. Filshie J, Hester J. Guidelines for providing acupuncture treatment for cancer patients—a peer-reviewed sample policy document. *Acupunct Med.* 2006;24(4):172–182.

53. Lewith G, Berman B, Cummings M, Filshie J, Fisher P, White A. Systematic review of systematic reviews of acupuncture published 1996–2005. *Clin Med.* 2006;6(6):623–625 [comment].

54. Ernst E, White AR. Prospective studies of the safety of acupuncture: a systematic review. *Am J Med.* 2001;110(6):481–485.

55. Filshie J. Safety aspects of acupuncture in palliative care. *Acupunct Med.* 2001;19(2):117–122.

56. Lu W, Dean-Clower E, Doherty-Gilman A, Rosenthal DS. The value of acupuncture in cancer care. In: Cohen L, Frenkel M, eds. *Integrative Medicine in Oncology: Hematology/Oncology Clinics of North America.* Philadelphia: Elsevier, Inc.; 2008.

57. Thomas RC, Hawkins K, Kirkpatrick SH, Mondry TE, Gabram-Mendola S, Johnstone PA. Reduction of lymphedema using complete decongestive therapy: roles of prior radiation therapy and extent of axillary dissection. *J Soc Integr Oncol.* 2007;5(3):87–91.

58. Ahles TA, Tope DM, Pinkson B, et al. Massage therapy for patients undergoing autologous bone marrow transplantation. *J Pain Symptom Manage.* 1999;18(3):157–163.

59. Stephenson NL, Weinrich SP, Tavakoli AS. The effects of foot reflexology on anxiety and pain in patients with breast and lung cancer. *Oncol Nurs Forum.* 2000;27(1):67–72.

60. Grealish L, Lomasney A, Whiteman B. Foot massage. A nursing intervention to modify the distressing symptoms of pain and nausea in patients hospitalized with cancer. *Cancer Nurs.* 2000;23(3):237–243.

61. Wilkinson S, Aldridge J, Salmon I, Cain E, Wilson B. An evaluation of aromatherapy massage in palliative care. *Palliat Med.* 1999;13(5):409–417.

62. Russell NC, Sumler SS, Beinhorn CM, Frenkel MA. Role of massage therapy in cancer care. *J Altern Complement Med.* 2008;14(2):209–214.

63. Myers CD. The value of massage therapy in cancer care. In: Cohnen L, Frenkel M, eds. *Integrative Medicine in Oncology: Hematology/Oncology Clinics of North America.* Philadelphia: Elsevier, Inc.; 2008.

64. Blanchard CM, Denniston MM, Baker F, et al. Do adults change their lifestyle behaviors after a cancer diagnosis? *Am J Health Behav.* 2003;27(3):246–256.

65. Baider L, Uziely B, De-Nour AK. Progressive muscle relaxation and guided imagery in cancer patients. *Gen Hosp Psychiatry.* 1994;16(5):340–347.

66. Sloman R. Relaxation and the relief of cancer pain. *Nurs Clin North Am.* 1995;30(4):697–709.

67. Moskowitz L. Psychological management of postsurgical pain and patient adherence. *Hand Clin.* 1996;12(1): 129–137.

68. Ross MC, Bohannon AS, Davis DC, Gurchiek L. The effects of a short-term exercise program on movement, pain, and mood in the elderly. Results of a pilot study. *J Holistic Nurs.* 1999;17(2):139–147.

69. Spiegel D. Psychosocial aspects of breast cancer treatment. *Semin Oncol.* 1997;24(1):36–47.

70. Walker L, Walker M, Odston K. Psychological, clinical and pathological effects of relaxation training and guided imagery during chemotherapy. *Br J Cancer.* 1999;80(1–2): 262–268.

71. Wallace KG. Analysis of recent literature concerning relaxation and imagery interventions for cancer pain. *Cancer Nurs.* 1997;20(2):79–87.

72. Richardson MA, Post-White J, Grimm EA, Moye LA, Singletary SE, Justce B. Coping, life attitudes, and immune responses to imagery and group support after breast cancer treatment. *Altern Ther Health Med.* 1997;3(5):62–70.

73. Turner-Cobb JM, Sephton SE, Koopman C, Blake-Mortimer J, Spiegel D. Social support and salivary cortisol in women with metastatic breast cancer. *Psychosom Med.* 2000;62(3):337–345.

74. Coker KH. Meditation and prostate cancer: integrating a mind/body intervention with traditional therapies. *Semin Urol Oncol.* 1999;17(2):111–118.

75. Massion AO, Teas J, Hebert JR, Wertheimer MD, Kabat-Zinn J. Meditation, melatonin and breast/prostate cancer: hypothesis and preliminary data. *Med Hypotheses.* 1995;44(1):39–46.

76. Arakawa S. Relaxation to reduce nausea, vomiting, and anxiety induced by chemotherapy in Japanese patients. *Cancer Nurs.* 1997;20(5):342–349.

77. Manyande A, Berg S, Gettins D, et al. Preoperative rehearsal of active coping imagery influences subjective and hormonal responses to abdominal surgery. *Psychosom Med.* 1995;57:177–182.

78. Syrjala KL, Chapko ME. Evidence for a biopsychosocial model of cancer treatment-related pain. *Pain.* 1995;61(1):69–79.

79. Troesch LM, Rodehaver CB, Delaney EA, Yanes B. The influence of guided imagery on chemotherapy-related nausea and vomiting. *Oncol Nurs Forum.* 1993;20(8):1179–1185.

80. Fawzy FI, Fawzy NW, Arndt LA, Pasnau RO. Critical review of psychosocial interventions in cancer care. *Arch Gen Psychiatry.* 1995;52:100–113.

81. Helgeson VS, Cohen S, Schulz R, Yasko J. Group support interventions for women with breast cancer: who benefits from what? *Health Psychol.* 2000;19(2):107–114.

82. Spiegel D, Bloom JR, Yalom I. Group support for patients with metastatic cancer. A randomized outcome study. *Arch Gen Psychiatry.* 1981;38:527–533.

83. Fawzy FI, Cousins N, Fawzy NW, Kemeny ME, Elashoff R, Morton D. A structured psychiatric intervention for cancer patients: I. Changes over time in methods of coping and affective disturbance. *Arch Gen Psychiatry.* 1990;47:720–725.

84. Helgeson VS, Cohen S, Schulz R, Yasko J. Education and peer discussion group interventions and adjustment to breast cancer. *Arch Gen Psychiatry.* 1999;56(4):340–347.

85. Richardson JL, Shelton DR, Krailo M, Levine AM. The effect of compliance with treatment on survival among patients with hematologic malignancies. *J Clin Oncol.* 1990;8:356–364.

86. Gordon JS. Mind–body medicine and cancer. In: Cohen L, Frenkel M, eds. *Integrative Medicine in Oncology: Hematology/Oncology Clinics of North America.* Philadelphia: Elsevier, Inc.; 2008.

87. Devine EC, Westlake SK. The effects of psychoeducational care provided to adults with cancer: meta-analysis of 116 studies. *Oncol Nurs Forum.* 1995;22(9): 1369–1381.

88. Newell SA, Sanson-Fisher W, Savolainen NJ. Systematic review of psychological therapies for cancer patients: overview and recommendations for future research. *J Natl Cancer Inst.* 2002;94(8):558–584.

89. Ernst E, Pittler MH, Wider B, Boddy K. Mind–body therapies: are the trial data getting stronger? *Altern Ther Health Med.* 2007;13(5):62–64.

90. Bower JE, Woolery A, Sternlieb B, Garet D. Yoga for cancer patients and survivors. *Cancer Control.* 2005;12(3):165–171.

91. Chandwani KD, Thornton B, Perkins GH, Arun B, Raghuram NV, Nagendra HR, Wei Q, Cohen L. Yoga improves quality of life and benefit finding in women undergoing radiotherapy for breast cancer. *J Soc Integr Oncol.* 2010;8(2):43–55.

92. Cohen L, Warneke C, Fouladi RT, Rodriguez MA, Chaoul-Reich A. Psychological adjustment and sleep quality in a randomized trial of the effects of a Tibetan yoga intervention in patients with lymphoma. *Cancer.* 2004;100(10):2253–2260.

93. Spiegel D, Moore R. Imagery & hypnosis in the treatment of cancer patients. *Oncology.* 1997;11(8):1179–1189.

94. Integration of behavioral and relaxation approaches into the treatment of chronic pain and insomnia. NIH Technology Assessment Panel on Integration of Behavioral and Relaxation Approaches into the Treatment of Chronic Pain and Insomnia. *JAMA.* 1996;276:313–318.

95. Zeltzer LK, Dolgin MJ, LeBaron S, LeBaron C. A randomized, controlled study of behavioral intervention for chemotherapy distress in children with cancer. *Pediatrics.* 1991;88(1):34–42.

96. Morrow GR, Morrell C. Behavioral treatment for the anticipatory nausea and vomiting induced by cancer chemotherapy. *N Engl J Med.* 1982;307:1476–1480.

97. Faymonville ME, Mambourg PH, Joris J, et al. Psychological approaches during conscious sedation. Hypnosis versus stress reducing strategies: a prospective randomized study. *Pain.* 1997;73(3):361–367.

98. Lang EV, Benotsch EG, Fick LJ, et al. Adjunctive non-pharmacological analgesia for invasive medical procedures: a randomised trial. *Lancet.* 2000;355(9214):1486–1490.

99. Lang EV, Berbaum KS, Faintuch S, et al. Adjunctive self-hypnotic relaxation for outpatient medical procedures: a prospective randomized trial with women undergoing large core breast biopsy. *Pain.* 2006;126(1–3):155–164.

100. Montgomery GH, Bovbjerg DH, Schnur JB, et al. A randomized clinical trial of a brief hypnosis intervention to control side effects in breast surgery patients. *J Natl Cancer Inst.* 2007;99(17):1304–1312.

101. Jellin JM. *Natural Medicines Comprehensive Database.* June 15, 2008. Available at: http://www.naturaldatabase.com. Accessed June 12, 2010.

102. Chambliss WG, Hufford CD, Flagg ML, Glisson JK. Assessment of the quality of reference books on botanical dietary supplements. *J Am Pharm Assoc (Wash DC).* 2002;42(5):723–734.

103. Sweet BV, Gay WE, Leady MA, Stumpf JL. Usefulness of herbal and dietary supplement references. *Ann Pharmacother.* 2003;37(4):494–499.

104. Walker JB. Evaluation of the ability of seven herbal resources to answer questions about herbal products asked in drug information centers. *Pharmacotherapy.* 2002;22(12):1611–1615.

105. *Cochrane Collaboration Steering Group: The Cochrane Collection.* June 15, 2008. Available at: http://www.cochrane.org. Accessed June 12, 2010.

106. Dickersin K, Manheimer E. The Cochrane Collaboration: evaluation of health care and services using systematic reviews of the results of randomized controlled trials. *Clin Obstet Gynecol.* 1998;41(2):315–331.

107. Basch E, Ulbricht C. *Natural Standard* [cited 2008]. June 15, 2008. Available at: http://www.naturalstandard.com. Accessed June 12, 2010.

108. NCI. *Office of Cancer Complementary & Alternative Medicine: CAM Information.* June 15, 2008. Available at: http://www.cancer.gov/cam/. Accessed June 12, 2010.

109. *Memorial Sloan-Kettering Cancer Center: About Herbs.* June 15, 2008. Available at: http://www.mskcc.org/aboutherbs. Accessed June 12, 2010.

110. *Oxford University–Bandolier: Evidence Based Thinking about Health Issues.* June 15, 2008. Available at: http://www.medicine.ox.ac.uk/bandolier/. Accessed June 12, 2010.

111. *The University of Texas MD Anderson Cancer Center: Complementary/Integrative Medicine Education Resources (CIMER).* June 15, 2008. Available at: http://www.mdanderson.org/cimer. Accessed June 12, 2010.

112. *Health on the Net Foundation. About Health on the Net.* June 15, 2008. Available at: http://www.hon.ch/global/. Accessed June 12, 2010.

113. Engel GL. The need for a new medical model: a challenge for biomedicine. *Science.* 1977;196(4286):129–136.

114. Quinten C, Coens C, Mauer M, et al. Baseline quality of life as a prognostic indicator of survival: a meta-analysis of individual patient data from EORTC clinical trials. *Lancet Oncol.* 2009;10(9):865–871.

115. Chlebowski RT, Blackburn GL, Thomson CA, et al. Dietary fat reduction and breast cancer outcome: interim efficacy results from the Women's Intervention Nutrition Study. *J Natl Cancer Inst.* 2006;98(24):1767–1776.

116. Pierce JP, Natarajan L, Caan BJ, et al. Influence of a diet very high in vegetables, fruit, and fiber and low in fat on prognosis following treatment for breast cancer: the Women's Healthy Eating and Living (WHEL) randomized trial. *JAMA.* 2007;298(3):289–298.

117. Pierce JP, Stefanick ML, Flatt SW, et al. Greater survival after breast cancer in physically active women with high vegetable–fruit intake regardless of obesity. *J Clin Oncol.* 2007;25(17):2345–2351.

118. Meyerhardt JA, Heseltine D, Niedzwiecki D, et al. Impact of physical activity on cancer recurrence and survival in patients with stage III colon cancer: findings from CALGB 89803. *J Clin Oncol.* 2006;24(22):3535–3541.

119. Meyerhardt JA, Niedzwiecki D, Hollis D, et al. Association of dietary patterns with cancer recurrence and survival in patients with stage III colon cancer. *JAMA.* 2007;298(7):754–764.

120. Doyle C, Kushi LH, Byers T, et al. Nutrition and physical activity during and after cancer treatment: an American Cancer Society guide for informed choices. *CA Cancer J Clin.* 2006;56(6):323–353.

121. World Cancer Research Fund in association with American Institute for Cancer Research. Food, Nutrition and the Prevention of Cancer: A Global Perspective. World Cancer Research Fund, Washington DC; 1997.

122. Litton JK, Gonzalez-Angulo AM, Warneke CL, et al. Relationship between obesity and pathologic response to neoadjuvant chemotherapy among women with operable breast cancer. *J Clin Oncol.* 2008;26(25):4072–4077.

123. Li CI, Daling JR, Porter PL, Tang MT, Malone KE. Relationship between potentially modifiable lifestyle factors and risk of second primary contralateral breast cancer among women diagnosed with estrogen receptor-positive invasive breast cancer. *J Clin Oncol.* 2009;27(32):5312–5318.

124. Frenkel M, Cohen L. Incorporating complementary and integrative medicine in a comprehensive cancer center. In: Cohen L, Frenkel M, eds. *Integrative Medicine in Oncology: Hematology/Oncology Clinics of North America.* Philadelphia: Elsevier, Inc.; 2008.

125. Tasaki K, Maskarinec G, Shumay DM, Tatsumura Y, Kakai H. Communication between physicians and cancer patients about complementary and alternative medicine: exploring patients' perspectives. *Psychooncology.* 2002;11(3):212–220 [see comment].

126. NIH Consensus Conference. Acupuncture. *JAMA.* 1998;280(17):1518–1524.

127. Alimi D, Rubino C, Pichard-Leandri E, Fermand-Brule S, Dubreuil-Lemaire ML, Hill C. Analgesic effect of auricular acupuncture for cancer pain: a randomized, blinded, controlled trial. *J Clin Oncol.* 2003;21(22):4120–4126.

128. Park J, Linde K, Manheimer E, Molsberger A, Sherman K, Smith C, et al. The status and future of acupuncture clinical research. *J Altern Complement Med.* 2008;14(7):871–881.

129. Jedel E. Acupuncture in xerostomia--a systematic review. *J Oral Rehabil.* 2005;32(6):392–396.

130. Garcia MK, Chiang JS, Cohen L, Liu M, Palmer JL, Rosenthal DI, Wei Q, Tung S, Wang C, Rahlfs T, Chambers MS. Acupuncture for radiation-induced xerostomia in patients with cancer: a pilot study. Head Neck. 2009;31(10):1360–1368.

131. Lee MS, Kim KH, Choi SM, Ernst E. Acupuncture for treating hot flashes in breast cancer patients: a systematic review. Breast Cancer Res Treat. 2009;115(3):497–503.

132. Crew KD, Capodice JL, Greenlee H, Apollo A, Jacobson JS, Raptis G, et al. Pilot study of acupuncture for the treatment of joint symptoms related to adjuvant aromatase inhibitor therapy in postmenopausal breast cancer patients. J Cancer Surviv. 2007;1(4):283–291.

133. Crew KD, Capodice JL, Greenlee H, Brafman L, Fuentes D, Awad D, et al. Randomized, blinded, sham-controlled trial of acupuncture for the management of aromatase inhibitor-associated joint symptoms in women with early-stage breast cancer. J Clin Oncol. 2010;28(7):1154–1160.

SECTION VII

Grief and End-of-Life Issues

An Overview of Grief

• Steven Thorney and Debra Sivesind

Grief-related issues impact us every day in our role as clinicians working in an oncologic setting. However, apart from the brief time spent with patients and their loved ones at the moment of death, oncology clinicians do not typically accompany the patient's family on its journey of grief, mourning, and bereavement. This is not a criticism, but simply a statement of reality in a world where patients' homes and communities are often dislocated from the tertiary centers in which they receive medical care.

In the vast world that lies between home and the point of medical care, the bulk of grief work has been played out beyond the reach of clinicians and researchers. We struggle to know just how long "normal grief and bereavement" should actually last, and we still await longitudinal studies that will validate the concept of the "stages of grief." However, it is vital that in our attempts to develop empirical norms and debate whether more pathological forms of grief belong as disease categories in the *Diagnostic and Statistical Manual of Mental Disorders* (DSM),[1] we recognize that grief will always be a part of the human experience.

We serve our patients and families well when we recognize that grief work has begun long before a person enters our clinical care. Journey into that private moment when a lump is felt or when bloody sputum is observed, and the realization settles in that "something's not right." Medical tests are run. The conversation comes days later. Fear and anxiety grip the heart as the words, "I want you to see an oncologist," are spoken. Grief is well under way

in this person's life as he or she fights projections into an unknown future: "How far along is the cancer? What will happen to my wife and children? I can't afford to be off from work. Will my insurance cover me? We had a vacation planned next week, and I'm going to ruin it all. Who'll take care of mom and dad? What did I do to deserve this? Why is this happening to me? I'm all alone and I had trouble just getting to my doctor's appointment. Who will care for me? Will this disease take my life? I'm afraid of pain. I'm afraid of dying."

Throughout the course of cancer care, it is important to recognize that these questions multiply for the patient and family as they address a myriad of psychosocial and spiritual concerns and the grief attached to them. As oncologic professionals, we can help people prepare for the potential "long haul" of grief and bereavement by assisting them through supportive presence, listening, and counsel, and by recognizing and addressing their current losses and the anticipatory grief of an unknown future. Further, clinicians serve patient and family well when risk factors for a complicated bereavement are recognized early and appropriate referrals made.

■ DEFINITIONS

Grief, bereavement, and mourning are used by some clinicians synonymously. Others draw distinctions among them. Rando[2] defines grief as the process of psychological, social, and somatic reactions to the perception of loss, thus implying that the grief process represents a continuous development involving many changes. Grief may be a reaction to many types of losses, and not limited to death. Each person's grief is unique and is shaped by one's particular perception of one's loss. Although Rando's[2] earlier work used the term mourning interchangeably with grief, mourning may be seen as having two meanings. The first is drawn from Bowlby's[3] psychoanalytic theory that views mourning as a wide array of intrapsychic processes prompted by loss, which are both conscious and unconscious. Rando's[4] later work defines a distinction between grief and mourning, the former relating to reactions to the perception of loss and the latter seen as incorporating initial grief as well as social-derived actions taken for the purpose of coping with and adaptation to the loss. Zisook et al[5] define grief as the emotional, behavioral, social, and functional responses to loss not necessarily related to death.

THE GRIEVING PROCESS

Types of Losses

We experience many losses throughout life; some are physical or tangible, such as the loss of a possession or a loved one. Psychosocial losses such as the ending of an important relationship or the loss of a job can produce very significant grief reactions.[2] Unfortunately, the impact of these psychosocial losses is often not appreciated, and grieving persons are left alone to navigate their grief experience.

Holmes and Rahe's[6] research in the 1960s heightened awareness that stressful life events can cause illness and are cumulative in nature. Likewise, unresolved, cumulative, physical, and psychosocial grief in our lives can hamper our ability to cope in constructive ways when confronted with the death of a loved one or when facing one's own death. Assessment and care of individuals encountered in the oncologic setting will include clarifying current, past, and ongoing losses. The clinician may then be able to assist the person in understanding healthy coping mechanisms that have sustained and guided him or her through previous losses and attenuate the maladaptive ones. Some of these varied types of losses are outlined below.

Material losses include such things as the loss of income, familiar surroundings, a way of life, or objects of significance.[16,53,57] Certainly, serious medical illness will inevitably produce significant financial stress that will necessitate changes in the patient's material life.

Relationship losses are those in which the opportunity to relate to self, others, or a higher power is lost or impaired.[2,16,53] Relationship losses also stem from death itself, retirement, layoffs, transfer, divorce, or chronic conditions.

Health losses and the attendant impact on self-esteem and body image occur with disfiguring surgery, the visual sight of a tumor, the loss of muscular or neurologic control, fatigue, weight loss or gain, hair loss, pain, and shortness of breath. All of these are reminders that life is not what it used to be.[16]

Role loss relates closely to relationship losses but with more emphasis on the shift of function within the family, workplace, or community environments.[53] It includes all those things one "used to do" and is now unable. These tasks may include paying the bills, caring for the children, mowing the lawn, and/or earning a living. Conversely, a loved one or friend who is now assuming these roles is adjusting to the stress of these new demands, the time commitment, perceived inadequacy, and possibly the fatigue and emotional sense of the unfairness of it all.

Systemic losses occur when systems change.[53] Anyone who has been through a layoff has an understanding of the grief and longing for the way it "used to be." Family systems have a unique, yet familiar pattern of functioning. When trauma, such as cancer, occurs, there is change and disruption within the system. Family members take on new and unfamiliar roles.

Dreams and hopes for the future can fade or evaporate in the face or wake of cancer.[16] The patient's view of God or core values may need to be reevaluated through the process of grieving. Baumeister[7] speaks of losses such as these as a breakdown in a person's "assumptive world." The assumptions held about the world are threatened by a major loss. One's sense of control and the predictability of events may change, resulting in isolation, brokenness, and loss of meaning.

Reactions to Loss

The reactions to loss are personal and individually unique. They may include a wide range of affective, physical, cognitive, spiritual, and behavioral reactions. These reactions fall into a wide highway of what can be considered "normal" grief. The intensity of any one or more of these reactions is conditioned by the significance of the loss to the individual's sense of self, personality, values, and outlook on the world. For example, the death of an elderly, distant relative to a protracted illness is likely to generate fewer disturbing reactions than, say, the loss of a spouse whose young children are still in the home.[16]

Grief reactions generally abate over time; however, there is no scholarly consensus on their duration within the normal course of the grieving process. Engel[8] and Lindemann[9] suggested a duration of weeks to months. Over time, grief counselors have changed their view of normal grief, lengthening its duration. Parkes[10] observed the chronic nature of grief and reported that after 13 months of bereavement the widows who were interviewed had difficulty experiencing pleasure and complained of being depressed, poorly adjusted, and still spending much of their time grieving.[5] For some individuals the second year of grief may be worse than the first in that social support diminishes, and the reality of the permanent absence of the loved one sinks to new levels within one's being. It has been affirmed in the literature that distressing, nonpathological grief reactions can occur for 2 or more years after the death of a loved one.[11–13] Other authors have found that aspects of nonpathological grief may be interminable, the "timeless" emotional involvement with the deceased representing a healthy adaptation to the loss.[14]

Needless to say, protracted periods of disorganization, confusion, searching, and yearning are distressing to individuals, not infrequently leading them to conclude that they are "going crazy."[15] Often, it is helpful for clinicians to normalize this and other grief reactions through attentive listening, reassurance and validation of feelings, and the provision of community resources. For members of affinity groups or a religious community, care and assistance may come through rituals, structures, beliefs, and support.

Anticipatory Grief

Great medical strides have been made against cancer. Some are now curable; others become a chronic disease with which one can live with quality, meaning, and purpose. Sadly, cancer also remains a lethal disease, which claims thousands of lives each year in this country alone.

Case example (fictitious) of anticipatory grief

Ted is a man in his thirties, married with two school-age children. He was diagnosed 2 years ago with a melanoma for which he received chemotherapy and has had no evidence of disease—until now. He and his wife, Judy, have arrived at a cancer center from their home 200 miles away for consideration of further curative treatment.

Ted's employer was quite understanding through his first courses of treatment. Paychecks continued to arrive, and medical insurance was maintained. This time, however, Ted has already been told that his position would need to be filled if he anticipates a protracted absence. He was advised that long-term disability may be needed. The potential loss of medical insurance looms as a threat to treatment options and financial well-being. Judy has already noticed Ted's increasing level of fatigue and has assumed some of his household roles.

Judy has worked in the home since the children were born. She taught middle school students following college graduation, but that was years ago. Their children are currently staying with her parents. While they have a supportive community of family and friends, none live nearby.

The extended family is not without financial and social means, but medical bills and the maintenance of two domiciles have stretched their now limited resources. Ted and Judy have received help from their church community, which has held fundraisers for them.

Ted has been told that his disease is widely metastatic. There is an investigational drug for which he qualifies, but the prognosis is not good. He has been told that he may only have a year's life expectancy if the treatment regimen goes well.

Ted and Judy's story is not unusual or surprising to any cancer clinician. They are grappling with a number of losses. Material loss is experienced in reduced income and possible job severance. Relationships have changed due to proximity. Disease-free health is a thing of the past. Judy is assuming new roles within the family unit and is considering future employment. Their hopes and dreams for the future are beginning to fade. Life, at times, seems bleak. In Ted and Judy's minds, this scenario is not the way "it is supposed to be." They have begun to question their faith in a beneficent God.

Anyone with the losses identified above is capable of generating one or more grief reactions as Ted and Judy seek to find meaning in life as their "assumptive world" is shaken. In an effort to maintain a sense of control and order in life, Baumeister[7] suggests that humans frequently assume a world that is fair and benevolent where good things happen to good people. The course of an illness like cancer can shatter such ideas as one is confronted with the fragility of life, its vulnerability, and one's powerlessness to affect change. The fundamental meaning in life is shaken.[2,16] In this world pain can be physical, psychological, and spiritual. Suffering is another way of describing the physical, psychological, and spiritual pain experienced as the center of one's being seems to be unraveling.[17]

Both patient and loved ones are faced with grieving the loss of their assumptive world, adjusting to and coping with life's new realities in the face of a potentially fatal disease. In addition, those who are to go on living struggle to envision a future without the loved one in it. These are among the challenges (and opportunities) encompassed by anticipatory grief. It is into this world that the oncologic clinician walks every day.

Rando[18] has written extensively on the topic of anticipatory grief and presents a case in more recent writing[4] for the use of the term, anticipatory mourning, arguing that grief is only one component among several in the anticipatory mourning experience. Further complicating the discussion, thanatologists have argued and debated the very merits and existence of anticipatory grief. Lindemann[9] suggests that the threat of the death of a loved one could initiate grief reactions including "depression, heightened preoccupation with the departed, a review of all forms of death which might befall him, and anticipation of the modes of readjustment which might be necessitated by it." These anticipatory reactions coupled with the emotional responses they engender can serve to moderate the intensity of grief experienced by the bereaved should death occur. Anticipatory grief (mourning) may also reduce the possibility of serious medical, psychological, and social reactions.[5,18,19] Lindemann[9] further observed that emotional detachment carried to the extreme can cause premature emotional and physical withdrawal by the caregiver, especially if death is prolonged or does not occur. Parkes[20] even questioned the concept of anticipatory grief, arguing that the emotional reaction to a terminal diagnosis is not grief with its sense of loss and desolation but rather a feeling of intense separation anxiety and fear. He concludes that anticipatory loss may have emotional implications different from those experienced after the loss.[5,20]

Rando[4,18] offers the following points on anticipatory grief:

- Anticipatory mourning is the phenomenon encompassing seven generic operations (grief and mourning, coping, interaction, psychosocial reorganization, planning, balancing conflicting demands, and facilitating an appropriate death) that, within the context of adaptational demands caused by experiences of loss and trauma, is stimulated in response to the awareness of life-threatening or terminal illness in oneself or a significant other and the recognition of associated losses in the past, present, and future.[4(p4)] It mandates a delicate balance of simultaneously holding onto, letting go of, and drawing closer to the dying loved one.[18(p35)]

- In the case of death through illness, anticipatory grief (mourning) has the potential to reduce or eliminate unfinished business, premature detachment, and poor communication with the dying person. Appropriate predeath interactions with the dying person may help to prevent postdeath grief complications.[18]

- Anticipatory grief (mourning) is multifaceted, involving numerous active processes of mourning, and should not be equated with postdeath grief. It does not automatically occur in the face of a terminal illness and is variable case by case as each caregiver will experience ambivalence, denial, and hope differently.[18]

- Anticipatory grief is a misnomer. One grieves not only for the anticipated loss of a loved one in the future, but also for past and present losses. Acknowledging that some view grief as a total detachment from the dying as opposed to detachment from one's previous hopes for the future with that person, Rando[18] asserts that anticipatory grief can go awry. Inappropriate, premature detachment can obstruct or block healthy interaction with the dying person.

- Anticipatory grief (mourning) is multidimensional and impacts the dying person and those with whom the person is emotionally involved. It encompasses the past, present, and future; and includes psychological, social, and physiological factors.[18]

- Anticipatory grief (mourning) for the caregiver presents a host of issues that may need to be addressed, including powerlessness, guilt, sorrows, depression, fear, anger, and uncertainty. The world that one knew may feel violated. There may be other, ongoing losses. Dealing with family disruptions, depletion of self in terms of energy, time, and finance, as well as balancing competing tasks may come into play.[18]

- Therapeutic anticipatory grief (mourning) engages three interdependent processes that build upon each other. The first is an individual, intrapsychic process in which the threat of the loss is gradually accommodated. Both affective and cognitive concerns are addressed, and the future is contemplated. The second is an interactional process. This includes intentional interaction with the dying person with the hopeful outcome of resolution of relationship issues. This interactional process includes the rendering of help to the dying person that serves to diminish feelings of uselessness. Finally, anticipatory grief (mourning) addresses and begins the renegotiation of familial and social processes.[18]

• Anticipatory grief (mourning) requires a balancing act on the part of the griever. Too much or too little can adversely impact the survivor's adjustment.[18]

"Normal Grief"

Beginning in infancy, the attachments made through relationships become the most significant aspect of our lives. A sense of wholeness is developed based on the perceived attitudes that develop from those relationships. Grief has the power to disrupt the life of a human being precisely because these attachments are broken. The experience of a broken attachment may also precipitate vulnerability in one's sense of wholeness.[21]

The Tasks of Grief

Pastoral theologian Oates[22] proposed a theory of grief in 1955. He identified common aspects in the grieving experience that included shock, numbness, the struggle of reality versus fantasy, an overwhelming flood of grief, selective memory, acceptance of the loss, and affirmation of moving on in life.

Since that time, numerous theorists have described grief as a process that includes specific stages.[23–25] Zisook (2009) emphasizes that these stages must not be taken too literally. Instead, they should be seen as a nonlinear, fluid process through which a person moves over the course of time. The most recent edition of the *Handbook of Psychiatry in Palliative Medicine*[5(p203)] proposes a conceptualization that grief be defined as "the permanent biopsychosocial response to the loss of an attachment figure" rather than a series of stages through which one moves. Within this conceptualization, numerous emotional and behavioral responses are outlined. Grief, whether conceived as specific tasks, fluid stages, or a permanent biopsychosocial response, evokes behavioral, cognitive, emotional, and spiritual states in human beings.[5,26]

Worden[26] discusses four tasks of mourning. In contrast to the "stages of grief" mentioned earlier, these four tasks are fluid as an individual moves through the experience of grief. The tasks of mourning include accepting the reality of the loss, working through the pain of grief, adjusting to an environment in which the deceased is missing, and emotionally relocating the deceased and moving on with one's life.[26]

The first part of the journey is accepting the reality that the person is dead and will not return. It is the acknowledgment that the deceased's reunion with this world is not possible. Behaviors the survivor may exhibit during this time include searching for the dead person, calling out to them, and perhaps even seeing the deceased during daily life activities.[26] In order to facilitate grieving persons' acceptance of their loss, Showalter[27] suggests that clinicians encourage the bereaved to name all of the losses incurred as a result of the death as a way of regaining control and coming to terms with its reality.

As an ego defense against the reality of a loss, denial is commonly employed by grieving persons. VanDuivendyk[28] asserts that this period is a gift that allows a person time to prepare for the truth by pushing away reality until one is ready to face the loss. In that sense, denial may be healthy. As an immature and inflexible defense, denial can also be maladaptive. A person might deny the reality of the loss or simply deny that death is irreversible. One might deny the meaning of a loss in an attempt to make the loss less significant than it actually is. An example would be choosing to believe "he wasn't a good dad," or "we weren't that close."[26,29] Accepting the reality of the loss takes time, because the adjustment is both intellectual and emotional. Persons may "know" that their loved one is dead, and yet years later instinctively pick up the phone to call the deceased to relay joyful news. Acceptance and denial may wax and wane over the course of the grieving process.[26]

Accepting the reality of the loss may be facilitated through a funeral service. The psychological benefits of a funeral lie in its confirmation of the reality of the death as well as setting the stage for acknowledgment and expression of feelings. In addition, recollections of the loved one stimulated at the funeral may accelerate healthy adjustments to the loss. Comments from friends and family are living memorials that help to integrate the image of the deceased. Social benefit is derived from funeral services in that the community is allowed to come together in a supportive way. The ritual, meaning, and structure of the funeral often serve to mitigate the loss of predictability and control that death engenders. It is a starting point for reintegrating the living into the community.[2] For some that community is religious where a common understanding of God or higher power provides strength, comfort, and hope for the future.

Working through the pain brought on by grief may be difficult and can affect individuals physically, psychically, socially, emotionally, and spiritually. There is an old adage, "the only way out of grief is through it." One may deny the pain, compartmentalize it, and pretend it is not there. The pain may be avoided through the use of alcohol and licit or illicit drug use. Others try to run from the loss by moving to a new location. Worden[26] asserts that acknowledging and working through the pain of grief is essential. Grief may manifest itself with other symptoms or maladaptive behaviors if this task is not accomplished. Parkes[10(p173)] was aware of this when he stated: "If it is necessary for the bereaved person to go through the pain of grief in order to get the grief work done, then anything that continually allows the person to avoid or suppress this pain can be expected to prolong the course of mourning."

Adjusting to an environment in which the deceased is missing is another task that may emerge about 3 months after death. The difficulty of the adjustment may be experienced when returning to an empty house, not having the phone answered when you call, reaching over in the middle of the night and finding no one there, raising children alone, or finding ways to make financial ends meet. There may be sleepless nights of pining, longing, and loneliness. One may begin to ask, "Who am I without this person?" and "In what do I really believe?" New roles will be adopted, and new skills will be learned.

Some bereaved people struggle in adapting to the loss by promoting their own helplessness and powerlessness, not developing new skills, and withdrawing from the world.[26] Over time, however, many people experience a growing sense of confidence, independence, and mastery of new tasks and skills, which are essential for adjusting to an environment in which the deceased is missing.[16]

Emotionally relocating the deceased and moving on with life is the last of the tasks described by Worden.[26] He describes the difficult task of finding the strength, energy, and courage necessary to give up the lost relationship and create new emotional attachments.

A simple visualization practice that may facilitate this process begins by asking participants to place one hand close in front of their eyes. Initially, all that can be seen is the hand, symbolizing the deceased and the grief the bereaved feels. As one slowly moves the hand away from the face, edges are perceived. As the fingers are slightly spread, one begins to see through the grief. The hand moves further from the face, and a world is recognized around the grief, a world in which one is a part and in which one can invest. Grief and the object of bereavement, symbolized by the hand and arm, are still attached though located in a different place. The grieving process is much the same. Space is created that allows the griever to form new attachments and experience love again.

Emotionally withdrawing from the deceased is not easy. Withdrawing may seem disloyal. The pain may be so intense that a vow is made to never love again. The counselor who comes alongside the bereaved faces the challenge of nurturing that person's reinvestment in the world and the people in it, coming to know that loving another does not mean that they loved the deceased less.[26]

Complications of Grief

Complicated grief (CG) is considered to be a prolonged reaction that goes beyond the expected response to the death of a loved one. It may lead to maladaptive behaviors and negative social and occupational functioning. It has also been associated with a higher rate of physical and mental health problems and even a higher mortality rate.[30–33]

In his classic work *Mourning and Melancholia*,[54] Freud discusses how individuals grieve and cope in different ways. He suggests that melancholia is a pathological reaction to the loss of a love attachment. These grief-stricken individuals have difficulty with integration of the loss and managing their external world. Freud, followed by other theorists, looked at love and attachment in relationships as an important factor in grief and loss. These ideas have had a lasting impact on the scientific study of grief and complications of grief.

Bowlby[34] looked at attachment seeking as an instinctive motivational system that begins at birth. Particular predisposing attachment styles may predict attachment-seeking behaviors throughout life. Bowlby[3,35] suggests that attachment behaviors that are repeated in life to fulfill otherwise unmet needs may lead to symptoms of CG when that bond is disrupted or lost.

Shear and Shair[36] postulate that it is important to know as much as possible about the characteristics of an adult attachment relationship to understand more precisely what is lost when a loved one dies. Attachment styles may be described as secure or insecure.

Insecure attachment styles may make an individual more vulnerable to separation distress later in life, leading to CG. An insecure attachment may be characterized by a feeling of uncertainty about the availability of an attachment figure. These attachments are characterized by higher-than-usual dependency needs in the relationship and higher anxiety and fear about separation. These personalities are prone to repeatedly attach to others in an unhealthy web that may result in the individual being unable to distinguish one's own thoughts and feeling from the other. Health care professionals may notice caregivers with compulsive caregiving styles, clinging, excessive dependency, and temperamental behaviors.[37] Other observable predeath family behaviors may include conflicted and hostile families, low levels of family cohesion, and a lack of expressiveness about thoughts and feelings.[38]

Relationships with stable secure attachments have been shown to be psychologically healthy and resilient.[39] A secure base in a relationship provides each individual to freely interact in the world, seek novelty, take risks, and explore the unknown. There is a natural confidence in the accessibility of the attachment figure and a sense of freedom and mutual independence. A bereaved individual from a secure attachment can more readily discuss attachment-related emotions and memories coherently and with good insight. He or she will react emotionally to the loss but is not as likely to feel overwhelmed by grief over time.

In consideration of attachment styles as a predictor of CG, there is a growing body of scientific literature that postulates an insecure, unhealthy attachment is more likely to lead to a persistent unresolved separation response. Identifying the maladaptive behaviors in bereaved individuals that occur as a result of unhealthy attachment styles would logically be a way to measure CG. The Inventory of Complicated Grief[40] is one tool that looks at this. A cluster of symptoms that include yearning, pining, and searching for the deceased and being stunned and unable to accept the reality of a loved one's death are all significant for the measurement of CG. Excessive anger and bitterness, along with prolonged difficulty moving on in life, may persist. This tool is a reliable self-report measure of CG at 6 months after the identified death. A score of 25 or more is considered to confirm a CG reaction. There have been more recent attempts to modify this tool and look at other factors to predict who may be at risk for CG. The World Health Organization (WHO) has advised palliative care providers of the need to provide support to caregivers after the death of a loved one.[41] It stands to reason that the more we know about the risk factors for CG predeath, the more likely therapeutic interventions

can be put into place earlier in the postdeath grief process (Tomarken et al,).[58]

Even though CG is not included in the DSM, a growing body of knowledge suggests between 10% and 25% of bereaved individuals experience CG.[36,43,44] These percentages suggest that 1 million individuals per year may experience CG.[45] There is ongoing debate about entering CG as a psychiatric disorder in the next edition of the DSM. In the current DSM edition,[1] enduring complications of grief are diagnosed as a major depressive episode (MDE), clinical anxiety, or posttraumatic stress disorder (PTSD).[46] Several studies have suggested that CG is a distinct disorder separate from the DMS-defined MDE, clinical anxiety, and PTSD and, if left untreated, may lead to long-lasting dysfunction.[43,44,47,48] This does not assume the idea that symptoms of CG are completely independent of the mental disorders mentioned, but that there should be a distinction made for reasons of diagnosis and treatment. Studies have demonstrated that symptoms of an MDE after a loss declined significantly with the use of an antidepressant, but other disturbing symptoms related to grief persisted.[40,49]

MDEs are not uncommon after the loss of a loved one and may affect as many as 25% of grieving individuals at 2 months postloss.[30] In developing criteria for CG, evidence suggests that symptoms assessed at 6 months postloss were more predictive of long-term complications than those assessed at 2 months. To allow individuals to suffer for 6 months before being considered for diagnosis and treatment seemed unethical.[43] It is therefore believed to be prudent to treat severe MDE at any time, and all cases of MDE after 2 months postloss even though CG is not considered "problematic" until 6 months.[5]

Suggestions for the treatment for grief-related syndromes are varied. As discussed earlier, the treatment for MDE should include the consideration of antidepressant therapy. The symptoms of CG may sometimes be resistant to antidepressant therapy; therefore, other treatment options should be considered. Shear and colleagues[45] used cognitive–behavioral therapy that directly addressed the trauma related to the loss to treat CG. They used exercises including repeated retelling of the story of the death and confronting previously avoided situations by encouraging imaginable conversations with the deceased. They showed that cognitive–behavioral therapy of this design was better than using supportive interpersonal psychotherapy for CG.

■ NONPHARMACOLOGIC INTERVENTIONS

The clinician's role in facilitating anticipatory grief, assessing for complicated bereavement, and offering community resources for grief is complex. Interventions might include:

- Open communication and honesty about treatment options and goals of care. Such communication contributes to symptom control, a sense of self-worth and self-control on the part of the patient and family, as well as helping to establish a therapeutic bond.[16]
- Encouragement of life review by facilitating reminiscing. Through these remembrances, meaning and purpose in life may be affirmed, forgiveness may be offered or received, and feelings may be shared.[50] Reminiscence is one of the ways in which the bereaved may recapture loving memories of the deceased prior to the illness.[51]
- Education about the process of anticipatory grief for the caregiver.
  - (a) Validation and normalization of ambivalent, conflicting feelings. For example, caregivers may experience guilt over wishing that the suffering would end. Other feelings may include sadness, anger, and hurt if the dying person begins to withdraw.
  - (b) Modeling behaviors for the caregivers such as sitting at the bedside, talking to and touching dying persons even if they are nonresponsive. Such behaviors on the part of the caregiver might mitigate feelings of uselessness.[51]
- Assessment for the risk of a complicated bereavement.
  - (a) Attentive listening and identification of the significance of losses a person is experiencing, including past, present, and future losses. Observation of adaptive and maladaptive coping styles.
  - (b) Utilization of a multidisciplinary approach that includes physician, nurse, social worker, counselor, and chaplain. This allows for the broadest understanding of family dynamics and observation of unhealthy attachment styles that may lead to CG.
  - (c) Planning of family meetings with the attending physician and members of the multidisciplinary team. These meetings allow for a common understanding of the disease process, provide an opportunity for the patient and family to express worries, fears, and concerns, and facilitate making short- and long-term plans. Family members may emerge with a greater sense of empowerment through knowledge, a sense of control, and a clearer sense of shared responsibility. In these meetings clinicians may observe family dynamics that predict maladaptive coping styles. Family members who are not present may alert the clinician to investigate their need for support.
  - (d) Observation of patterns of visitation, particularly watching for signs of detachment and absence on the part of significant others.
  - (e) Suggestion of follow-up with one's primary care physician.
- Facilitating grief work by using helpful techniques.
  - (a) Using evocative language—for example, using the word "death" or "died" may stimulate the expression of painful feelings and the acceptance of the reality of the loss.[26]
  - (b) Using symbols. Pictures, letters, clothing, or video tapes provide images and impressions of the deceased that may facilitate the bereaved speaking "to" the deceased and not "about" the deceased.[26]
  - (c) Encouraging writing a letter to the deceased. This may facilitate the expression of feelings and assist in bringing closure to unfinished business.[26]
  - (d) Encouraging drawing. Drawing may stimulate feelings and memories of the deceased. Children often respond well to this technique.[26]
  - (e) Setting up role play. Role play can be useful in anticipatory, normal, or CG as a way to build skills around situations that are feared or awkward to those grieving.[26]
  - (f) Using cognitive restructuring. This acknowledges that one's thoughts influence one's feelings. By assisting the bereaved to identify and express thoughts, particularly those that may be inaccurate, exaggerated, or irrational, the clinician may assist in ameliorating painful emotions.[26]
  - (g) Encouraging the creation of memory books. This may assist the bereaved in developing a realistic image of the dead person. A memory book may especially assist children as they reexperience grief at each developmental milestone.[26]
  - (h) Using guided visual imagery. Visualization may help by assisting the griever (whether in anticipation or postdeath) to picture the dying or deceased and say what needs to be said to that person. These voicings may include regrets and

disappointments as well as affirmations and expressions of love.[26]

- Encouraging the use of rituals.
  - (a) Facilitating expression of the grieving process through attention to rituals that symbolize transition, healing, and continuity.[52]
  - (b) Inquiring about religious beliefs and making referrals to clerics as appropriate.
  - (c) Rituals provide a way for individuals or groups to act out their grief through structured activities that help to overcome emptiness, provide a sense of self-control, release emotions, and channel grief within specific time frames, making overwhelming feelings more manageable.[2]
- Encouraging the use of community resources.
  - (a) Recognizing that the bulk of grief work is done outside of the medical community.
  - (b) Suggesting a visit to one's primary care physician to assess one's overall physical and emotional well-being.
  - (c) Identifying resources in the community that offer grief support: hospices, funeral homes, religious communities, American Cancer Society, and counseling centers.
- Identifying online resources such as:
  - (a) The Dougy Center (http://www.dougy.org);
  - (b) GriefNet (http://www.griefnet.org)
  - (c) Growth House, Inc (http://www.growthouse.org);
  - (d) Transformations (http://www.transformations.com).
- Identifying resources for those with complications of bereavement such as:
  - (a) Depression and Bipolar Support Alliance (http://www.dbsalliance.org);
  - (b) National Alliance on Mental Illness (http://www.nami.org);
  - (c) National Institute of Mental Health (http://www.nimh.nih.gov);
  - (d) National Mental Health Association (http://www.nmha.org).
- Offering educational events with and for community organizations that address grief needs.

■ THE CLINICIAN'S GRIEF

Clinicians working in oncology encounter grief every day. A clinician may choose to deny this reality, risking the professional burnout that comes from emotional detachment. By recognizing and embracing the myriad of losses encountered daily and seeking ways in which to find renewal, the professional may continue serving with compassion.

Confronting our own mortality is an important contribution to the well-being of those we encounter. Failing to examine our personal relationship to impermanence and loss will inevitably deaden our relationship to the stark realities confronted by our patients. Examples of self-care may include the completion of a will, advance directive, and desired funeral arrangement, or contemplation of phone calls to be made because of unfinished business. Also included is reflection on questions such as: What experiences and lessons shape your ideas about death and dying? What are your hopes and goals before life ends? What attitudes need adjustment? Attending the funeral of a patient may help. Experience the finality, the pain and sorrow, the finiteness and limitation, and the awareness of personal mortality. Within the workplace itself, grief among coworkers can be acknowledged in healthy ways through intentional time taken for expression of feelings, memorial services for patients and memory boards, or memory books for specific families.

KEY POINTS

- Grief is an expected human response to loss.
- Grief reactions are precipitated not only by loss due to death, but also by material, relational, health, role, systemic, and assumptive losses.
- Grief impacts people affectively, physically, cognitively, spiritually, and behaviorally.
- Anticipatory grief allows for the reality of the loss to be absorbed over time, the resolution of unfinished business, the review of one's assumptive world, and the consideration of future plans.
- CG is experienced by 10% to 25% of the bereaved population.
- CG is more likely to be experienced by bereaved individuals who have had unhealthy attachment lifestyles.
- Clinicians who address their mortality and attend to their grief may be less prone to compassion fatigue and burnout.

REFERENCES

1. American Psychiatric Association. *Diagnostic and Statistical Manual of Mental Disorders*. 4th ed, text revision. Washington, DC: Author; 2000.

2. Rando TA. *Grief, Dying, and Death*. Champaign, Ill: Research Press Company; 1984.

3. Bowlby J. *Attachment and Loss: Loss—Sadness and Depressive Symptoms*. Vol 3. New York, NY: Basic Books; 1980.

4. Rando TA. The six dimensions of anticipatory mourning. In: Rando TA, ed. *Clinical Dimensions of Anticipatory Mourning*. Champaign, Ill: Research Press; 2000.

5. Zisook S, Irwin SA, Shear MK. Understanding and managing bereavement in palliative care. In: Chochinov HM, Breitbart W, eds. *Handbook of Psychiatry in Palliative Medicine*. 2nd ed. New York, NY: Oxford University Press; 2009.

6. Holmes T, Rahe R. The Social Readjustment Rating Scale. *J Psychosom Res*. 1967;11(2):213–218.

7. Baumeister RF. *Meanings of Life*. New York, NY: Guilford Press; 1991.

8. Engel GL. Is grief a disease? *Psychosom Med*. 1961;23: 18–22.

9. Lindemann E. Symptomatology and management of acute grief. *Am J Psychiatry*. 1944;101:141–148.

10. Parkes CM. Psychosocial transitions: a field study. *Soc Sci Med*. 1971;5:101–115.

11. Harlow SD, Goldberg EL, Comstock GW. A longitudinal study of the prevalence of depressive symptomatology in elderly widowed and married women. *Arch Gen Psychiatry*. 1991;48:1065–1068.

12. Zisook S. Unresolved grief. In: Zisook S, ed. *Biopsychosocial Aspects of Bereavement*. Washington, DC: American Psychiatric Association; 1987.

13. Zisook S, Shuchter SR. Uncomplicated bereavement. *J Clin Psychiatry*. 1993;54(10):365–372.

14. Goin MK, Burgoyne RW, Goin JM. Timeless attachment to a dead relative. *Am J Psychiatry*. 1979;136:988–989.

15. Wolfelt A, Holping Dispel S. Common myths about grief. Available at: www.centerforloss.com. 2007. Accessed September 2010.

16. Storey P, Knight CF. *Alleviating Psychological and Spiritual Pain in the Terminally Ill*. 2nd ed. New York, NY: Mary Ann Liebert Inc; 2003.

17. Cassell EJ. *The Nature of Suffering and the Goals of Medicine*. New York, NY: Oxford University Press; 1991.

18. Rando TA. Living and learning the reality of a loved one's dying: traumatic stress and cognitive processing in anticipatory grief. In: Doka KJ, Davidson J, eds. *Living with Grief: When Illness is Prolonged*. Bristol, Pa: Taylor & Francis; 1997.

19. Fulton R, Fulton J. A psychosocial aspect of terminal care: anticipatory grief. *Omega*. 1971;2:91–99.

20. Parkes CM, Weiss RS. *Recovery from Bereavement*. New York, NY: Basic Books; 1983.

21. Switzer, DK. Grief and loss. In: Hunter RJ, ed. *Dictionary of Pastoral Care and Counseling*. Nashville, Tenn: Abingdon Press; 1990.

22. Oates W. *Anxiety in Christian Experience*. Philadelphia, Pa: The Westminster Press; 1955.

23. DeVaul RA, Zisook S, Faschingbauer TR. Clinical aspects of grief and bereavement. *Prim Care*. 1979;6(2): 391–402.

24. Glick IO, Weiss RS, Parkes CM. *The First Year of Bereavement*. New York, NY: John Wiley; 1974.

25. Pollock GH. The mourning–liberation process in health and disease. *Psychiatr Clin North Am*. 1987;10:345–354.

26. Worden JW. *Grief Counseling and Grief Therapy: A Handbook for the Mental Health Practitioner*. New York, NY: Springer Publishing Company; 1991.

27. Showalter SE. Coping with loss. *Am J Hospice Palliat Care*. 1996;13(5):46–48.

28. Vanduivendyk TP. *The Unwanted Gift of Grief*. Binghamton, NY: The Haworth Press; 2006.

29. Dorpat TL. Suicide, loss and mourning. *Life Threat Behav*. 1973;3:213–224.

30. Clayton, PJ. Bereavement and depression. *J Clin Psychiatry*. 1990;51(7):34–40.

31. Kaprio J, Koskenvuo M, Heli R. Mortality after bereavement: a prospective study of 95,647 widowed persons. *Am J Public Health*. 1987;77(3):283–287.

32. Prigerson HG, Bierhals AJ, Kasl SV, et al. Traumatic grief as a risk factor for mental and physical morbidity. *Am J Psychiatry*. 1997;154(5):616–623.

33. Zisook S, Shuchter SR, Sledge PA, et al. The spectrum of depressive phenomena after spousal bereavement. *J Clin Psychiatry*. 1994;55(4):29–36.

34. Bowlby J. *Attachment and Loss: Attachment*. Vol 1. New York, NY: Basic Books; 1969.

35. Bowlby J. *Attachment and Loss: Separation—Anxiety and Anger*. Vol 2. New York, NY: Basic Books; 1973.

36. Shear K, Shair H. Attachment, loss, and complicated grief. *Dev Psychobiol*. 2005;47(3):253–267.

37. Van Doorn C, Kasl S, Beery L, et al. The influence of marital quality and attachment styles on traumatic grief and depressive symptoms. *J Nerv Ment Dis.* 1998;186(9): 566–573.

38. Grassi L. Bereavement in families with relatives dying of cancer. *Curr Opin Support Palliat Care.* 2007;1:43–49.

39. Mikulincer M, Shaver PR, Pereg D. Attachment theory and affect regulation: the dynamics, development and cognitive consequences of attachment-related strategies. *Motiv Emotion.* 2003;27:77–102.

40. Prigerson HG, Maciejewski PK, Reynolds CF, et al. Inventory of complicated grief: a scale to measure maladaptive symptoms of loss. *Psychiatry Res.* 1995;59:65–79.

41. Johnson G, Abraham C. The WHO objectives for palliative care: to what extent are we achieving them? *Palliat Med.* 1995;9:123–137.

42. BrintzenhofeSzoc KM, Smith ED, Zabora JR. Screening to predict complicated grief in spouses of cancer patients. *Cancer Pract.* 1999;7(5):233–239.

43. Lichtenthal WG, Cruess DG, Prigerson HG. A case for establishing complicated grief as a distinct mental disorder in DSM-V. *Clin Psychol Rev.* 2004;6:637–662.

44. Simon NM, Shear KM, Thompson EH, et al. The prevalence and correlates of psychiatric comorbidity in individuals with complicated grief. *Compr Psychiatry.* 2007;48(5):395–399.

45. Shear K, Frank E, Houck PR, Reynolds CF. Treatment of complicated grief. *JAMA.* 2005;293(21):2601–2608.

46. Bonanno GA, Neria Y, Mancini A, Coifman KG, Litz B, Inse B. Is there more to complicated grief than depression and posttraumatic stress disorder? A test of incremental validity. *J Abnorm Psychol.* 2007;116(2):342–351.

47. Boelen PA, van den Bout J. Complicated grief, depression, and anxiety as distinct post loss syndromes: a confirmatory factor analysis study. *Am J Psychiatry.* 2005;162(11):2175–2177.

48. Prigerson HG, Bierhals AJ, Kasl SV, et al. Complicated grief as a disorder distinct from bereavement-related depression and anxiety: a replication study. *Am J Psychiatry.* 1996;153(11):1484–1486.

49. Pasternak RE, Reynolds CF, Schlernitzauer MA, et al. Open-trial nortriptyline therapy of bereavement-related depression in late life. *J Clin Psychiatry.* 1991;52: 307–310.

50. Lichter I, Mooney J, Boyd M. Biography as therapy. *Palliat Med.* 1993;7:133–137.

51. Doka KJ. When illness is prolonged: implications for grief. In: Doka KJ, Davidson J, eds. *Living with Grief: When Illness is Prolonged.* Bristol, Pa: Taylor & Francis; 1997.

52. Van der Hart O. *Rituals in Psychotherapy: Transition and Continuity.* New York, NY: Irvington; 1983.

53. Corr CA, Corr DM. Anticipatory mourning and coping with dying: similarities, differences, and suggested guidelines for helpers. In: Rando TA, ed. *The Clinical Dimensions of Anticipatory Mourning.* Champaign, Ill: Research Press; 2000.

54. Freud S. Mourning and melancholia. In: *Complete Psychological Works.* Vol 14. Standard ed. London: Hogarth Press; 1957.

55. Osterweis M, Solomon F, Green M, eds. *Bereavement: Reactions, Consequences, and Care.* Washington, DC: National Academy Press; 1984.

56. Parkes CM. *Bereavement: Studies of Grief in Adult Life.* New York, NY: International Universities Press; 1972.

57. Shuchter SR, Zisook S. The course of normal grief. In: Stroebe MS, Stroebe W, Hansson RO, eds. *Handbook of Bereavement: Theory, Research and Intervention.* Cambridge: Cambridge University Press; 1997.

58. Tomarken A, Holland J, Schachter S, et al. Factors of complicated grief pre-death in caregivers of cancer patients. *Psychooncology.* 2008;17:105–111.

Palliative Medicine and the Cancer Patient

• *David Hui and Eduardo Bruera*

■ INTRODUCTION

Despite significant progress in the treatment of cancer, approximately half of all cancer patients would eventually succumb to their disease, with one third of the deaths happening within 6 months of diagnosis.[1] Palliative care is an approach that improves the quality of life of patients and their families living with a life-threatening illness through the prevention and relief of suffering by means of early identification and impeccable assessment and treatment of pain and other problems, physical, psychosocial, and spiritual.[2] Good symptom management contributes not only to improving patients' quality of life, but also to supporting patients through intensive treatments. The 58th World Health Assembly[3] emphasizes that palliative care should be represented as one of the four pillars of modern oncology, alongside the disciplines of medical, radiation, and surgical oncology. Indeed, as patients with advanced cancer live longer as a result of advances in cancer therapy, the need for palliative care is only going to increase.

In this chapter, we shall discuss the structure, processes, outcomes, and challenges related to palliative care for advanced cancer patients. Specifically, we will address the various components of the palliative care team and organizational structure in the oncology setting. Following this, we shall review the key assessment and management strategies to physical, psychosocial, and existential distress in patients and their caregivers, and examine a number of palliative care–related outcomes. In the final

section, we shall highlight several key challenges faced by palliative care, and the potential solutions to overcoming these barriers.

■ STRUCTURE OF PALLIATIVE CARE

The Palliative Care Team

The nature of palliative medicine involves provision of care to patients with advanced disease who frequently experience complex symptoms and psychosocial issues. This necessitates a highly integrated interprofessional team with acquired expertise in symptom management, communication skills, and end-of-life decision making to provide comprehensive support to both patients and caregivers. A palliative care team typically consists of physicians, nurses, social workers, pharmacists, dieticians, chaplains, physiotherapists, and occupational therapists (Fig. 25-1). Depending on the local resources, other disciplines such as clinical psychologists, psychiatrists, music therapists, and art therapists may also contribute as part of the team.[4,5]

Because of the complex and ever-evolving needs of patients with advanced cancer, members of the palliative care team need to communicate frequently and regularly to share updated assessments, and to establish common goals of care and treatment plans. Good communication helps to ensure that the various aspects of care are addressed in a comprehensive manner, and that all members of the team communicate with patients

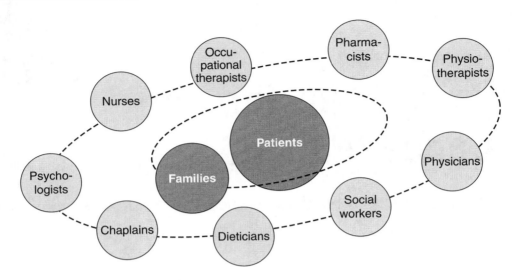

FIGURE 25-1. Interprofessional nature of palliative care. The multidisciplinary nature of palliative care allows the health care team to address patients' and their caregivers' physical, psychosocial, and existential needs in a holistic manner. Furthermore, excellent communication among team members (dotted line) allows the team to provide consistent messages, treatment plans, and direction of care.

and their families with a unified message to minimize confusion and iatrogenic distress. In particular, family meetings represent a powerful intervention that brings the patient, family, palliative care, and oncology teams together.[6]

The Palliative Care Settings

The organizational structure of palliative care is depicted in Figure 25-2, and may include an inpatient consultation service (mobile team), inpatient palliative care unit (PCU), and/or outpatient clinic. The backbone of inpatient palliative medicine is the consultation team, which receives referrals from inpatient oncology units and provides expert advice regarding symptom management, psychosocial support, transition of care, and discharge planning.

In some cancer centers, a PCU is available in which patients with advanced cancer can be admitted directly under palliative care. It represents an ideal setting for advanced cancer patients with severe physical, emotional, or existential distress, regardless of prognosis. One key advantage of a PCU is the ability to mobilize the interdisciplinary team, where patients and caregivers

can receive intensive supportive measures.[7-9] The PCU is a versatile machine designed to deliver personalized medicine tailored to the individual's needs. For patients who are dying, the PCU enables optimal symptom control, with a focus on comfort measures. For patients who are likely to go home, the PCU actively treats acute complications and symptoms related to the cancer and its treatments, and administers anticancer therapies. For patients who are going to hospice, the PCU represents a place of transition, both physically and psychologically, for them and their families. Thus, the PCU facilitates complex decision making and bridges the gap between acute care and the community (Fig. 25-2).

A third component of palliative care is the outpatient clinic, which provides consultation for patients from oncology clinics, and follow-up for patients recently discharged home from hospital. Compared with patients seen by palliative care in the inpatient services, patients who attend the outpatient clinic are generally not acutely ill, and are more likely to have a better performance status and a longer life expectancy. The outpatient clinic provides a unique setting where patients can be referred to palliative care earlier in the disease trajectory, enabling the team to provide longitudinal

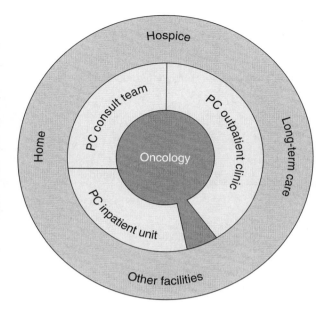

FIGURE 25-2. Structure of palliative care. Oncology service (innermost circle) is provided mainly through outpatient clinics, with a small proportion of patients requiring admission to the oncology inpatient unit for supportive measures or treatment administration. The palliative care service (middle circle) consists of inpatient consultation team, and in some cases palliative care unit and outpatient clinics, providing physical, psychosocial, and spiritual support. As patients get closer to the end of life, they may benefit from hospice services (outermost circle). Palliative care plays a critical role facilitating the transition from active treatment to end-of-life care.

follow-up, manage symptoms in a timely fashion, establish rapport with patients and their families, and facilitate a smooth transition of care over the course of illness.[10]

Palliative care and hospice care are frequently discussed together because they both focus on improving quality of life for patients with advanced disease; however, an important distinction should be made. The practice of palliative care is predominantly hospital based, while hospice delivers care in the community. Thus, patients seen by the palliative care team tend to be sicker, more likely in acute distress, and require more intensive management compared with hospice patients.[11] Furthermore, hospice predominantly focuses on end-of-life care, while palliative care is positioned to deliver care over the heterogeneous spectrum of disease from the time of diagnosis to death.[12]

■ THE PROCESSES OF PALLIATIVE CARE

In this section, we shall discuss the clinical assessment and management of physical, psychosocial, and existential distress. We will also address two critical clinical skills, communication and decision making in palliative care.

Management of Physical Distress

Patients with advanced cancer often have a high symptom burden as a result of progressive disease and/or antineoplastic treatments. For instance, patients with non-small cell lung cancer experience an average of 14 symptoms, while patients with small cell lung cancer report an average of 17 symptoms.[13] Another study using the Memorial Symptom Assessment Scale showed that advanced cancer patients have an average of 11 ± 6 symptoms.[14] While generation of sensory afferent input is an important determinant of symptom severity, how patients perceive and eventually express their symptoms can be modulated by various internal and external factors, including genetics, mental status, culture, social roles, expectations, understanding of the illness, personality, mood, setting, comorbid conditions, and rapport/trust in the health care team (Fig. 25-3).

Symptoms such as fatigue, pain, anorexia, constipation, and sleep disturbances are almost universally experienced by patients with advanced cancer, and frequently occur in clusters.[15,16] Dyspnea, nausea, diarrhea, and swelling may also occur, and can be very distressing to patients. Delirium is common among hospitalized patients, particularly those close to the end of life.[17,18] These physical symptoms not only impair patients' quality of life, but also affect their mobility and function, resulting in further distress in patients and their caregivers.[19]

Studies have demonstrated that patients tend to underreport their symptoms, which leads to underdiagnosis and undertreatment. Reasons for nondisclosure include fear of disease progression, apprehension that maximal treatment will not be offered, concern that they would be labeled as a complainer, belief that symptoms would not persist, and impression that no supportive treatments are available.[20] Thus, effective management of physical symptoms should begin with routine screening. Table 25-1 lists a number of well-validated instruments available for this purpose.[29] Positive items from screening should be followed by a focused history and physical to delineate the many factors contributing to a particular patient's symptom expression as outlined in Figure 25-3.

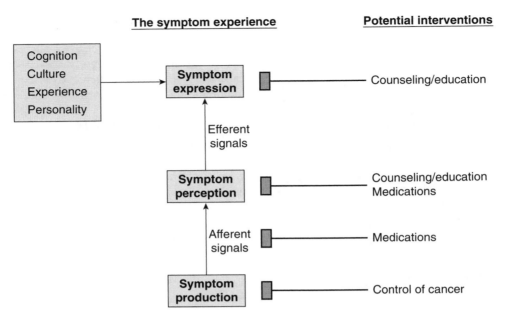

FIGURE 25-3. The pathway of symptom expression. Noxious stimuli result in neurotransmitter release, with subsequent activation of afferent neuronal pathways leading to the central nervous system. These signals are processed in the cerebral cortex, producing various sensations. However, how patients perceive and ultimately express their symptoms is dependent on many other factors, such as genetics, mental status, culture, social roles, expectations, understanding of the illness, personality, mood, setting, comorbid conditions, and rapport/trust in the health care team.

A detailed discussion of treatment of various symptoms is beyond the scope of this chapter. In addition to regular screening and good history taking, one key principle in management is involvement of the interdisciplinary team, as patients with advanced cancer seldom present with a single-dimension symptom. For instance, high doses of analgesia alone may not be effective in managing a patient with a high expression of pain if that patient also has severe emotional distress. Rather, the use of expressive counseling in conjunction with pain medications may be warranted.

Management of Psychosocial Distress

In addition to physical symptoms, advanced cancer is associated with many stressors, unpleasant feelings, and mood alterations, starting from the time of diagnosis to the time of death. According to the National Comprehensive Cancer Network, distress is defined as "a multifactorial unpleasant emotional experience of a psychological (cognitive, behavioral, emotional), social, and/or spiritual nature that may interfere with the ability to cope effectively with cancer, its physical symptoms and its treatment. Distress extends along a continuum, ranging from common normal feelings of vulnerability, sadness, and fears to problems that can become disabling, such as depression, anxiety, panic, social isolation, and existential and spiritual crisis."[30,31]

Emotional Reactions

Patients with advanced cancer frequently have to face bad news, such as abnormal investigation results, the need for further testing, disease progression, treatment failure, and lack of any further cancer treatment options. Patients' mood may also be negatively affected by the burden of physical symptoms, alterations in appearance, changes in bodily and sexual functions, and deterioration in performance status. End of life is associated with further distress as patients enter an irreversible phase of decline, with the impending loss of life compounded by existential concerns.

■ TABLE 25-1. Instruments for Symptom Screening and Assessments

Screening Tools	Description
Battery of symptoms	
Edmonton Symptom Assessment Scale (ESAS)[21]	Likert scale 1 to 10 for 10 symptoms including pain, fatigue, nausea, depression, anxiety, drowsiness, appetite, well-being, shortness of breath, and sleep
Global Distress Index of the Memorial Symptom Assessment Scale (MSAS-GDI)[22]	Likert scale 0 to 4 for 10 symptoms including lack of appetite, lack of energy, pain, drowsiness, constipation, dry mouth, sadness, worrying, irritability, and nervousness
Delirium	
Memorial Delirium Assessment Scale (MDAS)[23]	Likert scale 1 to 3 for 10 questions, including reduced level of consciousness, disorientation, short-term memory impairment, impaired digit span, reduced ability to maintain and shift attention, disorganized thinking, perceptual disturbance, delusions, decreased or increased psychomotor activity, and sleep–wake cycle disturbance. Higher scores suggest worse delirium (cutoff is traditionally defined as 7)
Mini-Mental State Examination (MMSE)[24]	Scored between 0 and 30 (normal). Key domains include orientation, repetition, recall, language use, comprehension, and basic motor skills
Alcoholism	
CAGE questionnaire[25]	4 questions including alcohol use, feeling to cut back, annoyed by others, feeling of guilt, and eye opener
Performance	
ECOG performance status[26]*	Simple and well-validated scale from 0 (normal) to 4 (bed bound)
Karnofsky performance status[27]	Scale from 0% (death) to 100% (normal function)
Palliative Performance Scale[28]	Modified from the Karnofsky performance status, with detailed description of ambulation, activity and evidence of disease, self-care, intake, and level of consciousness. Rating is from 0% (death) to 100% (normal function)

*Eastern Cooperative Oncology Group.

Despite the many challenges, patients with advanced cancer cope by maintaining a sense of hope, and, at times, heightened expectations for cancer treatments, clinical trials, and survival. However, as disease progresses on treatment, a sense of disillusionment and loss of direction may set in.[32]

Emotions commonly experienced by patients include shock, fear, anger, worry, anxiety, despair, grief, and denial. Given the circumstances, it is important to recognize that many of these feelings are normal, and may simply be monitored without specific interventions. However,

when these negative emotions become prolonged or significantly interfere with patients' daily function, it is important to provide the necessary support and counseling to alleviate undue psychological suffering.

Defensive and Coping Mechanisms

Patients utilize various defensive and coping strategies to deal with the many uncertainties and stressors associated with diagnosis, treatment, and progression of advanced cancer. Defense is defined as the conscious or subconscious avoidance of realities, while coping is an active problem-solving approach to dealing with issues.[33] Defensive mechanisms tend to be passive acts for suppressing/repressing emotions, and may include denial, withdrawal, rationalization (making up "logical" arguments), intellectualization (flight into reasons removing emotions), displacement, fantasy or wishful thinking, and engaging in addictive behaviors (eg, alcohol, illicit drugs). In comparison, coping mechanisms involve active engagement to deal with problem at hand, such as seeking social/religious support, discussing concerns with family, friends, or health care team, and applying various relaxation techniques.

Health care professionals can help patients to cope by supporting certain strategies that have worked for them in the past. Interference is generally not recommended if the coping strategies and defense mechanisms are adaptive to avoid disruption of a patient's emotional equilibrium. However, if and when these mechanisms become maladaptive and start to negatively affect a patient's daily function and decision-making capability, it is important to intervene clinically to minimize any further harm.[33]

Palliative care specialists and other health care professionals have an important role in helping patients to cope physically and emotionally during their illness. Clayton et al[34] highlighted a number of coping strategies that should be emphasized with patients and their families, which include (1) emphasizing what can be done, such as control of physical symptoms, emotional support, care, dignity, and practical logistics, (2) exploring realistic goals and helping patients to achieve them, and (3) discussing day-to-day living strategies.

Depression

The diagnosis of depression poses a particular challenge in advanced cancer patients, due to the fact that depressed mood is often a natural reaction to the multiple stressors while living with a life-limiting illness.[35] Furthermore, many of the physical symptoms that occur with depression, such as anorexia, weight loss, insomnia, and fatigue, are common at the end of life. However, when the sense of hopelessness, worthlessness, guilt, or grief becomes severe enough to interfere with daily function, active treatment for depression should be sought.

Prior to the diagnosis of depression in patients with advanced cancer, it is important to rule out various organic etiologies such as brain metastases and hypothyroidism. Hypoactive delirium also frequently mimics depression. History of any preexisting psychiatric disorders, alcohol abuse, and illicit substance use should also be noted, along with a detailed review of social history. All patients with suspected depression should be assessed for suicide risk. Advanced age, poor prognosis, lack of social support, sense of hopelessness, and delirium represent a number of important risk factors for suicide in cancer patients.[36]

Depression can be effectively treated using a combination of nonpharmacologic and pharmacologic measures. Exercise (eg, walking 30 minutes per day)[37] and exposure to bright light (eg, outdoors for 45 minutes per day)[38,39] both represent effective measures for improving mood and well-being, and should be encouraged.

In a *Cochrane* meta-analysis of advanced cancer patients with depressed mood but not yet been diagnosed with depression, psychotherapy is associated with a significant decrease in depression score compared with treatment as usual.[40] Different types of psychotherapy include supportive expressive counseling, cognitive behavioral therapy, and problem-solving therapy. While psychotherapy has not been studied in detail in advanced cancer patients diagnosed with major depressive disorder, it represents an important nonpharmacologic intervention for patients and an important skill for palliative care specialists.

Antidepressants such as tricyclic antidepressants (TCAs), selective serotonin reuptake inhibitors (SSRIs), and related agents can be useful.[41] The choice of medication depends on patients' symptoms. Patients with psychomotor agitation may be prescribed sedating medications such as mirtazapine and nortriptyline, while those with psychomotor retardation may benefit from fluoxetine. The effect of SSRIs may not be noticeable until 4 to 6 weeks; thus, patients with a short survival may benefit from more rapid-acting agents such as psychostimulants instead. Methylphenidate, dexamphetamine, methylamphetamine, and pemoline have demonstrated efficacy for the treatment of depression in far advanced cancer patients.[42] Patients with significant depression should be also referred to psychiatry for further management.

Anxiety

Physical, psychosocial, and existential stressors all contribute to anxiety in advanced cancer patients.[43] Thus, management of anxiety requires interdisciplinary interventions addressing specific contributing factors, including symptom management, supportive psychotherapy, and spiritual counseling. Relaxation techniques such as meditation and guided imagery may also be useful for some patients.

Benzodiazepines have been most commonly prescribed for anxiety, although evidence supporting its use is limited.[44] Other potential medications include antidepressants, buspirone, chlorpromazine, haloperidol, olanzapine, risperidone, hydroxyzine, methotrimeprazine, and thioridazine. Further research is required to determine the role of these agents for patients with advanced cancer.

Caregiver Support

In addition to holistic care for the cancer patient, palliative care places a particular emphasis on caregivers. This is because caregivers play a crucial role supporting their loved ones both physically and emotionally, and their well-being is often one of the key concerns for patients. Furthermore, many patients become delirious close to the end of life, necessitating substitute decision making. In these instances, the palliative care team works closely with patients' family caregivers to establish goals of care and end-of-life planning.[45]

The overall well-being of caregivers and patients is intricately linked. Caregivers are at risk of developing emotional distress, given the physical burden of providing care and the emotional burden of seeing their loved ones suffer. A recent study suggests that aggressive interventions at the end of life are associated with a higher risk of major depressive disorder in bereaved caregivers.[46] Family meetings can be useful in bringing patients, their caregivers, and the health care team on the same page. At the same time, split visits may be useful to discuss specific needs of caregivers, and strategies to help them prepare ahead.[47] Like patients, caregivers may also benefit from supportive psychotherapy.[48]

Another critical function of palliative care is the facilitation of anticipatory grief and bereavement in caregivers through education, counseling, and support. Caregivers should know that grieving is a natural process, and should be monitored for development of complicated grief.[49–51]

Understanding the Process of Dying

As the end of life approaches, it is important to educate patients and their families regarding the symptoms that are likely to occur, including being bedridden, delirium, and any other potentially distressing symptoms.[52] For instance, if family members were explained that death rattle is a natural process not associated with shortness of breath or patient distress, they may feel more at ease when it happens. By normalizing the process of dying, the palliative care team can help to lessen anxiety, reduce psychosocial suffering, and minimize emergency room visits. Moreover, patients and families can be better prepared logistically by anticipating their needs. Importantly, they should be reassured that the palliative care team is committed to providing continuity of care, and minimizing suffering through symptom optimization and holistic support.

Management of Existential Distress

The last few months of life represent one of the most stressful periods, yet one that also potentially carries the highest significance in life. If patients were relatively free from distress and have intact cognition, they may have the opportunity to reflect on their achievements, attempt closures with family and friends, define life's meaning, and prepare for the journey ahead. Indeed, some of the most important concerns for terminally ill cancer patients are existential in nature. These include "having a sense of hope," "knowing that my life has meaning and purpose," and "knowing that my life has been productive."[53] Spiritual issues such as "finding strength/comfort in my beliefs" are also important.

Thus, it is critical that the palliative care team helps alleviate suffering in its different forms, addresses patients' existential concerns, and facilitates a smooth transition. In this section, we shall discuss the concepts of suffering, total pain, hope, and meaning, and review practical measures to improve existential well-being.

Suffering and Total Pain

Dr Cassel[54] defines suffering as "the state of severe distress associated with events that threaten the intactness of the person." Living with advanced cancer, particularly at the end of life, inevitably involves variable degrees of physical, psychosocial, and existential suffering. One of the main goals of medicine is the relief of human suffering, although clinicians sometimes inadvertently introduce iatrogenic suffering through aggressive interventions, miscommunication, and missed therapeutic opportunities. Palliative medicine represents the discipline with acquired expertise aimed at minimizing suffering through comprehensive assessments and interprofessional teamwork.

Another concept similar to suffering is the idea of "total pain," defined as the sum of four components: physical, psychological, social, and spiritual.[55] This important framework highlights the complex interconnectedness between the body, mind, and spirit. For instance, a patient may rate his or her hip pain as 3 out of 10 due to the nociceptive input from bone metastasis, while another patient with similar level of noxious physical stimuli may rate his

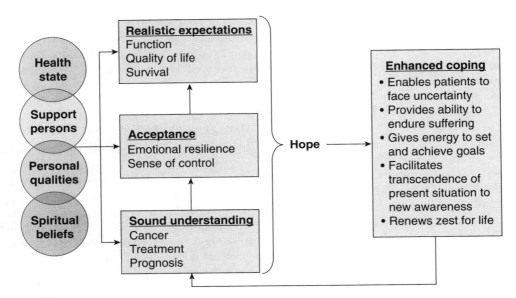

FIGURE 25-4. A conceptual model of hope. Authentic or essential hope is a process that requires (1) a clear understanding of the nature of disease, (2) emotional acceptance of the situation, and (3) the ability to set realistic goals. All of these steps are modulated by patients' physical, psychological, social, and spiritual state, in addition to personal preferences. Realistic hope can help patients cope better by developing new understanding and new awareness, which in turn could empower new hope. Health care professionals can help patients understand that they can have many different types of hopes at the same time.

or her pain as 10 out of 10 because of significant psychosocial (eg, recent divorce) or spiritual (eg, punishment from God) distress.[56] Pain of the first patient can easily be managed with analgesics, while pain of the second patient warrants comprehensive assessment with multidisciplinary input. The palliative medicine approach epitomizes an understanding of this complex relationship, and provides personalized care tailored to the individual's needs.

Hope and Meaning

Hope is defined as "a multidimensional dynamic life force characterized by a confident yet uncertain expectation of achieving a future good that, to the hoping person, is realistically possible and personally significant."[57] While hope is a future-oriented phenomenon, hoping is very much in the present. In a concept analysis, Johnson[58] identified 10 attributes of hope, including (1) positive expectation, (2) personal qualities with an inner strength and problem-solving approach to life, (3) spirituality, (4) goals, (5) comfort, (6) help/caring, (7) interpersonal relationships, (8) control, (9) legacy, and (10) life review.

Hope is a process that evolves with patients' comprehension of their illness. To foster realistic hope, patients need to have a clear understanding of their disease, along with emotional acceptance of their illness, from which they can derive realistic expectations and a sense of meaning (Fig. 25-4). It is important that patients know that they can hope for many things at the same time along the spectrum of hope.[34] In addition to hoping for a cure, patients and families can hope to live longer, enjoy a better quality of life, have the opportunities to complete important tasks, and achieve immortality. Specifically, immortality can be realized through surviving in the next generation, recognizing past contributions to society, and spiritual enlightenment.

The worry about destroying hope is one of the reasons for pursuing aggressive therapies and delaying end-of-life discussions. Yet, it is important to understand that essential hope is based on a good understanding and acceptance of reality. Palliative care can foster hope by many means. Specifically, all members of the palliative care team can help build and maintain realistic hope by providing optimal symptom control, being compassionate, communicating in a sensitive manner, providing supportive counseling, assisting patients to identify and accomplish specific tasks, and suggesting coping strategies.[34] Social workers are particularly well equipped to provide psychosocial and logistical support, while chaplains have an in-depth knowledge and experience to help patients explore their spirituality.

Life Review and Closure

Conduction of a life review is an important intervention to help patients foster hope, discover meaning, and, in the process, minimize suffering. Through reminiscing and self-reflection, patients have the opportunity to affirm their reasons for existence, arrive at resolutions, establish new understanding, and attain enlightenment. While life review can be conducted at bedside through daily interviews, dignity therapy represents a formal approach to perform a life review.[59] In a dedicated one-on-one session, a patient is asked specific questions about his or her life story, past accomplishments, and whether he or she has any specific messages for his or her family. The conservation is audiotaped, transcribed, edited, and subsequently read back to the patient within a few days. Dignity therapy has been found to decrease self-rated suffering and depression.[60]

While life review can help build a sense of meaning, the process of life closure can help bring a sense of peace about the end of life. It is important to encourage patients with far advanced cancer to get onto any uncompleted tasks sooner than later because the timing of death is unpredictable. Dr Byock[61] highlighted five things that patients need to say to loved ones before they die, including "Good bye," "Thank you," "I love you," "I am sorry," and "I forgive you." The palliative care team may contribute to life closure by assisting the patient to accomplish certain goals, such as bringing family members to see the patient for the last time.

Spirituality and Religiosity

Spirituality can be defined as "one's relationship with the transcendent questions that confront one as a human being and how one relates to these questions," whereas religion is "a set of texts, practices, and belief about the transcendent shared by a particular community."[62] Spirituality emerges as a dominant issue for almost all patients at the end of life.[53] Thus, health care professionals working with advanced cancer patients should be competent in addressing the spiritual aspects of care.[63]

While the great majority of advanced cancer patients have spiritual needs, few were asked about them, and even

■ **TABLE 25-2.** Tools for Spiritual History Taking

FICA[67]	SPIRIT[68]
Faith and beliefs	Spiritual belief system
Importance of spirituality to patient	Personal spirituality
Community of spiritual support	Integration with a spiritual community
Ask how the patient would like his or her spiritual needs to be addressed	Ritualized practices/restrictions
	Implications for medical care
	Terminal events planning

fewer had their spiritual needs addressed. Yet, spirituality and religiousness have practical clinical implications. Religiosity is associated with a higher likelihood of use of intensive life-prolonging medical care at the end of life.[64] Better spiritual support is associated with an improved quality of life and earlier referral to hospice,[65] while patients who reported that their spiritual needs were not met had lower self-rated quality of care and satisfaction with care.[66]

Members of the palliative care team should know how to take a spiritual history, to identify patients' religious coping strategies, and when to make a referral to pastoral care. Table 25-2 provides two simple mnemonics to initiate discussions regarding spiritual issues.[67,68] An in-depth discussion of spirituality can be found in Chapter 26.

Communication at the End of Life

In order to make sound decisions and foster realistic hope, patients need to have a clear understanding of their disease, the treatment options, and their prognosis. Yet, the literature suggests significant gaps in communication between patients and the health care team. For instance, a number of studies have demonstrated that one third of patients with metastatic lung cancer believe that their cancer is curable.[69,70] While denial likely plays an important role, these studies highlight the need for enhanced communication, regular assessments of patient's understanding, and decision-making aids.

Back et al[71] recently provided an excellent review of various communication issues related to end of life in cancer patients, including discussion of diagnosis, prognosis, treatment decisions, advance care planning, transition of care, and preparing for dying and death. The six-step "SPIKES" approach provides a useful framework for handling many of these difficult topics (Table 25-3).[72] When discussing prognosis, it is important to avoid quoting a specific number for survival. Rather, one should emphasize the uncertainties and provide a prognosis in terms of days, weeks, months, or years.

Although a small proportion of patients prefer their physicians not to share bad news with them directly, a great majority would like their physicians to be honest, realistic, and open about discussing end-of-life issues, provided that this happens at a time when they are ready.[73] The experienced clinician knows to share information at the appropriate moment and setting, and to customize it to the patient's intellectual understanding and emotional resilience. One communication technique is the "ask–tell–ask" approach, which involves asking the patient for permission before breaking bad news, and assessing whether he or she is ready for further information before proceeding.[71]

Decision Making at the End of Life

Patients with advanced cancer have to make numerous decisions regarding treatments, goals of care, and end-of-life planning. Many of these decisions are highly complex and emotionally charged. One of the key roles of the palliative care specialists is to help guide patients through the maze of difficult choices by providing individualized recommendations, taking into account the patient's preferences, health state, treatment options, and resources. It is important to note that clinical decision making is a continuous process with an ever-evolving content of discussion that reflects the changing health status and goals of the patient.

Patient Preferences in Decision Making

Patients differ in how much they want to participate in clinical decision making. Although the majority of patients prefer to make decisions in conjunction with their physicians, approximately 10% to 30% would favor their physicians making health care decisions on their behalf, while another 5% to 15% would rather make the decision with limited physician input. Studies have consistently demonstrated that physicians are unable to accurately predict how much patients want to participate in the decision-making process.[74–76] Thus, it is important to explicitly ask patients for their preference.

Transition of Care

As patients transition from active cancer treatments to end-of-life care, they have to face many difficult choices.

■ **TABLE 25-3. The SPIKES Approach to Effective Communication**[72]

Setting
Find a quiet, comfortable, and safe setting
Sit down with open posture
Speak to patient at eye level, slowly and gently
Ask the patient if he or she wants to be accompanied by family/friends during the discussion

Perception: what does the patient understand?
Explore patient's understanding of his or her illness and expectations

Information: how much information does the patient want to know?
"I have some bad news for you. Is it alright if I discuss the results with you today?"
"Some people like to know all details, while others only want to know the big picture. How would you like me to discuss the information with you?"

Knowledge: deliver information in a sensitive manner
Diagnosis: "Your biopsy results came back. The pathology report suggests that the cancer has returned"
Prognosis: "While none of us know how long exactly you will live, my best estimation is in terms of weeks"
Transition of care: "Considering another cycle of chemotherapy is an option. At the same time, planning ahead in case it does not work would also be helpful"

Empathic response
"This is a difficult time for you"
"It is normal for patients in similar situation to feel sad and loss of control. How are you feeling right now?"

Strategies
Take this opportunity to empower patients to define and achieve goals. Initiate discussions about important advance care planning issues such as philosophy of care, living will, and code status
Reassure patients your commitment to help and nonabandonment
Introduce other members of the interprofessional team, such as chaplain and social worker, who will be able to provide further support

Palliative care assists in this process by providing information, and physical and emotional support. There are numerous milestones along the cancer journey that signal the disease is advancing, and may serve as triggers for specific actions, such as advance care planning, palliative care involvement, and hospice referral. These "sentinel" events may include diagnosis of new metastasis, progressive disease while on standard treatment, declining performance status (from ECOG 2 to 3), extreme physical or emotional distress, and repeated hospital admissions. A better definition and recognition of these milestones may help streamline the process of transition.[77]

To facilitate a smooth transition, patients and their families should be presented with accurate clinical information, prognosis, realistic treatment options, and resources to help them plan ahead throughout the disease process, with frequent and regular follow-ups to reassess their understanding and goals as their cancer progresses.

Prognostication

In addition to the above transition of care milestones, patient's prognosis has important implications for many decisions, such as initiation of specific medications and avoidance of aggressive therapies. Hospice eligibility is based on a predicted survival of 6 months or less. As patients develop disease progression over time, knowing what to expect could provide them with a sense of control, and facilitate the process of advance care planning. Clinical prediction of survival is a prognosis formulated based solely on the clinician's knowledge and experience.[78] Although this intuitive estimation is associated with actual survival to a certain extent, clinicians tend to overestimate how long a patient will live, and be even more optimistic when communicating prognosis.[79,80]

A number of prognostic tools are available to increase the accuracy of prognostication in advanced cancer patients.[81–83] One of the most validated tools is the palliative prognostic score, which takes into account six variables: clinical prediction of survival, dyspnea, anorexia, Karnofsky performance status, leukocytosis, and lymphopenia.[84,85] A Web-based prognostic model of the Palliative Performance Scale is also available at http://web.his.uvic.ca/research/NET/tools/PrognosticTools/. It provides an estimated survival based on the Palliative Performance Scale, with further adjustments based on the patient's age, gender, and cancer diagnosis.[86]

Advance Care Planning

Pursuit of active cancer therapy should not prevent patients with advanced cancer from engaging in advance care planning and receiving palliative care services. However, patients and clinicians have the tendency to avoid discussing end-of-life issues until it is too late, as it is easier to just focus on cancer treatments.[87] When death approaches, many of the complex issues surrounding goals of care remain unresolved, which frequently lead to aggressive measures such as intensive care unit admissions, and significant distress in the unprepared patients and families.

Advance care planning is a process that involves superb communication and documentation. The palliative care team can help patients to better understand their prognosis, disease state, and reasons for planning ahead. Patients should be encouraged to "hope for the best, and plan for the worst," and be empowered to discuss their wishes with their families and friends. In addition to a will, patients should also prepare advance directives (living will) for heath-related matters, identify surrogates for substitute decision making, arrange durable power of attorney for financial matters, and complete out-of-hospital Do-Not-Resuscitate forms. Timely discussions of these matters can help bring peace of mind to patients and families, knowing that their wishes will be respected. Advance directives have also been shown to be associated with greater use of hospice and fewer reported concerns with communication.[88]

Hospice Referral

The decision to accept hospice care can be agonizing at times. Predictors of decreased utilization of hospice services include African American ethnicity, unmarried status, Charlson score >1, and higher education,[89] whereas African American ethnicity, less social support, worse functional status, and a greater burden of psychological symptoms are associated with increased perceived need for hospice services.[90] The main criterion for hospice referral in the United States is a prognosis of 6 months or less. Patients generally need to forgo life-sustaining measures such as chemotherapy prior to enrollment, as their care would be solely provided by hospices. This requirement is sometimes seen by patients and families as "giving up hope," and presents an unnecessary dilemma for those who desire both cancer treatments and quality of life measures. Patients and families should be made aware that the decision to accept hospice can be easily reversed, if they feel that the service is incompatible with their interest after a trial period.

While early access to hospice is an important indicator of quality of care,[91,92] studies have consistently demonstrated delayed referral to hospice services. In the United States, the median length of stay at hospice declined from 26 to 19 days between 1992 and 1998. Barriers to hospice referral include a fragmented health care system, lack of awareness of what hospices offer, and misconceptions about hospices.[93] Further education of health care professionals, patients, and their caregivers, along with refined hospice admission criteria and improved coordination, may increase access to this important service.

■ OUTCOMES OF PALLIATIVE CARE

According to the National Consensus Project,[94] palliative care is "both a philosophy of care and an organized, highly structured system for delivering care. The goal of palliative care is to prevent and relieve suffering and to support the best possible quality of life for patients and their families, regardless of the stage of the disease or the need for other therapies." A number of indicators of quality care have been established by the National Consensus Project,[94] National Quality Forum's *Preferred Practices for Palliative and Hospice Care*,[95] and the American Society of Clinical Oncology's (ASCO) *Quality Oncology Practice Initiative*.[96] All of these organizations emphasize the importance of achieving good pain and symptom control, avoidance of aggressive measures such as chemotherapy close to the end-of-life, and early hospice referral.

Research in the effectiveness of palliative care on improving quality of care and related outcomes is partly hampered by the heterogeneous definition of palliative care services and the limited methodological quality of published studies. Nevertheless, the cumulative evidence suggests a positive impact of palliative care on various clinical and administrative outcomes, including symptom control, patient and caregiver satisfaction, bereavement, avoidance of aggressive measures, and financial issues.

Symptom Control

A number of randomized controlled studies and systematic reviews support that palliative care is effective in reducing symptoms.[97] To date, several systematic reviews have examined the effectiveness of palliative care services.[98–102] All of these reviews highlighted the methodological limitations in the primary studies, but generally

supported that palliative care improves symptom control.[103] A meta-analysis also showed that palliative care is associated with significant improvement in pain (odds ratio [OR] 0.38, 95% confidence interval [CI] 0.23–0.64) and other symptoms (OR 0.51, 95% CI 0.30–0.88).[100]

Patient and Caregiver Satisfaction

Satisfaction is a novel outcome that captures various aspects of patients' and caregivers' experiences of end-of-life care. Higginson et al[100] performed a meta-analysis regarding the effect of palliative care interventions compared with conventional care, and reported no significant effects on patient satisfaction (OR 0.41, 95% CI 0.12–1.47) based on two small studies, but a significant impact on caregiver satisfaction (OR 0.57, 95% CI 0.03–0.96) based on three studies.[104] Enhanced family satisfaction with care is also supported by another systematic review.[98]

Avoidance of Aggressive Measures and Caregiver Bereavement

One of the key roles of palliative care is to provide excellent communication to facilitate transition of care. A number of palliative integrated care pathways have been shown to improve documentation of goals of care including resuscitation status,[105] decrease aggressive investigations,[106] and reduce emergency room and hospital visits.[107] Furthermore, end-of-life discussions have been found to be associated with less aggressive interventions, such as lower rates of ventilation, resuscitation, ICU admission, and earlier hospice enrollment, which in turn are associated with patient's improved quality of life and lower risk of major depressive disorder in bereaved caregivers.[46]

In a recent study of prostate cancer patients, hospice care has also been shown to decrease aggressive measures at the end of life, including ICU admissions, inpatient admissions, emergency room visits, stent or nephrostomy, cystoscopy, chemotherapy, and cardiopulmonary resuscitation.[89]

Financial Outcomes

Approximately one tenth of all health care expenditure is spent at the end of life.[108,109] Given that palliative care reduces aggressive interventions that are not only potentially futile but also highly expensive, it would make sense that palliative and hospice care can improve both the quality of care and cost of care. However, there are only a few studies on the economic aspect of care. A recent study compared the cost of patients receiving palliative care through a hospital consultation team to usual care, and found that palliative care involvement provides significant cost savings of $1696 to $4908 per admission and $279 to $374 per day.[110]

■ CHALLENGES OF PALLIATIVE CARE

Since Dr Cicely Saunders founded St. Christopher hospice in 1967, palliative care has evolved dramatically as a professional discipline in both infrastructure and knowledge base. However, many patients die in the United States without having received palliative care, suggesting that access to quality end-of-life care remains a challenge.[111]

In its 2001 report, the Institute of Medicine[77] identified eight key barriers to provision of effective palliative care, including the separation of palliative and hospice care from potentially life-prolonging treatment within the health care system, limited reimbursement for supportive care services, inadequate training of health care personnel in symptom management and other palliative care skills, and limited high-quality research. This section will highlight a number of societal, research, educational, and administrative barriers to the effective delivery of palliative care.

Societal Attitude on Death and Dying

Over the past decades, significant advances in medicine have improved both the quantity and quality of life in patients with advanced cancer. However, this has inadvertently shifted medicine from a profession of humanities to one driven by technology, associated with unrealistic expectations for cure.[112] Elimination of death becomes the only worthwhile goal clinically and academically. This death denial attitude has contributed to avoidance of open discussions regarding death and dying, transforming a natural process into a medical failure. A recent survey revealed that the term "palliative care" is associated with distress in health care professionals, and that they prefer to use the term "supportive care" instead.[113] This interesting finding reflects, to a certain extent, the continual stigma regarding death and dying.

At the individual patient level, death denial represents an obstacle to effective symptom management, advance care planning, discontinuation of "futile" treatments, and home death.[114] At the societal level, this attitude may also have contributed to a lack of public interest in and funding of clinical services, research, and education related to the end-of-life care.

More recently, we have witnessed a gradual but steady shift toward acceptance of palliative care, as a result of increased patient advocacy and pioneering research. For instance, the ASCO has put forth guidelines for provision of quality of end-of-life care, including avoidance of chemotherapy and access to hospice care close to the end of life.[115] Further recognition of the importance of palliative care and quality of life would hopefully accelerate the development of this field.

Research in Palliative Care

Despite a significant increase in the number of research studies over the past decade, much of the practice in palliative care is still based on empiric evidence. The relative paucity of high-quality research in palliative care can be attributed to a number of unique challenges, including patient characteristics, research design, infrastructure, and resources (Table 25-4).

The practice of evidence-based medicine mandates the translation of research findings into clinical practice. In addition to promoting research with practical significance, we need to develop up-to-date integrated care pathways and clinical practice guidelines to improve documentation, dissemination, and adoption of evidence into everyday practice.

Education in Palliative Care

The core competencies in palliative care—symptom control, communication, decision making, end-of-life care, and interprofessional teamwork—are fundamental to the delivery of high-quality care for patients with life-threatening diseases. Thus, all health care professionals working with advanced cancer patients should be competent with these skill sets. Yet, limited time is dedicated to palliative care–related issues in professional schools' training programs, resulting in a significant gap in knowledge about palliative care.

In a 1998 survey conducted by ASCO, 81% of oncologists who responded reported inadequate mentoring in discussing poor prognosis, 65% reported inadequate education about controlling symptoms, only 33% reported hearing lectures about palliative care issues during their oncology fellowship, and only 10% completed a rotation on a palliative care service or hospice. Ninety percent learned about palliative care through trial and error, whereas 38% said a significant source of education was a traumatic experience with a patient.[116,117] In a more recent

■ **TABLE 25-4.** Ten Barriers to Palliative Care Research and Potential Solutions

Barriers	Potential Solution
Patient accrual: Patient accrual is hampered by patients' frailty and vulnerability. Many patients are simply too weak, confused, or in too much distress to participate in studies	Study design needs to recognize frailty and minimize burden on patients and families
Patient interest: Patients are generally more interested in oncology trials than in symptom control studies	Focus on clinically important research questions Develop a structured approach to identify gaps in knowledge and areas of need
Patient retention: Limited survival of palliative care patients makes follow-up challenging, with a significant proportion of patients lost to follow-up	Study needs to be designed to capture key outcomes over a short period of time
Research terminologies: Lack of standardization of key terms contributing to heterogeneity of study	Consensus panel to define important terms in palliative care
Research methods: Many studies are underpowered, with variable quality of design	Increased training, resources, and infrastructure to enable high-quality research
Outcome measures: Many of the concepts in palliative care are abstract in nature (eg, communication, decision making, spirituality). Many of the outcomes in palliative care, such as symptoms, quality of life, and patient satisfaction, involve subjective measures, with few validated instruments' availability	Development and validation of new instruments Novel computerized adaptive design (eg, PROMIS) Standardization of instruments
Research personnel: There remain few palliative care specialists trained in research methodologies	Increased training of palliative care researchers
Research infrastructure: Limited palliative care clinical and research infrastructure in many hospitals	Improve infrastructure such as developing databases Collaborative effort with multicenter studies
Research funding: Limited resources from both public and private sources	Increase in funding dedicated to palliative care research
Translation to clinical practice: Slow distribution and adoption of research findings	Development of clinical guidelines to disseminate knowledge

survey of practicing medical oncologists, 69% reported that patients with advanced cancer constituted a major proportion of their practice. Almost 90% believed that medical oncologists should coordinate end-of-life care; almost over 40% felt that they were trained inadequately for this task.[118]

Given its relevance to clinical practice, palliative care should be integrated into the professional schools' educational curriculum through both didactic lectures and mandatory clinical rotations. Early exposure to palliative care would encourage more students to consider this field as a career and to contribute to this growing specialty. Furthermore, a sound understanding of palliative care issues in other health care professionals would facilitate integration of palliative care into other disciplines, enabling

timely access to quality palliative care for patients with advanced cancer.

Early Access to Palliative Care

Despite the general recognition that palliative care plays a crucial role for advanced cancer patients, the availability and degree of integration of palliative care is highly variable among hospitals and cancer centers across the United States.[111,119] Approximately half of all hospitals in the United States still do not have palliative care in place. When present, the quality of palliative care services is also heterogeneous, with varying degrees of availability of hospital consultation teams, PCUs, and outpatient clinics. To maximize the access and utilization of palliative care (Fig. 25-5), we need to overcome a number of

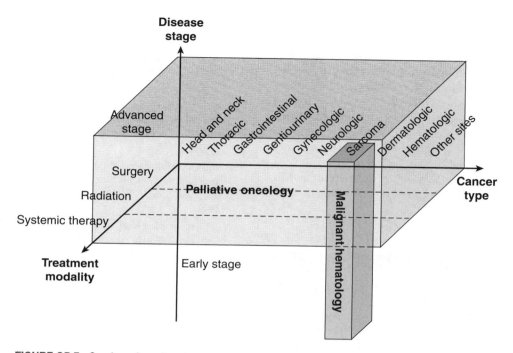

FIGURE 25-5. Overlap of services between palliative care and oncology. This three-dimensional diagram plots the patient population based on disease site (x-axis), treatment modality (y-axis), and disease state (ie, curable or advanced, z-axis). For instance, malignant hematologists (red box) primarily prescribe systemic therapy for patients with leukemia/lymphoma, from diagnosis to close to the end of life, while palliative care (green box) serves all cancer patients with advanced cancer from diagnosis of advanced disease to death. Thus, palliative care and oncology share many of the same patients. Early integration of palliative care into oncology services can help enhance the quality of life for patients with advanced cancer.

financial, infrastructural, professional, social, and educational barriers.

In addition to limited access to palliative care, patients tend to be referred to palliative and hospice care too close to the end of life,[120,121] while aggressive interventions such as cancer therapies are provided too close to death.[122–124] Late referrals to palliative care significantly decrease its effectiveness as a result of delayed symptom assessment and intervention, with limited time to establish a therapeutic relationship and to address important end-of-life issues.

Early incorporation of palliative care strategies in patients with advanced cancer has been shown to optimize symptom management,[97] facilitate psychosocial interventions,[125] enhance coordination of care, and facilitate patients' explicit transition from curative intent to palliative

intent.[126,127] This understanding led to the development of the comprehensive cancer care model, which integrates supportive care along with anticancer therapy from the time of diagnosis of advanced cancer.[128–130] ASCO has recently convened an expert panel to examine the progress toward comprehensive cancer care, and to outline the necessary steps for full integration of palliative care into oncology practice by 2020. The key recommendations were classified as policy, drug availability, education, integrative practice, and quality improvement.[117]

■ SUMMARY

The interconnected nature of physical, emotional, and spiritual well-being in patients with advanced cancer suggests that an interprofessional approach is essential to optimal patient management. Palliative care aims to improve the quality of life of cancer patients and families through early identification, assessment, and treatment of symptoms, and to minimize suffering through effective management of psychosocial and spiritual concerns. In this chapter, we outlined the structure, processes, and outcomes related to palliative care, and highlighted a number of challenges related to this evolving field. Further advances in palliative care research, enhanced training of oncologists and palliative care specialists, integrated clinical practice with early referrals, and improved patient education can all increase patients' access to quality palliative care.

KEY POINTS

- Patients with advanced cancer often experience significant physical symptoms, psychosocial concerns, and existential distress. The interconnectedness of these issues necessitates a highly integrated interprofessional approach.

- Palliative care aims to improve the quality of life of cancer patients and families through early identification, assessment, and treatment of symptoms, and to minimize suffering through effective management of psychosocial and spiritual concerns.

- Core competencies of palliative care include symptom management, psychosocial care, communication, complex decision making, and end-of-life care. Psychosocial issues particularly relevant to palliative care include depression, anxiety, expressive counseling, life review and closure, fostering hope, caregiver support, bereavement, and spiritual care.

- Early access to palliative care for patients with advanced cancer can help to optimize symptom control, improve quality of life and quality of care, increase caregiver satisfaction, and reduce health care costs.

- Further advances in palliative care research, enhanced training of oncologists and palliative care specialists, integrated clinical practice with early referrals, improved patient education, and increased funding are all needed to increase patients' access to quality palliative care.

REFERENCES

1. Ingham J. The epidemiology of cancer at the end of life. In: Berger A, Portenoy RK, Weissman DE, eds. *Principles and Practice of Supportive Oncology.* Philadelphia, Pa: Lippincott-Raven; 1998:749–765.

2. WHO. Pain relief and palliative care. In: *National Cancer Control Programmes: Policies and Managerial Guidelines.* 2nd ed. Geneva: World Health Organization; 2002: 83–91.

3. World Health Assembly. *WHA58.22 Cancer Prevention and Control.* Available at: http://www.who.int/gb/ebwha/pdf_files/WHA58/WHA58_22-en.pdf. Accessed July 30, 2009.

4. O'Connor M, Fisher C, Guilfoyle A. Interdisciplinary teams in palliative care: a critical reflection. *Int J Palliat Nurs.* 2006;12:132–137 [serial online].

5. Crawford GB, Price SD. Team working: palliative care as a model of interdisciplinary practice. *Med J Aust.* 2003;179:S32–S34 [serial online].

6. Yennurajalingam S, Dev R, Lockey M, et al. Characteristics of family conferences in a palliative care unit at a comprehensive cancer center. *J Palliat Med.* 2008;11:1208–1211 [serial online].

7. Lagman R, Rivera N, Walsh D, LeGrand S, Davis MP. Acute inpatient palliative medicine in a cancer center: clinical problems and medical interventions—a prospective study. *Am J Hosp Palliat Care.* 2007;24:20–28 [serial online].

8. Elsayem A, Swint K, Fisch MJ, et al. Palliative care inpatient service in a comprehensive cancer center: clinical and financial outcomes. *J Clin Oncol.* 2004;22:2008–2014 [serial online].

9. Lagman R, Walsh D, Heintz J, Legrand SB, Davis MP. A day in the life: a case series of acute care palliative medicine—the Cleveland Model. *Am J Hosp Palliat Care.* 2008;25:24–32 [serial online].

10. Ellis J, Lin J, Walsh A, et al. Predictors of referral for specialized psychosocial oncology care in patients with metastatic cancer: the contributions of age, distress, and marital status. *J Clin Oncol.* 2009;27:699–705 [serial online].

11. Bruera E, Neumann C, Brenneis C, Quan H. Frequency of symptom distress and poor prognostic indicators in palliative cancer patients admitted to a tertiary palliative care unit, hospices, and acute care hospitals. *J Palliat Care.* 2000;16:16–21 [serial online].

12. Fainsinger RL, Demoissac D, Cole J, Mead-Wood K, Lee E. Home versus hospice inpatient care: discharge characteristics of palliative care patients in an acute care hospital. *J Palliat Care.* 2000;16:29–34 [serial online].

13. Hopwood P, Stephens RJ. Symptoms at presentation for treatment in patients with lung cancer: implications for the evaluation of palliative treatment. The Medical Research Council (MRC) Lung Cancer Working Party. *Br J Cancer.* 1995;71:633–636.

14. Portenoy RK, Thaler HT, Kornblith AB, et al. Symptom prevalence, characteristics and distress in a cancer population. *Qual Life Res.* 1994;3:183–189 [serial online].

15. Walsh D, Rybicki L. Symptom clustering in advanced cancer. *Support Care Cancer.* 2006;14:831–836 [serial online].

16. Yamagishi A, Morita T, Miyashita M, Kimura F. Symptom prevalence and longitudinal follow-up in cancer outpatients receiving chemotherapy. *J Pain Symptom Manage.* 2009;37:823–830 [serial online].

17. Centeno C, Sanz A, Bruera E. Delirium in advanced cancer patients. *Palliat Med.* 2004;18:184–194 [serial online].

18. Del Fabbro E, Dalal S, Bruera E. Symptom control in palliative care—part III: dyspnea and delirium. *J Palliat Med.* 2006;9:422–436.

19. Bruera E, Bush SH, Willey J, et al. Impact of delirium and recall on the level of distress in patients with advanced cancer and their family caregivers. *Cancer.* 2009;115:2004–2012 [serial online].

20. Curt GA, Breitbart W, Cella D, et al. Impact of cancer-related fatigue on the lives of patients: new findings from the fatigue coalition. *Oncologist.* 2000;5:353–360.

21. Bruera E, Kuehn N, Miller MJ, Selmser P, Macmillan K. The Edmonton Symptom Assessment System (ESAS): a simple method for the assessment of palliative care patients. *J Palliat Care.* 1991;7:6–9 [serial online].

22. Portenoy RK, Thaler HT, Kornblith AB, et al. The Memorial Symptom Assessment Scale: an instrument for the evaluation of symptom prevalence, characteristics and distress. *Eur J Cancer.* 1994;30A:1326–1336 [serial online].

23. Breitbart W, Rosenfeld B, Roth A, Smith MJ, Cohen K, Passik S. The Memorial Delirium Assessment Scale. *J Pain Symptom Manage.* 1997;13:128–137 [serial online].

24. Folstein MF, Folstein SE, McHugh PR. "Mini-mental state". A practical method for grading the cognitive state of patients for the clinician. *J Psychiatr Res.* 1975;12:189–198 [serial online].

25. Ewing JA. Detecting alcoholism. The CAGE questionnaire. *JAMA.* 1984;252:1905–1907 [serial online].

26. Oken MM, Creech RH, Tormey DC, et al. Toxicity and response criteria of the Eastern Cooperative Oncology Group. *Am J Clin Oncol.* 1982;5:649–655 [serial online].

27. Schag CC, Heinrich RL, Ganz PA. Karnofsky performance status revisited: reliability, validity, and guidelines. *J Clin Oncol.* 1984;2:187–193 [serial online].

28. Anderson F, Downing GM, Hill J, Casorso L, Lerch N. Palliative Performance Scale (PPS): a new tool. *J Palliat Care.* 1996;12:5–11 [serial online].

29. Strasser F. Palliative care: evaluation instruments in daily clinical practice. *Ann Oncol.* 2006;17(suppl 10):x299–303 [serial online].

30. Vitek L, Rosenzweig MQ, Stollings S. Distress in patients with cancer: definition, assessment, and suggested interventions. *Clin J Oncol Nurs.* 2007;11:413–418 [serial online].

31. Holland JC, Andersen B, Breitbart WS, et al. *NCCN Clinical Practice Guidelines in Oncology. Distress Management.* Available at: http://www.nccn.org/professionals/physician_gls/f_guidelines.asp. Accessed July 30, 2010.

32. Cox K. Informed consent and decision-making: patients' experiences of the process of recruitment to phases I and II anti-cancer drug trials. *Patient Educ Couns.* 2002;46:31–38 [serial online].

33. Block SD. Perspectives on care at the close of life. Psychological considerations, growth, and transcendence at the end of life: the art of the possible. *JAMA.* 2001;285:2898–2905 [serial online].

34. Clayton JM, Hancock K, Parker S, et al. Sustaining hope when communicating with terminally ill patients and their families: a systematic review. *Psychooncology.* 2008;17:641–659.

35. Lloyd-Williams M, Reeve J, Kissane D. Distress in palliative care patients: developing patient-centred approaches to clinical management. *Eur J Cancer.* 2008;44:1133–1138 [serial online].

36. Chochinov HM. Depression in cancer patients. *Lancet Oncol.* 2001;2:499–505.

37. Mead GE, Morley W, Campbell P, Greig CA, McMurdo M, Lawlor DA. Exercise for depression. *Cochrane Database Syst Rev.* 2008;(4):CD004366 [serial online].

38. Golden RN, Gaynes BN, Ekstrom RD, et al. The efficacy of light therapy in the treatment of mood disorders: a review and meta-analysis of the evidence. *Am J Psychiatry.* 2005;162:656–662 [serial online].

39. Tuunainen A, Kripke DF, Endo T. Light therapy for non-seasonal depression. *Cochrane Database Syst Rev.* 2004;(2):CD004050 [serial online].

40. Akechi T, Okuyama T, Onishi J, Morita T, Furukawa TA. Psychotherapy for depression among incurable cancer

patients. *Cochrane Database Syst Rev.* 2008;(2):CD005537 [serial online].

41. Fulcher CD, Badger T, Gunter AK, Marrs JA, Reese JM. Putting evidence into practice: interventions for depression. *Clin J Oncol Nurs.* 2008;12:131–140.

42. Candy M, Jones L, Williams R, Tookman A, King M. Psychostimulants for depression. *Cochrane Database Syst Rev.* 2008;(2):CD006722 [serial online].

43. Roth AJ, Massie MJ. Anxiety and its management in advanced cancer. *Curr Opin Support Palliat Care.* 2007;1:50–56 [serial online].

44. Jackson KC, Lipman AG. Drug therapy for anxiety in palliative care. *Cochrane Database Syst Rev.* 2004;(1): CD004596.

45. Rabow MW, Hauser JM, Adams J. Supporting family caregivers at the end of life: "they don't know what they don't know". *JAMA.* 2004;291:483–491 [serial online].

46. Wright AA, Zhang B, Ray A, et al. Associations between end-of-life discussions, patient mental health, medical care near death, and caregiver bereavement adjustment. *JAMA.* 2008;300:1665–1673.

47. Radwany S, Albanese T, Clough L, Sims L, Mason H, Jahangiri S. End-of-life decision making and emotional burden: placing family meetings in context. *Am J Hosp Palliat Care.* 2009;26(5):376–383 [serial online].

48. Zaider T, Kissane D. The assessment and management of family distress during palliative care. *Curr Opin Support Palliat Care.* 2009;3:67–71 [serial online].

49. Penson RT, Green KM, Chabner BA, Lynch TJ Jr. When does the responsibility of our care end: bereavement. *Oncologist.* 2002;7:251–258 [serial online].

50. Hauser JM, Kramer BJ. Family caregivers in palliative care. *Clin Geriat Med.* 2004;20:671–688, vi [serial online].

51. Grassi L. Bereavement in families with relatives dying of cancer. *Curr Opin Support Palliat Care.* 2007;1:43–49 [serial online].

52. Morita T, Ichiki T, Tsunoda J, Inoue S, Chihara S. A prospective study on the dying process in terminally ill cancer patients. *Am J Hosp Palliat Care.* 1998;15:217–222.

53. Greisinger AJ, Lorimor RJ, Aday LA, Winn RJ, Baile WF. Terminally ill cancer patients. Their most important concerns. *Cancer Pract.* 1997;5:147–154 [serial online].

54. Cassel EJ. The nature of suffering and the goals of medicine. *N Engl J Med.* 1982;306:639–645 [serial online].

55. Saunders C. Introduction: history and challenge. In: Saunders C, Sykes N, eds. *The Management of Terminal Malignant Disease.* London, Great Britain: Hodder and Stoughton; 1993:1–14.

56. Delgado-Guay M, Parsons HA, Li Z, Palmer JL, Bruera E. Symptom distress in advanced cancer patients with anxiety and depression in the palliative care setting. *Support Care Cancer.* 2009;17:573–579 [serial online].

57. Herth K. Abbreviated instrument to measure hope: development and psychometric evaluation. *J Adv Nurs.* 1992;17:1251–1259 [serial online].

58. Johnson S. Hope in terminal illness: an evolutionary concept analysis. *Int J Palliat Nurs.* 2007;13:451–459.

59. Thompson GN, Chochinov HM. Dignity-based approaches in the care of terminally ill patients. *Curr Opin Support Palliat Care.* 2008;2:49–53 [serial online].

60. Chochinov HM, Hack T, Hassard T, Kristjanson LJ, McClement S, Harlos M. Dignity therapy: a novel psychotherapeutic intervention for patients near the end of life. *J Clin Oncol.* 2005;23:5520–5525 [serial online].

61. Byock I. *Dying Well: The Prospect for Growth at the End of Life.* New York, NY: Putnam/Riverhead; 1997.

62. Sulmasy DP. Spiritual issues in the care of dying patients: "… it's okay between me and god". *JAMA.* 2006;296:1385–1392 [serial online].

63. Lo B, Ruston D, Kates LW, et al. Discussing religious and spiritual issues at the end of life: a practical guide for physicians. *JAMA.* 2002;287:749–754 [serial online].

64. Phelps AC, Maciejewski PK, Nilsson M, et al. Religious coping and use of intensive life-prolonging care near death in patients with advanced cancer. *JAMA.* 2009;301:1140–1147 [serial online].

65. Balboni TA, Vanderwerker LC, Block SD, et al. Religiousness and spiritual support among advanced cancer patients and associations with end-of-life treatment preferences and quality of life. *J Clin Oncol.* 2007;25: 555–560.

66. Astrow AB, Wexler A, Texeira K, He MK, Sulmasy DP. Is failure to meet spiritual needs associated with cancer patients' perceptions of quality of care and their satisfaction with care? *J Clin Oncol.* 2007;25:5753–5757 [serial online].

67. Puchalski CM. Spirituality and end-of-life care: a time for listening and caring. *J Palliat Med.* 2002;5:289–294 [serial online].

68. Maugans TA. The SPIRITual history. *Arch Fam Med.* 1996;5:11–16 [serial online].

69. Chow E, Harth T, Hruby G, Finkelstein J, Wu J, Danjoux C. How accurate are physicians' clinical predictions of survival and the available prognostic tools in estimating survival times in terminally ill cancer

patients? A systematic review. *Clin Oncol (R Coll Radiol).* 2001;13:209–218 [serial online].

70. Mackillop WJ, Stewart WE, Ginsburg AD, Stewart SS. Cancer patients' perceptions of their disease and its treatment. *Br J Cancer.* 1988;58:355–358 [serial online].

71. Back AL, Anderson WG, Bunch L, et al. Communication about cancer near the end of life. *Cancer.* 2008;113: 1897–1910.

72. Baile WF, Buckman R, Lenzi R, Glober G, Beale EA, Kudelka AP. SPIKES—a six-step protocol for delivering bad news: application to the patient with cancer. *Oncologist.* 2000;5:302–311.

73. Parker SM, Clayton JM, Hancock K, et al. A systematic review of prognostic/end-of-life communication with adults in the advanced stages of a life-limiting illness: patient/caregiver preferences for the content, style, and timing of information. *J Pain Symptom Manage.* 2007;34:81–93 [serial online].

74. Bruera E, Sweeney C, Calder K, Palmer L, Benisch-Tolley S. Patient preferences versus physician perceptions of treatment decisions in cancer care. *J Clin Oncol.* 2001;19:2883–2885.

75. Bruera E, Willey JS, Palmer JL, Rosales M. Treatment decisions for breast carcinoma: patient preferences and physician perceptions. *Cancer.* 2002;94:2076–2080 [serial online].

76. Grunfeld EA, Maher EJ, Browne S, et al. Advanced breast cancer patients' perceptions of decision making for palliative chemotherapy. *J Clin Oncol.* 2006;24:1090–1098.

77. IOM, National Cancer Policy Board. *Improving Palliative Care for Cancer.* 1st ed. Washington, DC: Institute of Medicine; 2001.

78. Glare PA, Sinclair CT. Palliative medicine review: prognostication. *J Palliat Med.* 2008;11:84–103 [serial online].

79. Lamont EB, Christakis NA. Some elements of prognosis in terminal cancer. *Oncology (Huntingt).* 1999;13:1165–1170 [discussion 1172–1174, 1179–1180; serial online].

80. Christakis NA, Lamont EB. Extent and determinants of error in doctors' prognoses in terminally ill patients: prospective cohort study. *BMJ.* 2000;320:469–472 [serial online].

81. Glare P, Sinclair C, Downing M, Stone P, Maltoni M, Vigano A. Predicting survival in patients with advanced disease. *Eur J Cancer.* 2008;44:1146–1156 [serial online].

82. Maltoni M, Caraceni A, Brunelli C, et al. Prognostic factors in advanced cancer patients: evidence-based clinical recommendations—a study by the Steering Committee

of the European Association for Palliative Care. *J Clin Oncol.* 2005;23:6240–6248.

83. Stone PC, Lund S. Predicting prognosis in patients with advanced cancer. *Ann Oncol.* 2007;18:971–976.

84. Maltoni M, Nanni O, Pirovano M, et al. Successful validation of the palliative prognostic score in terminally ill cancer patients. Italian Multicenter Study Group on Palliative Care. *J Pain Symptom Manage.* 1999;17:240–247 [serial online].

85. Pirovano M, Maltoni M, Nanni O, et al. A new palliative prognostic score: a first step for the staging of terminally ill cancer patients. Italian Multicenter and Study Group on Palliative Care. *J Pain Symptom Manage.* 1999;17: 231–239 [serial online].

86. Lau F, Downing M, Lesperance M, Karlson N, Kuziemsky C, Yang J. Using the Palliative Performance Scale to provide meaningful survival estimates. *J Pain Symptom Manage.* 2009;38(1):134–144 [serial online].

87. Temel JS, McCannon J, Greer JA, et al. Aggressiveness of care in a prospective cohort of patients with advanced NSCLC. *Cancer.* 2008;113:826–833.

88. Teno JM, Gruneir A, Schwartz Z, Nanda A, Wetle T. Association between advance directives and quality of end-of-life care: a national study. *J Am Geriatr Soc.* 2007;55:189–194.

89. Bergman J, Saigal CS, Miller DC, et al. Hospice utilization by men dying of prostate cancer. *J Clin Oncol.* 27:15s, 2009 (suppl; abstr 9501).

90. Casarett DJ, Fishman JM, Lu HL, et al. The terrible choice: re-evaluating hospice eligibility criteria for cancer. *J Clin Oncol.* 2009;27:953–959 [serial online].

91. Earle CC, Landrum MB, Souza JM, Neville BA, Weeks JC, Ayanian JZ. Aggressiveness of cancer care near the end of life: is it a quality-of-care issue? *J Clin Oncol.* 2008;26:3860–3866.

92. Earle CC, Park ER, Lai B, Weeks JC, Ayanian JZ, Block S. Identifying potential indicators of the quality of end-of-life cancer care from administrative data. *J Clin Oncol.* 2003;21:1133–1138 [serial online].

93. Keating NL, Herrinton LJ, Zaslavsky AM, Liu L, Ayanian JZ. Variations in hospice use among cancer patients. *J Natl Cancer Inst.* 2006;98:1053–1059 [serial online].

94. National Consensus Project for Quality Palliative Care. *Clinical Practice Guidelines for Quality Palliative Care.* 2nd ed. Available at: http://www.nationalconsensusproject.org. Accessed July 30, 2010.

95. National Quality Forum. *A National Framework and Preferred Practices for Palliative and Hospice Care Quality.* Washington, USA: National Quality Forum; 2006.

96. Neuss MN, Desch CE, McNiff KK, et al. A process for measuring the quality of cancer care: the Quality Oncology Practice Initiative. *J Clin Oncol*. 2005;23: 6233–6239 [serial online].

97. Rabow MW, Dibble SL, Pantilat SZ, McPhee SJ. The comprehensive care team: a controlled trial of outpatient palliative medicine consultation. *Arch Intern Med*. 2004;164:83–91 [serial online].

98. Zimmermann C, Riechelmann R, Krzyzanowska M, Rodin G, Tannock I. Effectiveness of specialized palliative care: a systematic review. *JAMA*. 2008;299: 1698–1709 [serial online].

99. Lorenz KA, Lynn J, Dy SM, et al. Evidence for improving palliative care at the end of life: a systematic review. *Ann Intern Med*. 2008;148:147–159 [serial online].

100. Higginson IJ, Finlay IG, Goodwin DM, et al. Is there evidence that palliative care teams alter end-of-life experiences of patients and their caregivers? *J Pain Symptom Manage*. 2003;25:150–168 [serial online].

101. Critchley P, Jadad AR, Taniguchi A, et al. Are some palliative care delivery systems more effective and efficient than others? A systematic review of comparative studies. *J Palliat Care*. 1999;15:40–47 [serial online].

102. Salisbury C, Bosanquet N, Wilkinson EK, et al. The impact of different models of specialist palliative care on patients' quality of life: a systematic literature review. *Palliat Med*. 1999;13:3–17 [serial online].

103. Garcia-Perez L, Linertova R, Martin-Olivera R, Serrano-Aguilar P, Benitez-Rosario MA. A systematic review of specialised palliative care for terminal patients: which model is better? *Palliat Med*. 2009;23:17–22 [serial online].

104. Dy SM, Shugarman LR, Lorenz KA, Mularski RA, Lynn J; RAND-Southern California Evidence-based Practice Center. A systematic review of satisfaction with care at the end of life. *J Am Geriatr Soc*. 2008;56:124–129 [serial online].

105. Veerbeek L, van Zuylen L, Swart SJ, et al. The effect of the Liverpool Care Pathway for the dying: a multi-centre study. *Palliat Med*. 2008;22:145–151 [serial online].

106. Luhrs CA, Meghani S, Homel P, et al. Pilot of a pathway to improve the care of imminently dying oncology inpatients in a veterans affairs medical center. *J Pain Symptom Manage*. 2005;29:544–551 [serial online].

107. Dudgeon DJ, Knott C, Eichholz M, et al. Palliative care integration project (PCIP) quality improvement strategy evaluation. *J Pain Symptom Manage*. 2008;35:573–582 [serial online].

108. Emanuel EJ. Cost savings at the end of life. What do the data show? *JAMA*. 1996;275:1907–1914 [serial online].

109. Emanuel EJ, Emanuel LL. The economics of dying. The illusion of cost savings at the end of life. *N Engl J Med*. 1994;330:540–544 [serial online].

110. Morrison RS, Penrod JD, Cassel JB, et al. Cost savings associated with US hospital palliative care consultation programs. *Arch Intern Med*. 2008;168:1783–1790 [serial online].

111. Goldsmith B, Dietrich J, Du Q, Morrison RS. Variability in access to hospital palliative care in the United States. *J Palliat Med*. 2008;11:1094–1102 [serial online].

112. Zimmermann C, Rodin G. The denial of death thesis: sociological critique and implications for palliative care. *Palliat Med*. 2004;18:121–128 [serial online].

113. Fadul N, Elsayem A, Palmer JL, et al. Supportive vs. palliative care: what's in a name? A survey of medical oncologists and mid-level providers at a comprehensive cancer center. *Cancer*. 2009;115(9):2013–2021.

114. Zimmermann C. Death denial: obstacle or instrument for palliative care? An analysis of clinical literature. *Sociol Health Illn*. 2007;29:297–314 [serial online].

115. McNiff KK, Neuss MN, Jacobson JO, Eisenberg PD, Kadlubek P, Simone JV. Measuring supportive care in medical oncology practice: lessons learned from the Quality Oncology Practice Initiative. *J Clin Oncol*. 2008;26:3832–3837.

116. Hilden JM, Emanuel EJ, Fairclough DL, et al. Attitudes and practices among pediatric oncologists regarding end-of-life care: results of the 1998 American Society of Clinical Oncology survey. *J Clin Oncol*. 2001;19:205–212 [serial online].

117. Ferris FD, Bruera E, Cherny N, et al. Palliative cancer care a decade later: accomplishments, the need, next steps—from the American Society of Clinical Oncology. *J Clin Oncol*. 2009;27:3052–3058 [serial online].

118. Cherny NI, Catane R, European Society of Medical Oncology Taskforce on Palliative and Supportive Care. Attitudes of medical oncologists toward palliative care for patients with advanced and incurable cancer: report on a survey by the European Society of Medical Oncology Taskforce on Palliative and Supportive Care. *Cancer*. 2003;98:2502–2510 [serial online].

119. Coluzzi PH, Grant M, Doroshow JH, Rhiner M, Ferrell B, Rivera L. Survey of the provision of supportive care services at National Cancer Institute-designated cancer centers. *J Clin Oncol*. 1995;13:756–764 [serial online].

120. Cheng WW, Willey J, Palmer JL, Zhang T, Bruera E. Interval between palliative care referral and death

among patients treated at a comprehensive cancer center. *J Palliat Med.* 2005;8:1025–1032 [serial online].

121. Morita T, Akechi T, Ikenaga M, et al. Late referrals to specialized palliative care service in Japan. *J Clin Oncol.* 2005;23:2637–2644 [serial online].

122. Harrington SE, Smith TJ. The role of chemotherapy at the end of life: "when is enough, enough?". *JAMA.* 2008;299:2667–2678 [serial online].

123. Earle CC, Neville BA, Landrum MB, Ayanian JZ, Block SD, Weeks JC. Trends in the aggressiveness of cancer care near the end of life. *J Clin Oncol.* 2004;22:315–321 [serial online].

124. Emanuel EJ, Young-Xu Y, Levinsky NG, Gazelle G, Saynina O, Ash AS. Chemotherapy use among Medicare beneficiaries at the end of life. *Ann Intern Med.* 2003;138:639–643 [serial online].

125. Casarett D, Pickard A, Bailey FA, et al. Do palliative consultations improve patient outcomes? *J Am Geriatr Soc.* 2008;56:593–599 [serial online].

126. Meyers FJ, Linder J, Beckett L, Christensen S, Blais J, Gandara DR. Simultaneous care: a model approach to the perceived conflict between investigational therapy and palliative care. *J Pain Symptom Manage.* 2004;28:548–556 [serial online].

127. Meyers FJ, Linder J. Simultaneous care: disease treatment and palliative care throughout illness. *J Clin Oncol.* 2003;21:1412–1415 [serial online].

128. Lagman R, Walsh D. Integration of palliative medicine into comprehensive cancer care. *Semin Oncol.* 2005;32:134–138 [serial online].

129. Byock I, Twohig JS, Merriman M, Collins K. Promoting excellence in end-of-life care: a report on innovative models of palliative care. *J Palliat Med.* 2006;9:137–151 [serial online].

130. Byock I. Completing the continuum of cancer care: integrating life-prolongation and palliation. *CA Cancer J Clin.* 2000;50:123–132.

Health Care Professional Well-being

Health Care Professional Stress

• *James D. Duffy, Kenneth Sapire, and M. Alejandro Chaoul*

■ INTRODUCTION

Caring for cancer patients is challenging work. There can be very few professions that demand so much of their practitioners. It is important that we acknowledge this fact. Every day we are faced with clinical situations that demand both our professional expertise and our personal compassion. All of our patients are confronting a potentially life-threatening disease that, together with our intrusive therapies, very often produces tormenting physical symptoms and devastating psychosocial repercussions. Although our professional training may have prepared us well to master the technical challenges of our work, our professional schools have not prepared us to understand and navigate the human dimensions of our work as healers. Each of us has typically needed to find our own way through to navigating the experiential aspects of our work. Unfortunately, recent research demonstrates that despite our best efforts, the task of caring for cancer patients is exacting a substantial toll on our wellness and is also negatively impacting our ability to provide optimum care for our patients. As wounded healers, we often find ourselves emotionally and physically deplete and therefore unable to meet the needs of our patients, and ourselves. In this regard, recent research reveals a dispirited profession. Suicide rates for physicians are estimated to be as high as six times that of the general public, and 17% of physicians reported their mental health as fair or poor (more than twice the national average) and 46% described their medical practice as very or extremely stressful.[1-3]

This chapter reviews:

(a) some key concepts relating to wellness and stress in clinicians;
(b) recent research on the current state of health care provider wellness;
(c) the impact of health care provider stress and burnout on patient care;
(d) specific strategies to enhance health care provider wellness.

■ KEY CONCEPTS

It is important to understand several key concepts as they relate to wellness, that is, wellness, resilience, and burnout.

Wellness

Although there is currently no universally accepted definition for "wellness," there is a growing consensus that "wellness" is a multidimensional construct that describes a positive state (rather than simply the absence of illness). Dunn[4] has defined wellness as "an integrated method of functioning, which is oriented toward maximizing the potential of which the individual is capable. It requires that the individual maintain a continuum of balance and purposeful direction within the environment where he is functioning." Rather than being an "all or nothing" concept (like allopathic disease models), wellness describes a continuum and a movement to optimal well-being and human flourishing. The concept of wellness can sometimes be challenging to allopathic health care professionals who have a medical model that is constructed on a foundation of treating disease, and not supporting positive health. Since allopaths receive almost no training in recognizing and supporting the positive aspects of health, it is not surprising that they are not encouraged to nurture their own well-being. Most conceptual models of wellness describe different domains that represent distinct but synergistic aspects of the individual's relationship to various aspects of oneself and one's environment. Although each model may include different domains, all of them include the five domains of social, emotional, physical, intellectual, and spiritual wellness.[5] The synergistic and balanced interaction between these different domains will produce the individual's overall sense of well-being. Dysfunction within any one of these domains will therefore impact all other domains and will negatively impact on overall wellness, that is, no domain of wellness can be neglected if the individual or system wishes to continue to flourish. This integral approach provides us with an opportunity to examine how we are functioning across each domain and recognize our relative strengths and weaknesses. Each of these domains of wellness will now be reviewed with particular relevance to our work as oncology clinicians.

Social Wellness

Social wellness encompasses the quality and extent of interaction with others and the interdependence between the individual, others, the community, and nature.[6] Hettler[7] has defined social wellness as living in harmony with others with mutual respect. Support, satisfying relationships, trust, and intimacy are considered central to social wellness and the movement of individuals and systems toward integration between individual, society, and nature. Social wellness is the "the movement toward balance and interaction between the individual, society, and nature."[6] Durlak[8] has proposed that the core competencies necessary to achieve social wellness are (a) peer acceptance, (b) altruism, (c) attachments and bonding, (d) communication, (e) assertiveness, and (e) conflict resolution.

The modern health care professional faces daunting challenges when attempting to achieve social wellness. Indeed, in many respects our current health care systems appear to have been constructed with the specific intent of diminishing our social wellness—both as individuals and as a health care community. The modern clinician typically experiences unstable hierarchical relationships based on competition, distrust, and indirect communication. Our professional regulatory bodies have instituted harsh oversight mechanisms, and clinicians who admit that they are experiencing depression or severe stress are subject to intrusive investigations and increased supervisory oversight. Physicians who are plaintiffs in a malpractice suit are advised not to discuss the case with their peers, and even with their spouses. Communication between different health care professionals is typically poor and often contentious. As physicians and nurses move between different health care systems, most of our professional relationships are short-lived and superficial. The physician in private practice is likely to have very few opportunities for developing meaningful relationships with other clinicians, and his or her professional meetings have become organized around didactic presentations rather than opportunities for establishing and fostering long-term relationships with other clinicians.

Most clinicians now work in large hospitals and clinics distant from their home communities and seldom have an opportunity to interact with community or advocacy groups. Rather than viewing their hospitals as central to their identity, many of communities now view them as corporate interlopers whose goal is driven more by corporate financial bottom lines than by the welfare of the community.

The modern health care environment has been built around a distrust of nature and a belief in the sanctity of sterility. This is particularly true for modern oncology clinicians where many of our patients are immunocompromised and must be cared for under strict precautions. The 21st-century clinician works in a synthetic world of artificial materials, artificial light, and artificial smells—far detached from nature and the experience of one's relationship to nature. This isolation heightens our sense of disconnection from community and sharpens our sense of isolation.

Emotional Wellness

Hettler[7] described emotional wellness as the awareness and acceptance of a wide range of feelings in one's self and others, as well as an ability to constructively express, manage, and integrate feelings. He described an emotionally well person as flexible, open to development, able to function autonomously, and aware of his or her limitations. Such a person will establish relationships that are interdependent, committed, respectful, and trusting.[6]

Many of these attributes are contrary to what characterizes the modern physician. As a group, modern physicians tend to be very self-critical, and often have difficulty in expressing their feelings. This emotional constriction is fostered by the profession's support for objectivity and limited education in how to effectively manage the emotionally laden situations that are an inevitable part of being a physician. Oncology clinicians are repeatedly confronted with distressing situations that can quickly become overwhelming without the benefit of a supportive team. Poorly equipped to deal with these emotionally charged situations, and without the support of a team, oncology clinicians often shut down emotionally and develop a blind spot to the subjective aspects of their patient's experience. The dogged determination necessary to survive the training of a medical professional does not necessarily lend itself well to the flexibility necessary to navigate the uncertainties and personal challenges inherent to a clinical career. In addition, clinicians are often very self-critical and likely to internalize responsibility for poor clinical outcomes that are beyond their control. Finally, it is understandably a challenge for clinicians to maintain an optimistic and positive perspective on life when they live in a world colored by the suffering of their seriously ill and dying patients.

Physical Wellness

This has been defined by Hettler[7] as one's attention to physical self-care, activity level, nutritional needs, and the use of medical services. In this regard, health care professionals and particularly physicians are notoriously poor at caring for themselves. In a study of young Irish physicians, almost one third had not seen a general practitioner in the last 5 years, two thirds felt that they could not take time off when they were unwell, and almost one half believed they had neglected their own health.[9] McKevitt et al[9] reported that 80% of general practitioners and hospital doctors feel that they have to work through their episodes of medical illness. Physicians are also very bad at caring for one another and are unlikely to offer another physician assistance or intervene when they witness a colleague to be exhibiting evidence of physical or psychological distress. Once again, physicians are deterred from seeking help for their physical or psychological problems because most medical boards discriminate against physicians who must report these behaviors on the license applications.

Clinicians often have unhealthy lifestyles and must skip meals or work long hours without adequate sleep. Surveys indicate that doctors work an average of 50 to 60 hours per week—even when they are not working overnight shifts.[10]

Many health care organizations fail to provide adequate resources for their clinicians' wellness. Clinicians working in less-enlightened organizations must often forego their unused leave and may even be required to take vacation time in lieu of sick leave—even when they are suffering from a potentially contagious condition such as influenza.

Intellectual Wellness

This has been defined by Hettler[7] as the degree to which one's mind engages in creative and stimulating activities. This does not simply mean participating in intense academic intellectual pursuits but describes the participation in intellectual activity that is stimulating, creative, and energizing. Rather than being focused on one area of study, intellectual wellness requires enthusiastic exploration of a variety of intellectual pursuits, for example, the opera, philosophy, and travel. The key to intellectual wellness is balance and enthusiasm.

The intense competition for positions in health care professional schools requires that most clinicians have had to limit their intellectual horizons at an early age. Any interest in the arts must be quenched as aspiring young clinicians must master the biologic sciences and perform well on examinations that reward rote learning, and not creativity. This blinkered intellectual horizon is unlikely to widen for the clinician in practice. Required to demonstrate their competence in their respective specialties, clinicians must master an avalanche of new scientific data and are increasingly expected to demonstrate this competency on new board certifying examinations and recertifying examinations. Combined with their long hours, there is very little time available for most clinicians to pursue any intellectual pursuit beyond their particular area of clinical practice.

Spiritual Wellness

This has been defined by Hettler[7] as a worldview that gives unity and goals to thoughts and actions, as well as the process of seeking meaning, purpose in existence, and understanding one's place in the universe. Oncology clinicians inhabit a world in which their patients are confronting profound existential questions spawned by their illness and the sharp edge of their own mortality. Unfortunately, our professional schools have not prepared us for this challenge, and we must engage with our patients at the level of their biology—and not their spirit. In a world driven by cold scientific data and financial imperatives, it is becoming increasingly difficult for clinicians to discover the meaning in their work. The deepest sense of spiritual wellness is derived from our experience of connection to a transcendent purpose—something that is not easily discovered in the reductionist world view of modern medical science.

Resilience

Resilience should be an essential characteristic of any oncology clinician. It refers to the ability to successfully adapt to stressors, bounce back from setbacks, and maintain psychological well-being in the face of adversity.[11] There are two components to resilience, that is:

(a) *The ability to recover from adversity.* This does not necessarily describe a return to the status quo but describes the capacity to learn from the adversity and realign oneself to an overall higher level of functioning (even if one has acquired deficits as a result of the adverse event). Individuals, teams, and communities can exhibit resiliency. Oncology clinicians face adversity, directly or indirectly, on a daily basis. Our resilience enables us to absorb these challenges (such as the death of a patient) and return to our work each day with renewed commitment and enthusiasm.

(b) *Sustaining the pursuit of positive growth and flourishing.* Building upon an ecological model, Holling[11] has defined resiliency as the capacity to absorb perturbations and disturbances within the system. This requires the system to exhibit flexibility, learning, and responsivity, and to realign resources in synchrony with shifting internal and external realities. Resilient systems are therefore not static but display a dynamic fluidity that is constantly redefining its boundaries and its limitations. Survival is not sufficient for the resilient system—success is defined in terms of flourishing and the movement toward more sustainable ecosystems. Cancer can be viewed as an energetic system that has a short-lived exuberance but lacks the resiliency to maintain its long-term viability. Oncology clinicians are expected to spend a long career working with catastrophic medical situations. Unfortunately, most of our health care systems have failed to recognize the critical importance of developing resilient

health care communities that support both the long-term viability and flourishing of team members. This inevitably results in the burnout and demoralization of clinicians—and threatens the viability of the health care delivery system itself.

As the cornerstone for flexible and responsive systems, self-awareness is a critical component of resilient systems. Although simple cause and effect models may be sufficient to maintain closed homeostatic systems, the resilient system must possess more complex computations involving foresight, intentionally driven decisions, and dynamic interaction with other systems. Central to resilience is the system's shared commitment to a conscious or unconscious purpose, for example, survival of the ant colony or devotion to a higher purpose such as compassion. This essentially describes a "learning community" that is constantly appraising its own health and providing a feedback loop for integrating new information and adaptive responses. Although resilient systems must be sensitive to negative influences, they must be driven by positive aspirations and not by fear. The resilient health care community would facilitate communication across a nonhierarchical system that is organized around the common purpose of relieving the suffering of the community. Unfortunately, this does not describe our current profit-driven health care system.

Clinicians function as systems within the larger systems of their hospital, clinic, local community, country, and global ecosystem. It is therefore impossible to disarticulate the healer from these larger communities. Each system impacts the other. Our ancestor healers recognized the interdependence of all living systems and reminded us to first treat the community, then the patient, and then the disease. The environmental determinants of cancer are becoming increasingly clear—by failing to address this broader ecological disease, the modern oncologist is undermining both our own well-being and the ultimate sustainability of our entire ecosystem.

Burnout

Maslach et al[12] have proposed that burnout consists of three basic dimensions, that is:

- *Emotional exhaustion (EE)*—This describes the extent to which an individual feels emotionally burdened and exhausted by one's work. EE relates to high stress at work with feelings of personal depletion and being overextended. Individuals who are experiencing a high level of EE are likely to distance themselves from their patients, their families, and their coworkers. This emotional aloofness may be interpreted by others as a deliberate callousness, and not an innate inability of the person to make emotional connections with those around them. The health care professional with high EE is experienced by patients as cold and indifferent which undermines the empathic connection that is the foundation of any effective therapeutic relationship. "The health care professional with high EE is experienced by patients as cold and indifferent and this undermines the empathic connection that is the foundation of any effective therapeutic relationship". Clinicians with a high level of EE are likely to become irritable and critical of others—further alienating themselves from the relationships that are critical to their personal and professional well-being. Research suggests that high EE is correlated with dysfunctional organizations and the intense social interactions that are common in high-pressure health care organizations.[13]

- *Depersonalization (DP)*—This describes the extent to which a person has developed feelings of indifference and cynicism toward patients, the treatment plan and instructions given, or the service delivered in the work environment. DP relates to a poor callous attitude and response to situations.

- *Personal accomplishment (PA)*—This describes how fully a person is able to develop and acquire an innate sense of competency and personal achievement at work. Clinicians with a low level of PA typically feel that they are not able to provide adequate care for their patients and become overly self-critical and less likely to gain satisfaction from their work. This negative feedback loop will inevitably produce a downward spiral that further compounds the clinician's perceived stress and ability to develop mastery over the complex tasks inherent to modern health care. Low PA is most likely to manifest in situations where the clinician is overworked, does not have sufficient resources, and receives negative feedback from authority figures—unfortunately these are characteristics of many clinical oncology settings.

The Maslach Burnout Inventory (MBI) is the widely used and validated self-administered psychometric instrument that measures the individual's functioning within each of these three domains.[12]

How Common is Burnout among Oncology Clinicians?

Recent research has begun to shed light on the prevalence and determinants of burnout among clinicians. This growing database suggests wide variations in the prevalence and severity of burnout in different geographic regions and professional groups and also sheds some light on the predisposing factors to burnout. The first study in 1981 using the MBI in a sample of US physicians and nurses reported that one third of both groups reported high levels of EE, DP, and PA. The prevalence of burnout in US oncologists has been reported to be between 34% and 61.7%.[14,15,16]

One large multinational comparative study of 11,530 clinicians from Spain and several South American countries reported significant geographic differences in the prevalence of burnout. The prevalence of burnout in Spanish-speaking health care professionals from Spain and Argentina was 14% and 7.9%, respectively.[17] Professionals from Mexico, Ecuador, Peru, Columbia, Uruguay, Guatemala, and El Salvador had a remarkably low prevalence of burnout between 2.5% and 5.9%.[17] In this study, doctors (12.1%) and nurses (7.2%) had a significantly lower prevalence of burnout than their US counterparts. Emergency room doctors reported an incidence of 17%, internal medicine doctors 15.5%, and anesthesiologists and dermatologists had the lowest prevalence of 5%.[17]

Demographic variables among physicians that have been reported to increase the likelihood of burnout include:

- younger age;
- less clinical experience;
- single marital status;
- being a parent of young children.

Burnout among Nurses

Oncology nurses are being asked to care for sicker patients with shorter lengths of hospital stays. Unfortunately there are currently no data available on the prevalence of burnout in oncology nurses. Oncology nurses appear to experience higher rates of burnout than their colleagues in hospice, but do not appear to fare any worse than nurses working in other hospital departments (eg, ICU, general medical, HIV units).[18] Oncology nurses do report a higher level of emotional stress than their nursing colleagues.

Oncology nurses do however appear to experience less overall burnout than oncology physicians; however, they do score higher on measures of PA and also report more somatic symptoms than physician colleagues.[18]

Determinants of Burnout in Oncology Clinicians

Multiple organizational and personality factors have been correlated with a higher likelihood of developing burnout. Maslach[13] has proposed a model for understanding burnout as a consequence of the mismatch between the individual and his or her work environment. According to this model, the major work–life determinants of burnout are workload, control, reward, community, fairness, and values. Burnout is likely to occur when there is a mismatch between the individual's personal characteristics and his or her work environment in these domains.

Workload Several studies have reported excessive workload as a major contributor to burnout.[19,20,21] Excessive workload results in physical exhaustion, insufficient time to communicate with patients, insufficient personal time, and a disruption of work–life balance. Clinicians who are overworked experience diminished PA and diminished job satisfaction.

Control A key construct in organizational theory is the importance of matching authority and responsibility. Oncology clinicians typically work in high-stress environments where life and death decisions are commonplace. In this situation, clinicians who experience themselves as having no ability to shape their work conditions are likely to experience EE and diminished PA. Unfortunately, the growth of large health care delivery systems often disenfranchises individual clinicians and leaves them feeling like faceless cogs in an impersonal bureaucratic machine. Furthermore, oncology clinicians often treat incurable medical conditions that may render them feeling clinically inadequate and therefore challenging their sense of PA.

Reward This may be either in the form of tangible rewards such as salary and benefits or in more subjective forms such as job satisfaction and positive feedback from patients and coworkers. Once again, the emergence of large bureaucratic oncology delivery systems often leaves clinicians experiencing themselves as "provider numbers" who feel undervalued and unappreciated by their paymasters. Furthermore, these large systems inevitably erode the clinician–patient relationship that may result in clinicians receiving less positive feedback from their patients.

Community Individuals thrive within a supportive community that strengthens their sense of personal identity and provides a sense of connection to a purpose that extends beyond mundane individual ambitions. Unfortunately, although lip service is given to the importance of teamwork, most clinicians continue to communicate indirectly through the medical record and very seldom meet together with other members of the team. Indeed, within the pressure cooker that is modern health care, communication only occurs when it is motivated by disagreements or adverse outcomes. In this regard, clinicians who are facing a malpractice suit are given legal counsel not to discuss events with colleagues—further heightening their sense of alienation from the team. Furthermore, the modern clinician is likely to migrate between different organizations and often works at sites that are entirely disconnected from his or her home community. Interestingly, clinicians who are promoted to administrative positions within health care bureaucracy report increased job stress and higher levels of EE than other members of the team.

Fairness All members of the health care team should experience the system to be fair and equitable. Unfortunately, health care tends to be a hierarchical system, and clinicians are increasingly experiencing themselves as disenfranchised. Poor communication between team members typically compounds misperceptions and may drive a closed loop of escalating dissatisfaction and team dysfunction. Uncertainty or misunderstanding about changes in health care reimbursement fuels clinician suspicions about perceived unfair compensation.

Values Ideally, our actions should be aligned with our values. The vast majority of health care professionals entered their careers driven by altruistic, rather than selfish, ideals. Unfortunately, modern clinicians often experience themselves as being caught at the confluence of competing values. As employees and/or the recipients of impersonal third-party payers, clinicians are constantly challenged to provide effective and compassionate care for the lowest price. Academic clinicians are typically challenged to garner research funding while also being responsible for providing optimum and personalized care for their patients. Employees of for-profit health care companies must comply to an agenda that is ultimately driven by financial, rather than humanistic, priorities. Oncologists face the added challenge of aligning their values regarding futile and end-of-life care with those of their patients and their families. One would like to believe that clinicians' equanimity allows them to effectively and compassionately provide care that is consonant with whatever care their patient demands. In reality, however, it is often very difficult for clinicians to provide care that is not aligned with their own values. In this regard, in a study of oncologists and oncology nurses, Kash et al[22] reported that caring for dying patients and struggling with issues around Do Not Resuscitate orders were the major contributors of burnout.

Consequences of Burnout on Patient Care

Clinicians who are experiencing burnout are much more likely to leave the profession prematurely or repeatedly switch their employment site. This is becoming increasingly important given the increasing shortage of trained health care professionals. The cost to a health care facility of replacing a physician is estimated at $150,000 to $300,000, a figure that does not include the negative impact of staff turnover on the morale of staff and the trust of patients.[23]

Clinician burnout has a negative impact on the quality of care provided to patients. Physicians' level of job satisfaction has been demonstrated to have a negative impact on patient satisfaction, treatment adherence, and follow-through with lifestyle recommendations. Burnt-out physicians are more likely to make riskier treatment decisions and treatment errors. Among physicians describing themselves as experiencing high work-related stress, 50% felt that they were providing lower standards of medical care, with 7% reported serious mistakes and 2% to 4% reporting incidents that led directly to the death of a patient. Residents in training are most likely to experience work-related stress.[24] Shanafelt et al[25] reported that 75% of residents in their study met criteria for burnout. Those residents who met criteria for burnout were two to three times more likely to report that they had provided suboptimal care to their patients.

These data should raise the alarm and motivate clinicians and health care systems to address the rising tide of clinician burnout that is adversely affecting patient care.

■ COMPASSION FATIGUE

The concept of "compassion fatigue" among caregivers has recently garnered increasing attention. However, there is almost no empiric research to support the validity of compassion fatigue as a distinct syndrome. Figley[26] has suggested that compassion fatigue is "The natural consequent behaviors and emotions resulting from knowing about a traumatizing event experienced by a significant other and the stress resulting from helping or wanting to help a traumatized or suffering person." Rather than presenting a distinct syndrome, compassion fatigue appears to be akin to the EE and DP components of burnout. Controversy over definitional constructs aside, the concept of compassion fatigue highlights the importance of understanding and regulating our response to the suffering of our patients. In this regard, it is important to have a clear understanding of the nature and determinants of the key interpersonal processes that support our capacity to respond to the suffering of others. Compassion represents one's intention to be of benefit to others. It therefore does not make sense to describe "compassion fatigue." Empathy describes our cognitive and/or emotional perception of the other person's subjective state and requires that we are able to distinguish the boundary between our own experience and that of the other person. A failure to make this other/self boundary distinction will result in "emotional contagion" where we take on the experience of the other as oneself. Oncology clinicians who routinely work with patients in great emotional and physical distress must be able to maintain compassionate intention and empathic accuracy but must be careful not to become subject to emotional contagion. In order to accomplish this delicate balancing act, clinicians must become mindful of their relationship with themselves and their patients and develop the equanimity to skillfully balance their professional and personal emotional response to the suffering of their patients. Interestingly, as discussed below, recent research has demonstrated that mindfulness training is an effective approach to supporting physician wellness.

■ STRATEGIES FOR OPTIMIZING THE WELL-BEING OF ONCOLOGY CLINICIANS

The data and concepts reviewed above demonstrate that clinicians are currently experiencing very significant work-related stress that is negatively impacting their personal wellness *and* their ability to provide safe, compassionate, and effective care for their patients. Without immediate interventions, it is fair to suggest that the viability of our health care system is threatened. These interventions should be at both a personal and institutional level and will require novel approaches that are cognizant of complex systems approaches to resiliency and human flourishing.

Individual Approaches to Enhancing Clinician Wellness

- *Empower individuals to assume responsibility for change*: Health care professionals should be encouraged to assume personal responsibility for effecting changes in their lives that will support their flourishing. This empowerment must begin during their education and should be incorporated into their curriculum. Rather than being encouraged to become the passive recipients of an avalanche of medical facts, students should have an opportunity to explore and support their personal and professional development. As health care professionals we should be encouraged to "become the change" we are expecting in our patients and to model healthful lifestyles we would like our patients to pursue. Unfortunately, all too often, health care professionals perceive themselves to be the powerless victims of a health care industry that defines the nature and intention of their work. In many ways, we are "the canaries in the mineshaft," and our professional malaise reflects the same issues that are pervading our larger communities. As healers we need to become transformative agents for a culture that values wellness before illness and beg the process of transforming our communities by first changing ourselves. This is not an easy task—however, it must begin.

The place to start empowering ourselves is with clarifying our intention for our work—why did we decide to enter the healing profession? During times of self-doubt or extreme challenge, it is our intention that becomes the guiding star for our actions and our motivation to persevere.

The following quotation by the His Holiness the Dalai Lama[27] captures this ideal:

> No matter what is going on
> Never give up
> Develop the heart
> Too much energy in your country
> Is spent developing the mind
> Instead of the heart
> Be compassionate
> Not just to your friends
> But to everyone
> Be compassionate
> Work for peace
> In your heart and in the world
> Work for peace
> And I say again
> Never give up
> No matter what is going on around you
> Never give up

- *Become aware of wellness*: Most health care professionals live hectic lives. Running between our professional and personal responsibilities, we often develop unhealthy habits. Unfortunately, as described above, most of us pay very little attention to our wellness and will deprive ourselves of needed rest—even when we are sick.

It is important that we regularly take a moment to evaluate our own wellness. Atul Gawande[28] in his popular book *Checklists Manifesto: How to Get Thing Right* describes how effective simple checklists can be in identifying and avoiding problems before they become a catastrophe. Each of us should take time on a regular basis to take an inventory of our lives—and not wait until we are incapacitated. This requires honesty, courage, and most of all a genuine heartfelt compassion toward ourselves. As clinicians we often find it much easier to have compassion toward our patients than toward ourselves. However, unless we care for ourselves, we will be of limited benefit to others.

- *Identify domains of strength and weakness*: Sometimes, attempting to understand and rate our own wellness can be overwhelming. With so many different determinants of overall wellness, it can be difficult to tease out each of the factors in our lives that is supporting or detracting from our ability to flourish. One helpful approach is to utilize "the wheel of wellness"—this simple tool provides a simple schema for disentangling the complex tapestry that makes up our lives.[28] Completing a self-assessment of our health habits often provides us with unexpected insights into our current lifestyle and can become the foundation for developing an action plan for change.[28]

- *Food*: Most clinicians have received very little education in nutrition. This has important implications for the health of their patients and themselves. Given their busy lifestyles, clinicians often compromise on their diet and skip meals, or "eat on the run." Caffeine is often used as an energizer, and drug company–sponsored pizza and Chinese food can become the staple of our diet. Food can become a metaphor for taking control of our wellness and a doorway into establishing a more mindful relationship with our environment. One simple but effective approach to altering our diet is to adopt the anti-inflammatory diet pyramid described by Weil[30]

- *Mind*: The modern oncologist is bombarded with literally thousands of distractions each day, both at home and at work. Although much has been written about attention-deficit disorder as a medical condition, it is also reasonable to state that an inability to remain focused has become the central malady of the modern mind. The consequences of our scattered attention extend far beyond simple "forgetfulness." An increasing scientific database reveals a direct correlation between cognitive attentional state and inflammatory physiology. Consonant with this, several studies have reported that mindfulness meditation practices produce significant and sustained improvements in inflammatory markers, measures of autonomic stability, and emotional stability and flexibility.[31]

Mindfulness-based meditation interventions have been studie in numerous health care professional groups and have been demonstrated to produce improvements in mood, anxiety, burnout, quality of life, and self-compassion. In 2010, in a study of 70 primary care physicians who participated in an 8-week program that included mindfulness meditation, self-awareness exercises, and narrative writing, Krasner et al[32] reported significant and sustained improvements in (a) burnout, (b) mood, (c) conscientiousness, (d) emotional stability, and (e) empathy. The authors suggest that these improvements are associated with enhanced resiliency that helps physicians deal more effectively with the stress routinely encountered in their work as physicians.

These findings should motivate clinicians to adopt regular meditation practices. These programs (such as mindfulness-based stress reduction) are readily available within communities and are becoming increasingly popular among religious organizations.

- *Movement*: Unfortunately, many oncology clinicians must spend much of their day behind a desk and, after a hard day at work, feel too fatigued to participate in a regular exercise program. Having said this, it is crucial that clinicians incorporate some form of regular exercise into their daily routine. Simple things such as taking the stairs or taking a walk at lunchtime can be very helpful in improving one's wellness.

- Sleep hygiene: Many clinicians work long hours and/ or night shifts. This inevitability produces physiological changes that manifest as fatigue. The misalignment of the rhythmic circadian sleep cycle can lead to problems with an individual's ability to perform efficiently and also affects the metabolism of sleep hormones such as melatonin, and important sleep neurotransmitters. Sleep deprivation can clearly affect our ability to function socially and effectively at work with established links between job dissatisfaction, short sleeping time, and burnout associated with compromised mental health. This seemed to be more prominent in the female positions surveyed.[33] It is therefore important that we follow a regular sleep routine that includes at least 8 hours of unbroken sleep—unfortunately, this may not be possible in clinicians who are expected to be on call for long periods and may be awoken by their pagers at any time of the night!

- *Space*: Our environment has a profound effect on our physical and emotional well-being. A recent study in Hong Kong reported that residents who lived in areas of the city with nearby green space have significantly longer telomeres than matched city dwellers who did not have easy access to green spaces.[34] Several studies have demonstrated the impact of the hospital environment on several crucial measures of patient outcome, including mortality.[29,30,31]

Unfortunately, despite the mounting evidence linking the environmental ambience with health, most hospitals are impersonal synthetic environments. Clinicians who spend most of their waking hours in these environments will inevitably experience adverse physical and psychological effects. Whenever possible, we should attempt to introduce natural plant and light into our workspace, and take every opportunity to take a walk during lunchtime.

We should take an inventory of our home environment and clear clutter around our home as much as possible. The impact of toxic noise pollution, including violent television programming, should not be underestimated. Clinicians who spend most of their waking day working among seriously ill patients can clearly benefit from more positive entertainment than the crime shows and controversial news programming that fills our airwaves. "Beauty will save the world," said Frederich Nietchsze. It should become part of the everyday experience of every clinician.

- *Meaning*: In no other profession is meaning so easily accessed as in medicine. The oncology clinician lives on the sharp edge of existence with his or her patients and travels with them along a perilous journey that is signposted by profound existential questions. Unfortunately, our education has not prepared us for this task, and many of us find ourselves retreating to a world defined more by hard biological facts than by the challenging questions posed by human suffering. We may never discover the answers to these profound questions—we should however continue to keep them alive and explore them through our connection to a transcendent purpose discovered through our spiritual and/or religious life. Our intention for our work is central to this process, and each of us should strive to clearly define our motivations for our work as healers. During difficult times our clear intention will become a touchstone to guide us through that which allows us to identify the deeper purpose for our work.

- *Grief:* Oncology clinicians inevitably face repeated losses. Despite our best efforts, many of our patients will not survive their illness. We will also need to say goodbye to those patients who do recover. Many of these relationships are profound and forged through the cauldron of illness and suffering. Unfortunately, very little recognition is given to how painful these repeated losses can be, and the health team seldom takes an opportunity to acknowledge, share, and respect how the loss of every patient touches our lives. Formal and informal rituals may help to address this grief. Taking time at regular team meetings to acknowledge and process the loss of patients can be helpful. At an institutional level, regular (eg quarterly) memorial services for staff and families can be a powerful forum for supporting one another and validating our losses.

Institutional Approaches to Enhancing Clinician Wellness

Culture shapes behaviors. Although individual clinicians may develop their own strategies for supporting their wellness, each of them must work within a culture that exerts implicit and explicit constraints on one's wellness. Although most health care organizations claim to offer employee assistance programs, most of the resources offered are limited to an employee assistance program. Institutions should strive to align their stated values that emphasize the importance of core values of compassion, integrity, and respect and address this not just in the care of patients, but also as part of the relationship between employees at all levels of the organization.

Prioritizing Clinician Wellness

Unfortunately, most health care institutions fail to appreciate how their culture and environments can influence both the wellness of their clinicians and their patient outcomes. Physician distress is associated with increased absenteeism, the ordering of unnecessary diagnostic tests, less time spent with patients, increased staff turnover, and diminished patient satisfaction.

The direct correlation between physician stress and patient-related outcome strongly supports the introduction of measures of physician and staff wellness as quality indicators in health care systems. The development of valid objective measures of physician wellness (such as that developed by Arnetz[35]) allows for establishing longitudinal indicators that can be used to assess the impact of various institutionally driven initiatives. Although interventions aimed at improving physician wellness have proved to be effective in this regard, the link to improving patient quality of care has not yet been examined. Wallace et al[36] have described a model describing the linkages between physician wellness, patient outcomes, and health care system interventions (Fig. 26-1).

Once health care delivery systems have prioritized clinician wellness and have established quantitative measures of wellness, they can implement interventions that support a quality improvement cycle. The implementation of this model requires that these systems identify clinician wellness as a priority that warrants resource allocation.

Some of the numerous wellness strategies that could be implemented include:

- Support and empower the development of multidisciplinary teams.
- Facilitate healthy lifestyles through integrative systemwide initiatives such as healthy foods in the cafeteria, wellness coaches, educational materials, subsidized gym memberships, salary bonuses for employees who achieve target weight goals, and meditation programs.
- Create healthy environments based on natural materials, images, and sounds.
- Establish regular memorial ceremonies that recognize and appreciate those patients and staff who have passed away during the previous quarter.

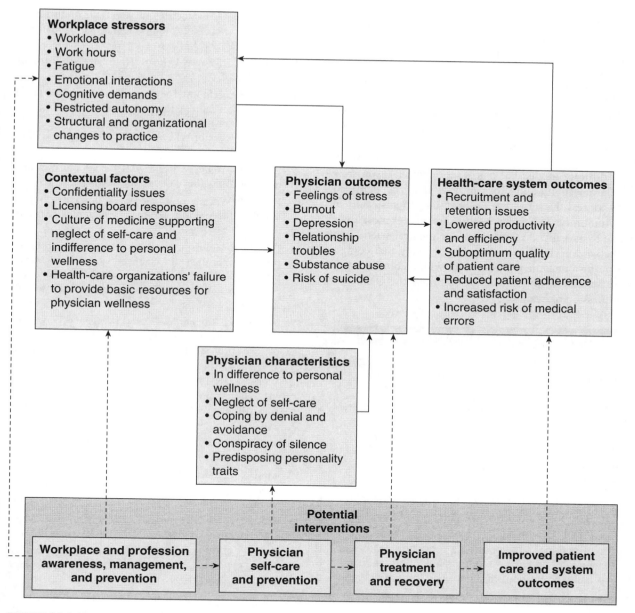

FIGURE 26-1. Linkages between physician wellness, patient outcomes, and health care system interventions. Reproduced with permission from Wallace et al.[36]

- Support sponsored charitable outreach programs with a partnership between the institution, staff, and community (eg, working together to improve the health care of an inner-city community or school).

- Pay attention to the small acts of support, for example, supporting staff lunches and celebrations, recognizing birthdays, and rewarding accomplishments with praise and tokens of appreciations.

- Celebrate successes such as patient quality goals, JCAHO, and/or Magnet Nursing Recognition.

■ SUMMARY

Modern health care is facing a crisis on many levels. These extend far beyond the financial bottom line and also include the declining morale of our health care professionals. The genesis of this declining morale is not to be found in inadequate funding but in the ascent of a health care model that places more emphasis on scientific objectivity and profit motives than on its mission to address the subjective needs of its patients, staff, and community. Any viable health care model must match the remarkable discoveries of our medical science with the wisdom that comes from recognizing that compassion for our patients must begin with a compassion for ourselves and those who have chosen the challenging profession of healing.

KEY POINTS

- ■ Health care professionals are experiencing very high levels of work-related stress distress and burnout.
- ■ Every clinician should enhance one's capacity for resilience (ie, one's ability to successfully adapt to stressors, bounce back from setbacks, and maintain psychological well-being in the face of adversity).
- ■ Clinician wellness has a very significant impact on health care quality and patient satisfaction.
- ■ Burnout is not an inevitable part of being an oncology clinician.
- ■ Mindfulness-based stress reduction programs have been shown to very significantly reduce clinician burnout and enhance job satisfaction.

REFERENCES

1. Cohen JS, Patten S. Well being in residency training: a survey examining resident physician satisfaction both within and outside of residency training and mental health in Alberta. *BMC Med Educ.* 2005;5:21.

2. Center C, Davis M, Detre T. Confronting depression and suicide in physicians: a consensus statement. *JAMA.* 2003; 289:3161–3166.

3. Henry J. OMA membership survey results confirm overwhelming level of frustration among Ontario physicians. *Ont Med Rev.* 2004;71:1–6.

4. Dunn HL. *High-level Wellness.* Thorofare, NJ: Charles B. Slack; 1997:4.

5. Myers JE, Luecht RM, Sweeney T. The factor structure of wellness: reexamining theoretical and empirical models underlying the Wellness Evaluation of Lifestyle (WEL) and the five-factor WEL. *Measure Eval Couns Dev.* 2004; 36:194–208.

6. Roscoe LJ. Wellness: a review of theory and measurement for counselors. *J Couns Dev.* 2009;87:216–226.

7. Hettler B. Wellness promotion on a university campus: family and community health. *J Health Promot Maintenance.* 1980;3:77–95.

8. Durlak JA. Health promotion as a strategy in primary prevention. In Cichetti J, Rappaport J, Sandler I, Weissberg RP, eds. *The Promotion of Wellness in Children and Adolescents.* Washington, DC: CWLA Press; 2000: 221–241.

9. McKevitt C, Morgan M, Dundas R, Holland WW. Sickness absence and 'working through' illness: a comparison of two professional groups. *J Public Health Med.* 1997;19:295–300.

10. Williams ES, Rondeau KV, Wiao Q, Francescutti LH. Heavy physician workloads: impact on physician attitudes and outcomes. *Health Serv Manage Res.* 2007;20:261–269.

11. Holling CS. Resilience and stability of ecological systems. *Annu Rev Ecol Systematics.* 1973;4:1–23.

12. Maslach C, EJackson S, Leiter MP. *Maslach Burnout Inventory Manual.* 3rd ed. Palo Alto, Calif: Consulting Psychologies Press; 1996.

13. Maslach C. Job burn out: new directions in research and intervention. *Curr Dir Psychol Sci.* 2003;12:189–192.

14. Demirci S, Yildirim YK, Ozsaran Z, Uslu R, Yalman D, Aras AB. Evaluation of burnout syndrome in oncology employees. *Med Oncol.* 2010;27(3):968–974.

15. Allegra CJ, Hall R, Yothers G. Prevalence of burnout in the US oncology population. *J Oncol Pract.* 2005;1(4): 140–147.

16. Whippen DA, Zuckrman EL, Anderson JW, Kamin DY, Holland JC. Burnout in the practice of oncology: results of a follow-up survey. *J Clin Oncol.* 2004;22(14S): 6053.

17. Grau A, Suner R, Garcia MM. Burnout syndrome in health workers and relationship with personal and environmental factors. *Gac Sanit.* 2005;19(6):463–470.

18. Bram PJ, Katz LF. A study of burnout in nurses working in hospice and hospice oncology settings. *Oncol Nurs Forum*. 1989;16:555–560.

19. Bragard I, Libert Y, Etienne AM, Merckaert I, Delvaux N, Marchal S, Boniver J, Klastersky J, Reynaert C, Scalliet P, Slachmuylder JL, Razavi D. Insight on variables leading to burnout in cancer physicians. *J Cancer Educ*. 2010 25(1):109–115.

20. Leiter MP, Frank E, Matheson TJ. Demands, values, and burnout: relevance for physicians. *Can Fam Physician*. 2009;55(12):1224–1225, 1225.

21. Arigoni F, Bovier PA, Mermillod B, Waltz P, Sappino AP. Prevalence of burnout among Swiss cancer clinicians, paediatricians and general practitioners: who are most at risk? *Support Care Cancer*. 2009;17(1):75–81.

22. Kash KM, Holland JC, Breitbart W, Berenson S, Daugherty J. Stress and burnout in oncology. *Oncology*. 2000;14:1621–1637.

23. Shi L. *Managing Human Resources in Healthcare Organizations*. 1st ed. Sudbury, Mass: Jones and Barrett Publishers; 2006.

24. Firth-Cozens J, Greenhaigh J. Doctors' perceptions of the links between stress and lowered clinical care. *Soc Sci Med*. 1997;44:1017–1022.

25. Shanafelt TD, Bradley KA, Wipf JW, Back AL. Burnout and self-reported patient care in an internal medicine residency program. *Ann Intern Med*. 2002;136:358–367.

26. Figley CR. Compassion fatigue: psychotherapists' chronic lack of self care. *J Clin Psychol*. 2002;58(11):1433–1441.

27. Tenzin Gyatso His Holiness the Dalai Lama. Primary source not known.

28. Gawande A. *The Checklist Manifesto*. New York, NY: Metropolitan Books; 2009.

29. Pace TW, Negi LT, Sivilli TI, Issa MJ, Cole SP, Adame DD, Raison CL. Innate immune, neuroendocrine and behavioral responses to psychosocial stress do not predict subsequent compassion meditation practice time. *Psychoneuroendocrinology*. 2010;35(2):310.

30. Witek-Janusek L, Albuquerque K, Chroniak KR, Chroniak C, Durazo-Arvizu R, Mathews HL. Effect of mindfulness based stress reduction on immune function, quality of life and coping in women newly diagnosed with early stage breast cancer. *Brain Behav Immun*. 2008;(6): 969–981.

31. Kiecolt-Glaser JK, Christian L, Preston H, Houts CR, Malarkey WB, Emery CF, Glaser R. Stress, inflammation, and yoga practice. *Psychosom Med*. 2010;(2):113–121.

32. Krasner MS, Epstein RM, Beckman H, et al. Association of an educational program in mindful communication with burnout, empathy, and attitudes among primary care physicians. *JAMA*. 2009;302(12):1284–1293.

33. Tokuda Y, Hayano K, Ozaki M, Bito S, Yanai H, Koizumi S. The interrelationships between working conditions, job satisfaction, burnout and mental health among hospital physicians in Japan: a path analysis. *Ind Health*. 2009;47(2):166–172.

34. Woo J, Tang N, Suen E, Leung J, Wong M. Green space, psychological restoration, and telomere length. *Lancet*. 2009;373(9660):299–300.

35. Arnetz BB. Psychosocial challenges facing physicians of today. *Soc Sci Med*. 2001;53:203–213.

36. Wallace JE, Lemaire JB, Ghali GA. Physician wellness. *Lancet*. 2009;374:1714–1721.

Index